CYSTIC FIBROSIS – RENEWED HOPES THROUGH RESEARCH

Edited by **Dinesh Sriramulu**

Cystic Fibrosis – Renewed Hopes Through Research
Edited by Dinesh Sriramulu

Published by InTech

Janeza Trdine 9, 51000 Rijeka, Croatia

Publishing Process Manager Romina Skomersic

Technical Editor Teodora Smiljanic

Cover Designer InTech Design Team

Additional hard copies can be obtained from orders@intechopen.com

Cystic Fibrosis – Renewed Hopes Through Research, Edited by Dinesh Sriramulu
p. cm.
ISBN 978-953-51-0287-8

For EU product safety concerns:
IN TECH d.o.o., Prolaz Marije Krucifikse Kozulić 3, 51000 Rijeka, Croatia,
info@intechopen.com or visit our website at intechopen.com.

Meet the editor

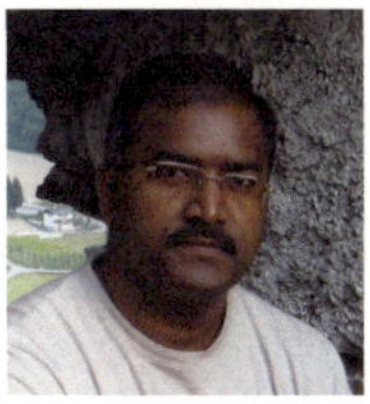

Dinesh D. Sriramulu, obtained his doctorate degree from the Technical University of Braunschweig, Germany. He started his research career at the Helmholtz Centre for Infection Research in Braunschweig, Germany in collaboration with the Karolinska Institutet, Stockholm, Sweden. His area of expertise is on the adaptation of bacteria towards diverse niches, from the human lung in the case of cystic fibrosis to the cattle rumen. He continued his research career at reputed institutions worldwide, like the University College Cork, Ireland; University of Medicine and Dentistry – New Jersey, USA; the Food and Drug Administration, Rockville, USA; University of Southern California, Los Angeles, USA; and the CIBIO, University of Trento, Italy. He published his research findings in various international peer-reviewed journals and presented his works at different international conferences. He serves as a peer-reviewer of a handful of scientific journals and as an expert referee for funding agencies.

Contents

Preface

The book 'Cystic Fibrosis – Renewed Hopes Through Research' emerged as a result of the contribution of interesting chapters by the experts in response to the invitation by Intech Open Access Publisher. This open-to-all initiative enables dissemination of scientific knowledge to a wide range of readers through an unrestricted access to book contents. Publication via virtual media enables constant update of information on a regular basis whenever appropriate.

Cystic fibrosis, also known as mucoviscidosis, is an autosomal recessive multi-system genetic disease that occurs predominantly among Caucasians. Though found highest among Irish population, the incidence of this disease among Africans and Asians, who are normally least-affected, is on the rise probably due to social aspects and it is also attributable to improved early diagnostic methods available. This disease is characterized by an abnormal transport of chloride and sodium across epithelium that leads to thickening of secretions mainly in the lungs, pancreas, liver and intestine. The multifarious nature of this disease pushes individuals with cystic fibrosis towards mortality.

Unlike in the classical textbook, the collection of chapters in this book explains the complexity of the disease, microbiology and immunological aspects, therapeutic options and disease management that encompasses topics from basic science to patient care. The contributors of chapters of this book are well-established members of the worldwide scientific community, which is focused on an ultimate goal of finding a cure for cystic fibrosis condition. Recent developments, in the study and treatment of disease organized in the form of chapters in the book, emphasizes the dominating role of interdisciplinary participation. Initial chapters of the book focused on topics dedicated to prognosis, radiology, gender differences and reproductive complications associated with the disease. It is followed by chapters on genetic, biochemical and molecular aspects of the disease target, the Cystic Fibrosis Transmembrane conductance Regulator protein channel. The collection of chapters under microbiology and immunology covers typical and atypical infections that are secondary in nature and one of the major causative of mortality of cystic fibrosis patients. A special emphasis has been given to therapeutic developments to include recent findings with respect to steps towards cure. This set of chapters show the inevitable need for an interdisciplinary approach in cystic fibrosis research. The final part of the book is dedicated to focus on the importance of management aspects in order to achieve success in the treatment of this complex disease and care of patients.

More recent findings, especially at the molecular level, have changed our knowledge and understanding about cystic fibrosis and have dramatically increased the life expectancy of the patients. Owing to the pleiotropic nature of cystic fibrosis condition, medical research should focus more on translational research, then finding a common cure for cystic fibrosis will be attainable in the near future. With this approach, a cohort- or patient-specific treatment strategy backed by an intense bench-to-bedside research flow is the only feasible option to cater to the needs of patients in order to lead, at least, a near-normal life. After all, by definition, "Health is a state of complete physical, mental and social well-being, and not merely the absence of a disease or infirmity."

On behalf of me and the publisher, we anticipate that this book will instill the interest of readers in understanding the clinical and social aspects of a complex disease such as cystic fibrosis.

I humbly thank the INTECH for appointing me as the Editor of this book and for publishing the same. I thank all the authors for their valuable contributions without which this book would not have been materialized. I would like to thank Helmholtz Centre for Infection Research – Braunschweig, Germany, which served as the knowledge centre for me to gain expertise in this field. Finally, I thank Dr. Lakshmy Dinesh for her continuous support in shaping various aspects of this book.

Dinesh D. Sriramulu
Helmholtz Centre for Infection Research, Braunschweig,
Germany

Part 1

Cystic Fibrosis – A Complex Syndrome

1

The Prognosis of Cystic Fibrosis – A Clinician's Perspective

Patrick Lebecque
Cliniques St-Luc, Université de Louvain, Brussels
Belgium

1. Introduction

Looking at the prognosis of Cystic Fibrosis (CF) from the clinician's point of view is very relevant. Median predicted survival age of CF increased from 6 months when the disease was first described (1938) to 12 years in 1970 and over 35 years in 2010 in the United States of America (Davis, 2006). Three types of factors weigh on this prognosis, which is conditioned by lung disease: factors linked to the quality of care management, to genetics and to the environment. It has been estimated from studies in twins and siblings that the relative influence of the latter two is roughly equivalent. Though pollution may have increased in certain areas, and lighter forms of CF are now being detected by neonatal screening and in clinics where nasal potential measurements are widely available, their impact is limited and can not account for the spectacular changes in life expectancy. Thus, this improvement is due essentially to a better care management. Quality of care is the main determinant of CF prognosis.

The question of prognosis is almost invariably the very first that parents of a newly diagnosed CF infant will ask their physician, whose task to answer in a sensitive and sensible fashion is by no means easy. This question is also at the heart of daily concerns of the clinician, who has to take its determinants into consideration not so much in view of their fascinating underlying mechanisms (e.g. modifier genes) but rather to the extent they can give grip to improved care.

2. How to express CF prognosis? Median predicted survival: Facts, limitations and hopes

CF is a serious disease, which reduces life expectancy. Parents have often already found on the internet the associated 'Median predicted survival', which is the estimated duration of time until 50% of a given population dies. This given number of years has the effect of a guillotine and haunts their thoughts. For CF patients in 2008, it was 37.4 years in the US (CFF Registry, 2008), 38.8 years in the UK (UK CF Registry, 2008) and 46.6 in Canada (44.8 years after excluding adult diagnoses) (Canadian CFF, 2008). However, for a number of methodological issues, it is difficult to compare results of national registries. Evaluating cohorts on the basis of the presence or absence of pancreatic insufficiency was recently suggested as a way to help to overcome some of the current limitations (Buzzetti *et al.*, 2009).

Limiting the analysis to patients homozygous for the *F508del* mutation could be even 'cleaner' (Zelin *et al.*, 2010; Lebecque *et al.*, 2010). It is important to note that over the past 60 years, median predicted survival has actually increased in a continuous fashion by almost 6 years every decade (Davis, 2006). Part of this improvement is probably linked to the increased detection of milder forms of the disease. As proposed for the comparison of registries, it would be interesting to study the data of only those patients homozygous for the *F508del* mutation. For four reasons developed below, this brutal landmark has limited value in an individual patient.

2.1 Cohort effects

Cohort survival curves consistently show that survival continues to improve with each successive birth cohort over the decades. However, this effect is not taken into account by current survival curves. As a result, advice based on the latter could be unduly pessimistic. This has led authors to model the trend observed in cohort survival curves and to extrapolate a median survival for recent cohorts. Accordingly, a median life expectancy of the order of 40 years was predicted for newborns in 1990 in the UK (Elborn *et al.*, 1991). This proved to be realistic and updated extrapolation for the birth cohort of the year 2000 predicts a median survival of 50 years (Dodge *et al.*, 2007). Recent work has further validated this approach (Jackson *et al.*, 2011).

2.2 Wide heterogeneity of the disease

Median predicted survival does not take into account the vast heterogeneity of CF. Yet the latter has long been recognized, even amongst patients homozygous for the *F508del* mutation (Kerem *et al.*, 1990; Johanssen *et al.*, 1991). When diagnosing a new patient carrying 2 CF-causing mutations, this variability renders precise individual prognosis almost always impossible.

2.3 Quality of life

The raw median predicted survival rate says nothing about quality of life. In CF, pulmonary function is often used as a surrogate for survival, with FEV_1 remaining the single most useful parameter (Kerem *et al.*, 1992). Though insensitive to early stages of the disease, spirometry is widely available, inexpensive, non-invasive and very reproducible. It can usually be performed from the age of 5 and upwards. FEV_1 has the advantage of reflecting pulmonary involvement, thereby conditioning prognosis, throughout the whole course of the disease. The rate of FEV_1 decline might be an even stronger surrogate for survival (Liou *et al.*, 2001; Schluchter *et al.*, 2002; Rosenbluth *et al.*, 2004).

Quality of life is at least as important as its length. For every human being, it is largely conditioned by how an individual handles the careful balance of renunciations, and accepts these. Its precise and fine perception inevitably escapes all questionnaires. Specific tools developed over the past 20 years cannot presume to its assessment but can help discern the impact of new treatment modalities and are increasingly being used in this context (Abbott *et al.*, 2011). This also implies that, given the choice between equally efficient treatments, the least invasive treatment and follow-up modalities are to be favoured (Wainwright *et al.*, 2011). Under close supervision and for adequately selected patients, home intravenous antibiotic treatment is a less disruptive alternative to hospital admissions. Though fatigue can be worse for home participants, home treatment has been associated to improvement in quality of life (Balaquer *et al.*, 2008). At all stages of this complex long-term disease, a holistic approach of the care management of both the patient and his family is essential (Bush *et al.*, 2006; Cohen-Cymberknoh *et al.*, 2011).

2.4 Hope for a curative treatment

Predicting survival of a disease based on the past and present data bypasses the possibility of discovering a cure. Despite all prognostic improvements linked to progress in follow-up and symptomatic treatment of CF, it remains imperative to discover a cure for respiratory disease of CF, for at least 3 reasons: i) current treatment is increasingly cumbersome, 'devouring' about 2 hours every day on average; ii) the cost of CF treatment is constantly rising, leading to fears that there may be increasing limitations as to its availability, even in richer countries; iii) some patients still experience a much more rapid FEV1 decline. The approach favoured today is that of the search for pharmacological agents capable of circumventing the consequences of genetic anomalies as determined by CFTR gene class mutations (Amaral, 2011; Rogan *et al.*, 2011). The principle is to interrupt 'the source' of the cascade of events that leads from an ionic transport anomaly in the respiratory epithelium to lung destruction. Treatment tailored to the type of mutation appears today reasonably within reach (Accurso *et al.*, 2010). Should this eventuality become a reality, the prognosis of patients still free of significant pulmonary lesions would be radically transformed.

3. Causes of death in CF

Over 95% of known causes of death in CF (including data following lung transplantations of CF patients) are linked to involvement of the respiratory system (CFF Registry, 2000). Amongst the specific and much rarer causes of death, feature complications of liver disease, dehydration and intestinal obstruction in countries where physicians have little knowledge of CF (Verma *et al.*, 2000).

4. Prognostic factors

A pragmatic way of looking at prognostic factors of CF is to distinguish those that are linked to the quality of care management and those on which care management has little (e.g. environmental factors) or no grip (genetic factors) (Wolfenden *et al.*, 2009). Figure 1 gives an overview of prognostic factors in CF.

Three aspects of the discussion are worth mentioning i) interactions between factors are numerous and their complex statistical evaluation study has probably been too shallow in many publications; ii) the evaluation of the role of certain less easily quantifiable factors, such as treatment adherence, escapes usual means of analysis; iii) our choice is to focus on factors that appear essential to a clinician. The complexity of interactions between the different factors is clearly illustrated by the example of the impact of passive smoking on respiratory function. Although the deleterious effects of passive smoking are well established, they vary according to CFTR genotype and certain alleles of modifying genes (Collaco *et al.*, 2008). Moreover, several studies demonstrated a link between passive smoking and socio-economic status (Smyth *et al.*, 1994).

One example of 'the clinician's choice' in the discussion is not to dwell on the often reported issue of a 'female disadvantage' (Rosenfeld *et al.*, 1997; Mehta *et al.*, 2010; Olesen *et al.*, 2010), which may not concern adult diagnosed CF patients (Nick *et al.*, 2010). Numerous hypotheses have been brought forward to account for it, without any practical impact to date. Furthermore, though this might have been achieved at the price of a higher burden of treatment in females (Olesen *et al.*, 2010), there is evidence that modern intensive treatment may result in similar key clinical parameters for the two genders (Verma *et al.*, 2008; Olesen *et al.*, 2010).

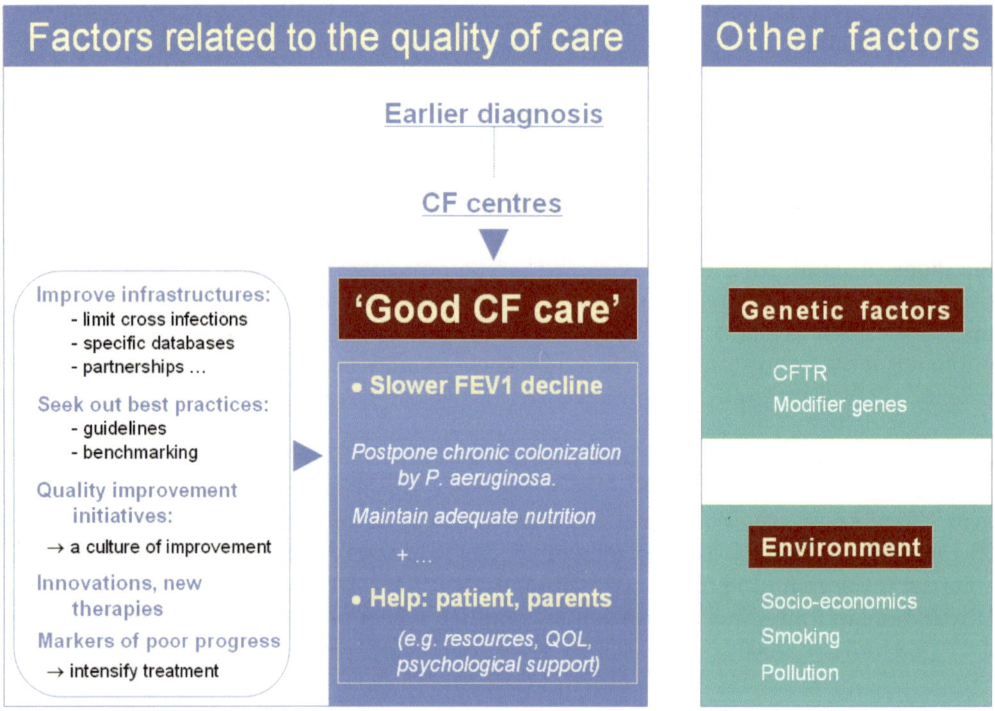

Fig. 1. Prognostic factors in CF

5. Good care management of CF

Early and mostly optimal management of CF is thus the principal reason for the improved prognosis observed over the past decades. Comprehensive follow-up and progress in symptomatic treatment proved essential. Antibiotics are the mainstay of CF therapy. In view of the complexity of this multisystemic and in many ways unique pathology, optimal management is only possible in truly specialized structures. Limiting the impact of economic status on treatment is an important issue. Most impressively, a pioneer clinician had already specifically stressed the importance of every single one of the above-named factors as early as 1974 (Crozier, 1974).

Taken in isolation and often combined to other factors (see discussion below), several complications can be linked to an accelerated rate of FEV_1 decline. Their awareness, prevention or early detection followed by optimal management carries the potential to reduce the rate of FEV_1 decline. This is well illustrated by the case for CF-related diabetes (CFRD) over the past 20 years. At one large CF centre, early detection and optimal management of CFRD resulted in a decrease on its impact on mortality and the disappearance of a sex difference in mortality (Moran *et al.*, 2009).

Two factors in particular, chronic airway colonisation by *Pseudomonas aeruginosa* (PA) and malnutrition, have such spontaneous prevalence and such prognostic impact, that their prevention constitutes one of the major objectives of CF care management.

Several medications have been associated to slowing down the rate of FEV_1 decline: dornase alpha (Konstan *et al.*, 2011), ibuprofen (Konstan *et al.*, 1995; Konstan *et al.*, 2007), azithromycin (Hansen *et al.*, 2005) and inhaled corticosteroids (De Boeck *et al.*, 2011). This does not mean that *all* patients will benefit from them. In addition, possible side-effects in the long-term have to be kept in mind (cf. e.g. ibuprofen). Also, it cannot be inferred that other drugs are necessarily ineffective: they may simply not have been subjected to appropriate studies, which occasionally may be due to commercial reasons or ethical concerns (e.g. physiotherapy).

5.1 Early diagnosis: CF newborn screening (NBS)

A number of studies using bronchoalveolar lavage (BAL) markers of infection and inflammation, lung function tests or computed tomography of the chest have documented that significant lung damage occurs very early in many, even asymptomatic, infants (Khan *et al.*, 1995; Ranganathan *et al.*, 2001; Davis *et al.*, 2007; Mott *et al.*, 2009). The results of two recent studies concerning very young infants who were investigated routinely after CF diagnosis by NBS are particularly striking (Sly *et al.*, 2009; Stafler *et al.*, 2011). Unsuspected positive cultures were found in 21-27% of them, there was evidence of airways inflammation with BAL neutrophilia in most patients and CT evidence of bronchial dilatation in 18.6%.

CF is a progressive disease for which symptomatic treatment has proven to have a real impact albeit of partial efficiency. So, starting treatment as early as possible is meaningful. CF NBS is now available throughout the USA and in many European countries. For those newborns carrying a genotype clearly associated with the disease, benefits of neonatal screening has long been proven in nutritional terms. Respiratory benefits have only recently been acknowledged (Accurso *et al.*, 2005; Rosenfeld *et al.*, 2010), as these were temporarily obscured by a publication indicating an increased risk of early chronic colonisation by PA in screened newborns (Farrell *et al.*, 2003). This increased risk was eventually linked to the lack of measures aiming to limit cross infections in that particular centre and subsequent studies failed to confirm it (Siret *et al.*, 2003; Sims *et al.*, 2005; Baussano *et al.*, 2006; Collins *et al.*, 2008). In countries with a high level of medical care, neonatal screening enables clinicians to diagnose CF in infants before the age of 2 months, with demonstrable benefits (Sims *et al.*, 2007).

5.2 The case for CF care centres

5.2.1 CF centres are necessary

CF NBS is universally coupled with immediate referral to a specialist centre. Guidelines and international consensus all emphasize this to be the key to efficiency for all CF programs

(Castellani *et al.*, 2009; Comeau *et al.*, 2007). Even outside the context of CF NBS, early referral to a specialist healthcare centre is considered as a major prognostic factor as highlighted in consensus reports on optimal management of CF (Littlewood, 2000; Kerem *et al.*, 2005; Colombo *et al.*, 2011). Though this has long been supported by a number of common sense reasons and has been mentioned as a model for the management of complex diseases (Schechter *et al.*, 2005), most published studies concerning the impact of this centralization on lung disease are either biased due to comparison with historical controls, and/or probably underpowered (Hill *et al.*, 1985; Nielsen *et al.*, 1988; Walters *et al.*, 1994; Collins *et al.*, 1999; Merelle *et al.*, 2001; Van Koolwijk *et al.*, 2002).

Two studies avoid these pitfalls. Mahadeva *et al.* compared two groups of adults who had either received continuous care from paediatric and adult CF centres (n=50) or had received neither paediatric nor adult centre care for their CF (n=36). Excluding body mass index as a covariate, FEV_1 was significantly better in the first group (Mahadeva *et al.*, 2000). More recently, a Belgian retrospective multicentre study clearly showed that earlier referral of children suffering from CF to specialist care was associated with significant pulmonary benefits (Lebecque *et al.* , 2009). Children referred 'early' (less than 2 years after diagnosis) had a better FEV_1 (86.7% pred. ± 19.4 *vs.* 77.2% ± 22.4, p=0.01) and a lower prevalence of PA (17.5% *vs.* 38.6 %, p<0.05) than carefully matched patients referred later.

5.2.2 CF centres might not be sufficient

Large differences between outcome variables obtained from the different centres have been recognized for a long time (Bauernfeind *et al.*, 1996) and are now drawing considerable attention as they may provide an opportunity to develop quality improvement initiatives. Striking illustrations of this outcome heterogeneity are provided by recent data from the 2007 US Registry (CFF Registry, 2007 - public data), allowing for comparisons between centres: i) mean FEV_1 (% predicted) for CF children aged 6-17 years ranged from 75 to 103% (national average: 92.6%, reference values: Wang & Hankinson) ii) the percentage of patients under 20 years of age with a BMI < 5th percentile ranged from 32 to 83% (national average: 52.7%) iii) MRSA infection rate ranged from 6 to 42% (national average: 21.2%). These differences persisted after taking into account socio-economic factors. Similar features can be derived from the CF German Registry where a quality management program with an overall coverage of 82% for the year of 2005 confirmed considerable differences between centres in terms of key parameters (Stern *et al.*, 2008). For instance, the percentage of children (6-18 years) with an FEV_1 above 80% of the predicted value ranged from 20 to 100% in centres treating less than 50 patients and from 35% to 100% in larger centres. Globally, the mean FEV_1 in this age group was 88% of the predicted value. A recent Belgian multicentre study confirmed the broad outcome differences between reference centres within this small country, where corresponding values for FEV_1 in children reportedly ranged from 74% to 95% predicted (Lebecque *et al.*, 2009) while the prevalence of *PA* (last visit of the year) ranged from 5 to 46% and the mean weight expressed as percentage of ideal body weight ranged from 88% to 100%.

5.2.3 Marked differences in clinical results between CF centres: Why?

One report of 18,411 patients followed in 194 North American centres in 1995 showed that close monitoring and heavier treatment (more frequent antibiotics in particular) clearly characterized those north-American centres with better clinical results (Johnson *et al.*, 2003). It is interesting to note that this more intensive management included two modalities which do not correspond to standard management: frequent prescription of nedocromil and more common prophylactic prescription of inhaled antibiotics, particularly in patients with still little pulmonary involvement. The use of nedocromil in CF is not well documented in the literature, neither is the potential of giving prophylactic inhaled antibiotics, which is discussed a little further in this chapter. Another North American study concerned 837 children aged 6 to 12 years (Padman *et al.*, 2007), whose CF centres were classified according to the children's FEV_1 values in 2003. The analysis also suggested that closer follow-up starting before the age of 3 years was characteristic of those centres with the best functional results. This 'more attentive and more active 'attitude' is in line with current standards of care, which are derived as much as possible from evidence-based medicine (Littlewood, 2000; Kerem *et al.*, 2005; Littlewood, 2005; Tiddens, 2009).

In 2002, the CFF launched an innovative Quality Improvement (QI) initiative, which included the vision statement that within 5 years, life expectancy of CF patients could be extended by 5-10 years through the consistent implementation of existing evidence-based clinical care (Quinton, 2007). However, evidence-based medicine has its limitations and possible stumbling blocks (Driever, 2002; Saarni *et al.*, 2004; Miles *et al.*, 2008; Shahar, 2008; Miles *et al.*, 2011), in particular when it concerns diseases as complex as CF for which numerous therapeutic modalities have simply not yet been adequately studied (Cheng *et al.*, 2000; David, 2001; Briggs *et al.*, 2006; Kraynack *et al.*, 2009). Best practice remains individualized in part, although a coherent foundation of evidence-based medicine is absolutely necessary.

One comparative study of 3 CF centres illustrates how even beside care standards, clinician intuition can lead to potentially judicious choices that deserve prospective studies. A better nutritional status was indeed linked to the prescription of dornase alpha (Pulmozyme ®) under the age of 2 years (Padman *et al.*, 2008), whereas the effects of Pulmozyme in this age group have only been reported in one limited study (Berge *et al.*, 2003) where 9 infants were given the drug for 2 weeks. The necessity to conceive and study new strategies stems from the fact that current ones are relatively powerless in preventing pulmonary lesions in early diagnosed infants (Stick *et al.*, 2009).

Information concerning the standards of CF care is widely available as are new drugs in rich countries. Differences in clinical results between various CF centres must therefore have a different origin. One can suspect subtle combinations of several factors resulting in small differences in interventionist attitudes. Beside adequate means i.e. infrastructures and human resources, optimal care requires a careful organisation (structure of the centre, coherence of attitudes, multiple fail safe systems etc.) necessitating considerable long-term thoughtful investment of all those involved.

5.2.4 Variability of outcomes in CF centres: Benchmarking as a right to patients

It is not possible for a CF clinic to function without landmarks. Specific databases prove to be very precious by giving immediate access to progress over time and by age group of essential parameters, thereby constituting a sort of 'compass' for measures that could be taken to improve care management. Although limiting the objective to FEV_1 improvement would be reductive, it clearly remains an essential parameter. The FEV_1 of patients aged 6-18 years old (Figure 2) is a particularly relevant landmark for the 3 following reasons: i) very few patients die or require transplantation prior to that age ii) a significant proportion of adults has not benefited from immediate specialized care iii) adolescence is a particularly high risk time period with regard to deterioration of respiratory function. Appropriate indicators to define nutritional outcomes are also necessary (Lai *et al.*, 2008). If they are to be used to compare CF centres, these indicators have to be adjusted for risk factors - which does not change the overall outcome variability of CF centres (Schechter *et al.*, 2002) - and several years should be taken into consideration, in order to appreciate their coherence and tendencies.

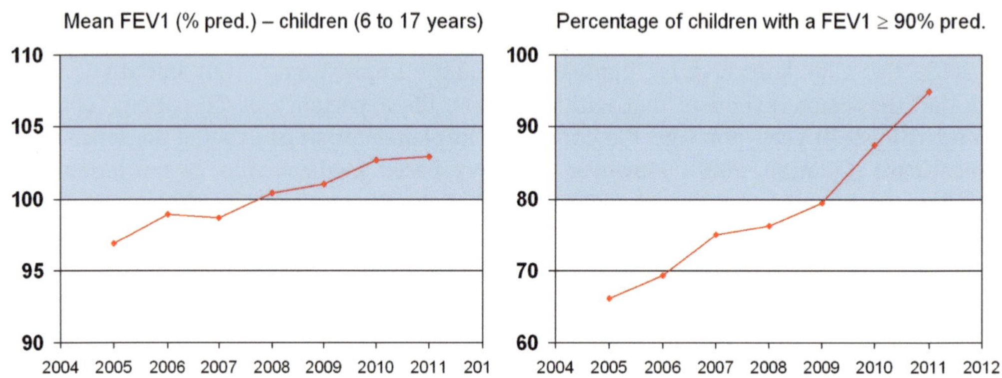

Fig. 2. Lung function in children followed-up at St Luc (last visit of the year, reference equations from Wang et al. for females through age 15 and males through age 17, and Hankinson et al. at older ages) (Wang et al., 1993; Hankinson et al., 1999).

The differences in mean FEV_1 observed in children from various CF centres can exceed 20% of predicted values. Recent data can help to perceive the implications of such differences: i) some centres now report a mean annual FEV_1 decline around 1% (Que, 2006) ii) in terms of FEV_1 (expressed in % pred.), improvements from baseline observed in two major randomized controlled trials of inhaled dornase alfa and tobramycin were less than 4% and 5% respectively (Fuchs *et al.*, 1994; Ramsey *et al.*, 1999) iii) in the USA, from 1990 to 2008, median FEV_1 at 12 years of age increased by 14 % predicted. Thus the prognostic significance of the differences between centres is major, also in terms of life expectancy. For this reason, public access to these data can be considered as a right to the patient and/or parents. In 2006, the outcomes data from the CF Foundation registry became public on the foundation's website, with an accompanying warning against simplistic interpretations. This choice bore witness to the priority given to the patients. Their health is at stake, and keeping them informed has to take precedence over the risk of embarrassing some physicians. In the USA, the fear that some patients may leave CF centres with average performance has not materialised: patients and their family maintain their trust once they realize that everything is done to improve results (Quinton, 2007).

5.2.5 'Good enough' care for CF does not exist: Towards a culture of improvement

Benchmarking, which is the process of identifying practices associated with the best results, may help to understand why certain centres obtain better clinical results. Not only can it be considered a right to the patients, it can also serve as an incentive to CF centres to increase their efforts to improve quality of care delivery. In the USA, most CF healthcare providers actually accepted it as a call to action (Schechter *et al.*, 2005). Public release of meaningful adjusted clinical outcomes data has been used in other fields of medicine, such as cardiac surgery, as a means to stimulate improvement efforts within the medical profession (Ferris *et al.*, 2010). Others have advocated 'softer' uses of benchmarking which do not require to be channelled via public data (Stern *et al.*, 2011). In the field of CF, benchmarking is not an easy task. It is possible when based on well-established CF registries but issues related to quality control and missing data obviously remain crucial (van der Ent, 2008). A number of methodological issues make it even harder to compare data from different countries. These include (but are not limited to) the population coverage level, the choice of reference equations, the type of subjects included in the registry (an increasing number of patients with milder forms of the disease are now being identified in some countries through wide access to CFTR gene sequencing and nasal potential difference measurements, or via CF NBS), a lack of uniform definitions of specific items (FEV_1 has been recorded as the last, the best, the mean or the average of the best value for each quarter of the year; normal FEV_1 has been defined as $\geq 80\%$ or $\geq 90\%$ of the predicted value in different registries) or of clinical conditions (hepatopathy, CF-related diabetes, pulmonary exacerbation), differences in age stratification (in the UK, adults are defined as patients ≥ 16 years old), inclusion or exclusion of lung transplanted patients ('another disease'), wide heterogeneity of CFTR mutations throughout the world, etc. There is indeed an obvious need for standardization in data collection if we are to compare different registries meaningfully. The ever present need to 'always try to do better' that animates so many clinicians and paramedics involved in caring for CF patients has led to the development of several QI initiatives. The latter have tended to improve key indices concerning either nutrition or respiratory function, but can also have other objectives such as a greater involvement of patients as partners in care, by sending them for example a copy of their own medical records (Treacy *et al.*, 2008). Guidelines and evidence-based medicine provide the directions in which changes for QI should be made. Various strategies can be put into place as part of these QI initiatives (Quinton, 2004; VandenBranden, 2004; Schechter, 2004; Quinton *et al.*, 2007; Britton *et al.*, 2008; Schechter *et al.*, 2010; Kraynack *et al.*, 2009; Quon *et al.*, 2011). They all rely on adequate infrastructures, the acknowledgement that changes are needed, relevant and quantifiable objectives identified on the basis of the centre's known clinical outcomes, the deployment of the necessary means and an objective evaluation of the various steps undertaken. Taking into consideration identified obstacles to optimal treatment (Zemanick *et al.*, 2010), trends of medication use over time (Konstan *et al.*, 2010), and the considerable differences in treatment practices (Borsje *et al.*, 2000) or in clinical approach between specialized CF centres (Kraynack *et al.*, 2011) could nurture reflection and help to identify and better discern the objectives and means to be put into place.

5.3 Tools and challenges

The range of responsibilities of a team dedicated to CF patients is vast, in keeping with the complexity of this chronic disease. Close and comprehensive follow-up enables an early start of an efficient symptomatic treatment. Guidelines and specific databases belong to those tools that are essential to the clinicians. The importance of the latter can not be overemphasized (Kerem *et al.*, 2005; Quinton *et al.*, 2007; Leal *et al.*, 2007; Tiddens, 2009).

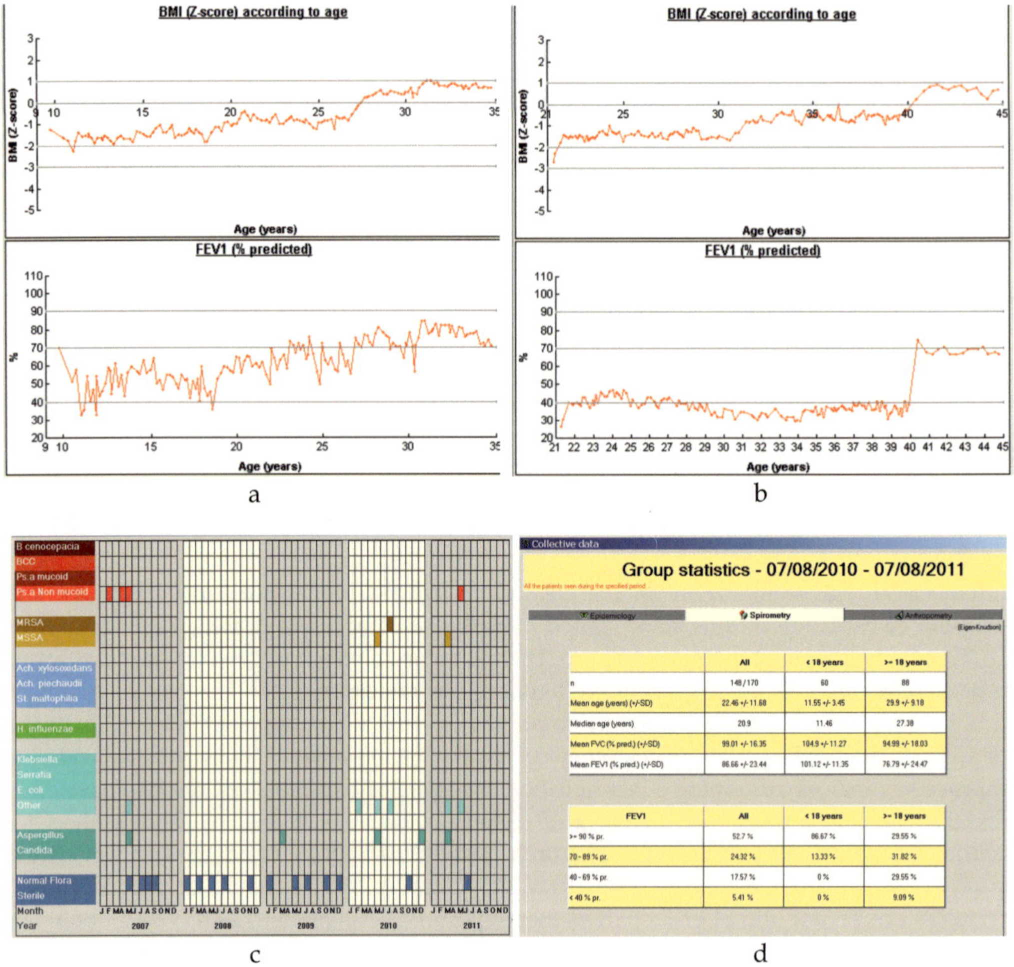

Fig. 3. Specific database provide instant access to critical information at the individual level and at the level of the clinic as a whole. *a*. Current treatment modalities occasionally lead to sustained very long-term improvement of both FEV_1 and BMI. *b*. They can also allow prolonged survival in stable conditions despite severe pulmonary lesions (this patient eventually benefited from a lung transplant following recurrent life-threatening haemoptysis). *c*: This screen summarize bacteriological findings of a given patient over 5 years, also allowing to determine at a glance the state of *Pseudomonas aeruginosa* infection according to a meaningful classification (Lee *et al.*, 2003). *d*: Instant access to key parameters at the scale of the whole clinic.

In the setting of the clinic, visualizing with a simple click trends of essential parameters such as FEV_1 or BMI can help the patient to fully understand the need for treatment modifications.

Regularly updated guidelines and in-depth reviews are essential resources. They cover most areas including standards of care (Kerem *et al.*, 2005), diagnosis (Farrell *et al.*, 2008), adult management (Yankaskas *et al.*, 2004), care of infants diagnosed by CF NBS (Accurso *et al.*, 2009; Sermet-Gaudelus *et al.*, 2010), nutrition (Sinaasappel *et al.*, 2002; CF Trust, 2002; Stallings *et al.*, 2008), antibiotic therapy (CF Trust, 2009), respiratory infections (Ramsey *et al.*, 2003), by *Pseudomonas aeruginosa* in particular (Döring *et al.*, 2000; Saiman *et al.*, 2003; Döring *et al.*, 2004; CF Trust , 2004; Hoiby *et al.*, 2005), microbiology laboratory standards (CF Trust 2010), pregnancy management (Edenborough *et al.*, 2008; Lau *et al.*, 2010) or complications such as Allergic BronchoPulmonary Aspergillosis (ABPA) (Stevens *et al.*, 2003), diabetes (Moran *et al.*, 2010), pneumothorax or haemoptysis (Flume *et al.*, 2010).

5.3.1 Challenge 1: Postpone chronic colonisation by *Pseudomonas aeruginosa*

The reasons for which PA has a predilection for the lungs of CF patients are still unclear (Gibson *et al.*, 2003). Its presence can often be detected early, at times within the first few months of life, even in the absence of any symptom. It will usually be isolated within the first 3 years (Burns *et al.*, 2001; Dakin *et al.*, 2002; West *et al.*, 2002; Hilliard *et al.*, 2007; Sly *et al.*, 2009; Stafler *et al.*, 2011). A prospective study has indicated that 90% of CF children aged 4 years and above presented at least 1 positive culture for PA (Li *et al.*, 2005). The early isolates of PA are generally non-mucoid and antibiotic susceptible. However, PA tends to colonise the airways of CF patients in a chronic, irreversible, fashion often associated to a change to a mucoid phenotype. At this stage, pulmonary function usually worsens and clinical symptoms become evident. Early detection of PA is crucial as there is a window of opportunity for effective eradication at this stage (Koch, 2002; Li *et al.*, 2005).

Chronic PA colonisation is associated with a lower FEV_1 in childhood (Kerem *et al.*, 1990), an accelerated rate of FEV_1 decline (Pamukcu *et al.*, 1995; Kosorok *et al.*, 2001; Emerson *et al.*, 2002), a shorter median life expectancy (CFF Registry, 1996; Emerson *et al.*, 2002) and much higher treatment costs (Baumann *et al.*, 2003). Preventing this colonisation is considered the most important challenge for the CF clinician, as it frequently determines the patient's future quality of life and long-term survival (CF Trust 2002; Koch, 2002). The current approach relies on two strategies (Frederiksen *et al.*, 1999): i) paying attention to segregate patients on bacteriological grounds in order to limit the risk of cross-infections (West *et al.*, 2002; Conway *et al.*, 2008), ii) early antibiotic treatment at the time of the first PA colonisation (Littlewood *et al.*, 1985; Valerius *et al.*, 1991; Frederiksen *et al.*, 1997; Lee *et al.*, 2004). A number of regimens have been evaluated (Stuart *et al.*, 2010) but there is no consensus about the best combination, dosage, or length of treatment course. An initial treatment protocol combining nebulised colistin with oral ciprofloxacin for 3 months is widely used. Combining this approach with intravenous antibiotics has also been reported, with a 5-year failure rate of only 12% (Douglas *et al.*, 2009). A prerequisite for this approach is a close bacteriological follow-up, with a time lapse between visits that cannot exceed 3 months. This interval is shorter (up to monthly) in many centres. An aggressive approach based on repeated BAL has not proven useful (Wainwright *et al.*, 2011). The 20% failure rate of the more commonly used approach (Frederiksen *et al.*, 1997; Lee *et al.*, 2004; Tacetti *et al.*, 2004) underlines the necessity to develop other intervention modalities.

It is paradoxical that prophylactic antibiotic therapy directed against PA has only been the subject of 1 retrospective study (Heinzl *et al.*, 2002) while prophylaxis against *Staphylococcus aureus*, whose threat is yet much easier to manage, has been investigated and hotly debated. The Austrian study was in fact very encouraging but the same group reported that long-term gentamicin inhalation in CF children was associated with reversible raised urinary N-acetyl-beta-D-glucosaminidase (NAG) activity, consistent with subtle subclinical renal tubular damage (Ring *et al.*, 1998). Tobramycin and amikacin however have lower renal toxicity than gentamicin and long-term use of high doses of inhaled tobramycin (TOBI) are now considered safe (Prober *et al.*, 2000). There are several theoretical arguments that make long-term inhaled prophylactic antibiotic therapy attractive (Lebecque *et al.*, 2008). Based on the use of low doses of Tobramycin or Amikacin, this approach has progressively been put into place at our centre over the past 20 years, and has probably contributed, along with other factors, to a distinctly low rate of chronic colonisation rate by PA in patients under 18 years of age (<5% for more than 10 years, according to Lee's definition) (Lee *et al.*, 2003).

5.3.2 Challenge 2: Maintain adequate nutrition

The poorer prognosis associated with being relatively underweight has long been recognized in CF children (Kraemer *et al.*, 1978). An overall parallelism exists between respiratory function and nutritional status progress over time (Zemel *et al.*, 2000; Steinkamp *et al.*, 2002; Konstan *et al.*, 2003; Milla, 2004; Pedreira *et al.*, 2005). While severe pulmonary disease seriously compromises the maintenance of a satisfactory nutritional status, proof of the opposite has also been demonstrated: maintaining a good nutritional status promotes respiratory function preservation. Evidence of the possible influence of maintaining a good nutritional status was first suggested by a comparison of the CF centres of Boston and Toronto (Corey *et al.*, 1988). In Toronto, CF patients had better respiratory function and were better fed, and the main difference in management appeared to be the lack of fat restriction in the Canadian hospital. Maintaining an adequate nutritional status has become a priority of CF care.

5.3.3 Many other challenges…

Early detection and adequate management of poor clinical course find their place here, along with appropriate management of complications, particularly those linked to an accelerated rate of FEV_1 decline as in ABPA (Kraemer *et al.*, 2006), diabetes (Milla *et al.*, 2000), gastro-esophageal reflux (Levy *et al.*, 1986), colonisation by *Burkolderia cenocepacia* (Ledson *et al.*, 2002; Courtney *et al.*, 2004) non-mucoid strains in particular (Zlosnik *et al.*, 2011), or by MRSA (Dasenbrook *et al.*, 2008). In the same vein it is worth insisting on the vulnerable period spanning from pre-adolescence to adolescence (Konstan *et al.*, 2007). The rate of FEV_1 decline is faster at that time, and the various reasons for which this is considered a risk period should especially mobilise the attention and energy of the care management teams (Segal, 2008). In the context of CF, ABPA diagnosis is often delicate, (de Almeida *et al.*, 2006; Thia *et al.*, 2009) as many features overlap with those of infective exacerbations in CF, but it is important: failing to recognize ABPA can lead to irreversible lesions, whereas overtreatment exposes the patient to deleterious side-effects of systemic corticosteroids.

The prevention of cross-infections is a daily preoccupation that predetermines the detailed organisation of the CF centres. One of the major challenges is to limit *Burkholderia cepacia complex* (BCC) infections. The prognostic significance of colonisation by *B. cenocepacia* is particularly dreaded, as its presence is associated to an accelerated rate of FEV_1 decline and a clinical picture that is often fatal (*cepacia* syndrome) (Isles *et al.*, 1984) and can affect patients up to then in very good health. In addition, *B. cenocepacia* is a cause for increased mortality following lung transplantation (Aris *et al.*, 2001; Boussaud *et al.*, 2008). Other germs of the BCC group such as B. *multivorans* or B. *dolosa* have a less gloomy effect on prognosis but have exceptionally also been associated to the occurrence of a *cepacia* syndrome (Zahariadis *et al.*, 2003; Blackburn *et al.*, 2004; Kalish *et al.*, 2006).

Several other essential factors are involved in global care management. There is no equivalent long-term illness to CF today in terms of the heavy burden of its symptomatic treatment. In a recent US study, adult patients - of whom only half had performed airway clearance - reported a mean time spent on treatment activities of 108 minutes per day (Sawicki *et al.*, 2009). Though very difficult to assess (Modi *et al.*, 2006), treatment adherence is undoubtedly a key issue in CF (Eakin et al, 2011) and requires permanent assessment and support (Pendleton, 2000). There is no magic recipe, but this subject has to be bridged at every consultation, in an open manner, with empathy and as part of a 'therapeutic alliance' (Lask, 1994; Cohen-Cymberknoh *et al.*, 2011). Another objective is to be able to propose psychological and/or social support in response to specific situations, either linked to the disease or impacting on treatment in real life.

5.3.4 Flags or indications for treatment intensification

Several clinical or biological markers have been associated with poorer outcome. Their main interest is that they can point to the need for reconsidering and optimizing symptomatic treatment. Some of these associations may appear simple common sense but the reality is often more complex: in-depth statistical analysis can reveal multiple independent factors and it is important to bear in mind that a statistically significant association is not equivalent to the demonstration of a causality link. For instance, a recent Canadian study showed that adult patients with CF who experienced at least 3 pulmonary exacerbations per year over a 3-year follow-up period were clearly high-risk patients, who warranted timely consideration for lung transplantation (de Boer *et al.*, 2011). However, such patients were more likely to be female and diabetic, two risk factors linked to poorer outcome. In addition, while frequent pulmonary exacerbations may predispose a patient to lung transplantation, patients on the list for lung transplants may be more aggressively treated, thereby appearing to have more exacerbations. Raised serum IgG levels (Wallwork *et al.*, 1974; Matthews *et al.*, 1980; Wheeler *et al.*, 1984; Proesmans *et al.*, 2011) and the presence of localized auscultation anomalies (Konstan *et al.*, 2007) also belong to the list of 'flags' for treatment intensification.

6. Environmental factors

6.1 Socioeconomic status

As for all chronic diseases, CF prognosis is more sombre in patients of poor socio-economic status (SES). In 1986, there were 113 deaths registered of CF patients in the UK. Median age of death was 17 years overall, but it was above 20 for patients whose parents had a non-manual job whereas it was below 10 for the others (Britton *et al.*, 1989). In a study of CF patients in the United States, the adjusted risk of death for indigent patients who qualified for Medicaid was 3.65 times higher than for those not receiving Medicaid. The average FEV_1 of Medicaid patients was less by 9.2% predicted than that of non-Medicaid patients, a difference which slightly increased by 0.54% per year of age (Schechter *et al.*, 1998). In a CFF study of 23,817 white patients diagnosed before the age of 18 years, a strong association was found between the median household income and the mortality rate. At 6 years of age, the absolute differences in mean FEV_1 and weight percentiles from the lowest to the highest income category were already very significant and they persisted into adulthood (O'Connor *et al.*, 2003). Furthermore, this study also clearly showed that the relationship between outcome and SES was incremental, rather than dichotomous and only affecting the most indigent. Though access to health insurance is much better in many European countries than in the US, the overall costs of CF treatment and follow-up are so high that patients with low SES are particularly at risk of inadequate resources and poor adherence. A better understanding of SES-related disparities and its causes is necessary to clarify the respective roles of a link between poverty and other environmental factors, health behaviours and limited access to optimal care. Low SES has recently been associated with lower health-related quality of life in CF patients and parents. After accounting for the effects of disease severity and SES, a negative effect of membership to a racial or ethnic minority on social and emotional functioning was also evident (Quittner *et al.*, 2010).

6.2 Exposure to smoking

Exposure to passive or active smoking has deleterious effects in healthy subjects and in patients with respiratory diseases. An accelerated rate of FEV_1 decline with age is documented in healthy adult smokers. Functional repercussions of passive smoking were assessed in a large study concerning 812 CF patients (Collaco *et al.*, 2008). Over a fifth of them (188, i.e. 23%) were exposed to passive smoking. At the age of 20, the mean FEV_1 of exposed patients was, independently of SES, 8% lower than that of non-exposed patients. This effect was even more pronounced in patients who were not homozygous for the *F508del* mutation, and was twice higher in patients who were also carriers of an unfavourable genotype with respect to the $TGF\beta_1$ modifier gene. Deleterious effects of active smoking should a priori be more severe but have not been investigated specifically in the context of CF. Exposure to smoking is a major environmental factor and screening for it should become routine practice in CF care as several pharmacological and non-pharmacological smoking cessation aids have proven their efficacy, the best results being obtained by combining modalities and tailoring therapy (Laniado-Laborin, 2010).

6.3 Other environmental factors

In a CF registry study, exposure to ozone and annual average exposure to particulate air pollution were both associated with an increased likelihood of pulmonary exacerbations. Exposure to particulate matter with an aerodynamic diameter of 2.5 µm or less was also associated with a decline in lung function (Goss *et al.*, 2004). Though environmental factors are not considered the main pathogenic factors in ABPA, experts have suggested that it may be worth examining the patient's environment in refractory cases (Stevens *et al.*, 2003). Altough the mechanisms are unclear, recent published evidence supports a link between climatic conditions (ambient temperature) and lung function in CF (Collaco et al., 2011). According to the authors, a hypothetical 18 year old white male with CF (Height: 175cm) with an FEV1 of 73.5% percent living in a cold climate would be expected to have an FEV1 of 66.1% had he resided in a 17 degree (Celsius) warmer climate.

Recreational use of marijuana is common in many countries. In a study of 173 adults, this drug was used by 20% of patients (Stern *et al.*, 1987). In the general population, such use has been associated with pulmonary manifestations (bronchitis, pneumothorax, apical bullae) (Tetrault *et al.*, 2007; Han *et al.*, 2010; Gao *et al.*, 2010) that could overlap clinical and radiological signs of CF, making it challenging to suspect them. Further studies seem warranted in this field.

7. Genetic factors

7.1 CFTR genotype

Depending on their repercussions on the synthesis of the CF Transmembrane conductance Regulator (CFTR) protein, mutations of the CF gene are usually classified into 5 groups (Welsh *et al.*, 1993). Mutations of classes I, II and III lead to the total or near-total absence of functional CFTR protein, whereas those of classes IV or V are associated to residual function of the CFTR protein, corresponding to a small % of normal activity. Pancreatic insufficiency is present in over 95% of patients carrying 2 class I, II or III mutations, whereas it is only rarely observed in patients carrying at least 1 class IV or V mutation (CF genotype-phenotype consortium, 1993; Koch *et al.*, 2001). Diabetes and severe hepatic involvement are 2 important CF complications that usually only occur in patients with exocrine pancreatic insufficiency. A recent study of 505 patients registered in Israel's databases did not observe a single case amongst 139 pancreatic sufficient patients (Augarten *et al.*, 2008). The relationship between CFTR genotype and the severity of the pulmonary involvement is much looser. On the whole, the genotype of patients carrying 2 mutations of class I, II or III is still considered high risk and is associated to earlier mortality than genotypes including at least 1 mutation of class IV or V ('low risk' genotypes) (Mc Kone *et al.*, 2006). Similarly, although their phenotype can be extremely variable, an overall more favourable prognosis has been associated to some mutations of class IV or V. Amongst the latter, there are mutations A455E (Gan *et al.*, 1995), 3849 +10kbC->T (Highsmith *et al.*, 1994; Duguépéroux *et al.*, 2005), 2789+5G->A (Duguépéroux *et al.*, 2005), D1152H (Musaffi *et al.*, 2006; Burgel *et al.*, 2010), R334W (Antinolo *et al.*, 1997), 3272-26A->G (Amaral *et al.*, 2001). The penetrance of the R117H mutation has convincingly been shown to be very low (Thauvin-Robinet *et al.*, 2009) and is modulated by the polypyrimidine variant in the intron 8 acceptor splice site (T7 or T5) in cis with R117H. However, FEV_1 at a given age can be extremely variable in patients sharing a same CFTR genotype and this is observed in patients homozygous for the *F508del* mutation as well as in patients carrying a "milder" genotype (Gan *et al.*, 1995). In practice, the link between CFTR genotype and severity of lung disease is not tight, making CFTR genotype most often of little value in predicting the prognosis at the individual level.

7.2 Modifier genes

Every clinician has in mind extreme examples of the heterogeneity of functional respiratory progress in CF patients, including amongst those that are homozygous for the *F508del* mutation. Though poorly compliant, chronically colonized by PA since adolescence and diabetic for 10 years, one 40 year-old patient keeps his FEV_1 above 80% of the predicted value whereas a young lady, with an optimal follow-up since birth and only occasionally *Aspergillus fumigatus* in sputum experiences a rapid functional decline from age 12 and requires a lung transplantation at 20. Environmental factors may play a role but admittedly such patients have to be either 'protected' for one or 'condemned' for the other, by particular allele combinations of modifier genes probably modulating the immune and inflammatory response in the lungs.

Family-based studies and especially comparisons of monozygous and dizygous twin pairs have proven fruitful in identifying and assessing the contribution of modifier genes in CF disease. Many studies in this field have yielded conflicting results and it is now realized that the repeatability of SNP–phenotype association studies with positive findings was low when less than 500 participants were included (Boyle, 2007). More recent studies are more powerful and use more sophisticated tools including whole-genome methods. Quite convincing evidence is now available that variants of at least 3 genes can be associated with lung disease severity in CF (Cutting, 2010): i) *MBL2*-deficient (10q) genotype: in normal subjects, mannose binding lectin (MBL) aids the phagocytosis of bacteria and deficiency in MBL seems to predispose to early infection with PA in CF ii) Increased $TGF\beta_1$ (19q) expression (Drumm *et al.*, 2005): this gene, which also modulates the risk for asthma and chronic obstructive pulmonary disease, encodes a cytokine playing a role in the regulation of inflammation and tissue remodelling iii) Increased *EDNRA* (4q) expression: Endothelin is a proinflammatory peptide and smooth muscle agonist which is increased in CF airways. Deleterious effects could be related to an impact on smooth muscle tone in the airways and/or vasculature (Darrah *et al.*, 2010). More recently, two loci causing variations in CF lung disease severity have been identified on chromosomes 11p and 20q respectively (Wright *et al.*, 2011). Variation in *TCF7L2* (10q) was reported to increase the risk of diabetes about threefold and even more in patients without previous treatment with systemic steroids (Blackman *et al.*, 2009). Variants of other genes are suspected to increase the risk of liver cirrhosis (Bartlett *et al.*, 2009) or meconium ileus. Further progress in the identification of modifier genes should result in an increased ability to predict severity of CF disease, and hopefully be accompanied by new perspectives for therapeutic intervention.

8. Conclusions

For patients, their relatives and also their carers, facing CF is often compared to running a long-distance race. It is also a team race, where no-one can let go. In terms of life expectancy, prognosis of the disease has been improving continuously since 40 years. However, it is almost always impossible to predict CF prognosis at the individual level. The quality of an early global care management is an essential prognostic determinant. Further progress in symptomatic CF treatment remains necessary, especially towards better prevention of respiratory involvement in early-diagnosed newborns and in the field of immunosuppression in lung transplantation. The discovery of a cure for the respiratory disease in CF would be a real breakthrough. A pharmacological approach tailored to the class mutations of the CFTR gene appears currently the most encouraging route in this direction.

Meanwhile, the essence of the carer's role today remains founded on these two maxims: 'Do not abandon the marathon' and 'Always try to do better'.

9. References

Abbott, J., Hart, A., Havermans T. *et al.* (2011). Measuring health-related quality of life in clinical trials in cystic fibrosis. *J Cyst Fibros.* Vol. 10, Suppl 2, pp 82-85.

Accurso, F., Sontag M. & Wagener J. (2005). Complications associated with symptomatic diagnosis in infants with cystic fibrosis. *J Pediatr.* Vol. 147, Suppl. 3, pp 37-41.

Accurso F., Rowe S., Clancy J. *et al.* (2010). Effect of VX-770 in persons with cystic fibrosis and the G551D-CFTR mutation. *N Engl J Med.* Vol. 363, No 21, pp 1191-2003.

Amaral, M., Pacheco P, Beck S. *et al.* (2001). Cystic fibrosis patients with the 3272-26A>G splicing mutation have milder disease than F508del homozygotes: a large European study. *J Med Genet.* Vol. 38, No 11, pp 777-783.

Amaral, M. (2011). Targeting CFTR: how to treat cystic fibrosis by CFTR-repairing therapies. *Curr Drug Targets* Vol. 12, No 5, pp 683-693.

Antinolo G., Borrego S, Gili M. *et al.* (1997). Genotype-phenotype relationship in 12 patients carrying cystic fibrosis mutation R334W. *J Med Genet.* Vol. 34, No 2, pp 89-91.

Aris R., Routh J, LiPuma J. *et al.* (2001). Lung transplantation for cystic fibrosis patients with Burkholderia cepacia complex. Survival linked to genomovar type. *Am J Respir Crit Care Med.* Vol. 164, No 11, pp 2102-2106.

Augarten A., Ben Tov A., Madgar I. *et al.* (2008). The changing face of the exocrine pancreas in cystic fibrosis: the correlation between pancreatic status, pancreatitis and cystic fibrosis genotype. *Eur J Gastroenterol Hepatol.* Vol. 20, No 3, pp 164-168.

Balaguer A. & González de Dios J. (2008). Home intravenous antibiotics for cystic fibrosis. *Cochrane Database Syst Rev.* CD001917.

Bartlett J., Friedman K, Ling S. *et al.* (2009). Genetic modifiers of liver disease in cystic fibrosis. *JAMA.* Vol. 302, No 10, pp 1076-1083.

Bauernfeind A., Marks M. & Strandvik B. (1996). Cystic fibrosis pulmonary infections: lessons from around the world. Birkhauser Verlag AG, Basel. ISBN-13: 978-3764350277

Baumann U., Stocklossa C., Greiner W. *et al.* (2003). Cost of care and clinical condition in paediatric cystic fibrosis patients. *J Cyst Fibros.* Vol. 2, No 2, pp 84-90.

Baussano I., Tardivo I., Belleza-Fontana R. *et al.* (2006). Neonatal screening for cystic fibrosis does not affect time to first infection with Pseudomonas aeruginosa. *Pediatrics.* Vol. 118, No 3, pp 888-895.

Berge M, Wiel E, Tiddens H. *et al.* (2003). DNase in stable cystic fibrosis infants: a pilot study. *J Cyst Fibros.* Vol. 2, No 4, pp 183-188.

Blackburn L., Brownlee K., Conway S. *et al.* (2004). 'Cepacia syndrome' with Burkholderia multivorans, 9 years after initial colonization. *J Cyst Fibros.* Vol. 3, No 2, pp 133-134.

Blackman S., Hsu S, Ritter S *et al.* (2009). A susceptibility gene for type 2 diabetes confers substantial risk for diabetes complicating cystic fibrosis. *Diabetologia* Vol. 52, No 9, pp 1858-1865.

Borowitz D., Robinson K., Rosenfeld M. *et al.* (2009). Cystic Fibrosis Foundation evidence-based guidelines for management of infants with cystic fibrosis. *J Pediatr.* Vol. 155, Suppl. 6, pp 73-93.

Boussaud V., Guillemain R, Grenet D *et al.* (2008). Clinical outcome following lung transplantation in patients with cystic fibrosis colonised with Burkholderia cepacia complex: results from two French centres. *Thorax.* Vol. 63, No 8, pp 732-737.

Borsje P, deJongste J, Mouton J *et al.* (2000). Aerosol therapy in cystic fibrosis: a survey of 54 CF centers. *Pediatr Pulmonol.* Vol. 30, No 5, pp 368-376.

Boyle M. (2007). Strategies for identifying modifier genes in cystic fibrosis. *Proc Am Thorac Soc.* Vol 4, No 1, pp 52-57.

Briggs T., Bryant M. & Smyth R. (2006). Controlled clinical trials in cystic fibrosis--are we doing better? *J Cyst Fibros.* Vol. 5, No 1, pp 3-8.

Britton J. (1989). Effects of social class, sex, and region of residence on age at death from cystic fibrosis. *BMJ.* Vol. 298, pp 483-7.

Britton L., Thrasher S. & Guttierez H. (2008). Creating a culture of improvement: experience of a pediatric cystic fibrosis center. *J Nurs Care Qual.* Vol. 23, No 2, pp 115-120.

Burgel P, Fajac I, Hubert D. *et al.* (2010). Non-classic cystic fibrosis associated with D1152H CFTR mutation. *Clin Genet.* Vol. 77, No 4, pp 355-64.

Burns J., Gibson R, McNamara S. *et al.* (2001). Longitudinal assessment of Pseudomonas aeruginosa in young children with cystic fibrosis. *J Infect Dis.* Vol. 183, No 3, pp 444-452.

Bush A. & Götz M. (2006). Cystic fibrosis. *Eur Respir Mon.* Vol. 37, pp 234–290.

Buzzetti R., Salvatore D., Baldo E. *et al.* (2009). An overview of international literature from cystic fibrosis registries: 1. Mortality and survival studies in cystic fibrosis. *J Cyst Fibros.* Vol. 8, No 4, pp 229-237.

Canadian CF Registry (2008), Available from http://www.fibrosekystique.ca/en/index.php

Castellani C., Southern K, Browlee K. *et al.* (2009). European best practice guidelines for cystic fibrosis neonatal screening. *J Cyst Fibros.* Vol. 8, No 3, pp 153-173.

CF Genotype-Phenotype Consortium (1993). Correlation between genotype and phenotype in patients with cystic fibrosis. *N Engl J Med.* Vol. 329, No 18, pp 1308-1313.

CFF Registry (1996), Cystic Fibrosis Foundation Patient Registry 1996 Annual Data Report. Bethesda, Maryland

CFF Registry (2000), Cystic Fibrosis Foundation Patient Registry 2000 Annual Data Report. Bethesda, Maryland

CFF Registry (2007), Cystic Fibrosis Foundation Patient Registry 2007 Annual Data Report. Bethesda, Maryland

CFF Registry (2008), Cystic Fibrosis Foundation Patient Registry 2008 Annual Data Report. Bethesda, Maryland Available from http://www.cff.org/research/ClinicalResearch/PatientRegistryRport/

CF Trust (2002). Nutritional management in cystic fibrosis.

CF Trust (2004). Pseudomonas aeruginosa infection in people with Cystic Fibrosis. Suggestions for Prevention and Infection Control.

CF Trust (2009). Antibiotic Treatment for Cystic Fibrosis.

CF Trust (2010). Laboratory Standards for Processing Microbiological Samples from People with Cystic Fibrosis.

Cheng K., Smyth R, Motley J. *et al.* (2000). Randomized controlled trials in cystic fibrosis (1966-1997) categorized by time, design, and intervention. *Pediatr Pulmonol.* Vol. 29, No 1, pp 1-7.

Cohen-Cymberknoh M., Shoseyov D. & Kerem E. (2011). Managing cystic fibrosis: strategies that increase life expectancy and improve quality of life. *Am J Respir Crit Care Med.* Vol. 183, no 11, pp 1463-1471.

Collaco J., Vanscoy L., Bremer L. *et al.* (2008). Interactions between secondhand smoke and genes that affect cystic fibrosis lung disease. *JAMA*. Vol. 299, No 4, pp 417-424.

Collaco J., McGready J., Green D. *et al.* (2011). Effect of temperature on cystic fibrosis lung disease and infections: a replicated cohort study. *PLoS One*. Vol. 6, No 11, e27784.

Collins C., MacDonald-Wicks L., Rowe S. *et al.* (1999). Normal growth in cystic fibrosis associated with a specialised centre. *Arch Dis Child*. Vol. 81, No 3, pp 241-246.

Colombo C. & Littlewood J. (2011). The implementation of standards of care in Europe: state of the art. *J Cyst Fibros*. Vol. 10, Suppl. 2, pp 7-15.

Comeau A., Accurso F., White T. *et al.* (2007). Guidelines for implementation of cystic fibrosis newborn screening programs: Cystic Fibrosis Foundation workshop report. *Pediatrics*. Vol. 119, No 2, pp e495-518.

Conway S. (2008). Segregation is good for patients with cystic fibrosis. *J R Soc Med*. Vol. 101, Suppl. 1, pp 31-35.

Corey M., Mc Laughlin F, Williams M. *et al.* A comparison of survival, growth, and pulmonary function in patients with cystic fibrosis in Boston and Toronto. *J Clin Epidemiol*. Vol. 41, No 6, pp 583-591.

Courtney J., Dunbar K, Mc Dowell A. *et al.* (2004). Clinical outcome of Burkholderia cepacia complex infection in cystic fibrosis adults. *J Cyst Fibros*. Vol. 3, No 2, pp 93-98.

Crozier D. (1974). Cystic fibrosis: a not-so-fatal disease. *Pediatr Clin North Am*. Vol. 21, No 4, pp 935-950.

Cutting G. (2010). Modifier genes in Mendelian disorders: the example of cystic fibrosis. *Ann N Y Acad Sci*. No. 1214, pp 57-69.

Dakin C., Numa A, Wang H. *et al.* (2002). Inflammation, infection, and pulmonary function in infants and young children with cystic fibrosis. *Am J Respir Crit Care Med*. Vol. 165, no 7, pp 904-910.

Darrah R., Mc Kone E., O'Connor C. *et al.* (2010). EDNRA variants associate with smooth muscle mRNA levels, cell proliferation rates, and cystic fibrosis pulmonary disease severity. *Physiol Genomics*. Vol. 41, No 1, pp 71-77.

Dasenbrook E., Merlo C., Diener-West *et al.* (2008). Persistent methicillin-resistant Staphylococcus aureus and rate of FEV1 decline in cystic fibrosis. *Am J Respir Crit Care Med*. Vol. 178, No 8, pp 814-821.

David T. (2001). Elusiveness of cystic-fibrosis treatment. *Lancet*. Vol. 357, p 633.

Davis P. (2006). Cystic fibrosis since 1938. *Am J Respir Crit Care Med*. Vol. 173, No 5, pp 475-482.

Davis S., Brody A., Emond M. *et al.* (2007). Endpoints for clinical trials in young children with cystic fibrosis. *Proc Am Thorac Soc*. Vol 4, No 4, pp 418-430.

de Almeida M., Bussamra M. & Rodrigues J. (2006). Allergic bronchopulmonary aspergillosis in paediatric cystic fibrosis patients. *Paediatr Respir Rev*. Vol. 7, No 1, pp 67-72.

De Boeck K., Vermeulen F., Wanyama S. *et al.* (2011). Inhaled corticosteroids and lower lung function decline in young children with cystic fibrosis. *Eur Respir J*. Vol. 37, No 5, pp 1091-1095.

de Boer K., Vandemheen K., Tullis E. *et al.* (2011). Exacerbation frequency and clinical outcomes in adult patients with cystic fibrosis. *Thorax* Vol. 66, No 8, pp 680-685.

Dodge J., Lewis P., Stanton M *et al.* (2007). Cystic fibrosis mortality and survival in the UK: 1947-2003. *Eur Respir J*. Vol. 29, No 3, pp 522-526.

Döring G., Conway S., Heijerman H. *et al.* (2000). Antibiotic therapy against Pseudomonas aeruginosa in cystic fibrosis: a European consensus. *Eur Respir J.* Vol. 16, No 4, pp 749-767.

Döring G., Hoiby N & Consensus study group. (2004). Early intervention and prevention of lung disease in cystic fibrosis: a European consensus. *J Cyst Fibros.* Vol. 3, no 2, pp 67-91.

Douglas T., Brennan S., Gard S. *et al.* (2009). Acquisition and eradication of P. aeruginosa in young children with cystic fibrosis. *Eur Respir J.* Vol. 33, no 2, pp 305-311.

Driever, M. (2002). Are evidenced-based practice and best practice the same? *West J Nurs Res.* Vol. 24, No 5, pp 591-597.

Drumm M., Konstan M., Schluchter M. *et al.* (2005). Genetic modifiers of lung disease in cystic fibrosis. N Engl J Med. Vol. 353, No 14, pp 1443-1453.

Duguépéroux I. & De Braekeleer M. (2005). The CFTR 3849+10kbC->T and 2789+5G->A alleles are associated with a mild CF phenotype. *Eur Respir J.* Vol. 25, No 3, pp 468-473.

Eakin M., Bilderback A., Boyle M. *et al.* (2011). Longitudinal association between medication adherence and lung health in people with cystic fibrosis. *J Cyst Fibros.* Vol. 10, No 4, pp 258-64. ISSN 1569-1993

Edenborough F., Borgo G., Knoop C. eta l. (2008). Guidelines for the management of pregnancy in women with cystic fibrosis. *J Cyst Fibros.* Vol. 7, Suppl. 1, pp 2-32.

Elborn J., Shale D. & Britton J. (1991). Cystic fibrosis: current survival and population estimates to the year 2000. *Thorax* Vol. 46, No 12, pp 881-885.

Emerson J., Rosenfeld M., McNamara S. *et al.* (2002). Pseudomonas aeruginosa and other predictors of mortality and morbidity in young children with cystic fibrosis. *Pediatr Pulmonol.* Vol. 34, No 2, pp 91-100.

Farrell P., Li Z., Kosorok M *et al.* (2003). Bronchopulmonary disease in children with cystic fibrosis after early or delayed diagnosis. *Am J Respir Crit Care Med.* Vol. 168, No 9, pp 1100-1108.

Farrell P., Rosenstein B., White T. *et al.* (2008). Guidelines for diagnosis of cystic fibrosis in newborns through older adults: Cystic Fibrosis Foundation consensus report. *J Pediatr.* Vol. 153, No 2, pp 4-14.

Ferris T. & Torchiana D. Public release of clinical outcomes data - Online CABG report cards. *N Engl J Med* 363: 1593-5.

Flume P., Mogayzel P., Robinson K. *et al.* (2010). Cystic fibrosis pulmonary guidelines: pulmonary complications: hemoptysis and pneumothorax. *Am J Respir Crit Care Med.* Vol. 182, No 3, pp 298-306.

Frederiksen B., Koch C. & Hoiby N. (1997). Antibiotic treatment at time of initial colonisation with Pseudomonas aeruginosa postpones chronic infection and prevents deterioration in pulmonary function in patients with cystic fibrosis. *Pediatr Pulmonol.* Vol. 23, No 5, pp 330–335.

Frederiksen B., Koch C. & Hoiby N. (1999) Changing epidemiology of Pseudomonas aeruginosa infection in Danish cystic fibrosis patients (1974-1995). *Pediatr Pulmonol.* Vol. 28, No 3, pp 159-166.

Gan K., Veeze H., van den Ouweland *et al.* (1995). A cystic fibrosis mutation associated with mild lung disease. *N Engl J Med.* Vol. 333, No 2, pp 95-99.

Gao Z., Wood-Baker R., Harle R. *et al.* (2010). "Bong lung" in cystic fibrosis: a case report. *J Med Case Reports*. Vol. 4, p 371.

Gibson R., Burns J. & Ramsey B. (2003). Pathophysiology and management of pulmonary infections in cystic fibrosis. *Am J Respir Crit Care Med*. Vol. 168, No 8, pp 918-951.

Goss C., Newsom S., Schildcrout J. *et al.* (2004). Effect of ambient air pollution on pulmonary exacerbations and lung function in cystic fibrosis. *Am J Respir Crit Care Med.* Vol. 169, No 7, pp 816-821.

Han B., Gfroerer J. & Colliver J. (2010). Associations between duration of illicit drug use and health conditions: results from the 2005-2007 national surveys on drug use and health. *Ann Epidemiol*. Vol. 20, No 4, pp 289-297.

Hankinson J., Odencrantz J., Fedan K. (1999). Spirometric reference values from a sample of the general U.S. population. *Am J Respir Crit Care Med.* Vol. 159, No 1, pp 79–87.

Hansen C., Pressler T., Koch C. *et al.* (2005). Long-term azitromycin treatment of cystic fibrosis patients with chronic Pseudomonas aeruginosa infection; an observational cohort study. *J Cyst Fibros*. Vol. 4, No 1, pp 35-40.

Heinzl B., Eber E, Oberwaldner B. *et al.* (2002). Effects of inhaled gentamicin prophylaxis on acquisition of Pseudomonas aeruginosa in children with cystic fibrosis: a pilot study. *Pediatr Pulmonol*. Vol. 33, No 1, pp 32-37.

Highsmith W., Burch L, Zhou Z. *et al.* (1994). A novel mutation in the cystic fibrosis gene in patients with pulmonary disease but normal sweat chloride concentrations. *N Engl J Med*. Vol. 331, No 15, pp 974-980.

Hill D., Martin A., Davidson G. *et al.* (1985). Survival of cystic fibrosis patients in South Australia. Evidence that cystic fibrosis centre care leads to better survival. *Med J Aust.* Vol. 143, No 6, pp 230-232.

Hilliard T., Sukhani S. Francis J. *et al.* (2007). Bronchoscopy following diagnosis with cystic fibrosis. *Arch Dis Child*. Vol. 92, No 10, pp 898-899.

Høiby N., Frederiksen B. & Pressler T. (2005). Eradication of early Pseudomonas aeruginosa infection. *J Cyst Fibros*. Vol. 4, Suppl. 2, pp 49-54.

Isles, A., McLusky I., Corey M. *et al.* (1984). Pseudomonas cepacia infection in cystic fibrosis: an emerging problem. *J Pediatr*. Vol. 104, No 2, pp 206-210.

Jackson A., Daly L., Kelleher C. *et al.* (2011). Validation and use of a parametric model for projecting cystic fibrosis survivorship beyond observed data: a birth cohort analysis. *Thorax*. Vol. 66, No 8, pp 674-679.

Johansen H., Nir M., Hoiby N. *et al.* (1991). Severity of cystic fibrosis in patients homozygous and heterozygous for delta F508 mutation. *Lancet*. Vol. 337, pp 631-634.

Johnson C., Butler S., Konstan M. *et al.* (2003). Factors influencing outcomes in cystic fibrosis: a center-based analysis. *Chest*. Vol. 123, No 1, pp 20-27.

Kalish L., Waltz D., Dovey M. *et al.* (2006). Impact of Burkholderia dolosa on lung function and survival in cystic fibrosis. *Am J Respir Crit Care Med*. Vol. 173, No 4, pp 421-425.

Kerem E., Corey M., Gold R. *et al.* (1990). Pulmonary function and clinical course in patients with cystic fibrosis after pulmonary colonization with Pseudomonas aeruginosa. *J Pediatr*. Vol. 116, No 5, pp 714-719.

Kerem E., Corey M., Kerem B. *et al.* (1990). The relation between genotype and phenotype in cystic fibrosis--analysis of the most common mutation (delta F508). *N Engl J Med*. Vol. 323, No 22, pp 1517-1522.

Kerem E., resiman J., Corey M. *et al.* (1992). Prediction of mortality in patients with cystic fibrosis. *N Engl J Med.* Vol. 326, No 18, pp 1187-1191.

Kerem E., Conway S., Elborn S. *et al.* (2005). Consensus Committee. Standards of care for patients with cystic fibrosis: a European consensus. *J Cyst Fibros.* Vol. 4, No 1, pp 7-26.

Khan T., Wagener J., Bost T. *et al.* (1995). Early pulmonary inflammation in infants with cystic fibrosis. *Am J Respir Crit Care Med.* Vol. 151, No 4, pp 1075-1082.

Koch C., Cuppens H., Rainisio M. *et al.* (2001). European Epidemiologic Registry of Cystic Fibrosis (ERCF): comparison of major disease manifestations between patients with different classes of mutations. *Pediatr Pulmonol.* Vol. 31, No 1, pp 1-12.

Koch C. (2002). Early infection and progression of cystic fibrosis lung disease. *Pediatr Pulmonol.* Vol. 34, No 3, pp 232-236.

Konstan M., Byard P. Hoppel C. *et al.* (1995). Effect of high-dose ibuprofen in patients with cystic fibrosis. *N Engl J Med.* Vol. 332, No 13, pp 848-854.

Konstan M., Butler S., Whol M. *et al.* (2003). Growth and nutritional indexes in early life predict pulmonary function in cystic fibrosis. *J Pediatr.* Vol. 142, No 6, pp 624 –630.

Konstan M., Scluchter M., Xue W. *et al.* (2007). Clinical use of Ibuprofen is associated with slower FEV1 decline in children with cystic fibrosis. *Am J Respir Crit Care Med.* Vol. 176, No 11, pp 1084-1089.

Konstan M., Morgan W., Butler S. *et al.* (2007). Risk factors for rate of decline in forced expiratory volume in one second in children and adolescents with cystic fibrosis. *J Pediatr.* Vol. 151, No 2, pp 134-139.

Konstan M., VanDevanter D., Rasouliyan L. *Et al.* (2010). Trends in the use of routine therapies in cystic fibrosis: 1995-2005. *Pediatr Pulmonol.* Vol. 45, No 12, pp 1167-1172.

Konstan M., Wagener J., Pasta D. *et al.* (2011). Clinical use of dornase alpha is associated with a slower rate of FEV1 decline in cystic fibrosis. *Pediatr Pulmonol.* Vol. 46, No 6, pp 545-553.

Kosorok M., Zeng L, West S. *et al.* (2001). Acceleration of lung disease in children with cystic fibrosis after Pseudomonas aeruginosa acquisition. *Pediatr Pulmonol.* Vol. 32, No 4, pp 277-287.

Kraemer R., Rüdeberg A., Hadorn B. *et al.* (1978). Relative underweight in cystic fibrosis and its prognostic value. *Acta Paediatr Scand.* Vol. 67, No 1, pp 33-37.

Kraemer R., Deloséa N., Ballinari P. *et al.* (2006). Effect of allergic bronchopulmonary aspergillosis on lung function in children with cystic fibrosis. *Am J Respir Crit Care Med.* Vol. 174, No 11, pp 1211-1220.

Kraynack N. & McBride J. (2009). Improving care at cystic fibrosis centers through quality improvement. *Semin Respir Crit Care Med.* Vol. 30, No 5, pp 547-558.

Kraynack N., Gothard M., Falletta L. *et al.* (2011). Approach to treating cystic fibrosis pulmonary exacerbations varies widely across us CF care centers. *Pediatr Pulmonol.* Apr 4. doi: 10.1002/ppul.21442. [Epub ahead of print]

Lai H. & Shoff S. (2008). Classification of malnutrition in cystic fibrosis: implications for evaluating and benchmarking clinical practice performance. *Am J Clin Nutr.* Vol. 88, No 1, pp 161-166.

Laniado-Laborin R (2010). Smoking cessation intervention: an evidence-based approach. *Postgrad Med.* Vol. 122, No 2, pp 74-82.

Lask B. (1994). Non-adherence to treatment in cystic fibrosis. *J R Soc Med*. Vol. 87, Suppl. 21, pp 25-27.

Lau E., Morarty C., Ogle R. *Et al.* (2010). Pregnancy and cystic fibrosis. *Paediatr Respir Rev*. Vol. 11, No 2, pp 90-94.

Leal T., Reychler G., Mailleux P. *et al.* (2007). A specific database for providing local and national level of integration of clinical data in cystic fibrosis. *J Cyst Fibros*. Vol. 6, No 3, pp 187-193.

Lebecque P., Leal T., Zylberberg K. *et al.* (2006). Towards zero prevalence of chronic Pseudomonas aeruginosa infection in children with cystic fibrosis. *J Cyst Fibros*. Vol. 5, No 4, pp 237-244.

Lebecque P., Leonard A., De Boeck K. *et al.* (2009). Early referral to cystic fibrosis specialist centre impacts on respiratory outcome. *J Cyst Fibros*. Vol. 8, No 1, pp 26-30.

Lebecque P, De Boeck K., Wanyama S. *et al.* (2010). CF Registries - plea for annual reports focusing on patients homozygous for the F508del mutation. *J Cyst Fibros*. Vol. 9, Suppl. 1, p 114 (A).

Ledson M., Gallagher M., Jackson M. *et al.* (2002). Outcome of Burkholderia cepacia colonisation in an adult cystic fibrosis centre. *Thorax*. Vol. 57, No 2, pp 142-145.

Lee T., Brownlee K., Conway S. *et al.* (2003). Evaluation of a new definition for chronic Pseudomonas aeruginosa infection in cystic fibrosis patients. *J Cyst Fibros*. Vol. 2, No 1, pp 29-34.

Lee T., Brownlee K., Denton M. *et al.* (2004). Reduction in prevalence of chronic Pseudomonas aeruginosa infection at a regional pediatric cystic fibrosis center. *Pediatr Pulmonol*. Vol. 37, No 2, pp 104-110.

Levy L., Durie P., Pencharz P. *et al.* (1986). Prognostic factors associated with patient survival during nutritional rehabilitation in malnourished children and adolescents with cystic fibrosis. *J Pediatr Gastroenterol Nutr* Vol. 5, No 1, pp 97–102.

Li Z., Kosorok M., Farrell P. *et al.* (2005). Longitudinal development of mucoid Pseudomonas aeruginosa infection and lung disease progression in children with cystic fibrosis. *JAMA*. Vol. 293, No 5, pp 581-588.

Liou T., Adler F., Fitzsimmons S. *et al.* (2001). Predictive 5-year survivorship model of cystic fibrosis. *Am J Epidemiol*. Vol. 153, No 4, pp 345-352.

Littlewood J., Miller M., Ghoneim A. *et al.* (1985). Nebulised colomycin for early pseudomonas colonisation in cystic fibrosis. *Lancet*. Vol. 1, p 865.

Littlewood J. (2000). Good care for people with cystic fibrosis. *Paediatr Respir Rev*. Vol. 1, No 2, pp 179-189.

Littlewood J. (2005). European cystic fibrosis society consensus on standards - a roadmap to "best care". *J Cyst Fibros*. Vol. 4, No 1, pp 1-5.

Mahadeva R., Webb K., Westerbeek R. *et al.* (1998). Clinical outcome in relation to care in centres specialising in cystic fibrosis: cross sectional study. *BMJ* Vol. 316, pp 1771-1775.

Matthews W., Williams M, Oliphint B. *et al.* (1980). Hypogammaglobulinemia in Patients with Cystic Fibrosis. *N Engl J Med*. Vol. 302, No 5, pp 245-249

McKone E., Goss C. & Aitken M. (2006). CFTR genotype as a predictor of prognosis in cystic fibrosis. *Chest*. Vol. 130, No 5, pp 1441-1447.

Mehta G., Macek M., Mehta A. *et al.* (2010). Cystic fibrosis across Europe: EuroCareCF analysis of demographic data from 35 countries. *J Cyst Fibros.* Vol. 9, Suppl. 2, pp 5-21.

Mérelle M., Schouten J, Gerritsen J. *et al.* (2001). Influence of neonatal screening and centralized treatment on long-term clinical outcome and survival of CF patients. *Eur Respir J.* Vol. 18, No 2, pp 306-315.

Miles A., Louglin M. & Polychronis A. (2008). Evidence-based healthcare, clinical knowledge and the rise of personalised medicine. *J Eval Clin Pract.* Vol. 14, No 5, pp 621-649.

Miles A. & Loughlin M. (2011). Models in the balance: evidence-based medicine versus evidence-informed individualized care. *J Eval Clin Pract.* Vol. 17, No 4, pp 531-536.

Milla C., Warwick W. & Moran A. (2000). Trends in pulmonary function in patients with cystic fibrosis correlate with the degree of glucose intolerance at baseline. *Am J Respir Crit Care Med.* Vol. 162, No 3 Pt 1, pp 891-895.

Milla C. (2004). Association of nutritional status and pulmonary function in children with cystic fibrosis. *Curr Opin Pulm Med* Vol. 10, No 6, pp 505–509.

Modi A., Lim C., Yu N. *et al.* (2006). A multi-method assessment of treatment adherence for children with cystic fibrosis. *J Cyst Fibros.* Vol 5, No 3, pp 177-185.

Moran A., Dunitz J. & Nathan B. *et al.* 2009. Cystic fibrosis–related diabetes: current trends in prevalence, incidence, and mortality. *Diabetes Care.* Vol. 32, No 9, pp 1626–1631

Moran A., Becker D., Casella S. *et al.* (2010). Epidemiology, pathophysiology, and prognostic implications of cystic fibrosis-related diabetes: a technical review. *Diabetes Care.* Vol. 33, No 12, pp 2677-2683.

Mott L., Gangell C., Murray C. *et al.* (2009). Bronchiectasis in an asymptomatic infant with cystic fibrosis diagnosed following newborn screening. *J Cyst Fibros.* Vol. 8, No 4, pp 285-287.

Mussaffi H., Prais D., Mei-Zahav M. *et al.* (2006). Cystic fibrosis mutations with widely variable phenotype: the D1152H example. *Pediatr Pulmonol.* Vol. 41, No 3, pp 250-254.

Nick J., Chacon C., Brayshaw S. *et al.* (2010). Effects of gender and age at diagnosis on disease progression in long-term survivors of cystic fibrosis. *Am J Respir Crit Care Med.* Vol. 182, No 5, pp 614-626.

Nielsen O., Thomsen B., Green A. *et al.* (1988). Cystic fibrosis in Denmark 1945 to 1985. An analysis of incidence, mortality and influence of centralized treatment on survival. *Acta Paediatr Scand.* Vol. 77, No 6, pp 836-841.

O'Connor G., Quinton H., Kneeland T. *et al.* (2003). Median household income and mortality rate in cystic fibrosis. *Pediatrics.* Vol. 111, No 4 Pt 1, pp e333-339.

Olesen H., Pressler T., Hjelte L. *et al.* (2010). Gender differences in the Scandinavian cystic fibrosis population. *Pediatr Pulmonol.* Vol. 45, No 10, pp 959-965.

Padman R., McColley S., Miller D. *et al.* (2007). Infant care patterns at epidemiologic study of cystic fibrosis sites that achieve superior childhood lung function. *Pediatrics.* Vol. 119, no 3, pp e531-537.

Padman R., Werk L., Ramirez-Garnica G. *et al.* (2008). Association between practice patterns and body mass index percentile in infants and young children with cystic fibrosis. *J Cyst Fibros.* Vol. 7, No 5, pp 385-390.

Pamukcu A., Bush A. & Buchdahl R. (1995). Effects of pseudomonas aeruginosa colonization on lung function and anthropometric variables in children with cystic fibrosis. *Pediatr Pulmonol.* Vol. 19, No 1, pp 10-15.

Pedreira C., Robert R., Dalton V. *et al.* (2005). Association of body composition and lung function in children with cystic fibrosis. *Pediatr Pulmonol.* Vol. 39, no 3, pp 276-280.

Pendleton D. The compliance conundrum in cystic fibrosis. *J R Soc Med.* Vol. 93, Suppl. 38, pp 9-13.

Prober C., Walson P. & Jones J. (2000). Technical report: precautions regarding the use of aerosolized antibiotics. Committee on Infectious Diseases and Committee on Drugs. *Pediatrics.* Vol. 106, No 6, p E89.

Proesmans M., Els C., Vermeulen F. *et al.* (2011). Change in IgG and evolution of lung function in children with cystic fibrosis. *J Cyst Fibros.* Vol. 10, No 2, pp 128-131.

Que C., Cullinan P. & Geddes D. (2006). Improving rate of decline of FEV1 in young adults with cystic fibrosis. *Thorax.* Vol. 61, No 2, pp 155-157.

Quinton, H. (2004). Using data to identify opportunities for change and to monitor progress. *Pediatr Pulmonol.* Vol. 38, Suppl. 27, pp 124-125.

Quinton H. & O'Connor G. (2007). Current issues in quality improvement in cystic fibrosis. *Clin Chest Med.* Vol. 28, No 2,pp 459-472.

Quittner A., Schechter M, Rasouliyan L. *et al.* (2010). Impact of socioeconomic status, race, and ethnicity on quality of life in patients with cystic fibrosis in the United States. *Chest.* Vol. 137, No 3, pp 642-650.

Quon B. & Goss C. (2011). A story of success: continuous quality improvement in cystic fibrosis care in the USA. *Thorax.* Aug 3. [Epub ahead of print]

Ranganathan S., Dezateux C., Bush A. *et al.* (2001). Airway function in infants newly diagnosed with cystic fibrosis. *Lancet.* Vol. 358, pp 1964-1965.

Ring E., Eber E., Erwa W. *et al.* (1998). Uinary N-acetyl-beta-D-glucosaminidase activity in patients with cystic fibrosis on long-term gentamicin inhalation. *Arch Dis Child.* Vol. 78, No 6, pp 540-543.

Rogan M. & Stoltz D. (2011). Cystic fibrosis transmembrane conductance regulator intracellular processing, trafficking, and opportunities for mutation-specific treatment. *Chest* Vol. 139, No 6, pp 1480-1490.

Rosenbluth D., Wilson K., Ferkol T. *et al.* (2004). Lung function decline in cystic fibrosis patients and timing for lung transplantation referral. *Chest* Vol. 126, No 2, pp 412-419.

Rosenfeld M., Davis R., Fitzsimmons S. *et al.* (1997). Gender gap in cystic fibrosis mortality. *Am J Epidemiol.* Vol. 145, no 9, pp 794-803.

Rosenfeld M., Emerson J., Mc Namara S. *et al.* (2010). Baseline characteristics and factors associated with nutritional and pulmonary status at enrollment in the cystic fibrosis EPIC observational cohort. *Pediatr Pulmonol.* Vol. 45, No 9, pp 934-944.

Saarni S. & Gylling H. (2004). Evidence based medicine guidelines: a solution to rationing or politics disguised as science? *J Med Ethics.* Vol. 30, No 2, pp 171-175.

Saiman L. & Siegel J. (2003). Infection control recommendations for patients with cystic fibrosis: Microbiology, important pathogens, and infection control practices to prevent patient-to-patient transmission. *Am J Infect Control.* Vol. 31, Suppl. 3, pp 1-62.

Sawicki G., Sellers D. & Robinson W. (2009). High treatment burden in adults with cystic fibrosis: challenges to disease self-management. *J Cyst Fibros*. Vol. 8, No 2, pp 91-96.

Schechter M., Shelton B., Margolis P. *et al.* (2001). The association of socioeconomic status with outcomes in cystic fibrosis patients in the United States. *Am J Respir Crit Care Med*. Vol. 163, No 6, pp 1331-1337

Schechter M. (2002). Demographic and center-related characteristics associated with low weight in pediatric CF patients. *Pediatr Pulmonol*. Vol. 34, Suppl. 24, p 331 (A)

Schechter, M. (2004). Key strategies for improving care. *Pediatr Pulmonol*. Vol. 38, Suppl. 27, pp 120-121.

Schechter M. & Margolis P. (2005). Improving subspecialty healthcare: lessons from cystic fibrosis. *J Pediatr*. Vol. 147, No 3, pp 295-301.

Schechter M. & Guttierez H. (2010). Improving the quality of care for patients with cystic fibrosis. *Curr Opin Pediatr*. Vol. 22, No 3, pp 296-301.

Schluchter M., Konstan M., Davis P. (2002). Jointly modelling the relationship between survival and pulmonary function in cystic fibrosis patients. *Stat Med*. Vol. 21, No 9, pp 1271-1287.

Segal, T. (2008). Adolescence: what the cystic fibrosis team needs to know. *J R Soc Med*. Vol. 101, Suppl 1, pp 15-27.

Sermet-Gaudelus I., Mayell S., Southern K. *et al.* (2010). Guidelines on the early management of infants diagnosed with cystic fibrosis following newborn screening. *J Cyst Fibros*. Vol. 9, No 5, pp 323-329.

Shahar E. (2008). Does anyone know the road from a randomized trial to personalized medicine? A review of 'Treating Individuals. From Randomized Trials to Personalised Medicine' *J Eval Clin Pract*. Vol. 14, No 5, pp 726-731.

Sims E., McCormick J., Mehta G. *et al.* (2005). Neonatal screening for cystic fibrosis is beneficial even in the context of modern treatment. *J Pediatr*. Vol. 147, Suppl. 3, pp 42-46.

Sims E., Clark A., McCormick J. *et al.* (2007). Cystic fibrosis diagnosed after 2 months of age leads to worse outcomes and requires more therapy. *Pediatrics*. Vol. 119, No 1, pp 19-28.

Sinaasappel M., Stern M., Littlewood J. *et al.* (2002). Nutrition in patients with cystic fibrosis: a European Consensus. *J Cyst Fibros*. Vol. 1, No 2, pp 51-75.

Siret D., Bretaudeau G., Branger B. *et al.* (2003). Comparing the clinical evolution of cystic fibrosis screened neonatally to that of cystic fibrosis diagnosed from clinical symptoms: a 10-year retrospective study in a French region (Brittany). *Pediatr Pulmonol*. Vol. 35, No 5, pp 342-349.

Sly P., Brennan S., Gangell C. *et al.* (2009). Lung disease at diagnosis in infants with cystic fibrosis detected by newborn screening. *Am J Respir Crit Care Med*. Vol. 180, No 2, pp 146-152.

Smyth A., O'Hea U., Williams G. *et al.* Passive smoking and impaired lung function in cystic fibrosis. *Arch Dis Child*. Vol. 71, No 4, pp 353-354.

Stafler P., Davies J., Balfour-Lynn I. *et al.* (2011). Bronchoscopy in cystic fibrosis infants diagnosed by newborn screening. *Pediatr Pulmonol*. Vol. 46, No 7, pp 696-700.

Stallings V., Stark L, Robinson K. *et al.* (2008). Evidence-based practice recommendations for nutrition-related management of children and adults with cystic fibrosis and pancreatic insufficiency: results of a systematic review. *J Am Diet Assoc.* Vol. 108, No 5, pp 832-839.

Steinkamp G. & Wiedemann B. (2002). Relationship between nutritional status and lung function in cystic fibrosis: cross sectional and longitudinal analyses from the German CF quality assurance (CFQA) project. *Thorax.* Vol. 57, No 7, pp 596-601.

Stern R., Byard P., Tomashefski J. *et al.* (1987). Recreational use of psychoactive drugs by patients with cystic fibrosis. J Pediatr. Vol. 111, no 2, pp 293-299.

Stern M., Wiedemann B., Wenzlaff P. *et al.* (2008). From registry to quality management: the German Cystic Fibrosis Quality Assessment project 1995 2006. *Eur Respir* J. Vol. 31, No 1, pp 29-35.

Stern M., Niemann M., Wiedemann B. *et al.* (2011). Benchmarking improves quality in cystic fibrosis care: a pilot project involving 12 centres. *Int J Qual Health Care.* Vol. 23, No 3, pp 349-356.

Stevens D., Moss R., Kurup V. *et al.* (2003). Allergic bronchopulmonary aspergillosis in cystic fibrosis--state of the art: Cystic Fibrosis Foundation Consensus Conference. *Clin Infect Dis.* Vol. 37, Suppl. 3, pp 225-264.

Stick S., Brennan S., Murray C. *et al.* (2009). Bronchiectasis in infants and preschool children diagnosed with cystic fibrosis after newborn screening. *J Pediatr.* Vol. 155, No 5, pp 623-628.e1

Stuart B., Lin J. & Mogayzel P. (2010). Early eradication of Pseudomonas aeruginosa in patients with cystic fibrosis. *Paediatr Respir Rev.* Vol. 11, No 3, pp 177-184.

Taccetti G., Festini F., Campana S. *et al.* (2004). Neonatal screening for cystic fibrosis and Pseudomonas aeruginosa acquisition. *J Pediatr.* Vol. 145, No 3, p 421.

Tetrault J., Krothers K., Moore B. *et al.* (2007). Effects of marijuana smoking on pulmonary function and respiratory complications: a systematic review. *Arch Intern Med.* Vol. 167, No 3, pp 221-228.

Thauvin-Robinet C., Munck A., Huet F. *et al.* (2009). The very low penetrance of cystic fibrosis for the R117H mutation: a reappraisal for genetic counselling and newborn screening. *J Med Genet.* Vol. 46, No 11, pp 752-758.

Thia L. & Balfour-Lynn I. (2009). Diagnosing allergic bronchopulmonary aspergillosis in children with cystic fibrosis. *Paediatr Respir Rev.* Vol. 10, No 1, pp 37-42.

Tiddens H. (2009). Quality improvement in your CF centre: taking care of care. *J Cyst Fibros.* Vol. 8, Suppl. 1, pp 2-5.

UK CF Registry (2008), Available from http://www.cftrust.org.uk/aboutcf/publications/cfregistryreports/

Treacy K., Elborn S., Rendall J. *et al.* (2008). Copying letters to patients with cystic fibrosis (CF): letter content and patient perceptions of benefit. *J Cyst Fibros.* Vol. 7, No 6, pp 511-514.

van Koolwijk L., Uiterwaal C., van der Laag J. *et al.* (2002). Treatment of children with cystic fibrosis: central, local or both? *Acta Paediatr.* Vol. 91, No 9, pp 972-977.

Valerius N., Koch C. & Høiby N. (1991). Prevention of chronic Pseudomonas aeruginosa colonisation in cystic fibrosis by early treatment. *Lancet.* Vol. 338, pp 725-726.

van der Ent C. (2008). Quality assessment: is the truth in the outcome? *Eur Respir J.* Vol. 31, No 1, pp 6-7.

Verma A., Dodd M., Haworth C. *et al.* (2000). Holidays and cystic fibrosis. *J R Soc. Med.* Vol. 93, Suppl. 38, pp 20-26.

Verma N., Bush A. & Buchdahl R. (2005). Is there still a gender gap in cystic fibrosis? *Chest.* Vol. 128, no 4, pp 2824-2834.

Wainwright C., Vidmar S., Armstrong D. *et al.* (2011). Effect of bronchoalveolar lavage-directed therapy on Pseudomonas aeruginosa infection and structural lung injury in children with cystic fibrosis: a randomized trial. *JAMA.* Vol. 306, No 2, pp 163-171.

Walters S., Britton J. & Hodson M. (1994). Hospital care for adults with cystic fibrosis: an overview and comparison between special cystic fibrosis clinics and general clinics using a patient questionnaire. *Thorax* Vol. 49, No 4, pp 300-306.

Wallwork J., Brenchley P, Mc Carthy J. *et al.* (1974). Some aspects of immunity in patients with cystic fibrosis. *Clin Exp Immunol.* Vol. 18, No 3, pp 303-320.

Wang X., Dockery D., Wypij D. *et al.* (1993). Pulmonary function between 6 and 18 years of age. *Pediatr Pulmonol* Vol. 15, No 2, pp 75-88.

Welsh M. & Smyth A. (1993). Molecular mechanisms of CFTR chloride channel dysfunction in CF. *Cell.* Vol. 73, No 7, pp 1251-1254.

West S., Zeng L., Lee B. *et al.* (2002). Respiratory infections with Pseudomonas aeruginosa in children with cystic fibrosis: early detection by serology and assessment of risk factors. *JAMA.* Vol. 287, No 22, pp 2958-2967.

Wheeler W., Williams M., Matthews W. *et al.* (1984). Progression of cystic fibrosis lung disease as a function of serum immunoglobulin G levels: a 5-year longitudinal study. *J Pediatr.* Vol. 104, no 5, pp 695-699.

Wolfenden L., Schechter M. (2009). Genetic and non-genetic determinants of outcomes in cystic fibrosis. *Paediatr Respir Rev.* Vol. 10, No 1, pp 32-36.

Wright F., Strug L, Doshi V. *et al.* (2011). Genome-wide association and linkage identify modifier loci of lung disease severity in cystic fibrosis at 11p13 and 20q13.2. *Nat Genet.* Vol. 43, No 6, pp 539-546.

Yankaskas J., Marshall B, Ebeling M. *et al.* (2004). Cystic fibrosis adult care: consensus conference report. *Chest.* Vol. 125, Suppl. 1, pp 1-39.

Zahariadis G., Lewy M. & Burns J. (2003). Cepacia-like syndrome caused by Burkholderia multivorans. *Can J Infect Dis.* Vol. 14, No 2, pp 123-125.

Zemanick E., Harris J., Conway S. *et al.* (2010). Measuring and improving respiratory outcomes in cystic fibrosis lung disease: opportunities and challenges to therapy. *J Cyst Fibros.* Vol. 9, No 1, pp 1-16.

Zemel B., Jawad A., Fitzsimmons S. *et al.* (2000). Longitudinal relationship among growth, nutritional status, and pulmonary function in children with cystic fibrosis: analysis of the Cystic Fibrosis Foundation National CF Patient Registry. *J Pediatr.* Vol. 137, no 3, pp 374-380.

Zlosnik J., Costa P., Brant R. *et al.* (2011). Mucoid and Nonmucoid Burkholderia cepacia Complex Bacteria in Cystic Fibrosis Infections. *Am J Respir Crit Care Med.* Vol. 183, No 1, pp 67-72.

Zolin A. (2010). Differences in disease severity of F508del homozygotes across European countries. *J Cyst Fibros.* Vol. 9, Suppl. 1, p 110 (A)

2

Radiological Features of Cystic Fibrosis

Iara Maria Sequeiros and Nabil A. Jarad
University Hospitals Bristol NHS Foundation Trust
United Kingdom

1. Introduction

With patients with cystic fibrosis (CF) living longer and reaching adulthood, conditions before not frequently encountered now play a larger role in the spectrum of CF related symptoms and complaints which continue to challenge clinicians in both outpatient and acute settings. It is in this context that the radiologist and different radiological imaging modalities can aid the clinician in order to establish an accurate diagnosis and steer appropriate treatment. In this chapter, we present a comprehensive review of common and not so common radiological features of both pulmonary and extra-pulmonary manifestations of CF.

With a huge variety of scans available at one's finger tips, or to be more precise, at the end of an electronic request form, it is vital that clinicians are familiar with the different existing imaging modalities, what information to expect from each one of them and the most appropriate scan to request to answer the specific clinical question, taking into consideration the patient's characteristics and needs- in other words, how to make best use of their Radiology Department. In this way, the required information can be obtained most rapidly and efficiently by using the correct test or tests performed in the correct order.

Chest radiographs are usually the exam of choice for the initial assessment and sequential follow-up of pulmonary disease in adult CF patients. It employs a very small dose of ionizing radiation and can be of great value in the detection of new infiltrates in acute infective exacerbations or diagnosing complications such as a pneumothorax. Plain radiography is also much used in patients complaining of acute abdominal pain, although findings can be non-specific and patients may require further imaging to characterize the abdominal pathology. An abdominal radiograph delivers a higher radiation dose and therefore should not be performed unnecessarily. Barium studies are not commonly used and it is believed that barium may cause obstruction in CF patients due to the thick intraluminal secretions. On the other hand, hypertonic oral contrast is used in some patients for the treatment of distal intestinal obstructive disease (DIOS). Air and contrast enemas continue to be used for the reduction of intussusception.

Ultrasound imaging does not carry any radiation hazard and has the added advantage of being relatively cheap and readily available. It can be useful in the chest in the assessment of pleural effusion or collection, but is most valuable for the evaluation of abdominal organs (e.g. liver, gallbladder, kidneys, spleen) and in patients with acute abdominal pain or suspected bowel pathology, such as DIOS, appendicitis or intussusception. The disadvantage of this modality is that it is completely operator dependent and sometimes images obtained are suboptimal due to patient related factors, such as obesity or overlying distended bowel gas.

Cross-sectional imaging techniques include computed tomography (CT) and magnetic resonance imaging (MRI). CT delivers high radiation - a chest CT is equivalent to over 200 chest radiographs in terms of radiation dose - and this needs to be considered, especially when dealing with young individuals such as CF patients. Chest CT imaging will be superior to plain radiograph in the assessment of initial or mild lung disease, in cases of poor clinical response when complications are suspected such as atypical mycobacteria infection and in pre-transplant evaluation. With the modern multi-detector CT scanners, the whole chest can be scanned in 10 to 20 seconds during a single breath-hold and therefore the exam is usually well tolerated even by the most breathless patient.

Much confusion is still seen when physicians request lung high resolution computed tomography (HRCT). The term high resolution implies a better quality scan, but in reality refers to 12 to 20 incremental ultra-thin 1 or 1.5mm thick image slices of the lung that are obtained at evenly spaced intervals through the chest and is indicated for the evaluation of diffuse interstitial or bronchial disease. It does not scan the whole volume of the chest and therefore is not appropriate for the assessment of lung nodules, malignancy, mediastinal lymphadenopathy or pleural disease, which are only fully imaged with a full lung volume spiral scan. HRCT increases the radiation dose delivered and should be limited to specific patients.

Abdominal CT imaging can be of great aid in the patient with acute abdominal pain in which the initial ultrasound scan was non-diagnostic. It is the scan of choice for the evaluation of the pancreas and therefore pancreatitis. MRI continues to be very expensive and not as accessible as CT. Its main indication is the assessment of hepatobiliary disease and cholangiopancreatography (MRCP). It is, as ultrasound, radiation free, but scans are sometimes prolonged and not always tolerated by those who are claustrophobic.

2. Pre-natal imaging

The use of radiological imaging in the aid of pre-natal diagnosis of CF and post-natal complications is well documented. Foetuses with CF have been associated with hyperechogenic foetal bowel detected by ultrasound during the second and third trimesters of pregnancy. Bowel is considered hyperechogenic if its echogenicity (brightness) is equal to or greater than that of the adjacent iliac bone (Al-Kouatly et al., 2001). Although this can be a normal finding, identified in 0.1-1.8% of foetuses, the risk of diagnosis of CF is greater if associated with bowel dilatation or the absence of an identifiable gallbladder (Hertzberg et al., 1996; Scotet et al., 2002).

3. The nose and sinuses

The upper airways are very frequently affected in CF, with over 75% of patients reporting some kind of sinus or nasal symptom such as nasal or sinus obstruction, nasal discharge, post-nasal drip and facial pain (Cepero et al., 1987). Sinusitis should be considered in all CF patients with nasal symptoms. A common cold is often suspected and can occur in CF patients, but when symptoms affect the CF patient only and no other member of the family, sinusitis is likely to be the cause. There is poor correlation between the severity of symptoms and imaging findings (Sakano et al., 2007). Indications for CT imaging include evaluation of the severity of the disease and pre-operative evaluation.

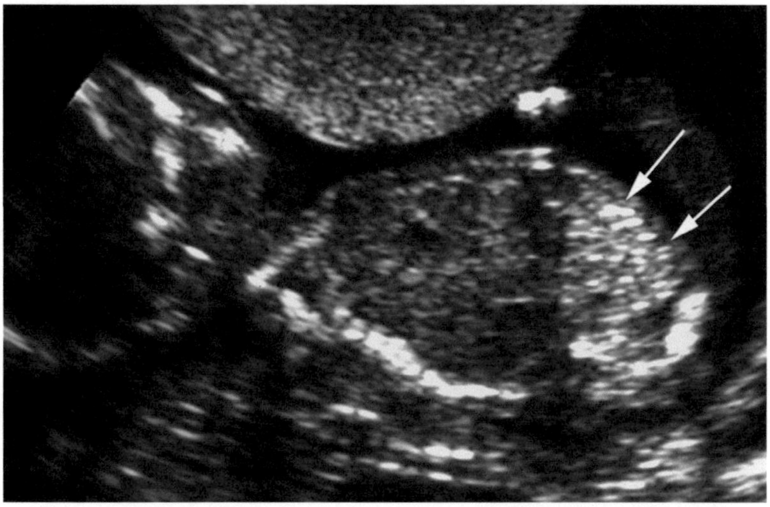

Fig. 1. Sagittal ultrasound view of a foetus with hyperechogenic bowel (arrows).

Imaging will reveal abnormalities even if not clinically manifested, such as small hypoplasic sinuses - often adult CF patients have no frontal sinus cavity - thickened nasal turbinates and thickened mucosa of the sinuses. Chronic inflammation and thickening of the mucosa of the nasal cavities and sinuses result in formation of inflammatory polyps and the accumulation of mucus in obstructed sinuses. Many patients undergo surgery to remove polyps and enlarge the outlet of obstructed sinuses, but relief tends to be temporary due to the recurrent nature of the disease.

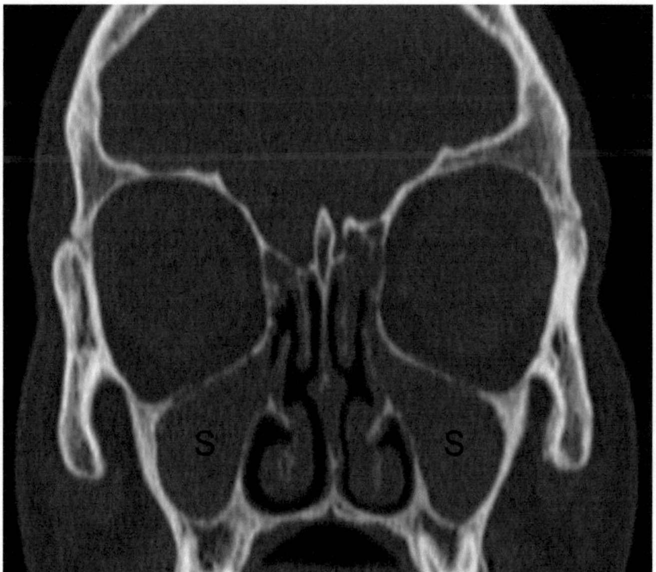

Fig. 2. Coronal CT image at the level of the nasal cavities showing complete opacification of the maxillary sinuses (S) in a case of recurrent sinusitis.

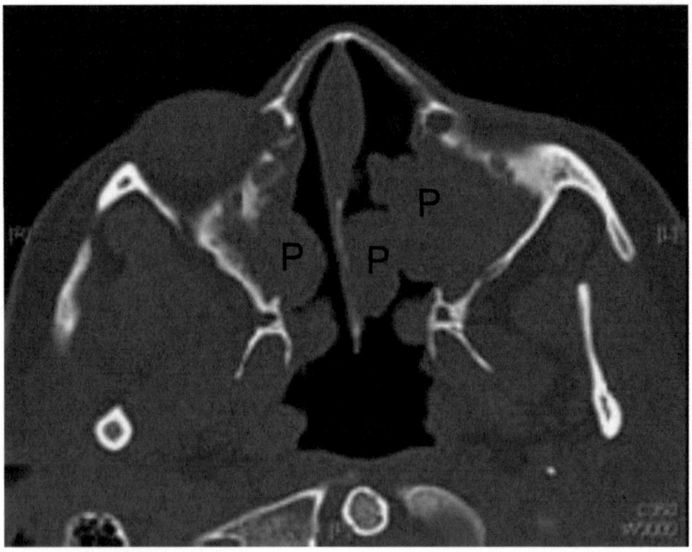

Fig. 3. Axial CT image at the level of the nasal cavities showing opacification of the maxillary sinuses and rounded densities in the nasal cavities (P) in a severe case of nasal polyposis.

4. Pulmonary manifestations

4.1 Bronchiectasis

Repeated chest infections are the hallmark of CF. These are usually associated with *Pseudomonas aeruginosa* or *Staphylococcus aureus* infection and clinically manifested by increased cough, sputum production, breathlessness and fatigue (Marshall, 2004). Classically CF initially affects the upper lobes, but severe cases will show diffuse bilateral disease affecting all of the lungs. Chest radiographs will reveal degrees of hyperinflation, dilated bronchi with thickened walls (cylindrical or cystic bronchiectasis) associated with well defined areas of air space opacification, as in lobar pneumonias, or nodules due to mucoid impaction, atelectasis, cavities and hilar lymphadenopathy. Pneumothorax is also frequently seen and can be recurrent (Hansell et al., 2005).

Chest radiographs are generally sufficient for regular clinical management and usually there is little visible radiographic change associated with clinical exacerbations. On the other hand it is now well established that CT imaging can give valuable information for the monitoring of disease progression and assessment of treatment response. Studies have shown a close relationship between HRCT findings and clinical and pulmonary functional evaluation of patients (Hansell et al., 2005). More severe cases may also show signs of right heart failure with pulmonary arterial hypertension and cor pulmonale.

4.2 Allergic bronchopulmonary aspergillosis

In patients with increased wheeze and asthma-type symptoms, and chest symptoms failing to improve despite antibiotic treatment, allergic bronchopulmonary aspergillosis (ABPA) should be suspected. Imaging can reveal transient and recurring areas of consolidation on chest radiographs, often due to atelectasis from mucoid plugging and bronchial obstruction, which subsequently improve after steroid therapy. Evaluation of ABPA in patients with CF is limited as imaging findings that are used to establish the diagnosis of ABPA in patients with asthma are common in patients with CF (Hansell et al., 2005).

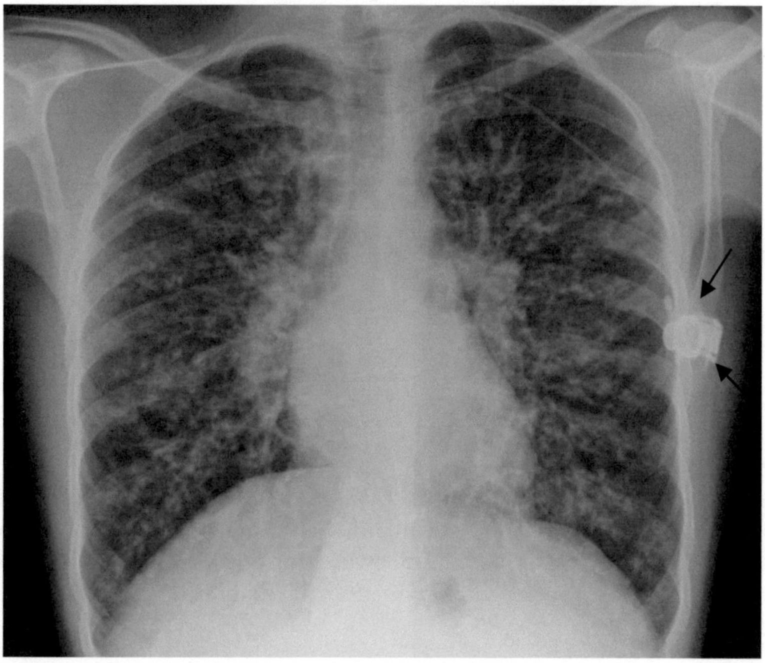

Fig. 4. Chest radiograph of a CF patient with hyperinflated lungs and severe bilateral and diffuse bronchiectasis seen as ring shadows and tram-track opacities that converge to the lung hila, which correspond to dilated thick walled bronchi. Note the port-a-cath device in the left chest wall and catheter in the distal superior vena cava used for the administration of intravenous antibiotics (arrows).

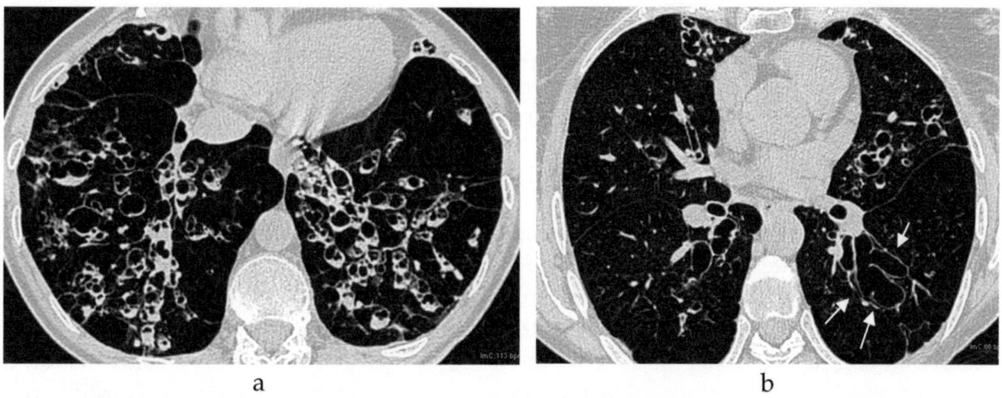

Fig. 5. Lung axial CT images demonstrating classic rounded cystic bronchiectasis throughout both lungs (fig. 5a) and varicose type bronchiectasis (arrows) (fig. 5b). The bronchi are dilated, thick walled and some contain mucus.

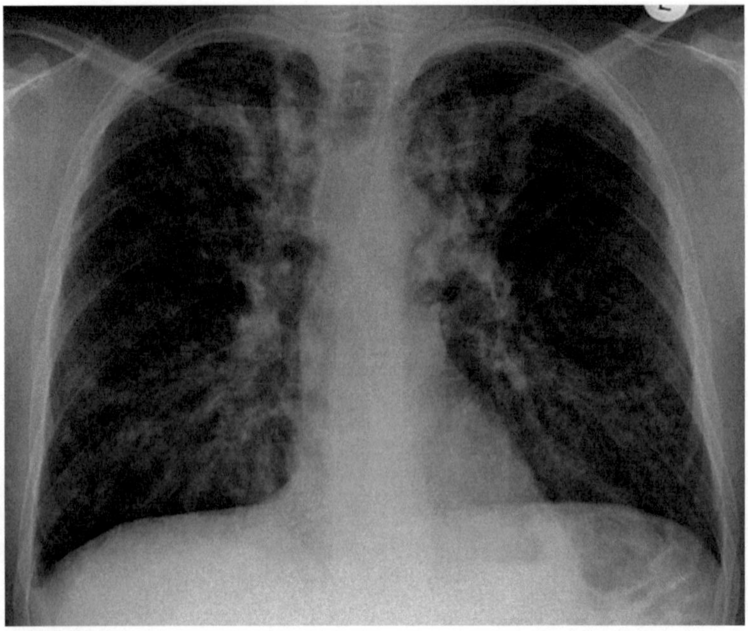

Fig. 6. Chest radiograph of CF patient with ABPA. There are bilateral widespread bronchiectasis, but the upper lobe bronchi are filled with mucus which was a new feature in comparison to previous radiographs. Clinical evaluation and elevated serum IgE and positive serum precipitins to Aspergillus confirmed the diagnosis of ABPA which improved with steroid treatment.

4.3 Non-tuberculous mycobacteria

Non-tuberculous (atypical) mycobacteria (NTBM) are increasingly isolated from CF patient's airways, although not always considered clinically significant. It is estimated that the lungs of 10% of adult CF patients are infected with NTBM. These bacteria consist of a range of organisms that differ in their virulence. Common varieties that infect CF lungs include *Mycobacterium fortuitum*, *Mycobacterium kansasii*, *Mycobacterium xenopi*, *Mycobacterium avium intracellulare* and *Mycobacterium cheloni* (*Mycobacteria abscessus*). *Mycobacterium abscessus* is especially important due to its high virulence, resistance to treatment and being one of the relative contra-indications for lung transplant.

Given the fact that chest symptoms in CF are common principally due to bronchiectatic lungs that are chronically infected with CF bacteria (mainly *P. aeruginosa*), determining the pathogenicity of NTBM is often challenging. In addition, the treatment of these bacteria is difficult with high rates of re-infection and recurrence, and long duration of treatment (12 to 18 months) that uses a combination of antibiotics often containing rifampicin, which is known to induce liver enzymes and therefore interferes with many CF drugs (antibiotics, insulin and contraceptive agents). For all these reasons, CF physicians seek confirmation of the pathogenesis of atypical mycobacteria prior to treatment. Mycobacteria is considered to play a role if the same species grows in the sputum on more than one occasion and symptoms persist after treating *P. aeruginosa*. Chest radiology using HRCT scans is therefore called upon to increase the degree of diagnostic certainty.

HRCT signs are often subtle and include one or more of the following: small centrilobular nodules and nodular changes in the periphery of the lungs, tree-in-bud opacities, new lung abscesses (Field et al., 2004; Olivier et al., 2003). Presence of one of more of these radiological signs together with chest and systemic symptoms that do not respond to anti-pseudomonas antibiotics would justify the start of treatment. Repeating the HRCT scan in 3 to 4 months after commencing the treatment is useful in showing radiological response.

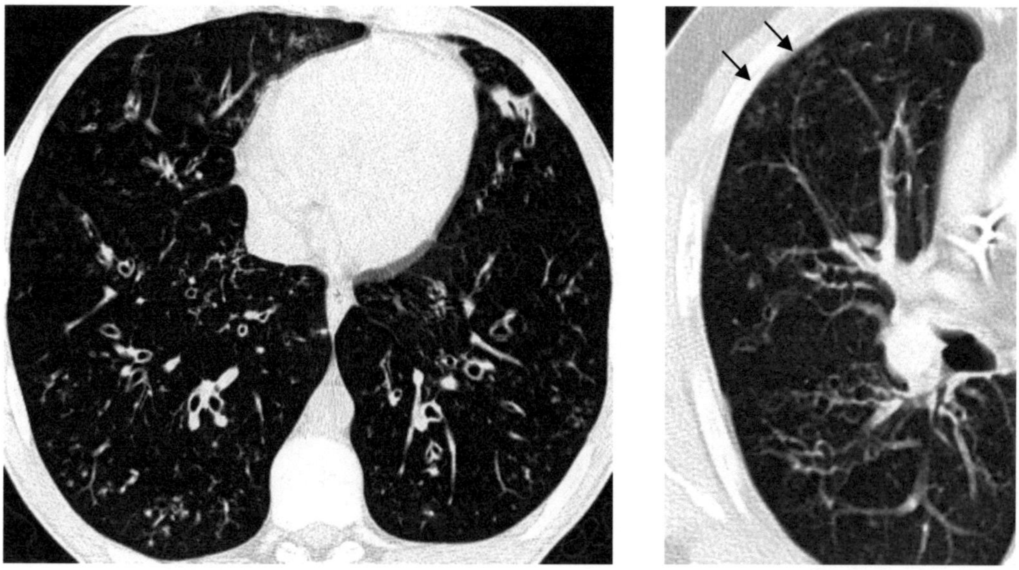

a b

Fig. 7. Lung axial CT image showing bronchiectasis, ground-glass and tree-in-bud opacities in both lung bases associated with non-tuberculous mycobacteria infection (fig. 7a). Close-up of tree-in-bud in the right middle lobe (arrows) (fig. 7b).

5. Abdominal manifestations

5.1 The pancreas

Autolysis of the pancreas due to viscous pancreatic enzymes and obstructed pancreatic ducts is known to start during intra-uterine life (Sturgess, 1984). This leads to fibrosis, atrophy and replacement of the pancreas by fat (Sequeiros et al., 2010) which clinically results in exocrine pancreatic insufficiency and malabsorption in up to 90% of patients (Rosenstein et al., 1998).

Pancreatitis can be the first manifestation of CF and is a rare complication among patients with CF with a reported incidence of approximately 1.24%. It mainly occurs during adolescence and young adulthood and is much more common among patients with preserved pancreatic tissue (De Boeck et al., 2005) and therefore considered pancreatic sufficient (10.3% of cases), but it can also occur among patients with pancreatic insufficiency (0.5% of cases). Pancreatitis is an important differential diagnosis that should be considered in the context of a CF patient presenting with acute abdominal pain.

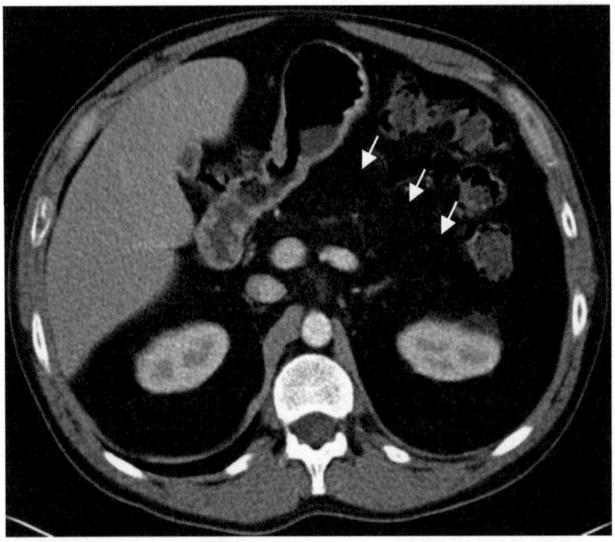

Fig. 8. Abdominal axial CT image of a CF patient at the level of the splenic vein showing the pancreas completely substituted by fat (arrows).

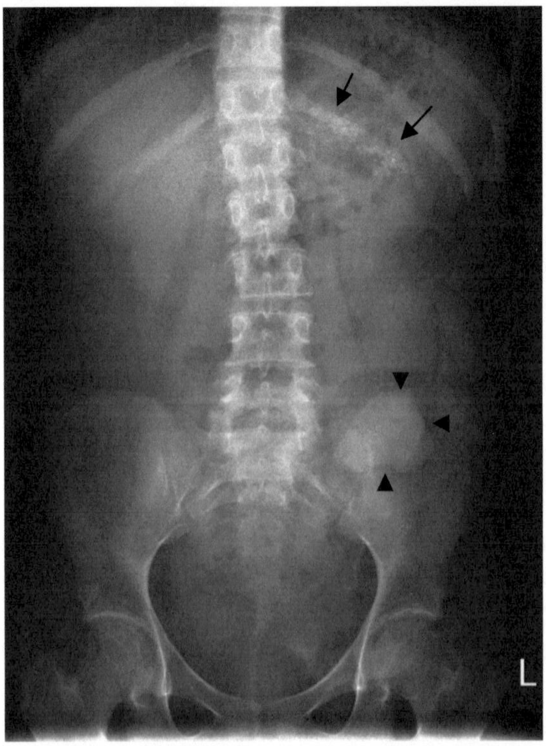

Fig. 9. Radiograph of the abdomen shows typical pancreatic calcifications secondary to CF related chronic pancreatitis in the left upper quadrant adjacent to the spine (arrows). Note the shadow in the left iliac fossa representing an ileostomy due to surgical management of previous bowel obstruction (arrow heads).

Pancreatic cysts are a relatively common finding in CF and can vary in size and number. Rarely, cysts can replace the entire pancreas in a condition called pancreatic cystosis, which can cause pain through mass effect (van Rijn et al., 2007). In such cases, surgical resection of the pancreas may be necessary.

5.2 Hepatobiliary disease

Hepatobiliary manifestations are common in CF and include fatty infiltration of the liver (steatosis), focal biliary cirrhosis with portal hypertension, microgallbladder and gallstones. Patients are more frequently asymptomatic, but liver disease is the second most common cause of death in CF (2.2% of deaths) and approximately 6-8% of individuals with CF have potentially fatal liver disease that requires liver transplantation (Genyk et al., 2001). It is thought to be a consequence of thickened secretions and abnormal bile flow within the liver causing bile duct obstruction. Signs of liver disease usually develop before or at puberty (Feigelson et al., 1993).

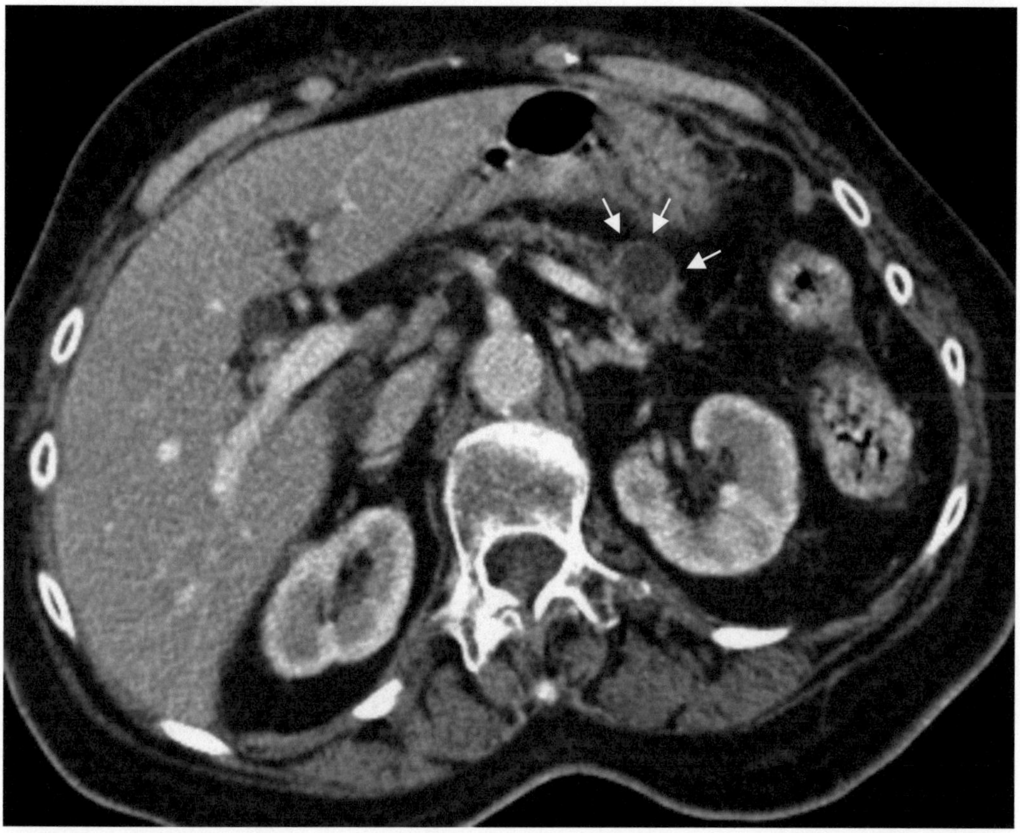

Fig. 10. Abdominal axial CT image at the level of the pancreas showing a small cyst in the tail of the pancreas (arrows).

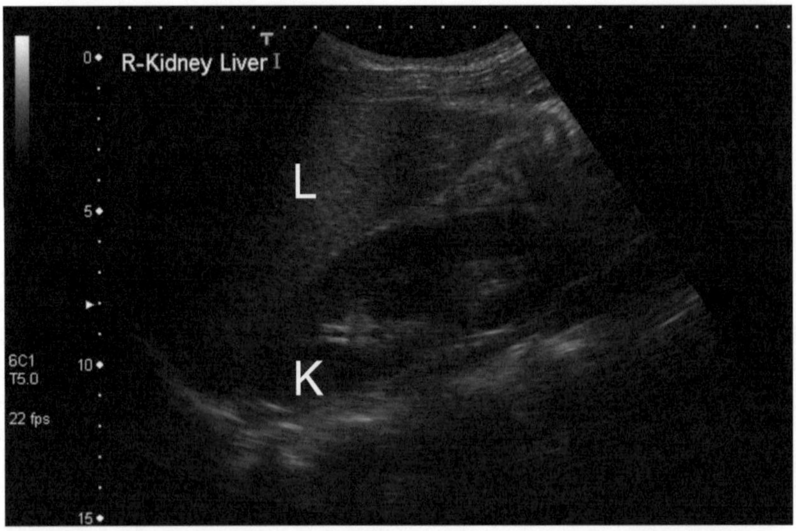

Fig. 11. Abdominal ultrasound image demonstrating echogenic (bright) liver due to diffuse fatty infiltration (L). A normal liver would look as dark as the adjacent right kidney (K).

Biliary calculi are present in 4-12% of patients. These are most commonly composed of cholesterol and thought to be a consequence of pancreatic insufficiency and the production of thick lithogenic bile (Agrons et al., 1996).

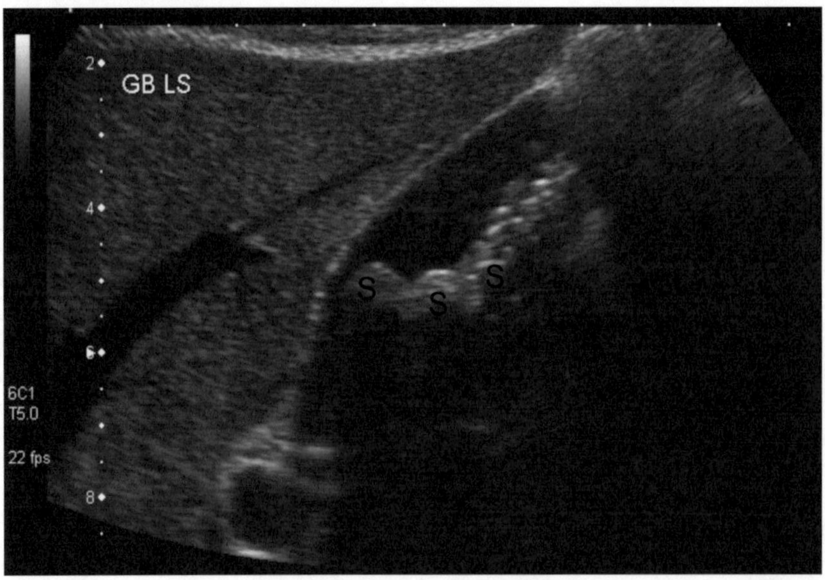

Fig. 12. Abdominal ultrasound image of a thin walled, non complicated gallbladder containing several stones (S).

Splenomegaly as a result of portal hypertension can be seen as massive enlargement of the spleen causing pain, dyspnoea and signs of hypersplenism and sometimes complicated with splenic infarcts or subcapsular haematomas.

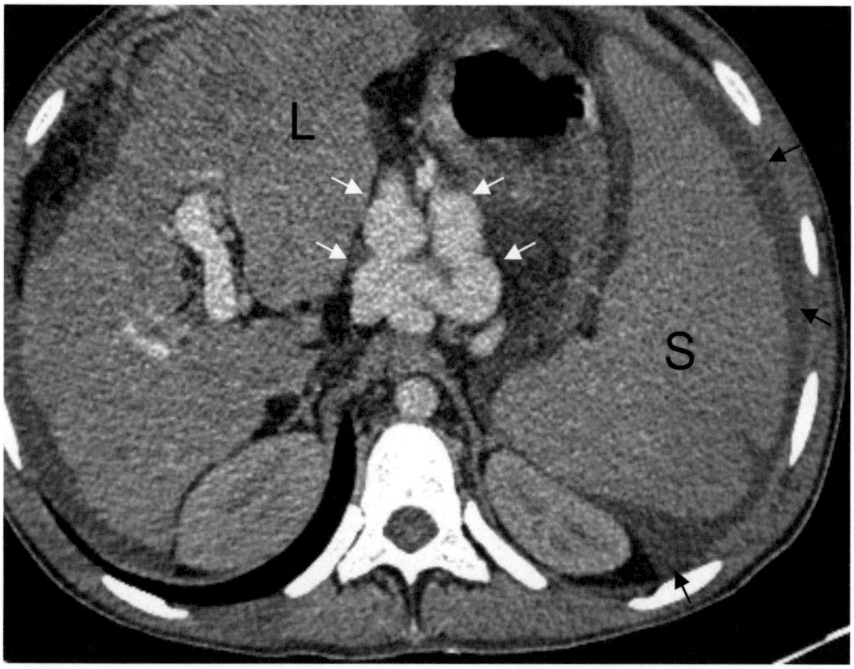

Fig. 13. Axial CT image of the abdomen showing a lobulated, macronodular cirrhotic liver (L), ascites (black arrows), splenomegaly (S) and varices (white arrows) due to portal hypertension.

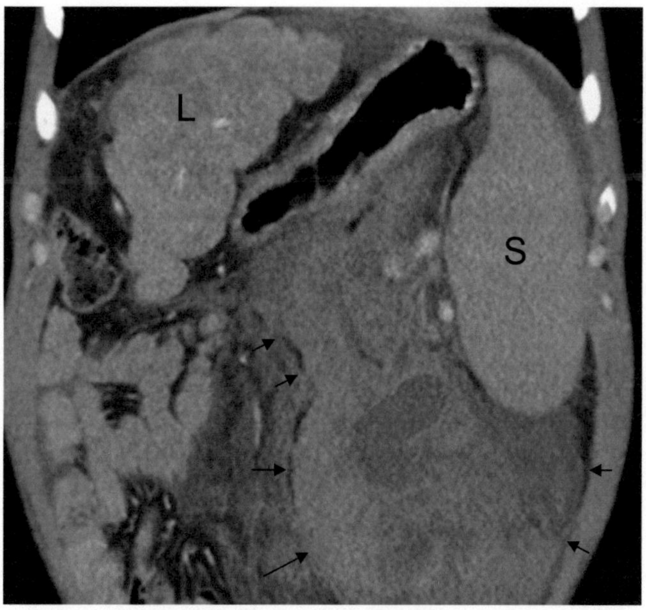

Fig. 14. Coronal CT image of the abdomen showing a large fatal spontaneous splenic haematoma (arrows) in a CF patient with severe portal hypertension and splenomegaly (S). Note the lobulated macronodular cirrhotic liver (L).

5.3 Meconium ileus

Bowel blockage of the newborn or meconium ileus is seen in 15-20% of neonates with CF and 25% of infants with meconium ileus prove to have CF (Hen et al., 1980). Meconium is composed of materials swallowed by the foetus during pregnancy, such as intestinal epithelial cells, mucus and amniotic fluid. In CF, mucus glands of the small intestine produce thick secretions and therefore the meconium sometimes becomes abnormally sticky and inspissated, causing a mechanical obstruction within the segment of the ileum. Classically, above the obstruction the bowel is greatly distended with fluid content, while below this level, the distal ileum and colon are collapsed. Soon after birth, usually in 24 to 48 hours, the newborn will present with abdominal distension and vomiting.

5.4 Distal intestinal obstructive syndrome

Distal intestinal obstructive syndrome or DIOS is the equivalent of meconium ileus in adults. It affects up to 15% of CF patients as a result of thickened intraluminal secretions, undigested food secondary to exocrine pancreatic insufficiency and impaired bowel motility (Speck & Charles, 2008). Patients complain of recurrent episodes of abdominal pain and distension, nausea and vomiting. Ultrasound imaging will reveal ditlated loops of small bowel containing "swirling" intraluminal echogenic material without forward propulsion motion in keeping with obstruction. Abdominal radiograph and CT show dilated small bowel loops with fluid levels and faecal material within the small bowel ("small bowel faeces").

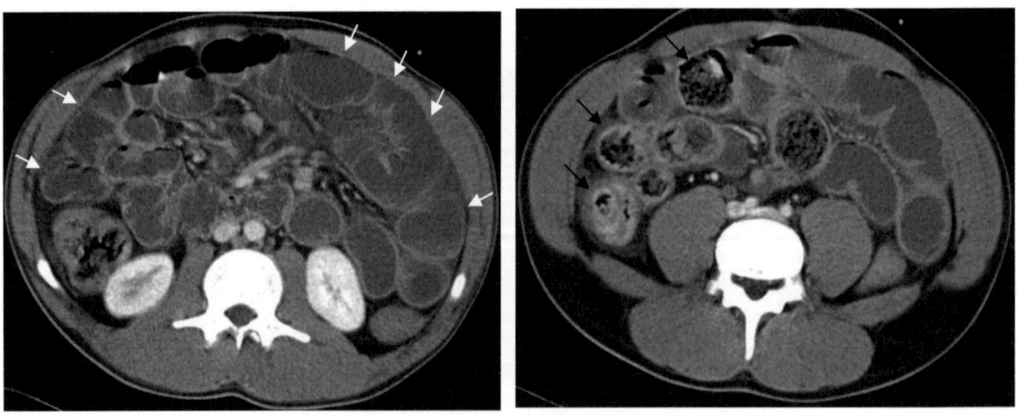

a b

Fig. 15. Axial CT scan of the abdomen of CF patient with acute abdominal obstruction after weeks of stopping to take exocrine pancreatic enzymes. Images show dilated loops of small bowel containing fluid (white arrows) (fig. 14a) and faecal material within the distal ileum in the right iliac fossa (black arrows) (fig. 14 b) - "small bowel faeces". Surgical intervention was necessary and revealed an obstructed ileum with inspissated secretions and undigested food.

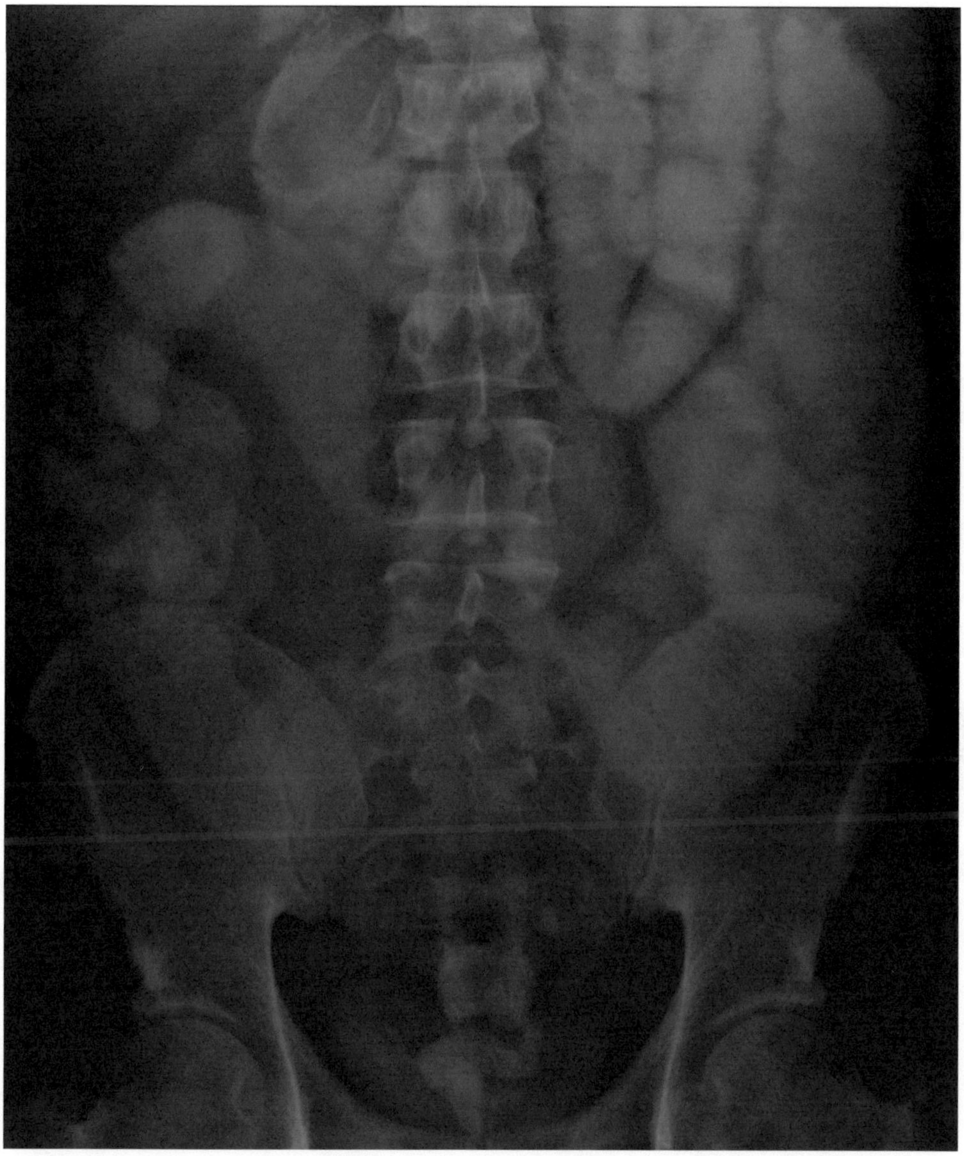

Fig. 16. CF patient with diagnosed DIOS managed clinically with hydration and oral hypertonic solution. Abdominal radiograph shows dilated loops of small bowel filled with ingested oral Gastrografin contrast agent.

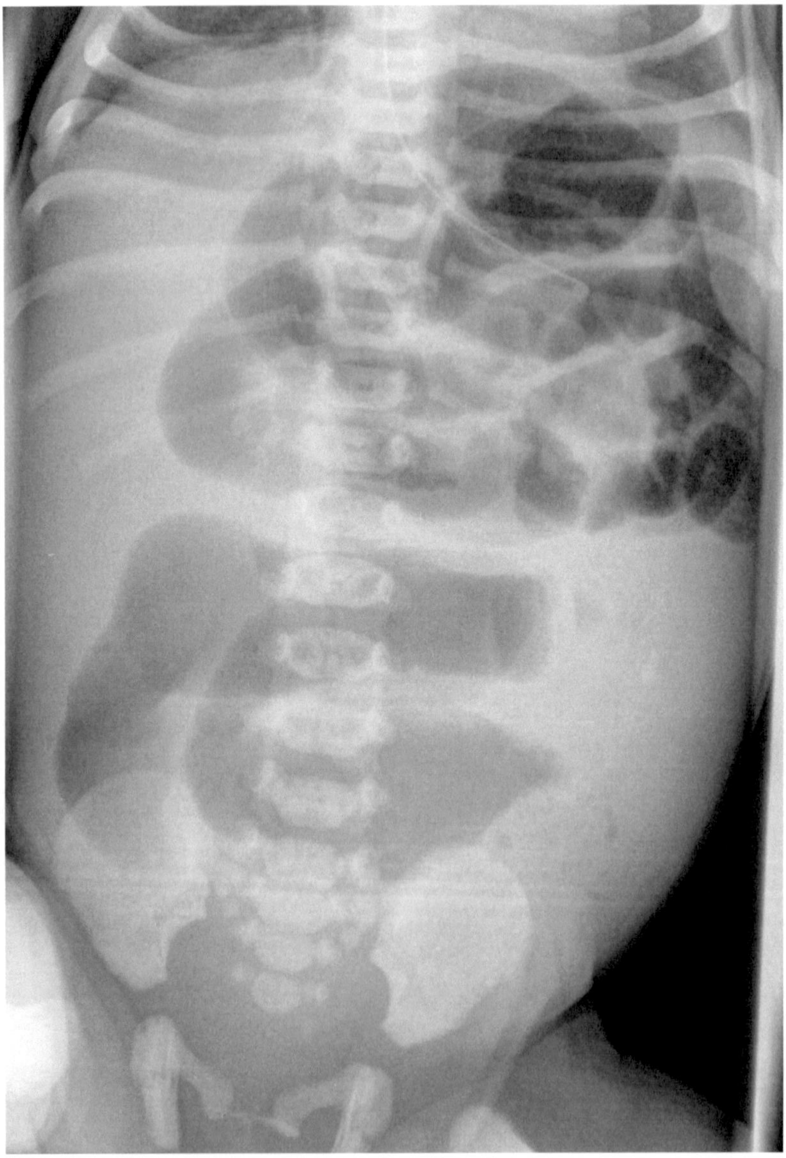

Fig. 17. Abdominal radiograph showing a pre-term infant with meconium ileus who was subsequently diagnosed with CF. He presented with marked abdominal distension at 3 days of life. There are markedly dilated loops of small bowel and no air is seen in the colon or rectum.

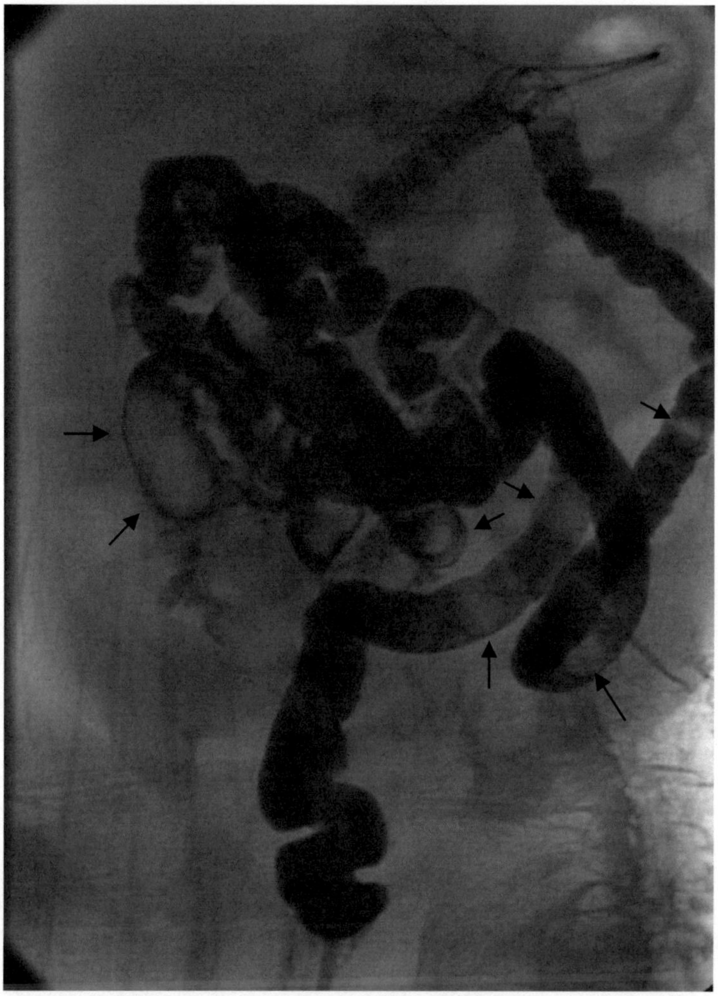

Fig. 18. Contrast enema in a neonate infant with meconium ileus. As is typical of the condition, the colon is small secondary to distal ileal obstruction and there is also small bowel dilatation. There are filling defects in the colon and terminal ileum representing meconium pellets (arrows).

5.5 Intussusception

Intussusception is more common in CF patients than in the general population and is seen in 1% of paediatric patients. It is rare in adulthood and comprises 5% of all intussusceptions and 1% of bowel obstructions (Nash et al., 2011). Intussusception can cause similar symptoms of acute abdominal pain as DIOS and is an important differential diagnosis that should be considered in acute obstruction as it may require surgical intervention, whilst DIOS is often managed non-surgically with hydration and oral hypertonic solutions (Speck & Charles, 2008). Intraluminal inspissated mucus, undigested food or enlarged lymphoid follicles can initiate an intussusception. Imaging reveals a bowel-within-bowel configuration which is pathognomonic of the condition (Gayer et al., 1998).

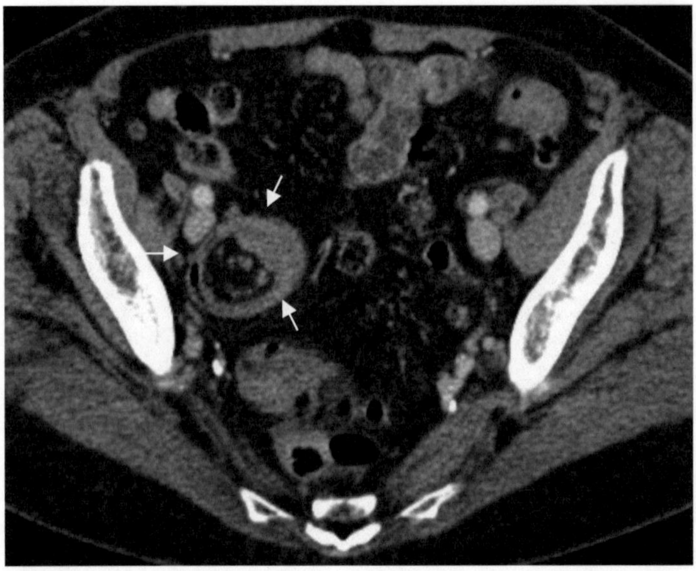

Fig. 19. Axial CT scan of the abdomen at the level of the iliac bones. Imaging reveals rounded structure with classic "bowel-within-bowel" configuration in the right iliac fossa in keeping with intussusception (arrows).

5.6 Fibrosing colonopathy

Fibrosing colonopathy is characterised clinically by right iliac fossa pain, where a thickened loop of bowel can sometimes be felt on clinical examination. It has been reported in association with children prescribed high strength pancreatic enzyme supplements, although the aetiology is not completely clear. Imaging has a limited role demonstrating non-specific large bowel wall thickening and final diagnosis is usually obtained with histology, which depicts submucosal fibrosis (Stacey et al., 1997).

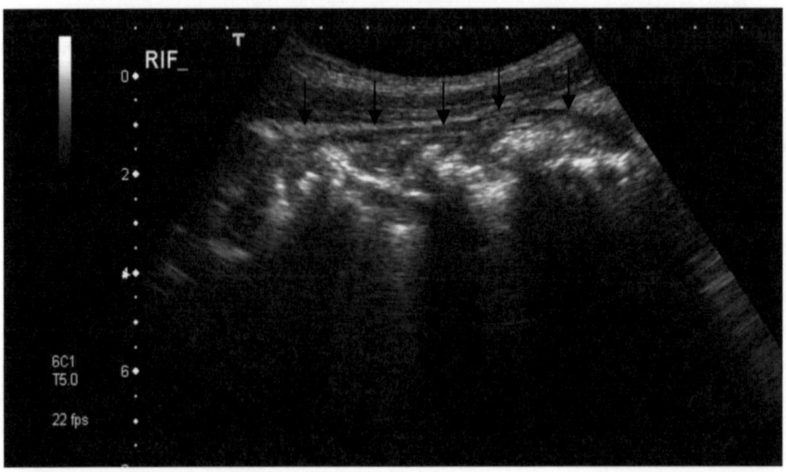

Fig. 20. Ultrasound image of the right iliac fossa showing a thick walled ascending colon (arrows) in a symptomatic CF patient.

5.7 Appendicitis

Appendicitis is relatively uncommon in CF, with a reported incidence of 1-2% compared to 7% in the general population. The cause of this is thought to be a protective effect of inspissated secretions against appendicitis (McCarthy et al., 1984). Although uncommon, it should always be considered in acute abdominal pain as a delayed diagnosis could result in subsequent rupture and abscess formation. Imaging features are similar to those seen in the general population.

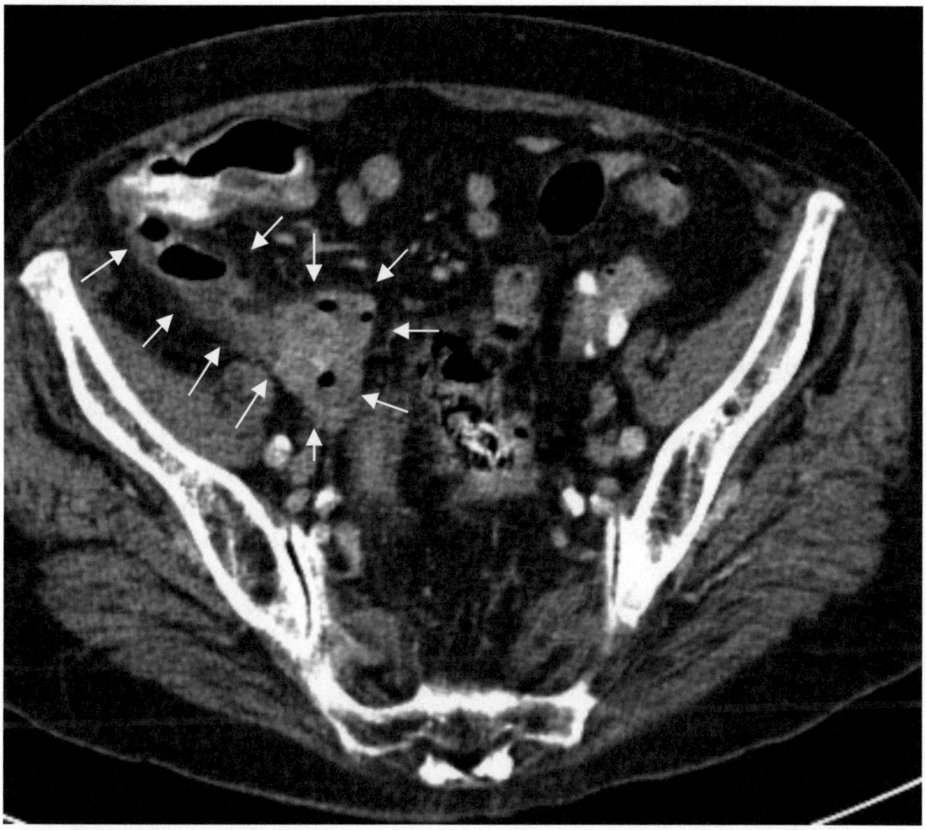

Fig. 21. Abdominal axial CT image at the level of the right iliac fossa showing a distended, thickened appendix with an associated collection (arrows) in acute appendicitis.

5.8 Nephrolithiasis

Nephrolithiasis is another important differential diagnosis of acute abdominal pain as there is a reported increased frequency of renal stone disease in CF in comparison to the general population (3-6.3% in CF patients versus 1-2% in age-matched controls) (Gibney & Goldfard, 2003). As with non CF patients, pain can affect the loin region or anywhere from the loin to the groin, and patients may also complain of haematuria and notice the voiding of tiny grains of stone. Initial assessment can be made with a CT of the kidneys, ureters and bladder (CT KUB) to confirm the diagnosis or with an ultrasound scan if obstruction and hydronephrosis is suspected in a patient with know nephrolithiasis.

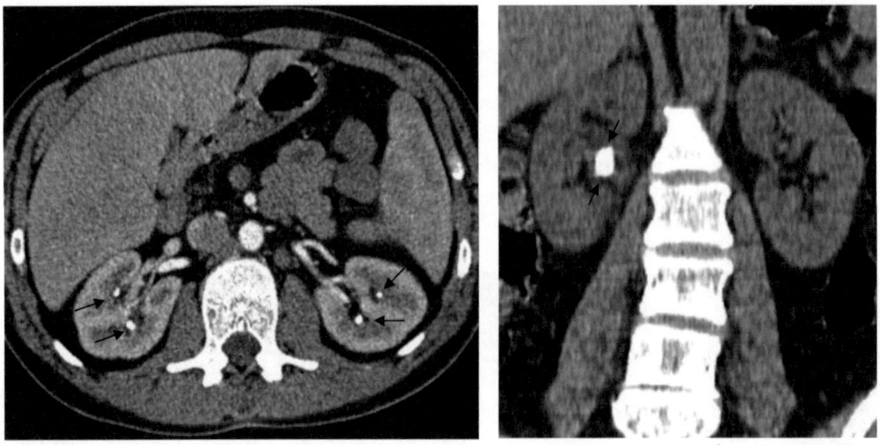

a b

Fig. 22. Axial CT scan of the abdomen of CF patient investigated for haematuria and recurrent abdominal pain with bilateral multiple kidney stones (arrows) (fig. 22a). Coronal CT scan of another patient showing a single stone in the right renal pelvis (arrows) (fig. 22b).

6. Hypertrophic pulmonary osteoarthropathy

This condition consists of a triad of clubbing, symmetric arthritis and periosteal new bone formation. Firstly associated with brochogenic carcinoma, it is also recognised in bronchiectasis, chronic lung inflammation and infection and CF, amongst others. Finger clubbing is the result of fibroelastic proliferation in the nail bed with thickening of the skin and subcutaneous tissues of the distal end of the fingers; synovitis leads to arthralgia and stiff swollen hands; periosteal new bone formation and cortical thickening affects long bones, more frequently the radius and ulna (Martinez-Lavin et al., 1993).

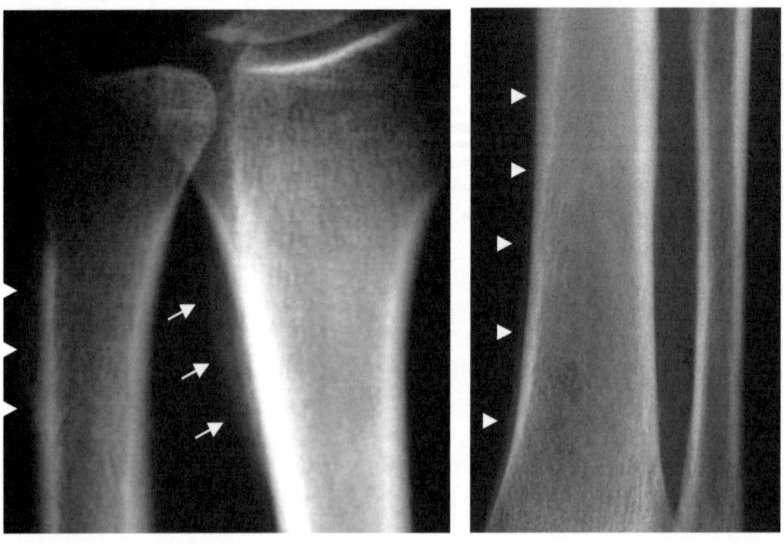

Fig. 23. Close-up radiographs of the distal long bones of the forearm and leg showing thickening of the cortical bone (arrows) as a result of chronic periostitis.

7. Conclusion

The lungs continue to account for the majority of CF complications and death, but with gastrointestinal complications becoming increasingly important and the ever growing availability of imaging facilities, clinicians and radiologists need to be aware of the larger spectrum of pathologies they might encounter and their radiological manifestations.

Imaging and close interaction between clinicians and radiologists is invaluable for the prompt and precise diagnosis of several CF related conditions. Some conditions can be diagnosed on the basis of imaging alone, avoiding unnecessary time wasting and invasive procedures, always reinforcing the necessity to maintain ionising radiation exposure to as low as reasonably achievable.

8. Acknowledgements

Dr Anthony Edey and Dr David Grier, Radiology Consultants, for kindly contributing with several images.

Kind thank you to all the cystic fibrosis patients of the Bristol Adult CF Centre for their generosity and resilience.

9. References

Agrons, GA., Corse, WR., Markowitz, RI., Suarez, ES., Perry, DR. (1996). Gastrointestinal manifestations of cystic fibrosis: radiologic-pathologic correlation. *Radiographics* 16: 871-893.

Al-Kouatly, HB., Chasen, ST., Streltzoff, J., Chervenak, FA. (2001). The clinical significance of fetal echogenic bowel. *Am J Obstet Gynecol* 185(5): 1035-1038.

Cepero, R., Smith, RJ., Catlin, FI., Bressler, KL., Furuta, GT., Shandera, KC. (1987). Cystic fibrosis - an otolaryngologic perspective. *Otolaryngol Head Neck Surg* 97(4): 356-360.

De Boeck, K., Weren, M., Proesmans, M., Kerem, E. (2005). Pancreatitis among patients with cystic fibrosis: correlation with pancreatic status and genotype. *Pediatrics* 115(4): e463-e469.

Feigelson, J., Anagnostopoulos, C., Poquet, M., Pecau, Y., Munck, A., Navarro, J. (1993). Liver cirrhosis in cystic fibrosis - therapeutic implications and long term follow up. *Arch Dis Child* 68: 653-657.

Field, SK., Fisher, D., Cowie, RL. (2004). Mycobacterium avium complex pulmonary disease in patients without HIV infection. *Chest* 126(2): 566-581.

FitzSimmons, SC., Burkhart, GA., Borowitz, D., Grand, RJ., Hammerstrom, T., Durie, PR., Lloyd-Still, JD., Lowenfels, AB. (1997). High-dose pancreatic-enzyme supplements and fibrosing colonopathy in children with cystic fibrosis. *N Engl J Med* 336: 1283-1289.

Gayer, G., Apter, S., Hofmann, C., Nass, S., Amitai, M., Zissin, R., Hertz, M. (1998). Intussusception in adults: CT diagnosis. *Clin Radiol* 53(1): 53-57.

Genyk, YS., Quiros, JA., Jabbour, N., Selby, RR., Thomas, DW. (2001). Liver transplantation in cystic fibrosis. *Curr Opin Pulm Med* 7(6): 441-447.

Gibney, EM., Goldfarb, DS. (2003) The association of nephrolithiasis with cystic fibrosis. Am J Kidney Dis 42(1): 1-11.

Hansell, DM., Armstrong, P., Lynch, DA., McAdams, HP. (2005). *Imaging of diseases of the chest, 4th edition* , Elsevier Mosby, Philadelphia.

Hen, J., Dolan, TF., Touloukian, RJ. (1980). Meconium ileus syndrome associated with cystic fibrosis and Hirschprung's disease. *Pediatrics* 66: 466-468.

Hertzberg, BS., Kliewer, MA., Maynor, C., McNally, PJ., Bowie, JD., Kay, HH., Hage, ML. (1996). Nonvisualization of the fetal gallbladder: frequency and prognostic importance. *Radiology* 199(3): 679-682.

Marshall, BC. Pulmonary exacerbation in cystic fibrosis. It's time to be explicit. (2004). *Am J Respir Crit Care Med* 169: 781-782.

Martinez-Lavin, M., Matucci-Cerinic, M., Jajic, I., Pineda, C. (1993). Hypertrophic osteoarthropathy: consensus on its definition, classification, assessment and diagnostic criteria. *J Rheumatol* 20(8): 1386-1387.

McCarthy, VP., Mischler, EH., Hubbard, VS., Chernick, MS., di Sant'Agnese, PA. (1984). Appendiceal abscess in cystic fibrosis. A diagnostic challenge. *Gastroenterology* 86(3): 564-568.

Nash, EF., Stephenson, A., Helm, EJ., Ho, T., Thippanna, CM., Ali, A., Whitehouse, JL., Honeybourne, D., Tullis, E., Durie, PR. (2011). Intussusception in adults with cystic fibrosis: a case series with review of the literature. *Dig Dis Sci* Jun 16 [Epub ahead of print].

Olivier, KN., Weber, DJ., Wallace Jr., RJ., Faiz, AR., Lee, JH., Zhang, Y., Brown-Elliot, BA., Handler, A., Wilson, RW., Schechter, MS., Edwards, LJ., Chakraborti, S., Knowles, MR., for the Nontuberculous Mycobacteria in Cystic Fibrosis Study Group. (2003). Non-tuberculous mycobacteria: multicentre prevalence study in cystic fibrosis. *Am J Respir Crit Care Med* 15: 828-834.

Rosenstein, BJ., Cutting, GR., and for the Cystic Fibrosis Foundation Consensus Panel. (1998). The diagnosis of cystic fibrosis: a consensus statement. *J Pediatr* **132**(4): 589-595.

Sakano, E., Ribeiro, AF., Barth, L., Neto, AC., Ribeiro, JD. (2007). Nasal and paranasal endoscopy computed tomography and microbiology of upper airways and the correlations with genotype and severity of cystic fibrosis. *Intl J Ped Otorhinol* 71: 41-50.

Scotet, V., De Braekeleer, M., Audrezet, MP., Quere, I., Mercier, B., Dugueperoux, I., Andrieux, J., Blayau, M., Ferec, C. (2002). Prenatal detection of cystic fibrosis by ultrasonography: a retrospective study of more than 346 000 pregnancies. *J Med Genet* 39(6): 443-448.

Speck, K., Charles, A. (2008). Distal intestinal obstructive syndrome in adults with cystic fibrosis: a surgical perspective. *Arch Surg* 143(6): 601-603.

Sequeiros, I., Hester, K., Callaway, M., Williams, A., Garland, Z., Powell, T., Wong, FS., Jarad, NA. (2010) MRI appearances of the pancreas in patients with cystic fibrosis: a comparison of pancreas volume in diabetic and non-diabetic patients. *Br J Radiol* 83: 921-926.

Sturgess, JM. (1984). Structural and developmental abnormalities of the exocrine pancreas in cystic fibrosis. *J Pediatr Gastroenterol Nutr* 3 Suppl 1:S55-66.

van Rijn, RR., Schilte, PP., Wiarda, BM., Taminiau, JA., Stoker, J. (2007). Case 113: Pancreatic cystosis. *Radiology* 243: 598-602.

3

The Cystic Fibrosis 'Gender Gap': Past Observations Present Understanding and Future Directions

Sanjay H. Chotirmall[1], Catherine M. Greene[1],
Brian J. Harvey[2] and Noel G. McElvaney[1]
[1]*Respiratory Research Division, Department of Medicine*
[2]*Department of Molecular Medicine, Royal College of Surgeons in Ireland*
Ireland

1. Introduction

Cystic Fibrosis (CF) is a systemic disease impacting upon several organ systems. These include gastrointestinal, reproductive, endocrine and pulmonary manifestations of which the latter contributes the heaviest burden of disease morbidity, mortality and impact on quality of life. The defective protein in the disease state is the Cystic Fibrosis Transmembrane Regulator (CFTR) that normally functions as an ion channel permitting intracellular chloride escape. Regulated by cyclic adenosine monophosphate (cAMP) and localized to the apical membrane of epithelial cells, CFTR's function is diminished or absent in CF precipitating a cycle of events including sodium hyper-absorption, mucus hypersecretion, impaired mucociliary clearance and pathogenic colonization with microorganisms. This in turn leads to the clinical picture of recurrent infections, bronchiectasis and airway destruction culminating in respiratory failure and premature death (Davis et al., 1996).

Several hundred mutations of the CFTR gene have been described with a sub-group causing disease. Differing mutations impact upon CFTR channel expression, localization and activity and in some cases a combination of these important functions. Dependent on these factors, CFTR mutations have been stratified into six distinct classes for example the class II ΔF508 mutation encodes a CFTR protein that is both defectively folded and processed resulting in disease (Rowe et al., 2005). Whilst the Republic of Ireland has both the highest incidence and carrier rates of CF worldwide, ΔF508 accounts for >95% alleles identified (Farrell, 2008).

An important long-standing observation in CF remains the fact that a gender dichotomy has been described. Females have poorer survival, worse lung function and earlier colonization with *Pseudomonas aeruginosa* when compared to males without adequate explanation. The following chapter will initially outline past epidemiological observations that have been made with regard to the CF 'gender gap' followed by our present understanding of potential explanations for these gender differences. A special focus on the major female sex hormone estrogen will be emphasized particularly its impact on the inflammatory and immune state within the female CF airway. Finally, directions for future basic science and clinical research in the area will be outlined.

2. Past observations

The female gender disadvantage has been observed in CF morbidity and mortality and is reported throughout the early literature. Differences encompass survival, lung function, frequency of infections and microbiological variation however despite investigation explanations have remained elusive. With the lack of adequate explanation persisting over the last decade, controversy has emerged as to whether such disparities in fact ever existed and if such variation could be explained by therapeutic factors or treatment differences alone that exist between countries and care centers worldwide.

The gender dichotomy outlined within early work in CF states that CF females have poorer survival, worse lung function and earlier colonization with *P. aeruginosa*. Early work by Corey *et al* (Corey & Farewell, 1996) assessing almost four thousand individuals with the disease from the Canadian registry illustrated that although regional differences in survival were identified that females had diminished survival of greater than five years when compared to males utilizing cohorts from both the 70's and 80's. The poorer survival in females was associated with poorer weight however the close inter-relation between declining pulmonary function, weight maintainence, gender and mortality was recognized and put forward for further investigation (Corey & Farewell, 1996). Similar results to these were uncovered from an Italian registry and then further confirmed in an independent United Kingdom assessment of mortality and survival in CF extending from 1947-2003 (Bossi et al., 1999; Dodge et al., 2007). In the early 90's, an important demographic shift in CF survival was noted. CF patients who previously were not surviving past childhood were now progressing to young adults. The proportion of adults with CF increased fourfold between the 70's and 90's together with a doubling of median survival from 14 to 28 years of age. Such changes in the age distribution of CF survival at this time provided clinicians further insight into the natural history of the disease that was previously unknown. Despite these improvements to CF survival, female patients continued to show a lower median survival age compared to males (25 versus 30 years of age in 1990) (FitzSimmons, 1993). Subsequent study involving >20,000 patients with CF and utilizing Cox proportional hazards regression analysis to compare age-specific mortality rates between genders again confirmed gender differences in median CF survival (25.3 versus 28.4 years for females versus males respectively) (Rosenfeld et al., 1997). Additionally, this work aimed to identify particular risk factors that may serve as potential explanatory variables for the observed gender related survival differences (Rosenfeld et al., 1997). Despite analysis using a variety of risk factors for death in CF including poor nutritional status, lung function, airway microbiology, pancreatic insufficiency, age at diagnosis, mode of presentation and race, none could account for the gender disparity identified further confirming the existence of a genuine 'gender gap' (Rosenfeld et al., 1997). Consequential to this and other works, it was unsurprising to note that gender was included as a major parameter in a predictive 5-year CF survivorship model developed to help both researchers and clinicians evaluate therapies, improve prospective study design, monitor practice patterns, counsel individual patients and aid determination of suitable candidates for lung transplantation (Liou et al., 2001).

A lack of explanation for such gender differences in CF disease together with a narrowing of this gap recently has ignited controversy with regard to whether the CF 'gender gap' ever existed. Some arguments have been put forward against the phenomena of the female disadvantage in CF which attempt to explain the gender differences based on therapeutic advances occurring over the last decade in the management of the disease. For instance, retrospective cross sectional analysis of annual assessment data from a single center has shown that during childhood and adolescence, the lung function and nutrition of CF patients should be equal between the genders and that individual clinic practice should be reviewed if a gender gap persists. The authors argue that prior studies that have shown poorer prognosis in CF females have generally combined data from several centers and that their aim was to determine whether with modern aggressive treatment of CF this gender difference remains when care is standardized within a single center (Verma et al., 2005). Whilst some of the arguments put forward by this work may be plausible, an important point to consider remains that the gender differences observed in CF were most clearly observed post-puberty and during adulthood and not during the adolescent years, the group assessed by this work. To lend further argument to this, recent data from an Italian registry confirmed the absence of a gender gap in CF survival however this assessment only included patients up to 16 years of age, too early to identify the previously described gender dichotomy (Viviani et al., 2011). As a result, one of the conclusions drawn from this dataset was that the emergence of mortality differences between the genders could not be excluded if this cohort was to be followed into adulthood, the timeframe of interest in older studies (Viviani et al., 2011). Additionally, although Olsen *et al* did acknowledge that females with CF are at higher risks of *P. aeruginosa* and *Burkholderia* colonization, require more intensified treatments with antibiotics and have greater rates of hospitalizations compared to males, they found no gender effect upon survival. It was again reiterated in the conclusions to this work that gender survival differences may in fact follow adolescence, the age group studied (Olesen et al., 2010).

To overcome some of the weaknesses in comparing CF survival data between institutions, a case mix adjustment method may be employed (O'Connor et al., 2002). Such a method accounts for baseline differences in both patient and disease characteristics and although no consensus with regards its use in CF currently exists, the characteristics utilized for such an adjustment should include those that differ across institutions and are associated with patient survival. By accounting for characteristics of disease severity that may be a consequence of treatment effectiveness, this analysis can abolish the argument put forward that improvements to treatment account for gender discrepancies observed in CF disease. Using such case mix adjustment methodologies, O'Connor *et al* have shown that female gender in CF remains associated with an increased risk of death (O'Connor et al., 2002). This conclusion is reached using a model encompassing patient and disease characteristics that are present at the time of diagnosis and not influenced by subsequent treatment strengthening the argument for the existence of a true 'gender gap'.

An alternative argument put forward to refute a true 'gender gap' is greater compliance to therapy among female patients with CF. Masterson *et al* studied adherence to infection control guidelines and medical therapy in a CF cohort and found that although age-related differences exist, gender was importantly not a significant factor for treatment adherence (Masterson et al., 2010).

In view of disagreement about the existence for gender variation in CF, a re-assessment for these differences was performed in early 2000, a time where survival rates were noted to have exponentially improved since the mid 80's. Although survival of both genders was discovered to have benefitted from this trend, females had consistently poorer survival rates compared to male patients re-iterating the existence of genuine gender differences (Kulich et al., 2003). This has been more recently confirmed by data published from our own Irish registry (Jackson et al., 2011). As a consequence, it is clear that female gender is a negative prognostic factor in CF - a finding illustrated across several countries, registries and CF care centers.

In addition to survival variances, differences in the acquisition and conversion of the major pathogen and colonizer *P. aeruginosa* have been described in CF. Females with CF acquire *P. aeruginosa* in advance of males and furthermore convert to their mucoid phenotype earlier conferring worse clinical outcomes (Demko et al., 1995). Longitudinal assessment of this organism in CF has shown a relatively short transition from no *P. aeruginosa* to non-mucoid *P. aeruginosa* however a much more prolonged period, sometimes over a decade preceding mucoid conversion. Transition to mucoid correlated with a deterioration in cough and chest radiography scores along with pulmonary function (Li et al., 2005).

Interestingly, an assessment specifically designed to evaluate whether earlier acquisition of *P. aeruginosa* by females in CF, the greater impact of the organism on lung function or a combination of both factors contributed to the poorer survival in females found that although acquisition of mucoid organism was associated with an increased rate of decline of pulmonary function in both genders males had consistently better FEV_1 (% predicted) and survival rates compared to females. This suggests that alternative factors and not *P. aeruginosa* alone contribute to the gender differences observed in female CF patients (Demko et al., 1995). Separate and independent analysis of the risk factors for initial acquisition of *P. aeruginosa* in children with CF identified by newborn screening found that female gender amongst others represents an important risk for early detection (Maselli et al., 2003). Further study has additionally shown that whilst chronic mucoid *P. aeruginosa* can have prognostic implications in disease outcomes, that female gender again remains an important risk factor for its early detection (Levy et al., 2008).

Whilst these past observations illustrate that gender differences are an important consideration in CF disease, they importantly do not explain why they exist. One important difference between genders and a potential avenue for exploration is the circulating female hormone estrogen. Estrogens are the primary female sex hormone and have fundamental roles during the menstrual cycle. They circulate in three forms: estrone (E_1), estradiol (E_2) and estriol (E_3), with E_2 being the predominant and most active form in the non-pregnant state. Both E_2 and progesterone fluctuations throughout the menstrual cycle have been implicated to impact upon pulmonary function however explanations to address such differences in CF remain lacking (Tam et al., 2011). Our group and others have conducted studies examining E_2 and its effects on infectious, inflammatory and immune consequences in the CF airway. Although such work remains ongoing, its results may provide insight for the first time into reasons for these fundamental gender differences that so far have not been adequately explained.

2.1 Pulmonary innate immunity

The lung constitutes a large surface of the body in contact with the outside environment. It is continuously exposed to a large number of airborne microbes or microbial molecules, and can also be confronted with pathogens approaching via the blood stream. A number of factors including lung structure and physiology and components of the pulmonary innate immune system interact to contribute to effective pulmonary defenses. Individual key factors of pulmonary innate immunity will be outlined following which the effects that E_2 may have on each component will be discussed. These include, but are not limited to the following:

2.1.1 Airway surface liquid (ASL)

The ASL is a protective layer of fluid that covers the airway epithelium. It contains electrolytes, soluble proteins and importantly provides an interface within which cilia can beat and move mucus up through the respiratory tract. The mucociliary escalator together with pulmonary surfactant provides a barrier material at the air-liquid interface of the lungs. Surfactant contains the surfactant proteins A (SP-A), SP-B, SP-C and SP-D which help to lower the surface tension and participate in innate immune defence.

2.1.2 Pattern recognition receptors (PRRs)

Toll-like receptors (TLRs) comprise a major family of PRRs that fulfil key roles in recognising, discriminating and responding to microbial infection (Greene & McElvaney, 2005). They are associated principally with macrophages and dendritic cells, however their expression is widespread and includes, but is not limited to cells of myeloid and lymphoid origin. TLRs are also expressed by pulmonary epithelial cells (Greene et al., 2005). Activation of TLRs by their cognate ligands can lead to induction of proinflammatory cytokine and antimicrobial peptide expression or up regulation of type 1 interferons. TLRs can also communicate with the adaptive immune response via modulation of cell adhesion and co-stimulatory molecules to induce longer term immunity and a range of non-microbial endogenous factors can also activate certain TLRs.

2.1.3 Antimicrobial proteins

A selection of antimicrobial peptides including the human beta-defensins (HBDs), cathelicidin/hCAP-18/LL-37, lactoferrin and lysozyme can be found in the respiratory tract. In addition to their direct bacterial killing activity some of these proteins also have anti-biofilm, anti-inflammatory and anti-viral properties (Rogan et al., 2006).

2.1.4 Proteases

In the healthy lung proteases fulfil basic homeostatic roles and regulate processes such as regeneration and repair. The principal classes of protease present in the lung are the serine, cysteinyl, aspartyl and metalloproteases. These can function to regulate processes as diverse as tissue remodelling, mucin expression, neutrophil chemotaxis and bacterial killing. Members of these protease classes orchestrate a diverse range of changes with respect to infection and inflammation in the lung (Greene & McElvaney, 2009).

2.1.5 Antiprotease protection in the lung

The activity of pulmonary proteases is regulated by antiproteases. There are three major serine antiproteases in the lung – alpha-1 antitrypsin, secretory leucoprotease inhibitor

(SLPI) and elafin. In addition to their anti-protease activities they also possess other intrinsic immunomodulatory, anti-inflammatory and antimicrobial properties (Greene & McElvaney, 2009).

2.2 Dysfunctional pulmonary innate immunity in cystic fibrosis

Pulmonary infection and inflammation in the CF lung are multifaceted processes. Defective chloride ion conductance due to mutant CFTR causes a decrease in the height of the ASL and an increase in both the volume and viscosity of mucus. The most important airway mucins are the secreted mucins, Muc5AC and Muc5B which are produced by goblet cells of the superficial airway epithelium. Their expression is increased in the CF lung and the overall composition of CF mucus is altered due to an increased content of macromolecules such as DNA, filamentous actin, lipids, and proteoglycans. Together these contribute to mucus plugging within the CF lung (Rose & Voynow, 2006; Voynow & Rubin, 2009). This also facilitates microbial colonisation with *P. aeruginosa, Staphylococcus aureus, Burkholderia cepacia, Prevotella* spp, *Candida* spp, and *Aspergillus* spp. One remarkable consequence of these events is an exaggerated influx of activated neutrophils into the lung. Due to the large numbers of infiltrating neutrophils higher than normal levels of neutrophil-derived reactive oxidant species and proteases are reached. The consequences of these events include (i) an imbalance in the lung's redox balance which can be further exaggerated due to reduced glutathione levels (Roum et al., 1993) that together lead to oxidative damage, and (ii) an imbalance in the normal protease-antiprotease balance due to the combined effects of oxidative inactivation of the normal anti-protease defences and the presence not only of excess neutrophil-derived but also bacterial-derived proteases (Greene & McElvaney, 2009).

Neutrophil elastase (NE) is the major protease released by neutrophils in the CF lung. It has significant effects (Kelly et al., 2008). Not only does it up regulate the expression of other proteases including metalloproteases and cysteinyl cathepsins (Geraghty et al., 2007), it can also inactivate certain serine antiproteases (elafin and SLPI) and abrogate their anti-inflammatory and immunomodulatory properties (Kelly et al., 2008; Weldon et al., 2009). In concert with proteinase-3, macrophage-derived metalloelastases and elastolytic proteases expressed by *P. aeruginosa,* NE can promote secretion of mucus and degrade surfactant proteins and antimicrobials. NE can also directly injure epithelial cells and reduce ciliary beat frequency, cleave haemoglobin, complement components and immunoglobulins and interfere with effective neutrophil killing of microbes (Kelly et al., 2008). NE also contributes not only to the intracellular killing of gram-negative bacteria by neutrophils but also, once released extracellularly, can play a role in bacterial killing by comprising a key component of neutrophil extracellular traps (NETs). NETs are involved in host defense (Brinkmann et al., 2004). They bind gram-positive and gram-negative bacteria and allow neutrophils to directly deliver high concentrations of serine proteases that degrade virulence factors and kill bacteria.

The high protease milieu of the CF lung can also impact deleteriously on antimicrobial protein activity. Defensins, lactoferrin, LL-37 and SLPI are all susceptible to proteolytic degradation particularly by cysteinyl cathepsins (Bergsson et al., 2009).

Pulmonary inflammation in CF is also mediated by proinflammatory molecules such as C5a, LTB4, ceramide, and the chemotactic tripeptide Proline-Glycine-Proline (Greene, 2010), which together contribute to the highly proinflammatory milieu in the CF lung. Furthermore the CF lung is a TLR agonist-rich milieu, represented by microbial-derived factors (bacterial, viral and fungal) and neutrophil elastase (NE), respectively (Greene et al., 2008). The chronic inflammatory phenotype evident in CF airway epithelial cells is likely due in large part to activation of TLRs (Greene et al., 2008). In the CF lung NE-induced activation of TLR signalling is mediated via EGFR ligand generation and EGFR activation (Bergin et al., 2008).

Overall the CF lung is highly prone to exaggerated inflammation. Although it is a neutrophil-rich environment, neutrophil degranulation and killing activity are dysfunctional. With inadequate anti-inflammatory mechanisms due to oxidation and proteolytic inactivation, incomplete resolution of infection occurs, bacterial biofilms remain established and infective exacerbations induce more severe symptoms. In females with CF these events may be further complicated due to gender-specific effects mediated in part by the female sex hormone estrogen which will now be discussed.

3. Present understanding

Estrogen, the predominant female hormone is released from the ovaries and subsequently circulates bound to sex hormone binding globulin (SHBG). Free E_2 interacts with its specific estrogen receptors (ERs) to affect human physiological responses. ERs are predominantly based in the cell cytoplasm however more recently, an association with the cell plasma membrane has been described (Levin, 2009). The major ERs are ERα and ERβ, which share structural similarities however can effect opposing responses based on tissue type and location (Weihua et al., 2003).

Traditional effector mechanisms associated with ERs are genomic where the hormone following binding to its receptor within the cell cytoplasm shuttles as a complex into the cell nucleus to induce gene transcription of estrogen-responsive genes (Metivier et al., 2006). Membrane associated ERs however act through non-genomic pathways that are more rapid affecting protein kinases and mobilizing intracellular calcium stores (Morley et al., 1992; Pedram et al., 2006; Pietras & Szego, 1975; Pietras et al., 2005; Razandi et al., 2000, 2004). Genomic and non-genomic pathways may interact with one another resulting in modification of gene transcription as the end-event.

ERs are distributed throughout the human body however proportions vary by organ system. In some settings, both receptors are expressed whereas in others one subtype predominates. For example, ERα is related to reproductive tissues, bone, liver and the kidney whilst ERβ is more abundant in the colon, bladder and lung. Its role in the lung, particularly one that is chronically inflammed is a subject of continuing research in the context of CF (Chotirmall et al., 2010). Emerging inflammatory, immune and microbiological data suggests a potential role for E_2 in the cause and course of chronic inflammatory lung diseases such as CF.

Over a monthly menstrual cycle, *in vivo* E_2 concentrations fluctuate with highest levels preceding ovulation with the lowest around menstruation. In view of its physiological role, ability to fluctuate in concentration, coupled to its capability to modulate cellular functions, responses and gene expression in those containing estrogen response elements (EREs), E_2

represents an attractive avenue for investigation in terms of the gender differences observed in CF disease.

Our current understanding of the role that E_2 plays within the female CF lung is driven by investigations focused on its effects upon the dysfunctional pulmonary innate immune system and specifically some of its key components as described above. One such component is the ASL which is already known to be compromised in the setting of CFTR dysfunction. Coakley *et al* (Coakley et al., 2008) have recently shown that in the setting of E_2 exposure ASL is further compromised by dehydration and an increased risk of infection and subsequent exacerbation during high circulating E_2 states. Therefore the two-week period of a single menstrual cycle where E_2 concentrations are highest represents a high risk time-frame of acquiring infection and promoting exacerbation (Coakley et al., 2008). To date however, this proposed relationship between E_2 concentration, menstrual cycle phase and infective exacerbations is yet to be illustrated by *in vivo* study and represents a future direction for clinical research.

We have added to the understanding of E_2's role within the innate immune system in CF by demonstrating that high circulating E_2 states confer a TLR hyporesponsiveness to a range of bacterial agonists manifested by an inhibition of IL-8 release. We found that the mechanism by which this phenomenon occurs is through ERβ-mediated upregulation of SLPI, an important anti-protease/anti-inflammatory described above that is widely expressed within the respiratory tract (Chotirmall et al., 2010). SLPI, in separate work has been shown to competitively inhibit NF-κB p-65 subunit binding to DNA inhibiting the transcription of NF-κB regulated genes such as IL-8 (Taggart et al., 2005). It is also important to note that in the non-CF context NF-κB has long been described to affect E_2 signaling pathways, for example within circulating monocytes or tissue macrophages E_2 can block LPS-induced NF-κB activity (Ghisletti et al., 2005). As we have demonstrated E_2 to have an anti-inflammatory role in the context of the female CF lung, we hypothesized that although an environment of chronic uncontrolled inflammation may be damaging over the course of lifelong disease, acute surges in inflammation particularly in the setting of an acute infection may in fact provide protection and play a crucial role in facilitating bacterial clearance. Our published data would suggest however that in CF females this acute inflammatory response to an infective exacerbation is blunted by the presence of circulating E_2 and when taken together with the compromised ASL, high circulating E_2 states create an environment prone to both acquisition of infection and a subsequently compromised response to it (Chotirmall et al., 2010). It is becoming clearer with studies such as those described that E_2 plays an important role in some of the observed gender differences in CF disease probably in tandem with other factors influencing clinical outcomes. One important offshoot from our work illustrating the hyporesponsive state induced by E_2 exposure is in potentially elucidating why anti-inflammatory agents such as the leukotriene B4 antagonist have been unsuccessful in clinical trial, in fact causing premature trial termination (trial registration: NCT00060801) owing to increased infection within the treatment arm (Schmitt-Grohe & Zielen, 2005). Despite this, it remains important to highlight that clinical benefit has been shown following use of high-dose Ibuprofen however mechanisms to explain these outcomes are still sought (Konstan et al., 1995). Notably, we detected ERβ to be the predominant ER within the CF airway by use of bronchial brushings obtained via bronchoscopy (Chotirmall et al., 2010). An increased ERβ expression is associated with oxidative stress and hypoxic conditions explaining why it probably predominates in the CF context (Chotirmall et al., 2010; Schneider et al., 2000).

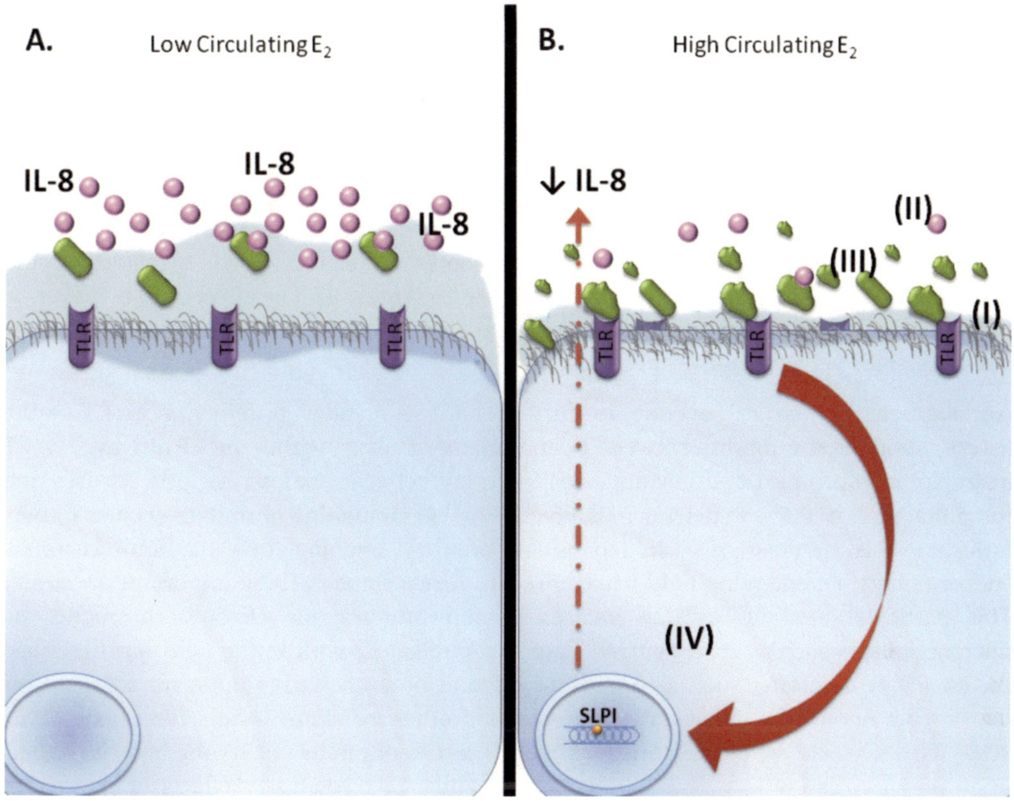

Fig. 1. The effect of 17β-estradiol (E_2) within the female CF airway. (A) In states of low circulating E_2 (luteal phase), a dehydrated airway surface liquid (ASL) overlies the CF female airway epithelium. Within the lumen, antimicrobials (pink) such as lactoferrin and neutrophil chemokines e.g. interleukin-8 (IL-8) are detected along-with potential *Pseudomonas aeruginosa* colonization. (B) During high circulating E_2 states (follicular phase), (I) a further disadvantaged and diminished ASL (Coakley et al; 2008) coupled with (II) an inhibitory effect and consequent dearth of anti-microbial peptides (Wang et al; 2010) combine to create an ideal environment primed for infection and exacerbation (III). (IV) Following infection, a blunted response to microbial agonists occur resulting in diminished luminal IL-8 and a hypo-responsive immune state (Chotirmall et al; 2010). These factors (I-IV) combine to confer an elevated risk of infection and subsequent exacerbation in the E_2 exposed CF airway.

More recent work additionally highlights a role for E_2 in *P. aeruginosa* infection. Proposed mechanisms include an enhanced Th17 regulated inflammatory response and suppression of innate antibacterial defences including the anti-microbial peptide lactoferrin (Wang et al., 2010). When assessed in unison, our work and others may provide an important mechanistic basis for some of the gender differences observed in CF disease. For instance, in CF, a dehydrated ASL overlies the female airway epithelium whilst within the lumen, antimicrobials and the neutrophil chemokines (e.g. IL-8, LTB4, C5a and Proline-Glycine-Proline) may be detected along with *P. aeruginosa* colonization. During high circulating E_2 states (follicular phase of the menstrual cycle), a further disadvantaged and diminished ASL (Coakley et al., 2008) coupled with impaired antimicrobial defences (Wang et al., 2010) combine to create an ideal environment primed for infection and exacerbation. Following infection, a blunted response to microbial agonists occurs resulting in diminished luminal IL-8 and a hypo-responsive immune state due to up-regulation of SLPI (Chotirmall et al., 2010). In tandem, these factors combine to confer an elevated risk of infection and subsequent exacerbation in the E_2 exposed CF airway (Figure 1). The effect of E_2 however on other antimicrobial peptides, proteases and anti-proteases within the pulmonary environment is yet to be fully established.

An alternate but critical avenue to further address gender differences in CF is by investigating the relationship between E_2 and microorganisms within the CF airway. The CF microbiome is complex and encompasses interplay between various bacteria, viruses and fungi that co-exist some to detrimental effect. Whether circulating hormones such as E_2 may influence this organism-rich milieu is an area of ongoing investigation. Microbial endocrinology, an emerging field has begun to address some of these important questions. This particular area of research focuses upon examining the effect of hormones on microorganisms such as *P. aeruginosa*. Thus far, published work in the field has described the effects of hormones such as noradrenaline and norepinephrine upon microorganisms that impact upon their adhesion proteins among other virulence factors (Freestone et al., 1999, 2008). Despite the crucial functions that E_2 carries out in its eukaryotic host, its impact upon prokaryotes are less clearly understood. Whilst E_2 mediates its effects in eukaryotes through its major receptors -α and -β, comparable structures have been sought within prokaryotes. Estrogen binding proteins have been identified in *P. aeruginosa* whilst *Escherichia coli* possesses enzymes with analogous homology to human ERs (Baker, 1989; Rowland et al., 1992; Sugarman et al., 1990). Additionally, it is known that *P. aeruginosa* actively breaks down E_2 to its major metabolite estriol (E_3) and whether such metabolites can impact upon microorganisms particularly in the CF context remains to be determined (Fishman et al., 1960). Importantly, certain fungi are capable of producing estrogenic-like substances termed myco-estrogens however, whether these have any relevance for pulmonary environment in CF remain undetermined.

4. Future directions

Our understanding of the role that E_2 may potentially play within the female CF airway has exponentially grown. Studies performed to date have implicated the hormone as a potential explanation for the long-observed gender differences in CF disease. With such advances to our understanding come further avenues for future exploration.

One such avenue is the role of modifying the endogenous concentration of E_2 to alleviate its detrimental effects. Use of the anti-estrogen agent Tamoxifen or the oral contraceptive pill (OCP) can achieve this albeit by differing mechanisms. Tamoxifen *in vitro* is able to re-instate the ASL to its pre-E_2 state confirming the importance of E_2 in mediating its negative effect (Coakley et al., 2008). Use of the OCP to modulate endogenous E_2 concentrations would be a preferred and safer option although no studies to date have examined use of the OCP in CF in terms of effects on ASL or infection frequency. Such studies will undoubtedly emerge in due course and may provide a valuable potential future therapeutic option for CF females.

Although E_2 in its most active form is the chosen compound for most studies to date, it must be considered that through its natural metabolic process that E_2 is broken down into metabolites such as E_3. Whether such metabolites have effects within the CF airway on immune, inflammatory or infectious consequences is another area for future focus. In terms of innate immunity, prior publications in the non-respiratory setting have shown that E_2 has a major influence on antimicrobial peptides such as lactoferrin, elafin and SLPI (Fahey et al., 2008).

Whilst we have shown in our work that E_2 up-regulates SLPI in CF bronchial epithelium, the effects of E_2 on other anti-microbials have yet to be fully established (Chotirmall et al., 2010). Furthermore, the functional consequence of E_2 exposure on the various anti-microbial peptides has not been addressed.

The complex effects of E_2 on inflammation continue to be deciphered and consequently ERβ agonists have emerged as anti-inflammatory candidates. The development of such a compound however remains a pharmacological challenge that the forthcoming decade should address. Other important estrogen-based chemical compounds include the estrogen dendrimer conjugate (EDC) that binds ERs but excludes them from accessing the cell nucleus and exerting genomic effects (Harrington et al., 2006). Future research utilizing compounds such as the EDC will evaluate the precise contributions of genomic versus non-genomic mechanisms in a variety of *in vitro* and *vivo* settings that will provide further insight into the mechanistic explanations for the gender disparities acknowledged.

Finally, an exciting new development in CF therapeutics is targeting of the basic genetic defect by the use of channel potentiators such as VX-770 (Accurso et al., 2010). Whether E_2 or gender appears to impact upon these emerging agents and their effects represents another exciting direction for both CF basic science and clinical research leading us into the next decade of CF care.

5. Acknowledgments

Funding for our cystic fibrosis research is gratefully acknowledged from the Higher Education Authority (HEA)-PRTLI Cycle 4, through a Molecular Medicine Ireland (MMI) Clinician-Scientist Fellowship Programme (CSFP) grant 2008-2011, the Irish CF Research Trust, the Medical Research Charities Group and the Health Research Board of Ireland, the Children's Medical and Research Centre, Crumlin Hospital and Science Foundation Ireland.

6. References

Accurso FJ, Rowe SM, Clancy JP, Boyle MP, Dunitz JM, Durie PR, Sagel SD, Hornick DB, Konstan MW, Donaldson SH, Moss RB, Pilewski JM, Rubenstein RC, Uluer AZ, Aitken ML, Freedman SD, Rose LM, Mayer-Hamblett N, Dong Q,Zha J, Stone AJ, Olson ER, Ordonez CL, Campbell PW, Ashlock MA & Ramsey BW. 2010. Effect of VX-770 in persons with cystic fibrosis and the G551D-CFTR mutation. *N Engl J Med.* Vol. 363, No. 21, pp1991-2003.

Baker ME. 1989. Similarity between tyrosyl-tRNA synthetase and the estrogen receptor. *FASEB J.* Vol. 3, No. 9, pp2086-8.

Bergin DA, Greene CM, Sterchi EE, Kenna C, Geraghty P, Belaaouaj A, Taggart CC, O'Neill SJ & McElvaney NG. 2008. Activation of the epidermal growth factor receptor (EGFR) by a novel metalloprotease pathway. *J Biol Chem.* Vol. 283, No. 46, pp31736-44.

Bergsson G, Reeves EP, McNally P, Chotirmall SH, Greene CM, Greally P, Murphy P, O'Neill SJ & McElvaney NG. 2009. LL-37 complexation with glycosaminoglycans in cystic fibrosis lungs inhibits antimicrobial activity, which can be restored by hypertonic saline. *J Immunol.* Vol. 183, No.1, pp543-51.

Bossi A, Battistini F, Braggion C, Magno EC, Cosimi A, de Candussio G, Gagliardini R, Giglio L, Giunta A, Grzincich GL, La Rosa M, Lombardo M, Lucidi V, Manca A, Mastella G, Moretti P, Padoan R, Pardo F, Quattrucci S, Raia V, Romano L, Salvatore D, Taccetti G & Zanda, M. 1992. [Italian Cystic Fibrosis Registry: 10 years of activity]. *Epidemiol Prev.* Vol. 23, No.1, pp5-16.

Brinkmann V, Reichard U, Goosmann C, Fauler B, Uhlemann Y, Weiss DS, Weinrauch Y & Zychlinsky A. 2004. Neutrophil extracellular traps kill bacteria. *Science.* 2004. Vol 5, No. 303(5663), pp1532-5.

Chotirmall SH, Greene CM, Oglesby IK, Thomas W, O'Neill SJ, Harvey BJ & McElvaney NG. 2010. 17Beta-estradiol inhibits IL-8 in cystic fibrosis by up-regulating secretory leucoprotease inhibitor. *Am J Respir Crit Care Med.* Vol. 182, No. 1, pp62-72.

Coakley RD, Sun H, Clunes LA, Rasmussen JE, Stackhouse JR, Okada SF, Fricks I, Young SL & Tarran R. 2008. 17beta-Estradiol inhibits Ca2+-dependent homeostasis of airway surface liquid volume in human cystic fibrosis airway epithelia. *J Clin Invest.* Vol. 118, No. 12, pp4025-35.

Corey M & Farewell V. 1996. Determinants of mortality from cystic fibrosis in Canada, 1970-1989. *Am J Epidemiol.* Vol. 143, No. 10, pp1007-17.

Davis PB, Drumm ML & Konstan MW.1996. State of the art: Cystic fibrosis. *Am J Respir Crit Care Med.* Vol. 154, No. 5, pp1229-56.

Demko CA, Byard PJ & Davis PB. 1995. Gender differences in cystic fibrosis: Pseudomonas aeruginosa infection. *J Clin Epidemiol.* Vol. 48, No. 8, pp1041-9.

Dodge JA, Lewis PA, Stanton M & Wilsher J. 2007. Cystic fibrosis mortality and survival in the UK: 1947-2003. *Eur Respir J.* Vol. 29, No. 3, pp522-6.

Fahey JV, Wright JA, Shen L, Smith JM, Ghosh M, Rossoll RM & Wira CR. 2008. Estradiol selectively regulates innate immune function by polarized human uterine epithelial cells in culture. *Mucosal Immunol.* Vol. 1, No.4, pp317-25.

Farrell PM. 2008. The prevalence of cystic fibrosis in the European Union. *J Cyst Fibros.* Vol. 7, No. 5, pp450-3.

Fishman J, Bradlow HL & Gallagher TF. 1960. Oxidative metabolism of estradiol. *J Biol Chem.* Vol. 235, pp3104-7.

FitzSimmons SC. 1993. The changing epidemiology of cystic fibrosis. *J Pediatr.* Vol. 122, No. 1, pp1-9.

Freestone PP, Haigh RD, Williams PH & Lyte M. 1999. Stimulation of bacterial growth by heat-stable, norepinephrine-induced autoinducers. *FEMS Microbiol Lett.* Vol. 172, No. 1, pp53-60.

Freestone PP, Sandrini SM, Haigh RD & Lyte M. 2008. Microbial endocrinology: how stress influences susceptibility to infection. *Trends Microbiol.* Vol. 16, No.2, pp55-64.

Geraghty P, Rogan MP, Greene CM, Boxio RM, Poiriert T, O'Mahony M, Belaaouaj A, O'Neill SJ, Taggart CC & McElvaney NG. 2007. Neutrophil elastase up-regulates cathepsin B and matrix metalloprotease-2 expression. *J Immunol.* Vol. 178, No. 9, pp5871-8.

Ghisletti S, Meda C, Maggi A & Vegeto E. 2005. 17beta-estradiol inhibits inflammatory gene expression by controlling NF-kappaB intracellular localization. *Mol Cell Biol.* Vol. 25, No. 8, pp2957-68.

Greene CM, Carroll TP, Smith SG, Taggart CC, Devaney J, Griffin S, O'Neill SJ & McElvaney NG. 2005. TLR-induced inflammation in cystic fibrosis and non-cystic fibrosis airway epithelial cells. *J Immunol.* Vol. 174, No. 3, pp1638-46.

Greene CM & McElvaney NG. 2005. Toll-like receptor expression and function in airway epithelial cells. *Arch Immunol Ther Exp (Warsz).* Vol. 53, No. 5, pp418-27.

Greene CM, Branagan P & McElvaney NG. 2008. Toll-like receptors as therapeutic targets in cystic fibrosis. *Expert Opin Ther Targets.* Vol. 12, No. 12, pp1481-95.

Greene CM & McElvaney NG. 2009. Proteases and antiproteases in chronic neutrophilic lung disease - relevance to drug discovery. *Br J Pharmacol.* Vol. 158, No. 4, pp1048-58.

Greene CM. 2010. How can we target pulmonary inflammation in cystic fibrosis? *Open Respir Med J.* Vol.4, pp18-9.

Harrington WR, Kim SH, Funk CC, Madak-Erdogan Z, Schiff R, Katzenellenbogen JA & Katzenellenbogen BS. 2006. Estrogen dendrimer conjugates that preferentially activate extranuclear, nongenomic versus genomic pathways of estrogen action. *Mol Endocrinol.* Vol. 20, No. 3, pp491-502.

Jackson AD, Daly L, Jackson AL, Kelleher C, Marshall BC, Quinton HB, Fletcher G, Harrington M, Zhou S, McKone EF, Gallagher C, Foley L & Fitzpatrick P. 2011. Validation and use of a parametric model for projecting cystic fibrosis survivorship beyond observed data: a birth cohort analysis. *Thorax.*Vol. 66, No. 8, pp674-9.

Kelly E, Greene CM & McElvaney NG. 2008. Targeting neutrophil elastase in cystic fibrosis. *Expert Opin Ther Targets.* Vol. 12, No. 2, pp145-57.

Konstan MW, Byard PJ, Hoppel CL & Davis PB. 1995. Effect of high-dose ibuprofen in patients with cystic fibrosis. *N Engl J Med.* Vol. 332, No. 13, pp848-54.

Kulich M, Rosenfeld M, Goss CH & Wilmott R. 2003. Improved survival among young patients with cystic fibrosis. *J Pediatr.* Vol. 142, No. 6, pp631-6.

Levin ER. 2009. Plasma membrane estrogen receptors. *Trends Endocrinol Metab.* Vol. 20, No. 10, pp477-82.

Levy H, Kalish LA, Cannon CL, Garcia KC, Gerard C, Goldmann D, Pier GB, Weiss ST & Colin AA. 2008. Predictors of mucoid Pseudomonas colonization in cystic fibrosis patients. *Pediatr Pulmonol.* Vol. 43, No.5, pp463-71.

Li Z, Kosorok MR, Farrell PM, Laxova A, West SE, Green CG, Collins J, Rock MJ & Splaingard ML. 2005. Longitudinal development of mucoid Pseudomonas aeruginosa infection and lung disease progression in children with cystic fibrosis. *JAMA.* Vol. 293, No. 5, pp581-8.

Liou TG, Adler FR, Fitzsimmons SC, Cahill BC, Hibbs JR & Marshall BC. 2001. Predictive 5-year survivorship model of cystic fibrosis. *Am J Epidemiol.* Vol. 153, No. 4, pp345-52.

Maselli JH, Sontag MK, Norris JM, MacKenzie T, Wagener JS & Accurso FJ. 2003. Risk factors for initial acquisition of Pseudomonas aeruginosa in children with cystic fibrosis identified by newborn screening. *Pediatr Pulmonol.* Vol. 35, No. 4, pp257-62.

Masterson TL, Wildman BG, Newberry BH & Omlor GJ. 2010. Impact of age and gender on adherence to infection control guidelines and medical regimens in cystic fibrosis. *Pediatr Pulmonol.* [Epub ahead of print].

Metivier R, Reid G & Gannon F. 2006. Transcription in four dimensions: nuclear receptor-directed initiation of gene expression. *EMBO Rep.* Vol. 7, No. 2, pp161-7.

Morley P, Whitfield JF, Vanderhyden BC, Tsang BK & Schwartz JL. 1992. A new, nongenomic estrogen action: the rapid release of intracellular calcium. *Endocrinology.* Vol. 131, No. 3, pp1305-12.

O'Connor GT, Quinton HB, Kahn R, Robichaud P, Maddock J, Lever T, Detzer M & Brooks JG. 2002. Case-mix adjustment for evaluation of mortality in cystic fibrosis. *Pediatr Pulmonol.* Vol. 33, No. 2, pp99-105.

Olesen HV, Pressler T, Hjelte L, Mared L, Lindblad A, Knudsen PK, Laerum BN & Johannesson M; Scandinavian Cystic Fibrosis Study Consortium. 2010. Gender differences in the Scandinavian cystic fibrosis population. *Pediatr Pulmonol.* Vol. 45, No. 10, pp959-65.

Pedram A, Razandi M & Levin ER. Nature of functional estrogen receptors at the plasma membrane. 2006. *Mol Endocrinol.* Vol. 20, No. 9, pp1996-2009.

Pietras RJ & Szego CM. Endometrial cell calcium and oestrogen action. 1975. *Nature.* Vol. 253(5490), pp357-9.

Pietras RJ, Levin ER & Szego CM. 2005. Estrogen receptors and cell signaling. *Science.* Vol. 7, No. 310(5745), pp51-3.

Razandi M, Pedram A & Levin ER. 2000. Plasma membrane estrogen receptors signal to antiapoptosis in breast cancer. *Mol Endocrinol.* Vol. 14, No. 9, pp1434-47.

Razandi M, Pedram A, Merchenthaler I, Greene GL & Levin ER. 2004. Plasma membrane estrogen receptors exist and functions as dimers. *Mol Endocrinol.* Vol. 18, No. 12, pp2854-65.

Rogan MP, Geraghty P, Greene CM, O'Neill SJ, Taggart CC & McElvaney NG. 2006. Antimicrobial proteins and polypeptides in pulmonary innate defence. *Respir Res.* Vol. 7, pp29.

Rose MC & Voynow JA. 2006. Respiratory tract mucin genes and mucin glycoproteins in health and disease. *Physiol Rev.* Vol. 86, No.1, pp245-78.

Rosenfeld M, Davis R, FitzSimmons S, Pepe M & Ramsey B. 1997. Gender gap in cystic fibrosis mortality. *Am J Epidemiol.* Vol. 145, No. 9, pp794-803.

Roum JH, Buhl R, McElvaney NG, Borok Z & Crystal RG. 1993. Systemic deficiency of glutathione in cystic fibrosis. *J Appl Physiol.* Vol. 75, No.6, pp2419-24.

Rowe SM, Miller S & Sorscher EJ. 2005. Cystic fibrosis. *N Engl J Med.* Vol. 352, No.19, pp1992-2001.

Rowland SS, Falkler WA Jr & Bashirelahi N. 1992. Identification of an estrogen-binding protein in Pseudomonas aeruginosa. *J Steroid Biochem Mol Biol.* Vol. 42, No. 7, pp721-7.

Schmitt-Grohe S & Zielen S. 2005.Leukotriene receptor antagonists in children with cystic fibrosis lung disease : anti-inflammatory and clinical effects. *Paediatr Drugs.* Vol. 7, No. 6, pp353-63.

Schneider CP, Nickel EA, Samy TS, Schwacha MG, Cioffi WG, Bland KI & Chaudry IH. 2000. The aromatase inhibitor, 4-hydroxyandrostenedione, restores immune responses following trauma-hemorrhage in males and decreases mortality from subsequent sepsis. *Shock.* Vol. 14, No. 3, pp347-53.

Sugarman B & Mummaw N. 1990. Oestrogen binding by and effect of oestrogen on trichomonads and bacteria. *J Med Microbiol.* Vol. 32, No. 4, pp227-32.

Taggart CC, Cryan SA, Weldon S, Gibbons A, Greene CM, Kelly E, Low TB, O'Neill SJ & McElvaney NG. 2005. Secretory leucoprotease inhibitor binds to NF-kappaB binding sites in monocytes and inhibits p65 binding. *J Exp Med.* Vol. 202, No.12, pp1659-68.

Tam A, Morrish D, Wadsworth S, Dorscheid D, Man SF & Sin DD. 2011. The role of female hormones on lung function in chronic lung diseases. *BMC Womens Health.* Vol. 11, No.24.

Verma N, Bush A & Buchdahl R. 2005. Is there still a gender gap in cystic fibrosis? *Chest.* Vol. 128, No.4, pp2824-34.

Viviani L, Bossi A & Assael BM; On behalf of the Italian Registry for Cystic Fibrosis Collaborative Group. 2011. Absence of a gender gap in survival. An analysis of the Italian registry for cystic fibrosis in the paediatric age. *J Cyst Fibros.* Vol. 10, No.5, pp313-7.

Voynow JA & Rubin BK. 2009. Mucins, mucus, and sputum. *Chest.* Vol. 135, No. 2, pp505-12.

Wang Y, Cela E, Gagnon S & Sweezey NB. 2010. Estrogen aggravates inflammation in Pseudomonas aeruginosa pneumonia in cystic fibrosis mice. *Respir Res.* Vol. 11, pp166.

Weldon S, McNally P, McElvaney NG, Elborn JS, McAuley DF, Wartelle J, Belaaouaj A, Levine RL & Taggart CC. 2009. Decreased levels of secretory leucoprotease inhibitor in the pseudomonas-infected cystic fibrosis lung are due to neutrophil elastase degradation. *J Immunol.* Vol. 183, No. 12, pp8148-56.

Weihua Z, Andersson S, Cheng G, Simpson ER, Warner M & Gustafsson JA. 2003. Update on estrogen signaling. *FEBS Lett.* Vol. 546, No. 1, pp17-24.

4

Cystic Fibrosis and Infertility

Maria do Carmo Pimentel Batitucci,
Angela Maria Spagnol Perrone and Giselle Villa Flor Brunoro
Federal University of Espírito Santo
Brazil

1. Introduction

Cystic fibrosis (CF) - or mucoviscidosis - is a common autosomal recessive inherited disease, affecting the whole body and causing progressive deficiencies. The name 'cystic fibrosis' refers to the characteristic scarring (fibrosis) and formation of cysts in the pancreas. The first anatomical and pathological description of the disorder was done by Landsteiner in 1905. In 1936, Fanconi et al. identified it as an autonomous illness, and in 1994 Farber et al. named it mucoviscidosis, due to the thick and viscous mucus secreted by the exocrine glands. It is accounted for by several clinical manifestations. Respiratory impairment is the most serious symptom (resulting from chronic infection in the lungs) and, though it is treatable, it is resistant to antibiotics and other medication. The large number of other symptoms include sinusitis, inadequate growth, diarrhoea and infertility, each of which is an effect of CF in other parts of the body. The mutated gene is transmitted by father and mother - although it may be that neither of them manifest the disease - and it is accounted for by the change in carrying ions through the membranes of the cells (Quinton et al., 1983). This compromises the function of the exocrine glands that produce thicker and hard-eliminating substances (mucus, sweat or pancreatic enzymes).

In 1953, Di Sant'Agnase et al. noted an increased sodium chloride rate eliminated through the sweat of patients with CF. Gibson and Cooke (1958) standardised the sweat test, which has become an important tool in the diagnosis of the disease. In 1958, Shwachman and Kulczucki designed a disease-severity assessment system. In 1985, the position of the CFTR gene was determined on the long arm of chromosome 7, q31 band, by restriction fragment linked polymorphism (Knowlton et al., 1985), and, in 1989, the full-length gene was sequenced (Collins, 1992).

The clinical manifestations of CF are primarily due to the obstruction of the ducts of organs (such as the lung and the pancreas) by thick, viscous secretions, changes in electrolytic concentrations, and the presence of abnormal contents. The primary cellular defect consists of a decreased or else absent expression of the CF transmembrane conductance regulator (CFTR) protein, which causes changes in chloride secretion. This protein is present in all endodermal and mesodermal cells, and it has been found in sweat glands, organs of the digestive system, and the airways' epithelium layer (Bargon et al., 1999). The primary defect causes dehydration of the airways, leading to an increased viscosity of mucus in the intercellular environment, and it predisposes the body to chronic bacterial infections

(Tummler et al., 1999). At birth, the lung is histologically normal, and the pathophysiological changes evolve with aging (Shwachman et al., 1970). CF leads to pulmonary bronchiectasis and atelectasis, compromising the bronchi and bronchioles and so causing pulmonary emphysema. The pancreas is the organ that presents the largest functional and structural changes (Rozov et al., 1991). The blockage of glandular ducts leads to malnutrition syndrome, biliary liver cirrhosis, intestinal obstruction, and gastroesophageal reflux. In newborn infants, the presence of ileum-meconium can mark the first manifestation of CF (Feingold et al., 1999). Exocrine insufficiency of the pancreas occurs in 95% of cases (Mousia-Arvanitakis, 1999) and results in a decrease or the absence of lipolytic, proteolytic and amylolytic enzymes in the pancreatic juice, leading to chronic diarrhoea with bulky, greasy and fetid faeces. As a result, malnutrition becomes evident, owing to the loss of calories and proteins through poor digestion (Reis e Damasceno, 1998). The blockage can also affect the biliary ducts - the thick bile leads to difficulties of drainage, and there may be a full blockage of the ducts which may evolve into cirrhosis (Kopel, 1992).

Advances in genetic engineering and the development of transgenic animals during the last decade of the twentieth century, in conjunction with the prospect of early diagnosis, has contributed to the provision of proper and effective treatments that can increase the quality of life of patients with CF.

1.1 Incidence

The incidence of CF varies according to ethnicity, ranging from 1 CF individual per 2,000 to 5,000 Caucasian live births in Europe, the United States and Canada, 1 CF individual per 15,000 African Americans, and from 1 CF individual per 40,000 live births in Finland (Brunechy, 1972). In Brazil, the estimated incidence for the southern region is closer to that of Central Europe's Caucasian population, whereas for other regions it reduces to 1 per 10,000 live births. This is despite the fact that there are variations in the frequency of mutations in different geographic regions, which would probably reflect a different prevalence of the disease (Raskum et al., 1993). In the US and in European countries, early diagnosis - before the first year of life - allows affected children to be promptly treated and monitored with regard to the variables that directly influence the prognosis of the disease, such as the follow-up of the weight and height curve, and the presence of upper airway colonisation by pathogens (which is closely related to worse prognosis).

In Brazil, since 2001, and with the approval of the National Newborn Screening Program and its introduction by the laboratory of the Ecumenical Foundation for Exceptional Protection (FEPE-PR, Portuguese acronym), CF screening has been implemented in the State of Parana. Before the establishment of the National Newborn Screening Program for CF, the data showed that the average age receiving a diagnosis of the disease ranged at around 1.6 years (Santos et al., 2005).

1.2 Genetics

The isolation of the CFTR is a result of many years of study on the part of numerous research groups. Situated in long arm of the chromosome 7, at band q31.3 (Heng et al., 1993), with 250 Kb, the region codifier of the CFTR consists in 27 exons. Most of the exons are far from one another by between 50 and 250 base pairs, except for exon 13 which has 723 base pairs of the genomic DNA. The CFTR protein has a molecular weight of 168,138 Da and it belongs to a transmembrane chloride ion channel superfamily protein, with 1,480 amino acids (Harris, 1992) present in apical membranes of those cells lining the surface of the gland tubes and the airways.

About 1,500 mutations have already been identified in the CFTR: the most frequent mutation is F508del, which is found in 30% of patients with CF (Zielenski, 2000). This mutation is caused by the deletion of three base pairs corresponding to the codon that translates a residue phenylalanine at position 508 of the CFTR polypeptide chain (Morral, 1994). Depending on ethnic groups in different geographic locations the relative frequency of this mutation vary among individuals affected by CF. In Northern Europe and North America, it reaches 70-90%; however it is less frequent in Southern Europe, where less of 50% of the CF chromosomes have this mutation (Morral et al., 1994).

The G542X mutation is considered to be the second most frequent mutation, and it accounts for 3.4% of alleles in CF (Tsui, 1992). At a molecular level, it leads to a replacement of nucleotides, which results in a stop codon at position 542 of the polypeptide chain, and thus the translation product is a non-functional peptide that will be degraded. According to the geographic location, the frequency of this mutation varies among the CF individuals. It may be found in the compound heterozygous with the ΔF508 mutation. Raskin et al. (1993) have noted the frequency of the G542X mutation in 5% of the Brazilian population.

The G551D mutation affects 2.4% of the chromosomes of the population of individuals with CF - in general - and it leads to a replacement of guanine for adenine in nucleotide 1784 and, as with the G542X mutation, it also is located in exon 11. In Brazil, it presents a frequency of 1% (Raskin et al., 1993). Other, less frequent, mutations include: W1282X, N1303K, R553X, R1162X, and R334W (with their incidence varying according to population). Table 1 shows the molecular changes, and consequences of the more common mutations in the cystic fibrosis gene (Tsui, 1992).

1.3 Treatment

Approximately 50% of affected individuals are diagnosed in the age range from zero to six years but this percentage goes to 90% for those aged zero to eight years. Since reinforced nutrition is associated with a better prognosis, the screening of newborn infants is indicated. CF is one of most studied genetic diseases under the new therapy approaches, such as gene therapy which aims to restore the CFTR function. Clinical trials of gene therapy have been performed with viral vectors and cationic lipids. Despite advances in our knowledge of the disease, there is no specific treatment for CF yet. Due to its multi-systemic and chronic character, its treatment should be performed in reference centres and with a multidisciplinary team. Patients responding well to the treatment showed a median survival which has been increasing year to year, from over two years in 1950 up to between thirty and forty years today (Ribeiro et al., 2002). It is necessary to establish a strong and uninterrupted treatment program which is addressed to the prophylaxis of infections and complications. It should be started as soon as possible and it should be individualised, taking into account its severity and the organs affected. Early treatment decreases the evolution of the pulmonary lesions, improves prognosis, and increases the chances of survival.

NAME	MUTATION	CONSEQUENCE
ΔF508	Deletion of 3pb between 1652 and 1655 of the exon 10	Deletion of Phe in codon 508
G542X	G→T in nt 1756 of exon 11	Gly→ stop code in codon 542
G551D	G→A in nt 1784 in exon 11	Gly→ Asp in codon 551
W1282X	G→A in nt 3978 of exon 20	Trp→ stop code in codon 1282
3905insT	Insertion of T after the nt 3905 of exon 20	Change the reading chart.
N1303K	C→G in nt 4041 of exon 21	Asn→Lys in codon 1303
3849+10kbC → T	C→T in a Eco RI fragment at the attachment 5′ of intron 19	ABERRANTE excision
R553X	C→T in nt 1789 of exon 11	Arg→ stop code in codon 553
621+1G→T	G→T in nt 1 of attachment 5′ of intron 4	Excision mutation
1717-1G→A	G→A in nt 1 of attachment 3′ of intron 10	Excision mutation
1078delT	Deletion of T in nt 1078 of exon 7	Change reading chart
2789+5G→A	G→A in nt 5 of end 5′ of intron 14b	Excision mutation
3849+4A→G	A→G in nt 4 of end 5′ of intron 19	Excision mutation
711+1G→T	G→T in nt 1 of attachment 5′ of intron 5	Excision mutation
R1162X	C→T in nt 3616 of exon 19	Arg→ stop code in codon 1162
1898+1G→A	G→A in nt 1 of attachment 5′ of intron 5	Excision mutation
R117H	G→A in nt 482 of exon 4	Arg→His in codon 117
3659delC	Deletion of C in nt 3659 of exon 19	Change the reading chart
G85E	G→A in nt 386 of exon 3	Gly→Glu in codon 85
2184delA	Deletion of A in nt 2184 of exon 13	Change the reading chart
Δ1507	Deletion of 3pb between nt 1648 and 1653 of exon 10	Deletion of IIe at codon 506 or excision mutation
R347P	G→C in nt 1772 of exon 7	Arg→Pro in codon 347
R560T	G→C in nt 1811 of exon 11	Art→Thr in codon 560 or excision mutation
A455E	C→A in nt 1496 of exon 9	Ala→Glu in codon 455
R334W	C→T in nt 1132 of exon 7	Arg→Trp in codon 334
S549R(T→G)	T→G in nt 1779 of exon 11	Ser→Arg in codon 549
Q493X	C→T in nt 1609 of exon 10	Gln→ stop code in codon 493
S549N	G→A in nt 1778 of exon 11	Ser→Asn in codon 549

Table 1. Table obtained from Tsui (1992).

Pseudomonas aeruginosa has been found in more than 80% of teenagers with CF (Dubouix et al., 2003). Once established in the airways, the *Pseudomonas aeruginosa* infection is not eradicated by antibiotics, which only reduce the number of the colonies of bacteria. In order to treat CF, antibiotics can be administered through oral, intravenous or inhalation routes - the choice of which route should be made according to demand, prophylaxis and maintenance.

Ribeiro et al. (2002) defined the main objective of the treatment of CF, namely: the continued education of patients and their relatives concerning the disease; prophylaxis of the infections with a full vaccination program; early detection and control of pulmonary infection; respiratory physiotherapy and the improvement of bronchial blockage; the correction of pancreatic insufficiency; nutritional support with guidelines for diet and vitamin supplementation; monitoring the progress of the disease and any complications; family genetic counselling; finally, the provision of any information to patients and relatives concerning any advances in knowledge of CF.

1.4 Genetic counselling

Genetic counselling is essential in order to improve the understanding of the medical, psychological and familial implications of the disease. This process consists of the following steps: the interpretation of the familial medical history so as to assess the possibility of any occurrence or recurrence of the disease; the provision of education on heredity, genetic tests, the management of the disease, prevention, resources and research; the offer of counselling so as to properly inform the patient of the risks of having an affected child and its future life chances (Resta et al., 2006). Thus, counselling involves confirmation of the diagnosis, the estimated risk of recurrence, the provision of information about the disease, offers of support, and assistance with the acceptance of the diagnosis. It also suggests the provision of proper treatment and the offer of alternatives for prevention, such as pre-natal diagnosis and pre-implantation diagnosis. The first step for effective genetic counselling is the confirmation of the diagnosis of the affected individual (Harper, 2000). The definitive diagnosis of the disease is done with clinical features and the increased concentration of electrolytes (chloride and sodium) in sweat. The presence of the disease may be supposed from an altered neonatal screening, before the onset of symptoms. The CF hereditary pattern is autosomal recessive (i.e. in order to manifest the disease, the individual should present a mutation in two of the alleles of the CFTR). Therefore, both of the parents of the affected individual are carriers (heterozygous), and the risk of the recurrence of a CF child at birth is 25%. The individual with CF may show the same mutation in both of the alleles (homozygous for certain mutations) or else different mutations in each of the alleles (compound heterozygous). Healthy individuals carrying the mutation in only one of the alleles are called heterozygous (Saraiva-Pereira et al., 2011).

With the increase in the life expectancy of CF patients, many women carrying the disease have had pregnancies, whereas the affected men had shown infertility secondary to the obstructive azoospermia; nonetheless they may also have children because of assisted reproduction techniques. The risk of a CF individual having affected children depends upon her/his partner - if the partner is a carrier of the disease, that risk is 50%. The frequency of carriers for CF within the general population varies according to ethnic origin. In Caucasian populations, the frequency of heterozygous varies from 1/25 to 1/30 individuals (Saraiva-Pereira et al. 2011). The main difficulties for the genetic counselling of CF are those cases in which clinical confirmation is uncertain or else those cases in which is not possible to detect carriers within the family.

2. CF and infertility

2.1 Clinical features of infertility in CF

CF is a genetic disorder caused by mutations in the Cystic Fibrosis Transmembrane Regulator (CFTR) gene (Kerem et al., 1989; Riordan et al., 1989; Rommens et al., 1989). The CFTR is an anion channel regulated by cAMP-dependent phosphorylation, and it is expressed in the apical membrane of epithelial cells of a wide variety of tissues, including the reproductive tracts. The physiological role of CFTR in reproduction and its involvement in the pathogenesis of reproductive diseases remains largely unknown (Chan et al., 2009). The CF disorder is characterised by altered chloride and the bicarbonate transport of secretory epithelial cells (Chan et al., 2006; Li et al., 2010; Quinton, 1990, 1999).

Approximately 97% CF men are sterile due to the congenital bilateral absence of the vas deferens (CBAVD) and obstructive azoospermia (Wong, 1998). It has been suggested that the absence of vas deferens might be related to the requirement of the CFTR function at the embryonic stage (Li et al., 2010). It was demonstrated that the expression of the CFTR is developmentally regulated: cultured epithelial cells from the human foetal vas deferens have been shown to express the CFTR (Harris et al., 1991). Therefore, it is conceivable that fluid secretion by the Wolffian duct is required for the normal development of vas deferens. When secretion is impaired in CF individuals, normal development might be interrupted and so lead to vas agenesis (Wong, 1998).

Clinically, CF patients present a spectrum of genital phenotypes ranging from normal fertility to severely unpaired spermatogenesis and CBAVD (Xu et al., 2007). The diagnosis of CBAVD is based on the presence of azoospermia in subjects with normal or small size testes, non-palpable vas deferens, the characteristic ultrasonography view, and changes in the physical and biochemical properties of ejaculate (Jarzabek et al., 2004). Male CF patients' semen is characterised by azoospermia, low volume, low or normal viscosity, and increased turbidity. Testicular specimens show active spermatogenesis, although 50% of the spermatozoa have malformed heads. The pre-meiotic spermatogonia in CF patients appear to be morphologically normal, whereas the post-meiotic spermatogenic stages show malformation or the impairment of nuclear division (Denning et al., 1968). Testicular biopsies of post-pubertal men with CF have shown abnormal histological findings, such as pathological spermatogenesis and an increased number of dysmorphic spermatozoa (Mak et al., 2000).

The investigation of CFTR expression in male reproductive tissues showed that CFTR was present in the epididymis and vas deferens throughout post-natal life. High levels of CFTR expression were found in the head of the epididymis, but a variable expression was seen in distal epididymis. No CFTR was detected in the human testis. Accordingly, it was suggested that the anomalies in spermatozoa described in CF adult patients may result from epididymal dysfunction (Tizzano et al., 1994). Primary cultures of rat epididymal epithelial cells demonstrated the functional expression of CFTR and its involvement in the regulation of chloride secretion and fluid formation in the epididymis (Wong, 1998). Under basal conditions, the epididymis generally reabsorbs fluid to concentrate sperm. However, the observation that neurohormonal factors stimulate CFTR-mediated chloride secretion by epididymal epithelia (Wong, 1998) suggests that epididymal fluid secretion may be stimulated so as to create the optimal fluid environment for sperm maturation, storage, and even transport during ejaculation (Chan et al., 2009). Approximately 18 % of non-clinical CF men with infertility due to a reduction of sperm quality, and 15 % men with azoospermia, have at least one mutation in the CFTR. The frequency of mutations in infertile males presents a significantly higher than expected 4 % of the CF carrier frequency within the population. This increased frequency of CFTR mutations in healthy men with reduced sperm quality, and in men with azoospermia without CBAVD, suggests that the CFTR protein might be involved in the process of spermatogenesis or sperm maturation, over and above playing a critical role in the development of the epididymal glands and the vas deferens (Van der Ven et al., 1996).

In order to fertilise eggs, mammalian sperm must acquire fertilising potential in the female reproductive tract through a process known as capacitation. Sperm capacitation is a prerequisite for the acrosome reaction, which is an exocytotic event releasing hydrolytic enzymes from the acrosome so as to enable spermatozoa to penetrate the egg investments and its plasma membrane (Jarzabek et al., 2004; Xu et al., 2007). Capacitation is associated with the elevation of intracellular pH and the hyperpolarisation of the sperm plasma membrane (Meizel & Deamer, 1978; Zeng et al., 1995). These events depend on extracellular bicarbonate, which activates adenylyl cyclase pathway producing cyclic adenosine monophosphate (cAMP) and various downstream cellular events (such as protein tyrosine phosphorylation) and results in sperm capacitation (Demarco et al., 2003; Xu et al., 2007).

As has been shown, CFTR secretes bicarbonate in the uterus and sperm, and its impairment leads to reduced sperm capacitation and the fertilising capacity of sperm (Wang et al., 2003; Xu et al., 2007). The interaction of the CFTR protein with its inhibitor or antibody significantly reduces sperm capacitation and associated bicarbonate-dependent events, including increases in intracellular pH, cAMP production, and membrane hyperpolarisation. The fertilising capacity of the sperm obtained from heterozygous CFTR mutant mice is also significantly lower compared with the wild-type. These findings suggest that sperm CFTR may be involved in the transport of bicarbonate important for sperm capacitation, and that CFTR mutations causing impaired CFTR function may lead to a reduced sperm fertilising capacity and male infertility other than CBAVD (Xu et al., 2007). A recent study showed that human sperm capacitation as facilitated by progesterone and acrossome reactions induced by recombinant human zona pellucida 3 peptides (rhuZP3) were both significantly inhibited by a CFTR inhibitor. In a group of fertile men, the percentage of spermatozoa expressing CFTR was significantly higher than that of the healthy and infertile men's group. In addition, the study showed that the presence of a CFTR inhibitor markedly depresses intracellular cAMP levels, sperm hyperactivation and the sperm penetration of zona-free hamster eggs (Li et al., 2010). Moreover, when spermatozoa from CF patients with CBAVD are used for intracytoplasmic sperm injection, fertilisation rates are not reduced, suggesting a specific defect in zona pellucid penetration or membrane fusion capacity in these spermatozoa (Silber et al., 1994; Li et al., 2010). CFTR appears to have a profound role in regulating sperm function (Chan et al., 2009).

In CF female patients, the cause of reduced fertility remains obscure. CFTR is expressed throughout the female reproductive tract in the cervix, oviduct, ovary, and uterus (Chan et al., 2002; Tizzano et al., 1994). CF has been associated with menstrual irregularities, including amenorrhea, irregular cycles, anovulation, smaller uteri, and delayed puberty (Johannesson et al., 1998; Stead et al., 1987). The absence of obvious anatomical abnormalities in the female reproductive tract - except for thick and tenacious cervical mucus with altered water and electrolyte content (Kopito et al., 1973) - has led to the general belief that abnormal mucus contributes to the reduced fertility of CF women by acting as a barrier to sperm passage (Chan et al., 2009). However, repeated and unsuccessful attempts with intrauterine insemination were also reported (Epelboin et al., 2001; Rodgers et al., 2000), suggesting that further abnormalities (such as inadequate fluid control throughout the rest of the reproductive tract) could also contribute to infertility in humans (Hodges et al., 2008).

As already noted, CFTR plays a crucial role in mediating uterine bicarbonate secretion and sperm capacitation, leading to the thought that CFTR bicarbonate secretion dysfunction might induce an impaired sperm fertilising capacity and reduced fertility in CF women. In a mouse sperm-endometrial epithelial cell co-culture system, it was demonstrated that endometrial epithelial cells possess a CFTR-mediated bicarbonate transport mechanism. A substantial decrease in apical fluid bicarbonate contents was observed after treatment with both blockers of CFTR and antisense oligonucleotides against CFTR when compared with the control. These results are consistent with the CFTR's mediating uterine bicarbonate secretion, and they indicate that defective CFTR might lead to impaired bicarbonate secretion in the uterus. *In vitro* fertilisation assays on zona-intact mouse eggs further demonstrated that the number of two-cell embryos obtained with sperm capacitated in a conditioned medium from CFTR antisense-treated endometrial cells was significantly reduced as compared with that obtained from sense-treated controls. Sperm capacitation and egg-fertilising ability depend - critically - on CFTR and bicarbonate content and defective CFTR-mediated bicarbonate secretion, and the lower fertilising capacity of sperm might also account for lower CF female fertility (Chan et al., 2009; Wang et al., 2003).

CFTR expression in the uterus is regulated by ovarian hormones with increasing expression in response to estrogen and decreasing expression in response to progesterone; this is a pattern that correlates with cyclic changes in uterine fluid (Zheng et al., 2004). Hormone changes have been observed in CF female adolescents, who displayed reduced estradiol and FSH levels (Reiter et al., 1981), and CF female adults, who displayed increased testosterone and reduced estradiol and progesterone levels, compared with age-matched controls (Johannesson et al., 1998). Interestingly, through observations in rodent uterus, CFTR was found to be co-expressed with the epithelial sodium channel (ENaC) in an out-of-phase fashion. With the maturation of ovarian follicles and the estrogen secretion phase, CFTR is highly expressed and ENaC is poorly expressed. Inversely, with corpus luteum activity and progesterone secretion, low CFTR expression and high ENaC expression are observed (Chan et al., 2002). This may explain maximal fluid secretion during the early phase of the oestrous cycle, when the level of oestrogen is at its highest. Similarly, at dioestrus, the attenuated fluid production with down-regulation of CFTR and increased reabsorption by up-regulation of ENaC may account for the disappearance of uterine fluid. These cyclic changes in CFTR and ENaC expression which result in uterine fluid volume variation have physiological significance. Maximal CFTR expression and - therefore - high uterine fluid production may lubricate the cervical and vaginal lumen for sperm movement towards the oviduct as well as sperm capacitation. Equally, low CFTR expression and - consequently - reduced fluid volume may enhance close contact on the endometrial surface, facilitating embryo implantation. Dynamic changes in the fluid microenvironment, particularly the fluid volume, in the female reproductive tract are dictated by CFTR expression, which is normally regulated by ovarian hormones throughout the cycle and accommodating various reproductive events. The impairment of CFTR expression may lead to the disturbance of the fluid environment, resulting in various pathological conditions and infertility (Chan et al., 2007; Chan et al., 2009).

Interestingly, abnormalities in the reproductive endocrine axis have been viewed as an indirect consequence of CF, though they have been largely ignored as possible contributors to observed female infertility (Stead et al., 1987). CFTR expression was found in the areas of the rat hypothalamus (thalamus and amygdale) which are involved in the regulation of sexual maturation and reproduction. CFTR might increase the acidification of synaptic vesicles, and thus play an important role in the central regulation of sexual maturation and fertility (Johannesson et al., 1997b). Delayed pubertal increments of serum gonadotropin and sex hormone levels in CF patients suggest a late maturation of the reproductive system (Reiter et al., 1981). Anovulatory women showed significantly lower luteal oestradiol and progesterone, but higher total testosterone concentrations when compared to healthy controls and the ovulatory CF women (Johannesson et al., 1998). In a mouse model, increased FSH levels were found in CFTR mutant females as a result of a decreased number of ovulatory follicles, leading to less estradiol production and a lack of feedback inhibition of FSH secretion. CF female mice exposed to exogenous hormones showed a correction of organ size and ovulation. These findings suggests that the CF reproductive organs can respond to gonadotropins, but that an impaired hypothalamic-pituitary-gonadal (HPG) axis may be a direct cause of reduced fertility in women with CF (Hodges et al., 2008; Johannesson et al., 1997b).

In CF women, late puberty and amenorrhea are common clinical findings due to the deficit in their nutritional status. It has also been suggested that the lack of ovulation is a consequence of malnutrition and catabolism. Clinically, the anovulatory women presented more profound essential fatty acid deficiency (EFAD) and hypersecretion of insulin during an oral glucose tolerance test compared to the ovulatory women (Johannesson et al., 1998). However, it was shown that menarcheal age was also delayed in CF females in good clinical and nutritional condition. Homozygous patients for the most common mutation - F508del - and those with a pathological glucose tolerance test (OGTT) showed the most delay in menarcheal age (Johannesson et al., 1997a). This may be explained by the fact that ovarian cells express insulin receptors that mediate gonadal steroid production. Experimental data has shown that insulin has a gonadotropic effect through different mechanisms, such as a direct effect on steroidogenic enzymes, the modulation of FSH or LH receptor number, synergism with FSH and LH, and nonspecific enhancement of cell viability (Porestky & Kalin, 1987). Insulin appears to be necessary for the ovary to reach its full steroidogenic potential. The difference observed in the insulin pattern in the pathological OGTT group might alter ovarian function and thereby cause further delay in sexual maturation (Johannesson et al., 1998). Polycystic ovaries were also described in CF women (Stead et al., 1987).

CFTR mutations were previously associated with Congenital Absence of Uterus and Vagina (CAUV). CF mutations might affect the normal embryological development of the Müllerian ducts. During the seventh week of gestation, the cranial end of the Müllerian duct is immediately adjacent to the Wolffian duct, and both ducts share a common basement membrane. The Wolffian duct then guides the caudal growth of the Müllerian ducts. By the ninth week of gestation, the Müllerian duct reaches the caudal end of the adjacent Wolffian duct. At this time, these ductal systems separate from each other, form separate basement membranes, and continue to develop independently (Ludwig, 1998). The interdependency of these two systems suggests that the same genetic factors may control the early development of both systems. Failure of the development of the Müllerian duct causes CAUV in females. The incidence of most common CFTR mutations found in patients with CAUV (8%) is twice that which is found in the general population (4%), but much less than the incidence of CFTR mutations in men with CBAVD (80%). This suggests that it is unlikely for CFTR mutations to cause CAUV in females as they cause CBAVD in some males. As such, the effect of the abnormal CFTR protein product on the Wolffian duct must occur at a time when the development of the Müllerian duct is no longer dependent on the Wolffian duct (Timmreck et al., 2003).

CF female patients have such pregnancy complications as premature labour and delivery and increased maternal and prenatal mortality due to severe maternal pulmonary infection and maternal weight loss (Cohen et al., 1980; Kent & Farquharson, 1993). However, the risk of the deterioration of health during pregnancy for females with CF is considered to be small, if good medical care is provided and if women are in a stable and good clinical condition (FitzSimmons et al., 1996).

There remain many unanswered questions as to the cause of infertility in CF, and the exact role of CFTR in reproductive physiology and the contribution of CFTR dysfunction to infertility in both sexes is far from understood (Chan et al., 2009).

2.2 CFTR mutations closely related to CF infertility

Infertility, or at least subfertility, in males with CF was first suspected in the 1960s (Denning et al., 1968; Radpour et al., 2008). Depending upon their molecular consequences, CFTR mutations may result in either a typical CF or else an atypical (often monosymptomatic) CF, such as congenital absence of the vas deferens (bi- or unilateral), bilateral ejaculatory duct obstruction, or bilateral obstructions within the epididymis (Jarzabek et al., 2004). Approximately 80% of CF male patients present CBAVD, a Wolffian duct anomaly (Radpour et al., 2008). Male infertility due to CBAVD has been shown to be commonly linked to CFTR mutations, and it is considered to be a genital form of CF or a CFTR-associated disease with incomplete CF expression (Dequeker et al., 2009; Kanavakis et al., 1998; Rave-Harel et al., 1997). Men with CBAVD are apparently healthy, with relatively normal lung and pancreatic functions. CBAVD appears to be a heterogeneous genetic condition, with many cases being mild forms of CF (DeBraekeleer and Férec, 1996).

Extensive studies have shown that patients with isolated CBAVD carry two CFTR mutations, usually in compound heterozygosity (Chillón et al., 1995; Claustres et al., 2000). Of isolated CBAVD patients, where the mutation is found on both CFTR, about 88% carry one severe mutation and one mild mutation, whilst the remaining 12% carry mild mutations on both CFTR (Claustres et al., 2000). This is in contrast to classical clinically CF patients, where about 88% of the CF patients carry severe mutations on both CFTR, whilst about 11% carry a severe mutation on one CFTR and a mild mutation on their second one (Claustres et al., 2000; Radpour et al., 2008). The most frequent CFTR mutation conferring a mild phenotype found in CBAVD patients is the 5T polymorphism (Chillón et al., 1995), which is an allele found at the polymorphic Tn locus in intron 8 of the CFTR, and which can be found as a stretch of 5, 7, or 9 thymidine residues at this locus. Less efficient splicing will occur when a lower number of thymidines are found, resulting in CFTR transcripts that lack exon 9 sequences (Chu et al., 1993; Radpour et al., 2008). Men with the 5T variant in the non-coding region of the gene will produce an abnormally low level of CFTR protein in the epididymis. However, there may be sufficient proteins for the prevention of disease in other organs (such as the lung and the gastrointestinal glands) normally affected by CF, which might explain why the lung and pancreas are normal in CBAVD, but the epididymis is not (DeBraekeleer and Férec, 1996; Jarzabek et al., 2004; Wong, 1998). The analysis of the level of correctly spliced RNA transcribed from the 5T allele in different tissues (nasal and epididymal epithelium) and its correlation with CF disease expression, has shown that in infertile males with normal lung function the level of correctly spliced transcripts found in the nasal epithelium was higher than the level found in the epididymal epithelium. It indicates that there is variability in the efficiency of the splicing mechanism both between different individuals and between different organs of the same individual. In many human monogenic diseases, high variability in disease expression is found among patients carrying the same genetic defect (Levy et al., 2010; Rave-Harel et al., 1997). The molecular basis for this variability has been suggested to be allelic heterogeneity, additional genetic loci, and/or environmental factors. Accordingly, allelic variants of genes involved in the splicing regulation might contribute to the different efficiencies of alternative splicing found amongst different individuals (Rave-Harel et al., 1997).

CFTR mutations may represent one of the most common abnormalities associated with male infertility, especially with CBAVD but also with obstructive azoospermia (Kanavakis et al., 1998). A screening of the entirety of the *CFTR* in males with CUAVD (congenital unilateral absence of vas deferens), CBAVD and obstructive azoospermia of the vas deferens, has shown that almost 64% of patients carry two *CFTR* mutations. The most frequent mutations observed amongst those patients were F508del (44.7%), T5 allele (36.2%), and R117H (19.1%) (Jézéquel et al., 2000). In a large French cohort study, the most frequent allele mutations identified in CBAVD male patients were F508del (21.7%), the 5T allele (16.3%) and R117H (4.4%), followed by D1152H (1.19%) and D443Y (0.93%). Two CFTR mutations (including the 5T allele) were present in 47.7% and one mutation in 24.6% of CBAVD patients, while no mutation was reported in the remaining 27.7%. Approximately 43.5% of patients with CBAVD carried one F508del allele, and 31.7% had at least one 5T allele. Altogether, at least one CFTR mutation was identified in 72.25% individuals with CBAVD (Claustres et al., 2000). In an Italian multicentric study, a molecular screening of the most common CFTR mutations in infertile couples was performed. CFTR mutations were detected in 4.6% of subjects, a percentage that overlaps with the general population carrier frequency. However, it was found a mutation-frequency of over 37% amongst CBAVD individuals and of 6% in males with non-obstructive azoospermia (Stuppia et al., 2005). In another study, the carrier status of CBAVD patients for the F508del mutation was screened and 57% were found to be carriers. Amongst these patients, 25% were later found to have compound heterozygotes for the F508del and R117H mutations (Williams et al., 1993). A study of the entire coding region of the CFTR of CBAVD patients found that 28.6% have mutations in both copies of the CFTR, 42.8% had one CFTR mutation, whilst in the remaining 28.6% no CFTR mutations were found (Kanavakis et al., 1998). These figures give an average of an eleven-fold increase of the carrier frequency compared to the population data on CFTR mutations in CBAVD patients. (Uzun et al., 2005). Amongst cases of obstructive azoospermia, 30% had one CFTR mutation whilst in the remaining 70% no mutations were found - this indicates an association between cases of obstructive azoospermia without CBAVD with CFTR mutations. The frequency of the IVS8(5T) allele was 14.3% for the CBAVD cases, which was three-fold higher than for normal chromosomes (Kanavakis et al., 1998). Similarly, another extensive analysis of the CFTR in CBAVD patients revealed that 42% of subjects were carriers of one CFTR allele and that 24% were compound heterozygous for CFTR alleles. The presence of only one CF allele in approximately 42% of CBAVD patients implies some role on the part of CF in CBAVD, although additional factors or genes are necessary for the development of CBAVD in those patients (Mercier et al., 1995; Van der Ven et al., 1996; Williams et al., 1993). The CFTR mutations commonly associated with male infertility are F508del, R117H, and the IVS8 (5T) polymorphism, each of which exhibit diverse frequencies among different cohorts (Van der Ven et al., 1996). Since the spectrum of CFTR mutations is markedly different amongst populations, the ethnic background of the patients should be taken into account so as to ensure that the most prevalent mutations appropriate to that particular population are included in the screening panel (DeBraekeleer & Férec, 1996). Altogether, the mutation-frequencies in infertile male patients are significantly higher than the expected carrier-frequencies in the general population (Van der Ven et al., 1996).

There are only a few studies on female CFTR mutation-frequency in the literature. It is generally assumed that fertility is reduced in CF women, although not as dramatically as in men. It was already proposed that CFTR mutations do not appear to be involved in female infertility (Morea et al., 2005) and CAUV condition (Radpour et al., 2008). The most common CFTR mutations - including the 5T allele - were tested in isolated CAUV female patients. These mutations were only found in 8% of the subjects, suggesting that it is unlikely that CFTR mutations cause CAUV in females (Timmreck et al., 2003). In a recent study, 24 women with altered fertility were screened for the F508del mutation. Amongst them, 37.5% showed reduced fertility without a known cause, 20.8% presented reduced fertility due to polycystic ovarian syndrome (although two of them demonstrated malformations of the reproductive tract), 37.5% had been pregnant previously although most of them had spontaneous abortions, and 8.3% presented early menopause. It was found that one patient who was a F508del mutation carrier and who had had an early menopause had also had a previous abortion. Unexpectedly - considering that Brazilian population is greatly mixed - the carrier frequency for the most common mutation in CF amongst infertile Brazilian women was similar to that of Caucasian populations. It was proposed that there are common clinical features between women with altered fertility and with CF women, and that CF mutations may be more frequent than expected amongst patients with fertility issues (Brunoro et al., 2010). Large cohort studies on CFTR mutation-frequency among infertile women are needed.

2.3 Considerations for CF mutation screening tests

According to the CF Mutation Database, around 20 mutations have individual worldwide frequencies greater than 0.1%, and can thus be considered to be common mutations (Lay-son et al., 2011). These common mutations vary by geographic and/or ethnic origin. Latin American countries have a high ethnic admixture and they show a wide distribution of 89 different mutations. Most of these mutations are frequent in Spain, Italy, and Portugal, and so is consistent with the origin of the European settlers. A few mutations found among Africans are also present in those countries which were part of the slave trade. This may be the result of the miscegenation of these populations. New mutations were also found which possibly originated in America (Pérez et al., 2007). As in most countries, F508del was the most common mutation detected, but in a lower proportion than the average frequency of 45-46% published for Latin-American countries (Keyeux et al., 2003; Pérez et al., 2007; Zielenski & Tsui, 1995), and the reported worldwide frequency of 66% (Lay-son et al., 2010; Zielenski & Tsui, 1995). The G542X mutation is the second most frequent mutation in Latin America, with a total frequency of 5.07%. N1303K, W1282X and R1162X are the next most frequent mutations, with variations from 0.59% to 3.95%. The frequency of the rest of the mutations varies from one country to another, but their overall frequencies are less than 1%, and could be considered to be rare in Latin America (Pérez et al., 2007). The carrier-rate and mutation-frequencies vary widely in different populations, and so screening tests with high detection-rates for CFTR mutations have to consider the population's ethnicity (Pieri et al., 2007).

There is increasing evidence that CFTR mutations may contribute etiologically to certain monosymptomatic disorders. Infertile men with isolate obstructive azoospermia may have mutations in the CFTR, many of which are rare in classical CF and not evaluated in most routine mutation screening. It was demonstrated that the routine mutation panel has failed to identify CFTR mutations and the IVS8-5T allele in 46% of CBAVD groups, 50% of CUAVD groups, and 79% of idiopathic epididymal obstruction groups. These results demonstrate that routine testing for CFTR mutations for infertile men may miss mild or rare gene alterations. The DNA sequence method detects more CFTR mutations than common mutation panels. This represents a significant problem because advances in assisted reproduction have allowed infertile male patients to conceive, raising the concern of transmitting - when present - pathogenic CFTR mutations onto progeny. The importance of accurate CFTR mutation detection in men with obstructive azoospermia and their partners has already been highlighted (Danzinger et al., 2004; Mak et al., 1999). Today, screening for a panel of CFTR mutations is offered to infertile men prior to in vitro fertilisation (IVF) or *intra cytoplasmic sperm injection* (ICSI), and includes only the most common mutations found amongst the CF patients of European and North American origin. The atypical CBAVD phenotype, however, is caused by milder mutations, most of them very rare or even not yet described, and thus not included in the panel of CF mutations usually screened. It was proposed that only an extensive CFTR screening can detect rare mutations that are not found by conventional screenings and commercial tests, and can thus improve the diagnosis and care of CF and CAVD as well as the prevention of new cases through the use of reproductive technologies (Pieri et al., 2007).

However, genetic testing should only be performed in the context of appropriate genetic counselling and laboratories should work in close association with clinical geneticists and reference laboratories so as to ensure that pertinent tests are performed and that proper information is provided to patients. There is no standard or preferred method, but laboratories should be aware of the limitations of their chosen method and they should know which mutations are not identified, whether the techniques are commercially available or else being developed within the laboratory. This means that individual laboratories should choose a method which is suited to their experience, workload, and scope of testing. In addition to the screen for frequent mutations, a complementary panel may be required to test population-specific mutations with a frequency above 1%. The knowledge of the ethnic or geographic origins of patients and their parents and grandparents is therefore important in order to determine the analysis to be performed (Dequeker et al., 2009). The knowledge of geographic or ethnic variations in the local population mutation-frequency is crucial so as to properly achieve effective genetic counselling and improve the cost-effectiveness of screening and diagnostic tests (Lay-son et al., 2011).

2.4 Ethical implications of genetic testing

According to the Patient Registry 2009 of the CF Foundation, USA there are growing numbers of CF adults 18 years of age and over. The percentage of CF patients aged 18 years or older has risen from 30% in 1990 to over 47% in 2009. It also have indicated that the median age of survival of patients with CF has risen from 27 years in 1985 to almost 36 years in 2009, leading to greater concern for the disease management of CF adults (Cystic Fibrosis Foundation Patient registry 2009: Annual data report, 2011). Coupled with an improved life expectancy, adult CF patients are more likely to seek independence from their families and pursue typical adult activities, such as attending college, entering serious relationships and pursuing careers (Modi et al., 2010). Issues related to sexual maturation, fertility, pregnancy and contraception have thus become important in the comprehensive care of CF patients (Tizzano et al., 1994). Fertility bears centrally to reproductive decision-making, determining whether natural conception is even an option or whether adoption or assisted reproductive technology must be considered (Hull & Kass, 2000). Along with the wish to conceive, CF parents and physicians confront major ethical issues regarding abortions, the premature termination of pregnancies, and possible arrangements in the event of morbidity or maternal mortality which should all be discussed prior to pregnancy (Barak et al., 2005).

There are still many paediatric CF clinics that continue to care for patients up to 18 years of age. Several studies have suggested that teenage patients and their parents have unmet information needs regarding the patient's sexual health. Usually, unplanned sex tends to be done without protection. An important priority for the CF team is to try to ensure that women with CF are aware of the risks of unplanned pregnancy. Collaboration between the family planning clinician and the teenager's CF physician is recommended (Roberts & Green, 2005). As such, reproductive counselling and reproductive health issues must be carefully addressed to CF adult patients (Hull & Kass, 2000; Sawyer, 1996). CF healthcare providers are an important source of information, and early discussion of sexual and reproductive health is indicated in paediatric settings for the adolescent patients, since a very high interest in future parenting is expressed by CF men. It has been suggested that there should be greater emphasis on infertility, semen analysis, and the prevention of sexually transmitted infections, backed with a greater focus on reproductive options within adult healthcare services (Sawyer et al., 2005).

In the 1980s, it was thought to be too risky for a woman with CF to get pregnant and that it was impossible for a man with CF to father a child. Nowadays, improvements in the nutrition and lung function of these patients make it possible for CF women to have a healthy pregnancy and baby. In 2009, the Patient Registry reported that 226 women with CF were pregnant. Successful outcomes can be achieved for both the CF mother and the child with careful patient assessment, combined with the integration of a multidisciplinary team, composed of the CF physician, the fertility specialist and the obstetrician (CF Foundation Patient registry 2009: Annual data report, 2011). Close follow-up of the maternal and foetal condition, along with careful monitoring of ventilation, immunology, diabetes, glucose tolerance and nutrition is important since all these parameters may be adversely affected in a CF pregnancy (Barak et al., 2005; Rodgers et al., 2000).

For CF men, advances in fertility medicine have given them the option to father children (CF Foundation Patient registry 2009: Annual data report, 2011). The use of assisted reproductive techniques (such as testicular micro-aspiration and intracytoplasmic sperm injection (ICSI)) has enabled testicular spermatozoa to fertilise ova without the need to be capacitated, or to undergo acrosome reaction or else penetrate and fuse it with the egg (Wong, 1998). A report on CF men that have undergone ICSI coupled with IVF showed that 62% of the couples successfully achieved pregnancy (McCallum et al., 2000). A group of CF azoospermia males were submitted to ICSI and 63% of the couples had clinical pregnancy (Hubert et al., 2006). However, before such measures are taken, genetic screening and counselling for the men and their partners should be mandatory in safeguarding their offspring from the risk of clinical CF (DeBraekeleer and Férec, 1996). Moreover, CF men should be informed about their own health and any long-term issues (such as the likelihood of premature death) and this information should be clearly shared with their partner (Hubert et al., 2006). In the case of CBAVD patients - a genital form of CF - most carry a severe CF-causing CFTR mutation and, therefore, have a 0.5% chance of transmitting the CFTR mutation to the child. Assuming a risk of 1/25 of the partner being a CF carrier, and that a carrier has a chance of 0.5% of transmitting the mutant CFTR to the child, the combined risk of CBAVD couples of having a CF child is 1/100 when compared with a risk of 1/2500 amongst general population (Radpour et al., 2008). The detection of a CFTR mutation in CF male patients and their spouses is crucial, since the presence of a CFTR mutation would present a high-risk situation whereas its absence would present a low-risk situation (DeBraekeleer and Férec, 1996). In cases of oligozoospermia, it is also ideal to screen both partners. It was also recommended that - if resources are stretched - amongst couples with a CBAVD male only the female needs to be routinely CF screened because, if she is negative, then the couple's residual risk of having a CF or CBAVD child will be reduced to 1:960 (Lewis-Jones et al., 2000). The reproductive options for the majority of CF men who are infertile include not having children, adoption, in vitro fertilisation with donor sperm, and microscopic epididymal sperm aspiration (MESA) coupled with in vitro fertilisation. There is also a complementary option, namely pre-implantation genetic diagnosis (PGD). PGD refers to the genetic testing of embryos created through IVF for the purpose of selecting embryos that would lead to the birth of a child unaffected by a detectable genetic defect. The notion of preventing a disease by preventing the birth of an individual with that disease is controversial. The CFF has no official position on this practice, and this type of decision is a personal choice to be made by the individual together with his/her physician (Davis et al., 2010).

3. Conclusion

The National Institutes of Health, USA recommends genetic counselling for any couple attempting assisted reproductive techniques where the man has CF or obstructive azoospermia and is positive for a CFTR mutation. It is important to analyse the clinical genetic conditions of the families by evaluating the full family history, by documenting the pregnancy and foetal, neonatal, and paediatric loss of life, as well as by cytogenetic studies of the couple and analysis for CFTR mutations. At this time, it is debatable whether it is better to perform the screening for mutations in the full gene or whether it is better to screening for typical local mutations of a population. It is also subject of debate if it is better to perform the screening for mutations in CF affected individuals only or also in their partner. All these choices have ethical and social implications and there may be better resolution with new population studies focused on the frequency of mutations in CF individuals with infertility. CF is now a disease of the adult population with many adult-specific issues. As such, adult CF patients must be treated by a well-trained interdisciplinary team of adult-care providers within the environment of the CF care network.

4. References

Barak, A., Dulitzki, M., Efrati, O., Augarten, A., Szeinberg, A., Reichert, N., Modan, D., Weiss, B., Miller, M., Katzanelson, D. & Yahav, Y. Pregnancies and outcome in women with cystic fibrosis. Isr Med Assoc J, Vol. 7, No. 2 (February 2005), pp. 95-98.

Bargon, J., Stein, J., Dietrich, C.F., Muller, U., Caspary,W.F., & Wagner, T.O. (1999). Gastrointestinal complications of adult patients with cystic fibrosis. *J Gastroenterol*, Vol. 37, No. 8, PP.739-749.

Brunoro, G.V., Wolfgramm, E.V., Louro, I.D., Degasperi, I.I., Busatto, V.C., Perrone, A.M., Batitucci, M.C. (2010). Cystic fibrosis Δf508 mutation screening in Brazilian women with altered fertility. Mol Biol Rep, November 2010, pp.1-4.

Brunecki, Z. The incidence and genetics of cystic fibrosis. (1972) *J. Med. Genet.*, Vol. 9, pp. 33-37, 1972.

Chan, L. N., Tsang, L.L., Rowlands, D.K., Rochelle, L.G., Boucher, R.C., Liu, C.Q. & Chan, H.C. (2002). Distribution and regulation of ENaC subunit and CFTR mRNA expression in murine female reproductive tract. *J. Membr Biol*, Vol. 185, No. 2, pp. 165–176.

Chan, H.C., Shi, Q.X., Zhou, C.X., Wang, X.F., Xu, W.M., Chen, W.Y., Chen, A.J., Ni, Y. & Yuan, Y.Y. (2006). Critical role of CFTR in uterine bicarbonate secretion and the fertilizing capacity of sperm. *Mol Cell Endocrinol*, Vol. 250, pp.106–113.

Chan, H.C., He, Q., Ajonuma, L.C. & Wang, X.F. (2007). Epithelial ion channels in the regulation of female reproductive tract fluid microenvironment: implications in fertility and infertility. Sheng Li Xue Bao, Vol. 59, No. 4 (August 2007), pp. 495-504.

Chan, H.C., Ruan, Y.C., He, Q., Chen, M.H., Chen, H., Xu, W.M., Chen, W.Y., Xie, C., Zhang, X.H. & Zhou, Z. (2009). The cystic fibrosis transmembrane conductance regulator in reproductive health and disease. J Physiol, Vol. 587, No. 10 (May 2009), pp. 2187-95.

Chillón, M., Casals, T., Mercier, B., Bassas, L., Lissens, W., Silber, S., Rommey, M.-C., Ruiz-Romero, J., Verlingue, C., Claustres, M., Nunes, V., Férec, C., & Estivill, X. (1995). Mutations in the cystic fibrosis gene in patients with congenital absence of the vas deferens. *N. Engl. J. Med*, Vol. 332, No. 22 (June 1995), pp. 1475–1480.

Chu, C.S., Trapnell, B.C., Curristin, S., Cutting, G.R. & Crystal, R.G. (1993). Genetic basis of variable exon 9 skipping in cystic fibrosis transmembrane conductance regulator mRNA. Nat Genet, Vol. 3, No. 2 (February 1993), pp. 151-156.

Claustres, M., Guittard, C., Bozon, D., Chevalier, F., Verlingue, C., Ferec, C., Girodon, E., Cazeneuve, C., Bienvenu, T., Lalau, G., Dumur, V., Feldmann, D., Bieth, E., Blayau, M., Clavel, C., Creveaux, I., Malinge, M.C., Monnier, N., Malzac, P., Mittre, H., Chomel, J.C., Bonnefont, J.P., Iron, A., Chery, M. & Georges, M.D. (2000). Spectrum of CFTR mutations in cystic fibrosis and in congenital absence of the vas deferens in France. Hum Mutat, Vol. 16, No. 2, pp. 143-56.

Cohen, L.F., Di Sant'Agnese, P.A. & Friedlander, J. (1980). Cystic fibrosis and pregnancy. A national survey. *Lancet*, Vol. 2, No. 8199 (October 1980), pp. 842–844.

Collins. F.S. (1992) Cystic Fibrosis. Molecular biology and therapeutic implications . *Science*, Vol. 256, pp. 774-779.

Cystic Fibrosis Foundation. (2011). Cystic Fibrosis Foundation Patient Registry 2009: Annual data report. 24.07.2011, Available from http://www.cff.org/LivingWithCF/QualityImprovement/PatientRegistry Report.

Danziger, K.L., Black, L.D., Keiles, S.B., Kammesheidt, A. & Turek, P.J. (2004). Improved detection of cystic fibrosis mutations in infertility patients with DNA sequence analysis. Hum Reprod, Vol. 19, No. 3 (March 2004), pp. 540-546.

Davis, L.B., Champion, S.J., Fair, S.O., Baker, V.L., Garber, A.M. (2010). A cost-benefit analysis of preimplantationpre-implantation genetic diagnosis for carrier couples of cystic fibrosis. *Fertil Steril*, Vol. 93, No. 6, pp. 1793-1804.

DeBraekeleer, M. & Férec, C. (1996). Mutations in the cystic fibrosis gene in men with congenital bilateral absence of the vas deferens. *Mol. Hum. Reprod*, Vol. 2, No. 9 (September 1996), pp. 669–677.

Demarco, I.A., Espinosa, F., Edwards, J., Sosnik, J., Vega-Beltra´ n, J.L., Hockensmith, J.W., Kopf, G.S., Darszon, A. & Visconti, P.E. (2003). Involvement of a Na^+/HCO_3^- Cotransporter in Mouse Sperm Capacitation. *J Biol Chem*, Vol. 278, No. 9 (February 2003), pp. 7001-7009.

Denning, C.R., Sommers, S.C., & Quigley, H.J. (1968). Infertility in male patients with cystic fibrosis. *Pediatrics*, Vol. 41, No. 1 (January 1968), pp. 7-17.

Dequeker, E., Stuhrmann, M., Morris, M.A., Casals, T., Castellani, C., Claustres, M., Cuppens, H., Des Georges, M., Ferec, C., Macek, M., Pignatti, P.F., Scheffer, H., Schwartz, M., Witt, M., Schwarz, M. & Girodon, E. (2009). Best practice guidelines for molecular genetic diagnosis of cystic fibrosis and CFTR-related disorders--updated European recommendations. Eur J Hum Genet, Vol. 17, No. 1 (January 2009), pp. 51-65.

DI Sant'Agnese, P.A.,Darling, R.C., Perera, G.A. & Schea, E. (1953). Abnormal electrolyte composition of sweat in fibrosis of the pancreas. *Pediatrics*, pp. 12:549.

Dubouix ,A., Campanac, C., Fauvel, J., Simon, M.F., Salles, J.P., Roques, C., Chap, H., Marty, N. (2003). Bactericidal properties of group IIa secreted phospholipase A(2) against *Pseudomonas aeruginosa* clinical isolates. *J Med Microbiol*, Vol. 52, No. 12 (December 2003), pp. 1039-1045.

Epelboin, S., Hubert, D., Patrat, C., Abirached, F., Bienvenu, T. & Lepercq, J. (2001). Management of assisted reproductive technologies in women with cystic fibrosis. *Fertil Steril*, Vol. 76, No. 6 (December 2001), pp. 1280–1281.

Fanconi, G., Uehlinger, E. & Knauer, C. (1936). Das Coeliakie-Syndrom bei angeborenem zystichem pâncreas fibromatose and bronkiektasen. *Wien Med Wochenschr*, Vol. 86, pp 753-756.

Farber, S. (1944). Pancreatic function and disease and early life. *Arch Pathol*, pp 37:238.

Feingoud, J. & Guilloud,-Bataille, M. (1999). Genetic comparisonsof patients with fibrosis cystic with or without meconium ileus. *Ann Genet*, Vol. 42, No. 3, pp. 147-150.

FitzSimmons, S.C., Fitzpatrick, S., Thompson, B., *Aitkin, M., Fiel, S., Winnie, G. & Hilman, B.* (1996). A longitudinal study of the effects of pregnancy on 325 women with cystic fibrosis. *Pediatr. Pulm.*, Vol. 13, pp. 99–101.

Gibson, L.E. & Cooke, R.E. (1959). A test for concentration of electrolytes in sweat in cystic fibrosis of the pancreas utilizing pilocarpine by iontophoresis. *Pediatrics,* Vol. 23, pp. 545-549.

Harper, P. (2000). *Practical Genetic Counselling*. 5th edition. Ed. Butterworth-Henemann. Cambridge.

Harris, A., Chalkley, G.C., Lankester, S.A. & Coleman, L.S. (1991). Expression of the Cystic Fibrosis gene in human development. *Development*, Vol. 113, No. 1 (September 1991), pp. 305-310.

Harris, A.(1992). Cystic fibrosis gene. *Brit. Med. Bull.* Vol. 48, pp. 736-753.

Heng, H.H.Q., Shi, X.M., Tsui, L.C. (1993). Fluorescence in situ hybridization mapping of the cystic fibrosis transmembrane conductance regulator (CFTR) gene to 7q31.3. *Cytogenet Cell Genet*, Vol. 62, pp. 108-109.

Hodges, C.A., Palmert, M.R. & Drumm, M.L. (2008) Infertility in females with cystic fibrosis is multifactorial: evidence from mouse models. *Endocrinology*, Vol. 14, No. 6 (June 2008), pp. 2790-2797.

Hubert, D., Patrat, C., Guibert, J., Thiounn, N., Bienvenu, T., Viot, G., Jouannet, P. & Epelboin, S. (2006). Results of assisted reproductive technique in men with cystic fibrosis. Hum Reprod, Vol. 21, No. 5 (May 2006), pp. 1232-1236.

Hull, S.C. & Kass, N.E. (2000). Adults with cystic fibrosis and (in)fertility: how has the health care system responded? J Androl, Vol. 21, No. 6 (November 2000), pp. 809-813.

Jarzabek, K., Zbucka, M., Pepiński, W., Szamatowicz, J., Domitrz, J., Janica, J., Wołczyński, S. & Szamatowicz, M. (2004). Cystic fibrosis as a cause of infertility. *Reprod Biol*, Vol. 4, No. 2 (July 2004), pp. 119-29.

Jézéquel, P., Dubourg, C., Le Lannou, D., Odent, S., Le Gall, J.Y., Blayau, M., Le Treut, A. & David, V. (2000). Molecular screening of the CFTR gene in men with anomalies of the vas deferens: identification of three novel mutations. Mol Hum Reprod, Vol. 6, No. 12 (December 2000), pp. 1063-1067.

Johannesson, M., Gottlieb, C. & Hjelte, L. (1997a). Delayed puberty in girls with cystic fibrosis despite good clinical status. *Pediatrics*, Vol. 99, No. 1 (January 1997), pp. 29–34.

Johannesson, M., Bogdanovic, N., Nordqvist, A.C., Hjelte, L. & Schalling, M. (1997b). Cystic fibrosis mRNA expression in rat brain: cerebral cortex and medial preoptic area. *Neuroreport*, Vol. 8, No. 2 (January 1997), pp. 535–539.

Johannesson, M., Landgren, B.M., Csemiczky, G., Hjelte, L. & Gottlieb, C. (1998). Female patients with cystic fibrosis suffer from reproductive endocrinological disorders despite good clinical status. *Human Reproduction*, Vol.13, No.8, pp.2092–2097.

Kanavakis, E., Tzetis, M., Antoniadi, T., Pistofidis, G., Milligos, S. & Kattamis, C. (1998). Cystic fibrosis mutation screening in CBAVD patients and men with obstructive azoospermia or severe oligozoospermia. Mol Hum Reprod, Vol. 4, No. 4 (April 1998), pp. 333-337.

Kent, N.E. & Farquharson, D.F. (1993). Cystic fibrosis in pregnancy. *Can Med Assoc J*, Vol. 149, No. 6 (September 1993), pp. 809–813.

Kerem, B.-S., Rommens, J.M., Buchanan, J.A., Markiewicz, D., Cox, T.K., Chakravarti, A., Buchwald, M. & Tsui, L.-C. (1989). Identification of the cystic fibrosis gene: genetic analysis. *Science*, Vol. 245, pp. 1073–1080.

Keyeux, G., Rodas, C., Bienvenu, T., Garavito, P., Vidaud, D., Sanchez, D., Kaplan, J.C. & Aristizábal, G. (2003). CFTR mutations in patients from Colombia: implications for local and regional molecular diagnosis programs. *Hum Mutat*, Vol. 22, No. 3 (September 2003), pp. 259.

Knowton, R.G., Cohen-Haguenauer, O. ,Van Cong, N. (1985). A polymorphic DNA marker linked to Cystic Fibrosis is located on chromosome 7. *Nature*, pp. 318: 380-382.

Kopito, L.E., Kosasky, H.J. & Shwachman, H. (1973). Water and electrolytes in cervical mucus from patients with cystic fibrosis. *Fertil Steril*, Vol. 24, No. 7 (July 1973), pp. 512–516.

Kopel, F. (1972). Gastrointestinal manifestations of cystic fibrosis. *Gastroenterology*, Vol. 62, pp.483-491.

Landsteiner, K. (1905). Darmverschluss durch eingedicktes meconium. *Zentrabl allg Path*, Vol. 6, pp. 903.

Lay-Son, G., Puga, A., Astudillo, P. & Repetto, G.M.; Collaborative Group of the Chilean National Cystic Fibrosis Program. (2011). Cystic fibrosis in Chilean patients: Analysis of 36 common CFTR gene mutations. J Cyst Fibros, Vol. 10, No. 1 (January 2011), pp. 66-70.

Levy, H., Cannon, C.L., Asher, D., García, C., Cleveland, R.H., Pier, G.B., Knowles, M.R. & Colin, A.A. (2010). Lack of correlation between pulmonary disease and cystic fibrosis transmembrane conductance regulator dysfunction in cystic fibrosis: a case report. J Med Case Reports, Vol. 4, pp. 117.

Lewis-Jones, D.I., Gazvani, M.R. & Mountford, R. (2000). Cystic fibrosis in infertility: screening before assisted reproduction: opinion. Hum Reprod, Vol. 15, No. 11 (November 2000), pp. 2415-2417.

Li, C.Y., Jiang, L.Y., Chen, W.Y., Li, K., Sheng, H.Q., Ni, Y., Lu, J.X., Xu, W.X., Zhang, S.Y. & Shi, Q.X. (2010). CFTR is essential for sperm fertilizing capacity and is correlated with sperm quality in humans. *Hum Reprod*, Vol. 25, No. 2 (February 2010), pp. 317-27.

Ludwig, K.S. (1998). The Mayer–Rokitansky–Küster syndrome, an analysis of its morphology and embryology. Part II: Embryology. *Arch Gynecol Obstet*, Vol. 262, No. 1-2, pp. 27–42.

Mak, V., Zielenski, J., Tsui, L.C., Durie, P., Zini, A., Martin, S., Longley, T.B. & Jarvi, K.A. (1999). Proportion of cystic fibrosis gene mutations not detected by routine testing in men with obstructive azoospermia. JAMA, Vol. 281, No. 23 (June 1999), pp. 2217-2224.

Mak, V., Zielenski, J., Tsui, L.C., Durie, P., Zini, A., Martin, S., Longley, T.B. & Jarvi, K.A. (2000). Cystic fibrosis gene mutations and infertile men with primary testicular failure. *Human Reproduction*, Vol. 15, pp. 436-439.

McCallum, T.J., Milunsky, J.M., Cunningham, D.L., Harris, D.H., Maher, T.A. & Oates, R.D. (2000). Fertility in men with cystic fibrosis: an update on current surgical practices and outcomes. Chest, Vol. 118, No. 4 (October 2000), pp. 1059-1062.

Meizel, S. & Deamer, D.W. (1978). The pH of the hamster sperm acrosome. *J Histochem Cytochem*, Vol. 26, pp.98–105.

Mercier, B., Verlingue, C., Lissens, W., Silber, S.J., Novelli, G., Bonduelle, M., Audrézet, M.P. & Férec, C. (1995) Is congenital bilateral absence of vas deferens a primary form of cystic fibrosis? Analyses of the CFTR gene in 67 patients. *Am. J. Hum. Genet*, Vol. 56, No. 1 (January 1995), pp. 272-277.

Modi, A.C., Quittner, A.L., & Boyle, M.P. (2010). Assessing disease disclosure in adults with cystic fibrosis: the Adult Data for Understanding Lifestyle and Transitions (ADULT) survey Disclosure of disease in adults with cystic fibrosis. *BMC Pulm Med*, Vol. 10, pp. 46.

Morea, A., Cameran, M., Rebuffi, A.G., Marzenta, D., Marangon, O., Picci, L., Zacchello, F. & Scarpa, M. (2005). Gender-sensitive association of CFTR gene mutations and 5T allele emerging from a large survey on infertility. Mol Hum Reprod, Vol. 11, No. 8 (August 2005), pp 607-614.

Morral, N., Bertranpetit, J., Estivill, X., Nunes, V., Casals, T., Gimenez, J. *et al.* (1994). The origin of the major cystic fibrosis mutation in European populations. *Nature Genet*, Vol. 7, pp. 169-175.

Mousia-Arvanitakis, J. (1999). Cystic fibrosis and the pancreas: recent scientific advances. *J Clin Gastroenterol*, Vol. 29, No. 2, pp. 138-142.

Oermann, C.M. (2000). Fertility in patients with cystic fibrosis. Chest, Vol. 118, No. 4 (October 2000), pp. 893-894.

Pérez, M.M., Luna, M.C., Pivetta, O.H. & Keyeux, G. (2007). CFTR gene analysis in Latin American CF patients: heterogeneous origin and distribution of mutations across the continent. J Cyst Fibros, Vol. 6, No. 3 (May 2007), pp. 194-208.

Pieri, P.C., Missaglia, M.T., Roque, J.A., Moreira-Filho, C.A. & Hallak, J. (2007). Novel CFTR missense mutations in Brazilian patients with congenital absence of vas deferens: counselling issues. Clinics, Vol. 62, No. 4 (August 2007), pp. 385-390.

Poretsky, L. & Kalin, M.F. (1987). The gonadotropic function of insulin. Endocr Rev, Vol. 8, No. 2 (May 1987), pp. 132-141.

Quinton, P.M. (1983). Chloride impermeability in cystic fibrosis. *Nature*, Vol 301, pp. 421-422.

Quinton, P.M. (1990). Cystic fibrosis: a disease in electrolyte transport. *FASEB J*, Vol. 4, pp. 2709–2717.

Quinton, P.M. (1999). Physiological basis of cystic fibrosis: a historical perspective. *Physiol Rev*, Vol. 79, No. 1 (January 1999), pp. S3–S22.

Radpour, R., Gourabi, H., Dizaj, A.V., Holzgreve, W. & Zhong, X.Y. (2008). Genetic investigations of CFTR mutations in congenital absence of vas deferens, uterus, and vagina as a cause of infertility. J Androl, Vol. 29, No. 5 (September 2008), pp. 506-13.

Raskin, S., Phillips III, J.A., Krishnamani, M. R. S., Jones, C., Parker, R.A. & Rozov, T. et al. DNA analysis of cystic fibrosis in Brazil by directed PCR amplification from Guthrie cards. (1993). *Am J Med Gen*, Vol. 46, pp. 665-669.

Rave-Harel, N., Kerem, E., Nissim-Rafinia, M., Madjar, I., Goshen, R., Augarten, A., Rahat, A., Hurwitz, A., Darvasi, A. & Kerem, B. (1997). The molecular basis of partial penetrance of splicing mutations in cystic fibrosis. *Am. J. Hum. Genet*, Vol. 60, No. 1 (January 1997), pp. 87–94.

Reis, F.J.C. & Damasceno, N. (1998). *Jornal de Pediatria*, Vol. 74 (Supl.1), PP. 76-94.

Ribeiro, J.D., Ribeiro, M.A.G.O., Ribeiro, A.F. (2002). *Jornal de Pediatria*, Vol. 78, Supl.2. S173.

Riordan, J.R., Rommens, J.M., Kerem, B.-S.; Alon, N., Rozmahel, R., Grzelczak, Z., Zielenski, J., Lok, S., Plavsic, N., Chou, J.-L., Drumm, M.L., Iannuzzi, M.C., Collins, F.S. & Tsui, L.-C. (1989). Identification of the cystic fibrosis gene: cloning and characterization of complementary DNA. *Science*, Vol. 245, pp. 1066–1073.

Roberts, S. & Green, P. (2005). The sexual health of adolescents with cystic fibrosis. J R Soc Med, Vol. 98, No. Suppl 45, pp. 7-16.

Rodgers, H.C., Knox, A.J., Toplis, P.J. & Thornton, S.J. (2000). Successful pregnancy and birth after IVF in a woman with cystic fibrosis. *Hum Reprod*, Vol. 15, No. 10 (October 2000), pp. 2152–2153.

Reiter, E.O., Stern. R.C. & Root, A.W. (1981). The reproductive endocrine system in cystic fibrosis. I. Basal gonadotropin and sex steroid levels. *Am J Dis Child*, Vol. 135, No. 5 (May 1981), pp. 422–426.

Resta, R., Biesecker, B.B., Bennett, R.L., Blum, S., Hahn, S.E., Strecker, M.N. &Williams, J.L. (2006). A new definition of Genetic Counselling. National Society of Genetic Counsellors' Task Force report. *J Genet Couns*. Vol. 15. No. 2, pp. 77-83.

Rommens, J.M., Iannuzzi, M.C. & Kerem, B.-S. (1989). Identification of Cystic Fibrosis gene: chromosome walking and jumping. *Science*, Vol. 245, pp.1059–1065.

Razov, T. (1991).Mucoviscidose (Fibrose Cística do pâncreas). *Revisões Pediátricas*, Projeto Áries.

Santos, G.P., Domingos, M.T., Wittig, E.O., Ried, C.A. & Rosário, N.A (2005). Neonatal cystic fibrosis screening program in the state of Paraná: evolution 30 months after implementation. *Jornal de Pediatria*, Vol. 81(3), pp. 240-244.

Saraiva-Pereira, M.L., Fitarelli-Kiehl, M. & Sanseverino, M.T.V. (2011). A Genética na Fibrose Ciística. *Rev HCPA*, Vol. 31, No. 2, pp. 160-167.

Sawyer, S.M. (1996). Reproductive and sexual health in adolescents with cystic fibrosis. *BMJ*, Vol. 313, pp. 1095-1096.

Sawyer, S.M., Farrant, B., Cerritelli, B. & Wilson, J. (2005). A survey of sexual and reproductive health in men with cystic fibrosis: new challenges for adolescent and adult services. Thorax, Vol. 60, No. 4 (April 2005, pp. 326-330.

Shwachman, H. & Kulesvecki, L.L. (1958). Long term study of 105 patients with cystic fibrosis: Studies made over a five to fourteen year period. *Am J Dis Child*, Vol. 96, pp. 6-15.

Shwachman, H., Redmond, A., Khaw, K.T.(1970). Studies in cystic fibrosis. Report of 130 patients diagnosed under 3 months of age over a 20 year period. *Pediatrics*, Vol.46, pp. 335.

Silber, S.J., Nagy, Z.P., Liu, J., Godoy, H., Devroey, P. & Van Steirteghem, A.C. (1994). Conventional in-vitro fertilization versus intracytoplasmic sperm injection for patients requiring microsurgical sperm aspiration. *Hum Reprod*, Vol. 9, No. 9 (September 1994), pp. 1705–1709.

Sokol, R.Z. (2001). Infertility in men with cystic fibrosis. *Curr Opin Pulm Med*, Vol. 7, No. 6 (November 2001), pp. 421–426.

Stead, R.J., Hodson, M.E., Batten, J.C., Adams, J. & Jacobs, H.S. (1987). Amenorrhoea in cystic fibrosis. *Clin Endocrinol*, Vol. 26, pp. 187–195.

Stuppia, L., Antonucci, I., Binni, F., Brandi, A., Grifone, N., Colosimo, A., De Santo, M., Gatta, V., Gelli, G., Guida, V., Majore, S., Calabrese, G., Palka, C., Ravani, A., Rinaldi, R., Tiboni, G.M., Ballone, E., Venturoli, A., Ferlini, A., Torrente, I., Grammatico, P., Calzolari, E. & Dallapiccola, B. (2005). Screening of mutations in the CFTR gene in 1195 couples entering assisted reproduction technique programs. Eur J Hum Genet, Vol. 13, No. 8 (August 2005), pp. 959-964.

Timmreck, L.S., Gray, M.R., Handelin, B., Allito, B., Rohlfs, E., Davis, A.J., Gidwani, G. & Reindollar, R.H. (2003). Analysis of cystic fibrosis transmembrane conductance regulator gene mutations in patients with congenital absence of the uterus and vagina. *Am J Med Genet*, Vol. 120A, No. 1 (July 2003), pp. 72–76.

Tizzano, E.F., Silver, M.M., Chitayat, D., Benichou, J.C. & Buchwald, M. (1994). Differential cellular expression of cystic fibrosis transmembrane regulator in human reproductive tissues. Clues for the infertility in patients with cystic fibrosis. *Am J Pathol*, Vol. 144, pp. 906–914.

Tummler, B., & Kiewitz, C. Cystic fibrosis: an inherited susceptibility to bacterial respiratory infections.(1999). *Mol Med Today*, Vol. 5, No. 8, pp. 351-358.

Uzun, S., Gökçe, S. & Wagner, K. (2005). Cystic fibrosis transmembrane conductance regulator gene mutations in infertile males with congenital bilateral absence of the vas deferens. Tohoku J Exp Med, Vol. 207, No. 4 (December 2005), pp. 279-285.

Van der Ven, K., Messer, L., Van der Ven, H., Jeyendran, R.S. & Ober, C. (1996). Cystic fibrosis mutation screening in healthy men with reduced sperm quality. *Hum Reprod*, Vol. 11, No. 3, pp. 513-517.

Wang, X.F., Zhou, C.X., Shi, Q.X., Yuan, Y.Y., Yu, M.K., Ajonuma, L.C., Ho, L.S., Lo, P.S., Tsang, L.S., Liu, Y., Lam, S.Y., Chan, L.N., Zhao, W.C., Chung, Y.W. & Chan, H.C. (2003). Involvement of CFTR in uterine bicarbonate secretion and the fertilizing capacity of sperm. *Nature Cell Biol* Vol. 5, No. 10 (October 2003), pp. 902–906.

Williams, C., Mayall, E.S., Williamson, R., Hirsh, A. & Cookson, H. (1993). A report on CF carrier frequency among men with infertility owing to congenital absence of the vas deferens. J Med Genet, Vol. 30, No. 11 (November 1993), pp. 973.

Wong, P.Y. (1998). CFTR gene and male fertility. Mol Hum Reprod, Vol. 4, No. 2 (February 1998), pp. 107-110.

Xu, W.M., Shi, Q.X., Chen, W.Y., Zhou, C.X., Ni, Y., Rowlands, D.K., Yi Liu, G., Zhu, H., Ma, Z.G., Wang, X.F., Chen, Z.H., Zhou, S.C., Dong, H.S., Zhang, X.H., Chung, Y.W., Yuan, Y.Y., Yang, W.X. & Chan, H.C. (2007). Cystic fibrosis transmembrane conductance regulator is vital to sperm fertilizing capacity and male fertility. *Proc Natl Acad Sci USA*, Vol. 104, No. 23, pp. 9816-9821.

Zeng, Y., Clark, E.N. & Florman, H.M (1995). Sperm membrane potential: hyperpolarisation during capacitation regulates zona pellucida-dependent acrosomal secretion. *Developmental Biology*, Vol. 171, No. 2, pp. 554-563.

Zheng, X.Y., Chen, G.A. & Wang, H.Y. (2004). Expression of cystic fibrosis transmembrane conductance regulator in human endometrium. *Hum Reprod*, Vol. 19, No. 12 (December 2004), pp. 2933– 2941.

Zielenski, J. & Tsui, L.C. (1995). Cystic fibrosis: genotypic and phenotypic variations. Annu Rev Genet, Vol. 29, pp. 777-807.

Zielenski, J. Genotype and phenotype in cystic fibrosis. (2000). *Respiration*, No. 67, pp. 117-133.

Part 2

CFTR – Genetics and Biochemistry

5

The Genetics of CFTR: Genotype – Phenotype Relationship, Diagnostic Challenge and Therapeutic Implications

Marco Lucarelli, Silvia Pierandrei, Sabina Maria Bruno and Roberto Strom
Dept. of Cellular Biotechnologies and Haematology - Sapienza University of Rome Italy

1. Introduction

Cystic fibrosis (CF; OMIM 602421, see OMIM link in the website section) is the most common lethal genetic disease of the Caucasian population, with a very variable prevalence, from 1/25000 to 1/900, depending on the geographical region (O'Sullivan & Freedman, 2009; Riordan, 2008). CF is caused by mutations of the cystic fibrosis transmembrane conductance regulator (CFTR) gene (Kerem et al., 1989; Rommens et al., 1989; Zielenski et al., 1991) (see Ensembl link in the website section), which encodes for a transmembrane multifunctional protein expressed mainly in epithelia (Trezise et al., 1993a; Yoshimura et al., 1991b) but also in several cell types of nonepithelial origin (Yoshimura et al., 1991a). It is an ATP- and cAMP-dependent Cl^- channel with the main function performed at the apical membrane of epithelial cells. This function is the Cl^- ion secretion in the colon and airways, or its reabsorption in sweat glands (Riordan, 2008; Vankeerberghen et al., 2002). In the lung, the main targeted organ of CF, an additional crucial function performed by CFTR is the regulation of the epithelial Na^+ channel (ENaC) activity. The exact mechanism of CFTR – ENaC interaction is not completely understood and contrasting evidences exist about the role of ENaC in CF. The most reliable vision of the basic defect is that, in the airway epithelia of CF patients, a CFTR deficiency causes an anomalous dual ion transport associated to an altered water absorption (Mall et al., 1998; Stutts et al., 1995; Berdiev et al., 2009) that, in turn, leads to sticky mucus and impaired mucociliary clearance (Donaldson et al., 2002; Matsui et al., 1998). The immune response greatly contributes to increased mucus viscosity through bacterial lysis and DNA release, as well as through immune cell death in the airways. Bacterial infections and inflammation produce bronchial obstruction, bronchiectasis, atrophy and, eventually, lung insufficiency. A probably non-exhaustive list of other CFTR functions includes: the bicarbonate secretion (Kim & Steward, 2009); the regulation of several other ionic channels and of the ion composition of intracellular compartments, as well the control of intracellular vesicle transport (Vankeerberghen et al., 2002); antibacterial activity exerted by epithelial cells (Pier et al., 1997; Schroeder et al., 2002) and macrophages (Del Porto et al., 2011; Di et al., 2006); maintenance of a correct level of hydration, essential for a physiologic development of male reproductive apparatus (Dube et al., 2008; Patrizio & Salameh, 1998; Trezise et al., 1993a), testis, pancreas, liver and intestine (O'Sullivan & Freedman, 2009; Ratjen & Doring, 2003); critical role in spermatogenesis (Trezise et al., 1993a; Trezise et al., 1993b; Xu et al., 2011b), sperm fertilizing capacity (Xu et al., 2007) and inflammatory response (Belcher & Vij, 2010; Buchanan et al., 2009; Campodonico et al., 2008; Mattoscio et al., 2010). The phenotypic severity of CF is essentially referable to CFTR residual function (Estivill, 1996; Zhang et al., 2009) that in turn depends on a combination of variables acting on the CFTR gene, transcript and/or protein, as well as to the action of variables external to CFTR. Random variability and the effect of the environment also influence the final phenotype (Figure 1). Depending on this complex situation, clinical manifestations of CF are highly variable. Some mono- or oligo-symptomatic phenotypes, namely the CFTR-related disorders (CFTR-RD), should have to be distinguished from poly-symptomatic classic CF (Dequeker et al., 2009). Nearly all male CF patients and several CFTR-RD male subjects show obstructive azoospermia due to congenital bilateral absence of the vas deferens (CBAVD); over 80% of CF patients show pancreatic insufficiency. The clinical history of CF patients is characterized by progressive, age-dependent, multiresistant bacterial infections of the lung, where the main pathogens are *Pseudomonas aeruginosa, Staphylococcus aureus, Haemophilus influenzae,* and the *Burkholderia cepacia* complex. Lung colonization causes the clinical decline, characterized by respiratory impairment, that is the main cause of morbidity and mortality. Despite advances in the treatment of CF, there is no definitive cure, the survival median of CF patients being at present limited to approximately 40 years .

2. The genetics of cystic fibrosis

The CFTR gene is located on the long arm of chromosome 7 (7q31.2), spans about 250 kb and contains 27 exons (Zielenski et al., 1991). The most common transcript is 6128 bases long and it is translated to a protein of 1480 aminoacids. The CFTR is under control of an housekeeping-type promoter with a time- and tissue-specific regulated expression established by alternative transcription start sites and/or alternative splicing (Vankeerberghen et al., 2002). CF is a monogenic autosomal recessive disease. Affected subjects have both the alleles mutated. When the same mutation is present on both alleles they are called homozygotes, whereas when different mutations are present on the 2 alleles they are called compound heterozygotes. A carrier of only 1 mutation on 1 allele has no clinical symptoms but has a genetic risk. Two carriers have a high risk of 1/4 (25%) of having an affected child and a risk of 1/2 (50%) of having a healthy carrier child, with a residual probability of 1/4 (25%) of having a healthy non-carrier child. In a given population, the frequency of couples at high risk depends on the frequency of carrier individuals. The prevalence of CFTR mutations and carrier frequency, as well as the incidence of CF, are highly variable depending on geographical region and ethnic group. The disease is very common among Europeans and white Americans with an incidence of about 1/3000 (about 1/27 carriers), whereas the incidence is lower in African Americans (1/17000) and Asian Americans (1/30000). It is uncommon in Africa and Asia with, for example, an incidence as low as 1/350000 in Japan. A comprehensive analysis of worldwide CF incidence and ethnic variations is available (Bobadilla et al., 2002; O'Sullivan & Freedman, 2009).

The basic view of the CF genetics explained above is complicated by biological variability, gene network and technical limitations in the mutational search. A more complex view is reported below.

2.1 Maturation, protein domains and mutational classes

The CFTR gene codes for a symmetric transmembrane protein of 1480 aminoacids that belongs to the family of ATP-binding cassette transporters (ABC transporters). The CFTR protein undergoes a complex transport and maturation process within the cell (Rogan et al., 2011; Vankeerberghen et al., 2002). Through an initial co-translational transport, the polypeptide is included in the membranes of the endoplasmic reticulum (130 kDa form) and is N-glycosylated (150 kDa form). By interacting with chaperones the polypeptide assumes the correct folding with a relatively low efficiency of about 25%, the remainder being degraded by the proteasome. Then it is transported to Golgi apparatus where, after further glycosylation, it becomes the mature CFTR (170 kDa form). It is then transported to the cell membrane where it performs its multiple functions, with a half-life of about 12 to 24 h. The CFTR protein exists in a cAMP-regulated dynamic condition of endocytosis and recycling in clathrin-coated vesicles. Finally it is degraded within lysosomes. After this complex pathway to intracellular and plasma membranes and owing to its multiple functions, the CFTR protein contains a number of different domains, each functionally specialized (Rogan et al., 2011; Vankeerberghen et al., 2002). Its NH_2-end interacts with the SNARE-proteins Syntaxin 1A (STX1A) and synaptosome-associated protein of 23 kDa (SNAP23) (Peters et al., 2001; Tang et al., 2011). The first (TMD1) and the second (TMD2) transmembrane domains, both consisting of six transmembrane helices, form the physical pore through the membrane. The nucleotide binding domains 1 (NBD1) and 2 (NBD2), functionally interacting, contain the sites for ATP binding and hydrolysis. The ATP binding to NBD1 site initiates channel activity, whereas the ATP binding to NBD2 site allows the formation of the intramolecular NBD1 - NBD2 tight heterodimer that turns the channel in a stable open state; the hydrolysis of the ATP bound at NBD2 starts the disruption of the heterodimer interface and finally leads to channel closure (Gadsby et al., 2006). The regulatory domain (R) contains most of the PKA, PKC and PKG phosphorylation sites and has a regulatory role in channel opening/closing. The ATP binding is allowed only after channel activation by PKA-dependent phosphorylation of the R domain. It also interacts with the SNARE protein Syntaxin 8 (STX8) (Bilan et al., 2004). The COOH-end interacts with PDZ domains of the CFTR-associated protein 70 (CAP70) (Wang et al., 2000a), of the Na^+/H^+ exchanger regulatory factor (NHERF, which in turn interacts with ezrin) (Seidler et al., 2009) and of the CFTR associated ligand (CAL) (Cheng et al., 2002). It also interacts with the α1 AMP-activated protein kinase (AMPK) (Hallows et al., 2000) and contains an internalization signal (Prince et al., 1999) and a binding site for the AP-2 adaptor complex (Weixel & Bradbury, 2000), needed for correct endocytosis.

CFTR mutations are at the present grouped into 6 classes (Table 1), according to their effects on transcription, cellular processing, final localization and quantitative level of functional protein (Amaral & Kunzelmann, 2007; O'Sullivan & Freedman, 2009; Rogan et al., 2011; Vankeerberghen et al., 2002). Class I identifies mutations with a complete lack of protein production. Usually they are nonsense mutations, severe splicing mutations (which produce only aberrant mRNA), small or large deletions or insertions. They act by generating in-frame or frameshift premature stop codons. The unstable transcripts and/or proteins formed are rapidly degraded or retain no functionality. In the class II are grouped protein trafficking defects based on ubiquitination and increased degradation, within the endoplasmic reticulum, of the misfolded protein. These are processing/maturation defects that severely decrease the protein quantity in the apical membrane, although often in a tissue-specific manner. In class III are included mutations leading to defective regulation that impair channel opening. Although the CFTR protein is able to reach the apical membrane, it is not properly activated by ATP or cAMP. The effect is a decrease or absence of functional CFTR protein. In class IV are grouped the defects of reduced Cl^- transport through CFTR. In this case the CFTR is present at the apical membrane but it is unable to properly sustain the Cl^- flux. Most of mutations included in classes II, III or IV are missense ones, that produce different degrees of CFTR impairment in reaching the cell apical membrane or in functioning although correctly localized. In some cases, however, also small deletions or insertions can be found. Class V mutations are splicing defects that cause a reduction of wild-type CFTR mRNA. At variance from the splicing mutations belonging to class I, the splicing mutations grouped in this class V do not completely abolish the correctly spliced form. Mutations of class VI decrease the stability of CFTR or affect the regulation of other channels. They can be missense mutations but also nonsense mutations possibly generating overdue stop codons, that allow the production of a protein that retains a partial Cl^- transport ability but is unable to correctly regulate other proteins.

2.2 The significance of genetics for personalized therapies

The increased knowledge about CFTR derived from over 20 years of basic and applied researches. This allowed both the development of symptom-based treatments, already in use, that greatly enhanced the life quality and lifespan of patients and the actual possibility of more effective personalized therapies. As well, a promise of primary defect correction also arose. As the most severe clinical aspect is respiratory impairment, the target tissue of these therapies is the pseudostratified epithelia of airways. A normalization of ion and water transport in respiratory epithelium can be achieved with the correction of less than 25% of the airway epithelial cells (Farmen et al., 2005; Johnson et al., 1992; Zhang et al., 2009). To classify a CFTR mutation in a functional class has recently become meaningful for a restoring strategy based on drugs acting on specific functional impairment (the so-called mutation-specific therapy) (Amaral & Kunzelmann, 2007; Becq et al., 2011; Kerem, 2005; Rogan et al., 2011) (Table 1). Particularly studied are the in-frame premature termination codons (class I). In general, many kind of tumours and more than a third of genetic diseases are originated by premature termination codons (Frischmeyer & Dietz, 1999). Also in CF, about 20% of affected subjects have at least 1 mutation that is an in-frame premature termination codon. Aminoglycoside antibiotics have shown to be useful to suppress in-frame premature termination codons by read-through and production of full-length CFTR protein (although a wrong aminoacid is inserted in each individual protein) allowing the targeting of class I mutations. The rationale of this approach is that a population of CFTR proteins each with a different wrong aminoacid will show an overall functionality greater than a population of identically truncated CFTR proteins. In this regard, recent findings, although not specifically obtained for CF, highlighted a surprisingly therapeutic potentiality for ribonucleoproteins. The authors (Karijolich & Yu, 2011) demonstrated the possibility, in vitro and in yeast, of the conversion of uridine into pseudouridine, a chemical transformation known as pseudouridylation. As all three translation termination codons contain a uridine residue at first position and the pseudouridylated nonsense codons code for serine, threonine tyrosine or phenylalanine, this may be a tool for converting nonsense into sense codons. Also in this case a wrong aminoacid will be inserted, although within a reduced choice of 4 aminoacids. Notably, the ribonucleoprotein complex used by the authors contain a RNA guide able to target the complex to a specific nonsense mutation. Chemical, molecular or pharmacological chaperones, usually called correctors (of trafficking), have been reported to be useful, by promoting protein folding and stabilizing CFTR structure, in the targeting of class II mutations. By increasing the activation of mutated CFTR correctly localized at the apical membrane and/or by extending its half-life, some drugs act as potentiators (of function) and are suitable for the targeting of class III, IV and V mutations. Class VI mutations may be targeted by either potentiators or suppressors of in-frame termination codons. Extensive lists of promising compound are available (Amaral & Kunzelmann, 2007; Becq et al., 2011; Rogan et al., 2011). For an up-to-date description of CF clinical trials see, in the website section, the links to the U.S. National Institutes of Health Clinical trials registry and database, and to the U.S. CF Foundation drug development pipeline.

The topic of mutational classes and personalized therapy is not devoid of problems. Some mutations produce multiple effects and should be classified in multiple classes. An emblematic example is the CFTR worldwide most common mutation, the F508del, a deletion of phenylalanine at position 508 of the CFTR protein. It is a class II mutation, because most of the protein is degraded within the endoplasmic reticulum; a small proportion of it reaches however the apical membrane where it behaves as a class III mutation, with only a limited capacity to bind ATP. In addition, the F508del protein has shown a decreased stability and an enhanced degradation also in post-endoplasmic reticulum compartments (Sharma et al., 2001), a behaviour that would point to the mutational class VI. It is in general quite difficult to classify a mutation without specific experimental studies aimed to its functional characterization. Due to the complexity of such studies, they have been performed only for a very limited number of the over 1800 sequence variations found in the CFTR gene. On the other hand, only in a limited number of cases it is possible to infer, by a theoretical approach, a relationship between the functional impairment and the protein domain where the mutation is located, as well a relationship between a specific DNA sequence variation and the class it should belong to. For example, although most of class III mutations localize in the R, NBD1 or NDB2 domains and most of class IV mutations localize in TMD1 or TMD2, if a missense mutation in these domains has been found, it cannot be assumed that the effect will effectively correspond to class III or IV, since that mutation might have a prevalent effect on protein trafficking and should therefore be classified as class II. Likewise, only for nonsense and frameshift mutations it is possible to reasonably assume a direct classification in class I, while for all other kinds of mutations it is very difficult to recognize the mutational class just from DNA sequence variation. For example, for splicing mutations it can be hazardous to deduce the possible amount of anomalous splicing only by software analysis, since just a limited amount of wild type mRNA would cause the shift of that mutation from class I to class V. Taking into account these considerations, although the class-specific personalized therapeutic approach can be at the moment applied only to a limited amount of CFTR mutations, its enhancement is foreseeable when the gap between the knowledge of the structure and the effect of a mutation will be filled by increasing numbers of mutation-specific functional studies.

Gene therapy would be the resolutive therapeutic intervention. Although, since the discovery of CFTR gene in 1989 more than 30 clinical trials of gene therapy have been undertaken, no gene therapy has been so far approved for clinical use (Conese et al., 2011; Davies & Alton, 2011; Griesenbach & Alton, 2011). The problems arose from the repeated administration of adenovirus- and adeno-associated virus-based vectors shifted the approaches to lentiviral vectors and non-viral strategies, as well as cell therapy. The evidence that a lot of work is still to be done in laboratory to optimize gene therapy tools arose. Two opposite approaches can be distinguished in gene therapy: the gene augmentation and the gene targeting. By the former approach, the entire wild-type CFTR gene, producing a normal gene function, is introduced into the cell without the need to know the specific CFTR mutation. On the contrary, the latter approach is a mutation-specific gene therapy strategy, as only the zone of mutation is targeted in situ, allowing the correction of the mutated zone of the gene. A recent study (Auriche et al., 2010) of gene augmentation in CF used the entire CFTR locus, including regulatory regions, cloned and delivered by a bacterial artificial chromosome (BAC), a non-viral vector. The possibility to obtain a physiologically regulated CFTR expression and activity, also of Pseudomonas internalization, in an in vitro cellular system has been demonstrated. The control of CFTR activity by naturally occurring regulatory elements appeared a critical aspect to obtain a physiologic CFTR expression pattern, to be taken under consideration in the planning of gene augmentation strategies. By the gene targeting, the corrected gene remains regulated by its endogenous regulatory machinery maintaining its physiologic expression pattern. Recent researches (Gruenert et al., 2003; Sangiuolo et al., 2008; Sangiuolo et al., 2002) applied to CF an intriguing gene targeting strategy, the Small Fragment Homologous Replacement (SFHR), that exchange a wild-type corrector DNA fragment with the endogenous mutated sequence, through a still undefined mechanism probably based on homologous recombination. Both approaches have to be enhanced before clinical application. The main difficulties encountered in the BAC approach are efficient manipulation and delivering to the proper cell population. The main hitches with SFHR are the low reproducibility and recombination efficiency, ranging from 0.01% to 5% (Gruenert et al., 2003). In both cases additional studies are needed to clarify the respective driving molecular mechanisms, to ameliorate our applicatory ability.

Mutation class	Functional effect	Kind of mutations	Mutation-specific therapy
I	Complete lack of protein production	Premature stop codons by: - nonsense - severe splicing - small or large deletions or insertions	Suppressors of in-frame premature termination codons
II	Processing and/or maturation protein defects	- missense - small deletions or insertions	Correctors (chemical, molecular or pharmacological chaperones)
III	Defective regulation of channel opening	- missense - small deletions or insertions	Potentiators
IV	Reduced Cl^- transport	- missense - small deletions or insertions	Potentiators
V	Reduction of wild-type mRNA	- partial splicing	Potentiators
VI	Protein decreased stability or impaired ability of other channel regulation	- missense - nonsense (overdue stop codons)	Potentiators or suppressors of in-frame overdue termination codons

Table 1. Classes of CFTR mutations and possible personalized therapeutic interventions.

2.3 The complexity and sources of variability in the genotype – Phenotype relationship of the CF and CFTR-RD

Separation of classic CF from CFTR-RD only represents a starting attempt to organize the great clinical variability of CF (Bombieri et al., 2011; Dequeker et al., 2009; Estivill, 1996; Noone & Knowles, 2001). In fact, within classic CF are usually grouped both poly-symptomatic and oligo-symptomatic forms greatly differing in the involvement of lung, pancreas, liver, sweat gland and reproductive apparatus (to consider only the main CF targets). Not easier is the task of categorizing the even more heterogeneous oligo- and mono-symptomatic CFTR-RD. In this regard CFTR mutations have been linked to a wide series of pathologies: obstructive azoospermia for CBAVD (Claustres, 2005; Cuppens & Cassiman, 2004; Stuhrmann & Dork, 2000); non-obstructive azoospermia, reduced sperm quality and spermatogenesis defects (Boucher et al., 1999; Dohle et al., 2002; Jakubiczka et al., 1999; Jarvi et al., 1998; Mak et al., 2000; Pallares-Ruiz et al., 1999; van der Ven et al., 1996); male hypofertility due to idiopathic seminal hyperviscosity (Elia et al., 2009; Rossi et al., 2004); female hypofertility due to thick cervical mucus (Gervais et al., 1996; Hayslip et al., 1997); neonatal hypertrypsinaemia with normal sweat test (Castellani et al., 2001a; Gomez Lira et al., 2000; Narzi et al., 2007; Padoan et al., 2002); idiopathic pancreatitis (Castellani et al., 2001b; Gomez Lira et al., 2000; Maire et al., 2003; Pallares-Ruiz et al., 2000); pulmonary diseases (Bombieri et al., 1998; Bombieri et al., 2000); disseminated bronchiectasis (Girodon et al., 1997; Pignatti et al., 1995); chronic rhinosinusitis (Raman et al., 2002; Southern, 2007; Wang et al., 2000b); nasal polyposis (Kerem, 2006; Pawankar, 2003); metabolic alkalosis, hypochloremia, hyponatriemia, hypokalemia and dehydration (Augusto et al., 2008; Kerem, 2006; Leoni et al., 1995; Priou-Guesdon et al., 2010; Salvatore et al., 2004); primary sclerosing cholangitis, biliary cirrhosis and portal hypertension (Collardeau-Frachon et al., 2007; Gallegos-Orozco et al., 2005; Girodon et al., 2002; Kerem, 2006; Sheth et al., 2003). Several CFTR-RD are still debated, as the involvement of CFTR mutations is often inferred from small case series or even isolated case reports, as well for controversial results (as for example for non-CBAVD male reproductive defects). In addition, in several cases only one mutated allele could be found by quite non homogeneous methodological approaches of mutational search. This raises the troublesome question whether it should be assumed that 2 mutated alleles are indeed present, but the mutational search protocol applied was unable to identify both of them, or if the possibility of CFTR-RD arising in heterozygotes might also be taken into consideration. Rather than an approach for categories, a vision of a mosaic of different clinical manifestations combined in a peculiar way in each patient, overall constituting a continuous gradient of disease clinical severity, seems to better reflect the reality.

Only a rough correspondence between mutational classes and clinical outcome can be found with, for example, more severe phenotypes generated by the combination of class I and class III mutations and milder phenotypes originated by class IV and V. The variability is however so high that clinicians usually do not use genotypes for prognosis. The problem of the relationship between genotype and phenotype in CF can be partitioned in, at least, 2 steps (Figure 1). The first step concerns the production of a CFTR protein with reduced functionality starting from a mutated CFTR genotype. The second step concerns the clinical manifestations that originate owing to the protein malfunction. It is generally accepted that the clinical severity of CF and CFTR-RD is correlated with the residual function of CFTR

(Estivill, 1996; Zhang et al., 2009). It is easy to collocate high (almost physiological) levels of CFTR protein at the same end of the spectrum of the strictly mono-symptomatic patients and very low (almost absent) levels to the other end, where the poly-symptomatic patients with severe clinical manifestations are ideally collocated. Within these extreme conditions, it is however very difficult to link the values of CFTR residual activity to the severity of clinical manifestations. This not only because of the lack of systematic studies, but also for the difficulty of measuring in a real quantitative manner both the CFTR residual function and the clinical severity. Although CFTR mutated genotypes responsible for intermediate levels of residual activity often consist of a classic mutation on one allele and a mild mutation, retaining some CFTR activity, on the other allele, also the link between a specific mutated genotype and its effect on the protein functionality is elusive. Again, also in this case, the lack of systematic functional studies, addressing in vitro the effect of the mutated genotype on the protein cellular fate, have greatly hampered the knowledge at this level.

Several sources of variability influence both steps and make the overall picture unclear (Figure 1).

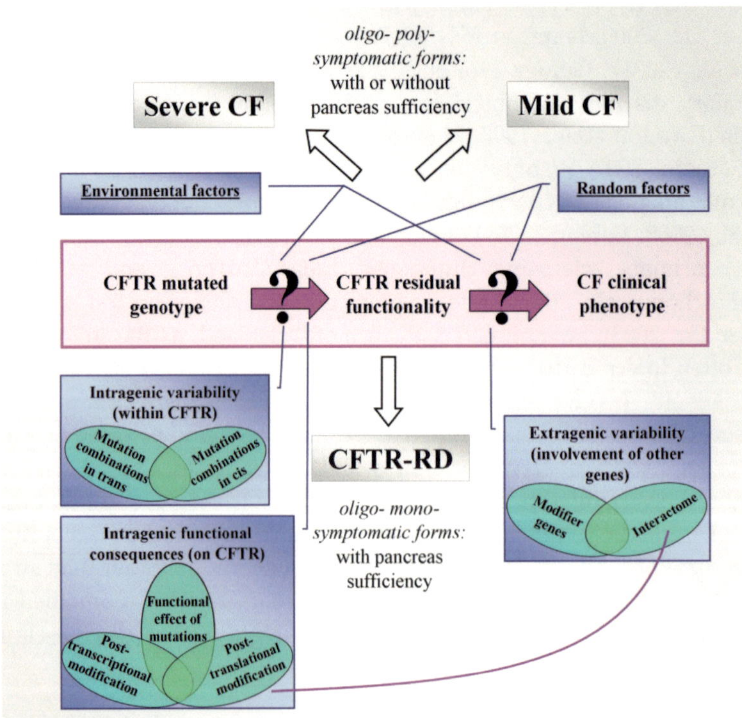

Fig. 1. The variability determinants of the genotype - phenotype relationship in CF and CFTR-RD.

The first step (from mutated genotype to residual function) is mainly influenced by structural and functional intragenic (CFTR-depending) variability. The structural intragenic variability is due to the large number of mutations and to the even larger number of their combinations both in trans, to originate homozygous and compound heterozygous genotypes, and in cis, with more than one mutation on the same allele to form the complex alleles. Trans and cis variability may also combine leading, for instance, to genotypes with 2 complex alleles and 4 different mutations each belonging to a different mutational class. The functional intragenic variability is due on one side to the variable impairment effect of mutations and, on the other side, to the influence of both post-transcriptional and post-translational modifications, possibly with overlapping effects and interacting mechanisms. The second step (from residual function to clinical phenotype) is more likely to be influenced by extragenic variability due to genes different from CFTR. Modifier genes can indeed modulate the original effect of CFTR mutations (Collaco & Cutting, 2008; Cutting, 2010; Merlo & Boyle, 2003; Salvatore et al., 2002; Slieker et al., 2005), as evidenced by the high phenotypic variability found in some subjects with identical CFTR mutated genotypes. Reciprocal influence between modifier genes and interactome (Wang et al., 2006), as well as an effect of interactome on intragenic functional variability, might also influence this step. Furthermore, it should be taken under consideration that the CFTR levels physiologically required can be tissue-specific, with only some organs affected despite the same CFTR residual function (Estivill, 1996). For example, the male reproductive apparatus appears as the most sensitive district to CFTR impairment, as nearly all men with CF (lower levels of functional CFTR) exhibit also CBAVD while, on the contrary, men with only CBAVD (higher level of functional CFTR) do not have other organs targeted. Superimposed to these genetic sources of variability the powerful role of environmental and random factors on both steps should not be undervalued. Due to these sources of variability, the genotype - phenotype relationship in CF is still poorly understood (Salvatore et al., 2011) with, therefore, our diagnostic, prognostic and therapeutic abilities severely limited.

3. Complex alleles and modifier genes

3.1 The relevance of complex alleles

The least addressed aspect of CFTR intragenic structural variability probably is the involvement of complex alleles, with two (or more) mutations in cis (on the same allele). Unfortunately, the most widely used protocols for a mutational search within the CFTR gene are designed only with the aim of finding the first two mutations on different alleles; additional mutations, possibly in cis with the already found mutations, may escape detection. The result is that the mutated genotypes of CF subjects with varying clinical presentations may appear identical, despite the presence of unfound complex alleles that might explain the divergent phenotypes. Undetected complex alleles may have important consequences. For example, if 2 already known disease-causing mutations have been found on both alleles (also on the allele with an in cis undetected additional mutation), the consequences will be an unclear genotype - phenotype relationship with prognostic failure. If at least 1 sequence variation with unclear functional significance in cis with an undetected additional disease-causing mutation has been found, a diagnostic error and/or misclassification of the sequence variation will arise. A systematic experimental search for complex alleles has not yet been undertaken. Probably for this reason only few complex alleles have been found so far and their prevalence is unknown. A probably non exhaustive list of CFTR complex alleles at the moment known is reported in Table 2. They have been more frequently found in patients with CF than CFTR-RD. Only in some cases an in vitro functional characterization has been performed, with the consequence that only in a limited number of these alleles it is possible to distinguish the relative functional contribution of

Complex allele	Bibliographic source
[R75Q;S549N]	Consortium for CF genetic analysis database
[$(TG)_mT_5$;2184insA]	Consortium for CF genetic analysis database
[129G>C;R117H]	Consortium for CF genetic analysis database
[F508del;R553Q]	(Dork et al., 1991);(Teem et al., 1993)
[3732delA;K1200E]	Consortium for CF genetic analysis database
[F508C;S1251N]	(Kalin et al., 1992)
[F508del;R553M]	(Teem et al., 1993)
[R117H;$(TG)_mT_n$]	(Kiesewetter et al., 1993; Massie et al., 2001; Peckham et al., 2006)
[125G>C;R75X]	Consortium for CF genetic analysis database
[R297Q;$(TG)_mT_n$]	Consortium for CF genetic analysis database
[R668C;3849+10kbC>T]	Consortium for CF genetic analysis database
[deleD7S8 (CFTR 3' 500 kb); F508del]	(Wagner et al., 1994)
[1716G>A;L619S]	Consortium for CF genetic analysis database
[405+1G>A;3030G>A]	Consortium for CF genetic analysis database
[G576A;R668C]	(McGinniss et al., 2005; Pignatti et al., 1995)
[$(TG)_mT_5$;A800G]	(Chillon et al., 1995)
[L88X;G1069R]	(Savov et al., 1995)
[S912L;G1244V]	(Clain et al., 2005; Savov et al., 1995)
[R334W;R1158X]	(Duarte et al., 1996)
[R347H;D979A]	(Clain et al., 2001; Hojo et al., 1998)
[-102T;S549R(T>G)]	(Romey et al., 1999)
[R74W;D1270N]	(Fanen et al., 1999)
[G628R;S1235R]	(Mercier et al., 1995; Wei et al., 2000)
[R117C;$(TG)_mT_n$]	(Massie et al., 2001)
[M470V;S1235R]	(Wei et al., 2000)
[I148T;3199del6]	(Rohlfs et al., 2002)
[S1235R;$(TG)_mT_5$]	(Feldmann et al., 2003)
[L24F;296+2T>G]	Consortium for CF genetic analysis database
[W356_A357del;V358I]	(McGinniss et al., 2005)
[V562I;A1006E]	(McGinniss et al., 2005)
[R352W;P750L]	(McGinniss et al., 2005)
[1198_1203delTGGGCT;1204G>A]	(McGinniss et al., 2005)
[V754M;*CFTR*dele3_10,14b_16]	(Niel et al., 2006)
[F508del;I1027T]	(Fichou et al., 2008)
[R74W;R1070W;D1270N]	(de Prada et al., 2010)
[$(TG)_{11}T_5$;A1006E]	(Tomaiuolo et al., 2010)
[R117L;L997F]	(Lucarelli et al., 2010)

Nucleotide notation: A = adenine, C = cytosine, G = guanine, T = thymine.
Aminoacid notation: A = alanine, C = cysteine, D = aspartic acid, E = glutamic acid, I = isoleucine, K = lysine, E = glutamic acid, , F = phenylalanine, G = glycine, L = leucine, M = methionine, N = asparagine, H = histidine, P = proline, Q = glutamine, R = arginine, S = serine, T = threonine, V = valine, W = tryptophan, X = stop codon (nonsense).
The link to the Consortium for CF genetic analysis database is reported in the website section.

Table 2. Complex alleles of CFTR (in chronological order of discovery).

each mutation. They often result in a combination of two mild mutations that, if isolated, cause CFTR-RD but if combined in cis originate CF. In some cases there is one main mutation whose phenotypic effect is worsened by a second sequence variation that may even be a neutral variant if isolated, such as F508C , R74W , S912L or M470V. Also variants that have a suppressive effect when in cis but originate a hyperactive CFTR when combined in trans, as for example the M470 and R1235, have been described. On the other hand, the finding of complex alleles also in CFTR-RD suggests the possibility that an additional mutation in cis may even lead to a lessening of the phenotypic severity (Mercier et al., 1995). This effect has been demonstrated for -102T, R553Q, R553M and R334W. The situation is further complicated by the fact that some CFTR polymorphisms, combined in specific haplotypes, may have at least CFTR-RD as phenotypic consequences (Steiner et al., 2004; Steiner et al., 2011).

3.2 The relevance of modifier genes

A small fraction of CF patients and a higher amount of CFTR-RD subjects remain with no CFTR mutations, also when high sensitivity methods of mutational search are used. In addition, CF and CFTR-RD patients with the same mutated CFTR genotypes often show divergent phenotypes. Also some intriguing cases have been reported: an unaffected sister who inherited the same CFTR alleles, without mutations, of her CF brother (Mekus et al., 1998) and two CF sibs, with no CFTR mutation found, who had inherited different parental CFTR allele (Groman et al., 2002). This suggested that genes different from CFTR may cause CF or CFTR-RD. The involvement of other genes in the definition of these phenotypes is relevant for the comprehension of both the molecular pathogenesis and the genotype - phenotype relationship. However, the widest action of the modifier genes probably is to modulate the CF final clinical phenotype in patients with both CFTR mutations found. Even more important, the modifier genes can represent excellent therapeutic targets, as they are able, by definition, to modify the clinical outcome of the disease but they are not mutated (on the contrary to the CFTR). A so-called bypassing approach has been proposed to correct the CF ionic imbalance by stimulating alternative ionic pathways that might compensate the impaired CFTR (Amaral & Kunzelmann, 2007). At present a comprehensive list of these genes does not exist and little is known about their effects and molecular mechanisms of action, as well as about their exact kind of interaction, if any, with the CFTR. Several putative modifier genes have been reported (Collaco & Cutting, 2008; Cutting, 2010; Merlo & Boyle, 2003; Slieker et al., 2005) to influence the second step, from CFTR residual functionality to clinical outcome. On the other hand, microRNA, known to exert a post-transcriptional regulation, have recently been shown to potentially influence the CFTR protein levels (Gillen et al., 2011; Xu et al., 2011a). Together with complex alleles, it is these genes that most probably represent the greatest source of variability in CF. Furthermore, modifier genes show tissue-specific levels of activity, that combine with equally tissue-specific CFTR levels, thus amplifying the complexity of the network. They may also influence the different CFTR functions, even in a tissue-specific manner. One of the most interesting gene complex proposed as CF modifier is the epithelial Na^+ channel (ENaC).

3.2.1 The ENaC genes

The human functional ENaC is composed of 3 subunits coded by 3 genes with sequence similarities: α (SCNN1A gene) (Voilley et al., 1994), β (SCNN1B gene) and γ (SCNN1G gene)

(Voilley et al., 1995). The ENaC protein has the functional properties of a Na^+ channel with high Na^+ selectivity, low conductance and amiloride sensitivity. It is expressed in human epithelial cells that line the distal renal tubule, distal colon and several exocrine glands; an ENaC-mediated amiloride-sensitive electrogenic Na^+ reabsorbtion has been documented in the upper and lower airways (Hummler et al., 1996). Genetic diseases are caused by either loss- or gain-of-function mutations in the ENaC genes: loss-of-function mutations in one of the three subunits cause pseudohypoaldosteronism type I (PHA-I) (Chang et al., 1996) characterized by severe renal dysfunction, arterial hypotension and reduced reabsorbtive capacity of both kidney and lung; gain-of-function mutations in either SCNN1B or SCNN1G are responsible for Liddle's syndrome, a severe form of hypertension (Shimkets et al., 1994). Interestingly, some PHA-I patients, without CFTR mutations, also exhibit CF-like lung symptoms, such as recurrent bacterial infection of the airways (Hanukoglu et al., 1994).

Because of the involvement of both CFTR and ENaC in the physiologic dual ion transport, it was supposed that also ENaC deregulation and/or molecular lesions might sustain CF or CFTR-RD. There are indeed experimental evidences validating this hypothesis. The over-expressing β-ENaC mouse model has CF-like pulmonary symptoms, with morbidity and mortality partially reduced by preventive treatment with amiloride, an inhibitor of the ENaC channel (Zhou et al., 2008). Wild type CFTR has been shown, in a heterologous cellular system and in polarized primary human bronchial epithelial cultures, to prevent the proteolitic stimulation of ENaC, thus downregulating Na^+ absorption (Gentzsch et al., 2010). Enhanced expression of all the 3 ENaC genes was shown in the nasal epithelium of CF patients (Bangel et al., 2008). In human bronchial epithelial cells, the CFTR regulates the functional surface expression of endogenous ENaC, by influencing its trafficking (Butterworth, 2010; Rubenstein et al., 2011). However, also experimental evidences against a direct involvement of ENaC and/or of CFTR - ENaC interaction in CF pathogenesis have been provided. According to one study (Joo et al., 2006), CF airway submucosal glands do not display ENaC-mediated fluid hyperabsorption, differently from the ciliated cells of the airway surface. Another study (Nagel et al., 2005) evidenced that human CFTR fails to inhibit the human ENaC channel in a heterologous experimental system of Xenopus oocytes. Finally, no increased sodium absorption has been found in newborn $CFTR^{-/-}$ pigs, an animal model with features resembling those of human CF disease (Chen et al., 2010). The differences between CF and CFTR action in humans and pigs, the fact that the study has been conducted only shortly after birth and that CF patients have a mutated CFTR and not a $CFTR^{-/-}$, should however be taken into account. Following the above considerations, mutational search in the ENaC genes have been performed in CF and CFTR-RD patients. Both, loss-of-function (Huber et al., 2010; Sheridan et al., 2005) and gain-of-function (Mutesa et al., 2008; Sheridan et al., 2005) mutations have been found in the SCNN1B gene of CFTR-RD patients. Several variants of SCNN1B and SCNN1G have been also found in bronchiectasis patients, some of them with only one CFTR mutation. A significantly increased prevalence of ENaC rare polymorphisms have been found in CFTR-RD patients (Azad et al., 2009), with some of these variants producing alterations of ENaC activity (Azad et al., 2009; Huber et al., 2010). The bulk of these data allows to ascribe to ENaC some roles in CF and/or CFTR-RD. This is reinforced also by the findings of physical and functional co-regulatory interactions between SNARE proteins (in particular Syntaxin 1A) and both the CFTR and ENaC (Peters et al., 2001). It is likely that wild-type ENaC is deregulated by the mutated CFTR. Moreover, ENaC genes can also act as additional mutated genes either when only one or no copy of CFTR is mutated (the ENaC genes behaving as concomitant pathogenetic factors with respect to CFTR) or when both copies of the CFTR gene are mutated (the ENaC genes as modifiers, modulating the CF phenotype). Little is known about the prevalence and kind of mutations, as well as about the role of other kind of ENaC alterations, such as transcriptional modifications. This last point is quite intriguing considering that a deregulation of ENaC, rather than mutations of it, seems more frequently the main pathogenic mechanism. The topic of the regulation of ENaC activity further increases the complexity of the puzzle, as multiple biochemical and cellular pathways are involved in the lung (Bhalla & Hallows, 2008; Butterworth, 2010; Eaton et al., 2010; Edinger et al., 2006; Gaillard et al., 2010; Gentzsch et al., 2010). However, little is known about the tissue-specific expression of ENaC and the coordinated transcriptional regulation of the 3 SCNN1 genes. The structure of these genes suggested a role for DNA methylation. The SCNN1G gene has 2 CpG islands in its promoter region and exon 1 (Auerbach et al., 2000; Zhang et al., 2004), the SCNN1B gene has 1 CpG island in its promoter and exon 1 (Thomas et al., 2002) and the SCNN1A gene has a high density of CpG sites, that are however not organized in a CpG island (Ludwig et al., 1998). In effect, experimental evidences suggest that DNA methylation can control transcription of the SCNN1G gene (Zhang et al., 2004).

In general, the search for new genes involved in genetic diseases, in addition to the identification and characterization of new pathogenetic mechanisms, allows the identification of new therapeutic targets. The functional interaction between CFTR and ENaC evidenced by the vast majority of experimental data makes ENaC genes attractive therapeutic targets, since it looks easier to attempt the correction of the regulation of wild type ENaC than the correction of the mutated CFTR. The ENaC gene activity repression has been tempted by amiloride, with partially contrasting results obtained in humans (Burrows et al., 2006) and animal models (Zhou et al., 2008). Also RNA interference seems a valuable and specific tool (Caci et al., 2009; Yueksekdag et al., 2010). The experimental evidences that ENaC genes undergo a DNA methylation-dependent transcription, raised new therapeutic opportunity in epigenetics and chromatin remodelling.

4. The genetics, biochemistry and clinics in the diagnosis of CF

Due to the wide range of signs and symptoms, CF and CFTR-RD diagnosis is difficult, particularly in infancy. On the other hand, CF early diagnosis, revealing pancreas insufficiency, preventing malnutrition and allowing a prompt treatment of lung infections, improves both lifespan and quality of life. In addition, it allows the early selection of high risk couples. For these reasons, neonatal screening programs have been activated worldwide (Castellani & Massie, 2010; Lai et al., 2005; Southern et al., 2007). The most used neonatal screening procedure is based on a single or double dosages (at birth and later on, between the third and fifth week of life) of immunoreactive trypsinogen (IRT), possibly combined with a I level mutational analysis (Castellani et al., 2009; Narzi et al., 2002). In addition to CF newborns, it has been demonstrated that also CFTR-RD newborns are selected by the screening programs (Boyne et al., 2000; Castellani et al., 2001a; Massie et al., 2000; Narzi et al., 2007; Padoan et al., 2002). In a part of newborns positive to the neonatal screening, only one or even no CFTR mutation, sometimes linked to borderline sweat test values, are found. This raises diagnostic uncertainty (Parad & Comeau, 2005) and provides evidence that some carriers are selected by neonatal screening (Castellani et al., 2005; Laroche & Travert, 1991;

Scotet et al., 2001). A common effect of the introduction of CF neonatal screening is the progressively increasing number of CF diagnoses performed each year by screening and the decreasing number of diagnoses performed by symptoms. By definition, neonatal screening selects a lot of false positive subjects and, consequently, is not a diagnostic procedure. On the other hand, also several other pathologies different from CF have a positive sweat test, as well as some CF and a lot of CFTR-RD subjects have a borderline or even negative sweat test. In some cases measurements of the nasal potential difference and/or intestinal Cl^- flux appear to be quite useful procedures. Taking into account also the highly variable clinical manifestations of CF and CFTR-RD, some of which superimposable to those of other pathologies, it became clear that none of this measurements alone allows a full diagnosis of CF or CFTR-RD. For these reasons, as stated by recent general (Farrell et al., 2008), neonatal screening-oriented (Castellani et al., 2009; Mayell et al., 2009; Sermet-Gaudelus et al., 2010), sweat test-oriented (Green & Kirk, 2007; Legrys et al., 2007) and genetic-oriented (Castellani et al., 2008; Dequeker et al., 2009) guidelines, the diagnosis of CF and CFTR-RD may only be made by a coordinated evaluation of clinical, biochemical and genetic data (Figure 2 upper part). In the last years genetic assessment has been clearly emerging as the most crucial point. In fact if 2 CF or CFTR-RD disease-causing mutations on the different alleles are found, a reliable diagnosis can be defined. Both the finding of the CFTR mutations and their functional interpretation are however very critical points, as described below.

4.1 The technical complexity of the mutational search in the CFTR gene

Over 1500 CFTR mutations and 300 polymorphisms are at moment known (in the website section see the links to the Consortium for CF genetic analysis database and to the human gene mutation database (HGMD)). The F508del is the worldwide most common mutation, accounting, on average, for about 60% of mutated alleles in northern European and North American populations. Few other single mutations account for more than about 5%. In addition the frequencies of CFTR mutations are very different depending on the geographical area (Bobadilla et al., 2002; O'Sullivan & Freedman, 2009). The simplest approach of mutational search would be to define a panel of mutations to be included in a rapid and low-cost test allowing a direct search. However, the high genetic heterogeneity has at least 2 consequences that limit such an approach. First, it is impossible to establish a general mutational panel applicable worldwide; second, the allelic detection rate, also of geographical optimized mutational panels, rarely exceeds the 80% and often is quite lower (Bobadilla et al., 2002; O'Sullivan & Freedman, 2009; Tomaiuolo et al., 2003). The detection rate is the genetic equivalent of the laboratory operative characteristics called diagnostic sensitivity. In this case it represents the proportion of mutated alleles that the specific genetic test is able to evidence. The practical consequence of a limited detection rate is that in case of a negative test, the presence of a mutation not included in the analyzed panel of mutations can not be excluded. A widely accepted approach of mutational search is the multistep one. Usually, methods of I, II and III levels are recognized (Figure 2 lower part). The I level methods are based on the search panels of the most common CFTR mutations by entry-level techniques. They are the most commonly used methods worldwide. However, due to technical and cost limitations, they show a low detection rate as at best they search for the most common CFTR mutations of the specific geographical area. At the moment commercial methods able to search near all CFTR mutations of specific geographic areas are not available. The I level genetic tests are therefore of limited prognostic and diagnostic usefulness, particularly in CFTR-RD subjects with borderline clinical and/or biochemical values. In this case, the use of methods with higher detection rate are fundamental to resolve uncertain diagnoses. The II level methods are scanning procedures usually able to analyze all the exons, adjacent intronic zones and proximal 5'-flanking of the CFTR gene. In last years, several enhanced methods specific for CFTR scanning have been developed as for example denaturing gradient gel electrophoresis (Costes et al., 1993; Fanen et al., 1992), single-strand conformation polymorphism and heteroduplex analysis (Ravnik-Glavac et al., 1994), denaturing high pressure liquid chromatography (D'Apice et al., 2004; Le Marechal et al., 2001; Ravnik-Glavac et al., 2002), and re-sequencing (Lucarelli et al., 2002; Lucarelli et al., 2006). Due to the progressively reducing costs of the re-sequencing and to the need of further characterization by re-sequencing of positive findings of other scanning techniques, the re-sequencing has become the most used II level method. However, no mutational scan technique able to detect all the CFTR mutations exists. Also the re-sequencing, at the moment the method of mutational search with the highest detection rate, is able to select about 97% of CFTR mutations. The remaining 3% of alleles carry mutations not identified. These may be large deletions, completely intronic mutations that may reveal cryptic exons and mutations in the distal 5'-flanking as well as 3'-UTR zones. Although little is known about the geographical variability of the prevalence of this kind of mutations, due to their overall limited amount and to the extended analysis of the CFTR gene, the re-sequencing shows not only a higher, but also a more constant detection rate than mutational panel-based techniques. Automated protocol of re-sequencing, as well as software templates for automated analysis of re-sequencing data (Ferraguti et al., 2011), have also greatly reduced the time and efforts needed for both the experimental and data processing phases. It should be clear that the use of scanning techniques may raise the problem of functional interpretation of sequence variations found. In fact, whereas the mutational panels are usually planned as to include only disease-causing CFTR mutations, by using scanning procedures also sequence variations not previously characterized from functional point of view may be selected. This may complicate the genetic counselling. The III level methods should be aimed to the search for large deletions, full intronic and distal 5'-flanking, as well as 3'-UTR, mutations. In practise, commercially available products only exist either for the search of most common CFTR large deletions or for the CFTR scanning for gene dosage (gain or loss of genetic material). Although full intronic, distal 5'-flanking and 3'-UTR mutations are assessable by re-sequencing, only recently some efforts have been done to value the pathogenetic contribution of these kind of mutations to CF and CFTR-RD. Whatever technique based on PCR and/or hybridization is applied, the possibility that polymorphisms within the primer/probe recognition sequence may interfere with the pairing reactions should be taken under consideration. So, also if the detection rate is kept to a maximum by including all the 3 levels of mutational search, a full assessment of mutations is virtually impossible to reach, due to the likely, even if small, decrease in analytical sensitivity.

The practical application of this multistep approach changes depending on its use in subjects with disease suspect for diagnostic purposes or in general population subjects for genetic risk lowering. In the first case it is reasonable to progressively go through the levels up to the finding of 2 CFTR mutations on different alleles. If no mutation is found (or at least 1 mutation is not found) even at the III level, the genetic test contributes to a reasonable exclusion of the CF or CFTR-RD diagnosis. On the contrary, in the second case, since it can be difficult to apply all mutational search levels to each subject checking its carrier status, an appropriate genetic residual risk is usually chosen and the mutational search with the suitable detection rate is performed.

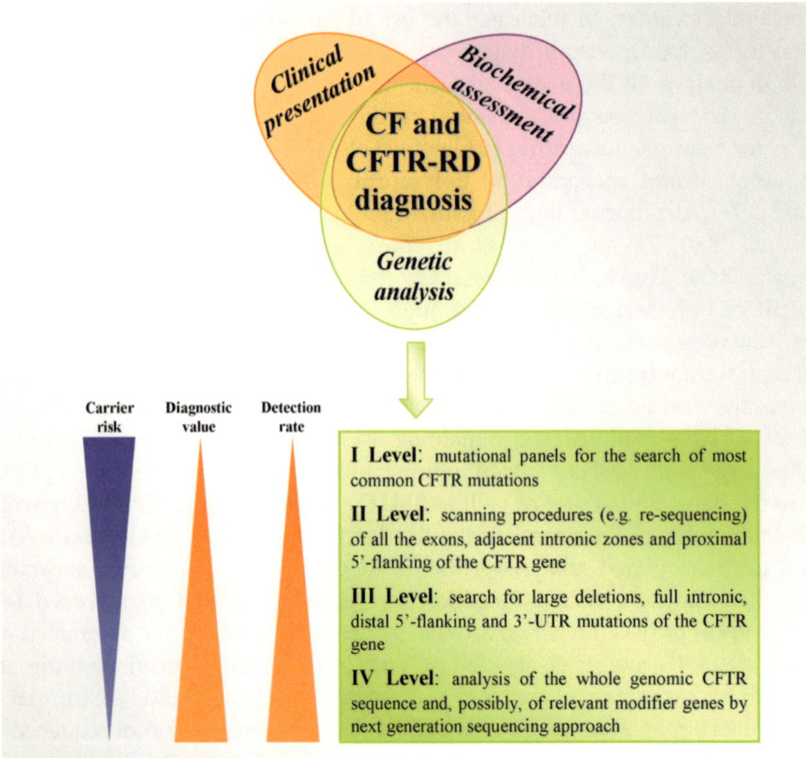

Fig. 2. The genetic analysis, biochemical assessment and clinical presentation contribute to the diagnosis of CF. The multistep genetic approach allows a progressive increase of detection rate and diagnostic value of the test in subjects with CF or CFTR-RD suspect, as well as a progressive decrease of carrier risk in general population subjects.

Usually, no scanning techniques are applied for genetic risk lowering , also because of the possibility to select sequence variations hardly valuable from a pathogenetic point of view. The use of the I level mutational panel approach to assess the genetic risk raises 4 possibilities. If both members of the couple are positive to the mutational search, the risk for an affected child is 1/4 (25%). If both members of the couple are negative the residual risk is so low that no other action is required, although it should be kept in mind that the risk is not zero and this should be made clear to the couple by the genetic counselling. For example, with a carrier frequency of 1/27 and a detection rate of the applied mutational panel of about 85%, the couple residual risk of having an affected child, with CFTR mutations different from those analyzed, if the genetic tests are both negative is about 1/120000. An intermediate residual risk arises when one member of the couple is carrier or CF. In these cases, considering the same above carrier frequency and detection rate, the risk is, respectively, of about 1/700 and 1/350. In these cases, in addition to the genetic counselling clarifying that a concrete risk exists, a possible extension of mutational search to further lower the genetic risk may be taken under consideration for the negative partner.

Following the above considerations, the often incomplete genetic characterization of CF and CFTR-RD patients is due to technical limitations; this constitute a further obstacle to our understanding of the genotype - phenotype relationship. An emblematic example of this are undetected complex alleles. Patients who do not undergo full mutational assessment, have discordant sweat test and/or clinical outcome, but show at a first mutational search apparently identical CFTR mutated genotypes, should undergo the search for complex alleles. The rising, within the last years, of parallel sequencing, also called next generation sequencing (NGS) (Su et al., 2011), allows to identify a possible IV level in the CFTR mutational search (Bell et al., 2011) (Figure 2 lower part). The possibility to study and analyze data of the whole genomic CFTR sequence (including introns, distal 5'-flanking and 3'-UTR zones) by massive re-sequencing, in an almost complete automated single run-based manner, will be a real possibility within next years. The NGS also has the potentiality to simultaneously study the genetics of modifier genes and, in general, of CFTR interactome to obtain a full assessment of genetic variability determining the final phenotype. If this kind of approach will be able to completely replace the multistep approach actually used is only matter of costs, investment and, finally, commercial choices. Several websites deal with CF and CFTR genetics, from diagnostic and quality assessment point of view, for example those of the European CF thematic network and of the European CF society (links reported in website section).

5. Conclusion

The comprehension of the gene network involved in CF and CFTR-RD is increasing. This is coupled with the enhancement of mutational search methodologies that allow the search for a continuously increasing number of mutations and sequence variations in the CFTR gene and in several other CF-related genes. The huge amount of structural data has to be supported by proper functional studies of single mutations, sequence variations, complex alleles and haplotypes. Only this will produce a full comprehension of genes and their molecular lesions cooperating in the definition of the final CF and CFTR-RD phenotypes, allowing full diagnosis and prognosis. As well, this will also allow the actual clinical use of mutation-specific therapies. When, in the mid-term, this objectives will be reached, the effect-oriented therapy now used will be turned into a cause-oriented therapy (Figure 3).

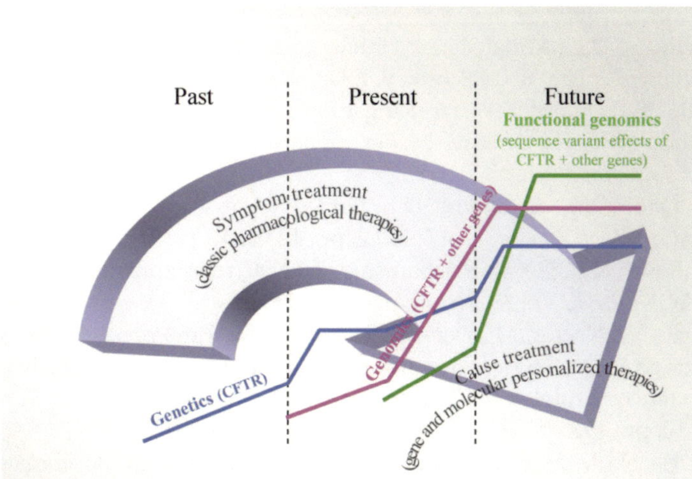

Fig. 3. A genetic-oriented view of CF and CFTR-RD therapy perspectives. The increasing knowledge about genetics, genomics and functional genomics change the therapy.

6. References

Amaral, M.D. & Kunzelmann, K. (2007). Molecular targeting of CFTR as a therapeutic approach to cystic fibrosis. *Trends Pharmacol.Sci.,* Vol.28, No.7, pp. 334-341.

Auerbach, S.D.; Loftus, R.W.; Itani, O.A. & Thomas, C.P. (2000). Human amiloride-sensitive epithelial Na^+ channel gamma subunit promoter: functional analysis and identification of a polypurine-polypyrimidine tract with the potential for triplex DNA formation. *Biochem.J.,* Vol.347 Pt 1, pp. 105-114.

Augusto, J.F.; Sayegh, J.; Malinge, M.C.; Illouz, F.; Subra, J.F. & Ducluzeau, P.H. (2008). Severe episodes of extra cellular dehydration: an atypical adult presentation of cystic fibrosis. *Clin.Nephrol.,* Vol.69, No.4, pp. 302-305.

Auriche, C.; Di Domenico, E.G.; Pierandrei, S.; Lucarelli, M.; Castellani, S.; Conese, M.; Melani, R.; Zegarra-Moran, O. & Ascenzioni, F. (2010). CFTR expression and activity from the human CFTR locus in BAC vectors, with regulatory regions, isolated by a single-step procedure. *Gene Ther.,* Vol.17, No.11, pp. 1341-1354.

Azad, A.K.; Rauh, R.; Vermeulen, F.; Jaspers, M.; Korbmacher, J.; Boissier, B.; Bassinet, L.; Fichou, Y.; Des, G.M.; Stanke, F.; De, B.K.; Dupont, L.; Balascakova, M.; Hjelte, L.; Lebecque, P.; Radojkovic, D.; Castellani, C.; Schwartz, M.; Stuhrmann, M.; Schwarz, M.; Skalicka, V.; de, M., I; Girodon, E.; Ferec, C.; Claustres, M.; Tummler, B.; Cassiman, J.J.; Korbmacher, C. & Cuppens, H. (2009). Mutations in the amiloride-sensitive epithelial sodium channel in patients with cystic fibrosis-like disease. *Hum.Mutat.,* Vol.30, No.7, pp. 1093-1103.

Bangel, N.; Dahlhoff, C.; Sobczak, K.; Weber, W.M. & Kusche-Vihrog, K. (2008). Upregulated expression of ENaC in human CF nasal epithelium. *J.Cyst.Fibros.,* Vol.7, No.3, pp. 197-205.

Becq, F.; Mall, M.A.; Sheppard, D.N.; Conese, M. & Zegarra-Moran, O. (2011). Pharmacological therapy for cystic fibrosis: from bench to bedside. *J.Cyst.Fibros.,* Vol.10 Suppl 2, pp. S129-S145.

Belcher, C.N. & Vij, N. (2010). Protein processing and inflammatory signaling in Cystic Fibrosis: challenges and therapeutic strategies. *Curr.Mol.Med.,* Vol.10, No.1, pp. 82-94.

Bell, C.J.; Dinwiddie, D.L.; Miller, N.A.; Hateley, S.L.; Ganusova, E.E.; Mudge, J.; Langley, R.J.; Zhang, L.; Lee, C.C.; Schilkey, F.D.; Sheth, V.; Woodward, J.E.; Peckham, H.E.; Schroth, G.P.; Kim, R.W. & Kingsmore, S.F. (2011). Carrier testing for severe childhood recessive diseases by next-generation sequencing. *Sci.Transl.Med.,* Vol.3, No.65, pp. 65ra4.

Berdiev, B.K.; Qadri Y.J. & Benos, D.J. (2009). Assessment of the CFTR and ENaC association. *Mol. Biosyst.,* Vol.5, No.2, pp. 123-127.

Bhalla, V. & Hallows, K.R. (2008). Mechanisms of ENaC regulation and clinical implications. *J.Am.Soc.Nephrol.,* Vol.19, No.10, pp. 1845-1854.

Bilan, F.; Thoreau, V.; Nacfer, M.; Derand, R.; Norez, C.; Cantereau, A.; Garcia, M.; Becq, F. & Kitzis, A. (2004). Syntaxin 8 impairs trafficking of cystic fibrosis transmembrane conductance regulator (CFTR) and inhibits its channel activity. *J.Cell Sci.,* Vol.117, No.Pt 10, pp. 1923-1935.

Bobadilla, J.L.; Macek, M., Jr.; Fine, J.P. & Farrell, P.M. (2002). Cystic fibrosis: a worldwide analysis of CFTR mutations--correlation with incidence data and application to screening. *Hum.Mutat.,* Vol.19, No.6, pp. 575-606.

Bombieri, C.; Benetazzo, M.; Saccomani, A.; Belpinati, F.; Gile, L.S.; Luisetti, M. & Pignatti, P.F. (1998). Complete mutational screening of the CFTR gene in 120 patients with pulmonary disease. *Hum.Genet.*, Vol.103, No.6, pp. 718-722.

Bombieri, C.; Claustres, M.; De, B.K.; Derichs, N.; Dodge, J.; Girodon, E.; Sermet, I.; Schwarz, M.; Tzetis, M.; Wilschanski, M.; Bareil, C.; Bilton, D.; Castellani, C.; Cuppens, H.; Cutting, G.R.; Drevinek, P.; Farrell, P.; Elborn, J.S.; Jarvi, K.; Kerem, B.; Kerem, E.; Knowles, M.; Macek, M., Jr.; Munck, A.; Radojkovic, D.; Seia, M.; Sheppard, D.N.; Southern, K.W.; Stuhrmann, M.; Tullis, E.; Zielenski, J.; Pignatti, P.F. & Ferec, C. (2011). Recommendations for the classification of diseases as CFTR-related disorders. *J.Cyst.Fibros.*, Vol.10 Suppl 2, pp. S86-102.

Bombieri, C.; Luisetti, M.; Belpinati, F.; Zuliani, E.; Beretta, A.; Baccheschi, J.; Casali, L. & Pignatti, P.F. (2000). Increased frequency of CFTR gene mutations in sarcoidosis: a case/control association study. *Eur.J.Hum.Genet.*, Vol.8, No.9, pp. 717-720.

Boucher, D.; Creveaux, I.; Grizard, G.; Jimenez, C.; Hermabessiere, J. & Dastugue, B. (1999). Screening for cystic fibrosis transmembrane conductance regulator gene mutations in men included in an intracytoplasmic sperm injection programme. *Mol.Hum.Reprod.*, Vol.5, No.6, pp. 587-593.

Boyne, J.; Evans, S.; Pollitt, R.J.; Taylor, C.J. & Dalton, A. (2000). Many deltaF508 heterozygote neonates with transient hypertrypsinaemia have a second, mild CFTR mutation. *J.Med.Genet.*, Vol.37, No.7, pp. 543-547.

Buchanan, P.J.; Ernst, R.K.; Elborn, J.S. & Schock, B. (2009). Role of CFTR, Pseudomonas aeruginosa and Toll-like receptors in cystic fibrosis lung inflammation. *Biochem.Soc.Trans.*, Vol.37, No.Pt 4, pp. 863-867.

Burrows, E.; Southern, K.W. & Noone, P. (2006). Sodium channel blockers for cystic fibrosis. *Cochrane.Database.Syst.Rev.*, Vol.3, pp. CD005087.

Butterworth, M.B. (2010). Regulation of the epithelial sodium channel (ENaC) by membrane trafficking. *Biochim.Biophys.Acta*, Vol.1802, No.12, pp. 1166-1177.

Caci, E.; Melani, R.; Pedemonte, N.; Yueksekdag, G.; Ravazzolo, R.; Rosenecker, J.; Galietta, L.J. & Zegarra-Moran, O. (2009). Epithelial sodium channel inhibition in primary human bronchial epithelia by transfected siRNA. *Am.J.Respir.Cell Mol.Biol.*, Vol.40, No.2, pp. 211-216.

Campodonico, V.L.; Gadjeva, M.; Paradis-Bleau, C.; Uluer, A. & Pier, G.B. (2008). Airway epithelial control of Pseudomonas aeruginosa infection in cystic fibrosis. *Trends Mol.Med.*, Vol.14, No.3, pp. 120-133.

Castellani, C.; Benetazzo, M.G.; Tamanini, A.; Begnini, A.; Mastella, G. & Pignatti, P. (2001a). Analysis of the entire coding region of the cystic fibrosis transmembrane regulator gene in neonatal hypertrypsinaemia with normal sweat test. *J.Med.Genet.*, Vol.38, No.3, pp. 202-205.

Castellani, C.; Cuppens, H.; Macek, M., Jr.; Cassiman, J.J.; Kerem, E.; Durie, P.; Tullis, E.; Assael, B.M.; Bombieri, C.; Brown, A.; Casals, T.; Claustres, M.; Cutting, G.R.; Dequeker, E.; Dodge, J.; Doull, I.; Farrell, P.; Ferec, C.; Girodon, E.; Johannesson, M.; Kerem, B.; Knowles, M.; Munck, A.; Pignatti, P.F.; Radojkovic, D.; Rizzotti, P.; Schwarz, M.; Stuhrmann, M.; Tzetis, M.; Zielenski, J. & Elborn, J.S. (2008). Consensus on the use and interpretation of cystic fibrosis mutation analysis in clinical practice. *J.Cyst.Fibros.*, Vol.7, No.3, pp. 179-196.

Castellani, C.; Gomez Lira, M.; Frulloni, L.; Delmarco, A.; Marzari, M.; Bonizzato, A.; Cavallini, G.; Pignatti, P. & Mastella, G. (2001b). Analysis of the entire coding region of the cystic fibrosis transmembrane regulator gene in idiopathic pancreatitis. *Hum.Mutat.*, Vol.18, No.2, pp. 166.

Castellani, C. & Massie, J. (2010). Emerging issues in cystic fibrosis newborn screening. *Curr.Opin.Pulm.Med.*, Vol.16, No.6, pp. 584-590.

Castellani, C.; Picci, L.; Scarpa, M.; Dechecchi, M.C.; Zanolla, L.; Assael, B.M. & Zacchello, F. (2005). Cystic fibrosis carriers have higher neonatal immunoreactive trypsinogen values than non-carriers. *Am.J.Med.Genet.A*, Vol.135, No.2, pp. 142-144.

Castellani, C.; Southern, K.W.; Brownlee, K.; Dankert, R.J.; Duff, A.; Farrell, M.; Mehta, A.; Munck, A.; Pollitt, R.; Sermet-Gaudelus, I.; Wilcken, B.; Ballmann, M.; Corbetta, C.; de, M., I; Farrell, P.; Feilcke, M.; Ferec, C.; Gartner, S.; Gaskin, K.; Hammermann, J.; Kashirskaya, N.; Loeber, G.; Macek, M., Jr.; Mehta, G.; Reiman, A.; Rizzotti, P.; Sammon, A.; Sands, D.; Smyth, A.; Sommerburg, O.; Torresani, T.; Travert, G.; Vernooij, A. & Elborn, S. (2009). European best practice guidelines for cystic fibrosis neonatal screening. *J.Cyst.Fibros.*, Vol.8, No.3, pp. 153-173.

Chang, S.S.; Grunder, S.; Hanukoglu, A.; Rosler, A.; Mathew, P.M.; Hanukoglu, I.; Schild, L.; Lu, Y.; Shimkets, R.A.; Nelson-Williams, C.; Rossier, B.C. & Lifton, R.P. (1996). Mutations in subunits of the epithelial sodium channel cause salt wasting with hyperkalaemic acidosis, pseudohypoaldosteronism type 1. *Nat.Genet.*, Vol.12, No.3, pp. 248-253.

Chen, J.H.; Stoltz, D.A.; Karp, P.H.; Ernst, S.E.; Pezzulo, A.A.; Moninger, T.O.; Rector, M.V.; Reznikov, L.R.; Launspach, J.L.; Chaloner, K.; Zabner, J. & Welsh, M.J. (2010). Loss of anion transport without increased sodium absorption characterizes newborn porcine cystic fibrosis airway epithelia. *Cell*, Vol.143, No.6, pp. 911-923.

Cheng, J.; Moyer, B.D.; Milewski, M.; Loffing, J.; Ikeda, M.; Mickle, J.E.; Cutting, G.R.; Li, M.; Stanton, B.A. & Guggino, W.B. (2002). A Golgi-associated PDZ domain protein modulates cystic fibrosis transmembrane regulator plasma membrane expression. *J.Biol.Chem.*, Vol.277, No.5, pp. 3520-3529.

Chillon, M.; Casals, T.; Mercier, B.; Bassas, L.; Lissens, W.; Silber, S.; Romey, M.C.; Ruiz-Romero, J.; Verlingue, C.; Claustres, M. & . (1995). Mutations in the cystic fibrosis gene in patients with congenital absence of the vas deferens. *N.Engl.J.Med.*, Vol.332, No.22, pp. 1475-1480.

Clain, J.; Fritsch, J.; Lehmann-Che, J.; Bali, M.; Arous, N.; Goossens, M.; Edelman, A. & Fanen, P. (2001). Two mild cystic fibrosis-associated mutations result in severe cystic fibrosis when combined in cis and reveal a residue important for cystic fibrosis transmembrane conductance regulator processing and function. *J.Biol.Chem.*, Vol.276, No.12, pp. 9045-9049.

Clain, J.; Lehmann-Che, J.; Girodon, E.; Lipecka, J.; Edelman, A.; Goossens, M. & Fanen, P. (2005). A neutral variant involved in a complex CFTR allele contributes to a severe cystic fibrosis phenotype. *Hum.Genet.*, Vol.116, No.6, pp. 454-460.

Claustres, M. (2005). Molecular pathology of the CFTR locus in male infertility. *Reprod.Biomed.Online.*, Vol.10, No.1, pp. 14-41.

Collaco, J.M. & Cutting, G.R. (2008). Update on gene modifiers in cystic fibrosis. *Curr.Opin.Pulm.Med.*, Vol.14, No.6, pp. 559-566.

Collardeau-Frachon, S.; Bouvier, R.; Le, G.C.; Rivet, C.; Cabet, F.; Bellon, G.; Lachaux, A. & Scoazec, J.Y. (2007). Unexpected diagnosis of cystic fibrosis at liver biopsy: a report of four pediatric cases. *Virchows Arch.*, Vol.451, No.1, pp. 57-64.

Conese, M.; Ascenzioni, F.; Boyd, A.C.; Coutelle, C.; De, F., I; De, S.S.; Rejman, J.; Rosenecker, J.; Schindelhauer, D. & Scholte, B.J. (2011). Gene and cell therapy for cystic fibrosis: from bench to bedside. *J.Cyst.Fibros.*, Vol.10 Suppl 2, pp. S114-S128.

Costes, B.; Fanen, P.; Goossens, M. & Ghanem, N. (1993). A rapid, efficient, and sensitive assay for simultaneous detection of multiple cystic fibrosis mutations. *Hum.Mutat.*, Vol.2, No.3, pp. 185-191.

Cuppens, H. & Cassiman, J.J. (2004). CFTR mutations and polymorphisms in male infertility. *Int.J.Androl*, Vol.27, No.5, pp. 251-256.

Cutting, G.R. (2010). Modifier genes in Mendelian disorders: the example of cystic fibrosis. *Ann.N.Y.Acad.Sci.*, Vol.1214, pp. 57-69.

D'Apice, M.R.; Gambardella, S.; Bengala, M.; Russo, S.; Nardone, A.M.; Lucidi, V.; Sangiuolo, F. & Novelli, G. (2004). Molecular analysis using DHPLC of cystic fibrosis: increase of the mutation detection rate among the affected population in Central Italy. *BMC.Med.Genet.*, Vol.5, pp. 8.

Davies, J.C. & Alton, E.W. (2011). Design of gene therapy trials in CF patients. *Methods Mol.Biol.*, Vol.741, pp. 55-68.

de Prada, M.A.; Butschi, F.N.; Bouchardy, I.; Beckmann, J.S.; Morris, M.A.; Hafen, G.M. & Fellmann, F. (2010). [R74W;R1070W;D1270N]: a new complex allele responsible for cystic fibrosis. *J.Cyst.Fibros.*, Vol.9, No.6, pp. 447-449.

Del Porto, P.; Cifani, N.; Guarnieri, S.; Di Domenico, E.G.; Mariggio, M.A.; Spadaro, F.; Guglietta, S.; Anile, M.; Venuta, F.; Quattrucci, S. & Ascenzioni, F. (2011). Dysfunctional CFTR alters the bactericidal activity of human macrophages against Pseudomonas aeruginosa. *PLoS.ONE.*, Vol.6, No.5, pp. e19970.

Dequeker, E.; Stuhrmann, M.; Morris, M.A.; Casals, T.; Castellani, C.; Claustres, M.; Cuppens, H.; Des, G.M.; Ferec, C.; Macek, M.; Pignatti, P.F.; Scheffer, H.; Schwartz, M.; Witt, M.; Schwarz, M. & Girodon, E. (2009). Best practice guidelines for molecular genetic diagnosis of cystic fibrosis and CFTR-related disorders--updated European recommendations. *Eur.J.Hum.Genet.*, Vol.17, No.1, pp. 51-65.

Di, A.; Brown, M.E.; Deriy, L.V.; Li, C.; Szeto, F.L.; Chen, Y.; Huang, P.; Tong, J.; Naren, A.P.; Bindokas, V.; Palfrey, H.C. & Nelson, D.J. (2006). CFTR regulates phagosome acidification in macrophages and alters bactericidal activity. *Nat.Cell Biol.*, Vol.8, No.9, pp. 933-944.

Dohle, G.R.; Halley, D.J.; Van Hemel, J.O.; van den Ouwel, A.M.; Pieters, M.H.; Weber, R.F. & Govaerts, L.C. (2002). Genetic risk factors in infertile men with severe oligozoospermia and azoospermia. *Hum.Reprod.*, Vol.17, No.1, pp. 13-16.

Donaldson, S.H.; Poligone, E.G. & Stutts, M.J. (2002). CFTR regulation of ENaC. *Methods Mol.Med.*, Vol.70, pp. 343-364.

Dork, T.; Wulbrand, U.; Richter, T.; Neumann, T.; Wolfes, H.; Wulf, B.; Maass, G. & Tummler, B. (1991). Cystic fibrosis with three mutations in the cystic fibrosis transmembrane conductance regulator gene. *Hum.Genet.*, Vol.87, No.4, pp. 441-446.

Duarte, A.; Amaral, M.; Barreto, C.; Pacheco, P. & Lavinha, J. (1996). Complex cystic fibrosis allele R334W-R1158X results in reduced levels of correctly processed mRNA in a pancreatic sufficient patient. *Hum.Mutat.*, Vol.8, No.2, pp. 134-139.

Dube, E.; Hermo, L.; Chan, P.T. & Cyr, D.G. (2008). Alterations in gene expression in the caput epididymides of nonobstructive azoospermic men. *Biol.Reprod.*, Vol.78, No.2, pp. 342-351.

Eaton, D.C.; Malik, B.; Bao, H.F.; Yu, L. & Jain, L. (2010). Regulation of epithelial sodium channel trafficking by ubiquitination. *Proc.Am.Thorac.Soc.,* Vol.7, No.1, pp. 54-64.

Edinger, R.S.; Yospin, J.; Perry, C.; Kleyman, T.R. & Johnson, J.P. (2006). Regulation of epithelial Na^+ channels (ENaC) by methylation: a novel methyltransferase stimulates ENaC activity. *J.Biol.Chem.,* Vol.281, No.14, pp. 9110-9117.

Elia, J.; Delfino, M.; Imbrogno, N.; Capogreco, F.; Lucarelli, M.; Rossi, T. & Mazzilli, F. (2009). Human semen hyperviscosity: prevalence, pathogenesis and therapeutic aspects. *Asian J.Androl,* Vol.11, No.5, pp. 609-615.

Estivill, X. (1996). Complexity in a monogenic disease. *Nat.Genet.,* Vol.12, No.4, pp. 348-350.

Fanen, P.; Clain, J.; Labarthe, R.; Hulin, P.; Girodon, E.; Pagesy, P.; Goossens, M. & Edelman, A. (1999). Structure-function analysis of a double-mutant cystic fibrosis transmembrane conductance regulator protein occurring in disorders related to cystic fibrosis. *FEBS Lett.,* Vol.452, No.3, pp. 371-374.

Fanen, P.; Ghanem, N.; Vidaud, M.; Besmond, C.; Martin, J.; Costes, B.; Plassa, F. & Goossens, M. (1992). Molecular characterization of cystic fibrosis: 16 novel mutations identified by analysis of the whole cystic fibrosis conductance transmembrane regulator (CFTR) coding regions and splice site junctions. *Genomics,* Vol.13, No.3, pp. 770-776.

Farmen, S.L.; Karp, P.H.; Ng, P.; Palmer, D.J.; Koehler, D.R.; Hu, J.; Beaudet, A.L.; Zabner, J. & Welsh, M.J. (2005). Gene transfer of CFTR to airway epithelia: low levels of expression are sufficient to correct Cl^- transport and overexpression can generate basolateral CFTR. *Am.J.Physiol Lung Cell Mol.Physiol,* Vol.289, No.6, pp. L1123-L1130.

Farrell, P.M.; Rosenstein, B.J.; White, T.B.; Accurso, F.J.; Castellani, C.; Cutting, G.R.; Durie, P.R.; Legrys, V.A.; Massie, J.; Parad, R.B.; Rock, M.J. & Campbell, P.W., III (2008). Guidelines for diagnosis of cystic fibrosis in newborns through older adults: Cystic Fibrosis Foundation consensus report. *J.Pediatr.,* Vol.153, No.2, pp. S4-S14.

Feldmann, D.; Couderc, R.; Audrezet, M.P.; Ferec, C.; Bienvenu, T.; Desgeorges, M.; Claustres, M.; Mittre, H.; Blayau, M.; Bozon, D.; Malinge, M.C.; Monnier, N.; Bonnefont, J.P.; Iron, A.; Bieth, E.; Dumur, V.; Clavel, C.; Cazeneuve, C. & Girodon, E. (2003). CFTR genotypes in patients with normal or borderline sweat chloride levels. *Hum.Mutat.,* Vol.22, No.4, pp. 340.

Ferraguti, G.; Pierandrei, S.; Bruno, S.M.; Ceci, F.; Strom, R. & Lucarelli, M. (2011). A template for mutational data analysis of the CFTR gene. *Clin.Chem.Lab Med.,* Vol.49, No.9, pp.1447-1451

Fichou, Y.; Genin, E.; Le, M.C.; Audrezet, M.P.; Scotet, V. & Ferec, C. (2008). Estimating the age of CFTR mutations predominantly found in Brittany (Western France). *J.Cyst.Fibros.,* Vol.7, No.2, pp. 168-173.

Frischmeyer, P.A. & Dietz, H.C. (1999). Nonsense-mediated mRNA decay in health and disease. *Hum.Mol.Genet.,* Vol.8, No.10, pp. 1893-1900.

Gadsby, D.C.; Vergani, P. & Csanady, L. (2006). The ABC protein turned chloride channel whose failure causes cystic fibrosis. *Nature,* Vol.440, No.7083, pp. 477-483.

Gaillard, E.A.; Kota, P.; Gentzsch, M.; Dokholyan, N.V.; Stutts, M.J. & Tarran, R. (2010). Regulation of the epithelial Na^+ channel and airway surface liquid volume by serine proteases. *Pflugers Arch.,* Vol.460, No.1, pp. 1-17.

Gallegos-Orozco, J.F.; Yurk, E.; Wang, N.; Rakela, J.; Charlton, M.R.; Cutting, G.R. & Balan, V. (2005). Lack of association of common cystic fibrosis transmembrane conductance regulator gene mutations with primary sclerosing cholangitis. *Am.J.Gastroenterol.*, Vol.100, No.4, pp. 874-878.

Gentzsch, M.; Dang, H.; Dang, Y.; Garcia-Caballero, A.; Suchindran, H.; Boucher, R.C. & Stutts, M.J. (2010). The cystic fibrosis transmembrane conductance regulator impedes proteolytic stimulation of the epithelial Na^+ channel. *J.Biol.Chem.*, Vol.285, No.42, pp. 32227-32232.

Gervais, R.; Dumur, V.; Letombe, B.; Larde, A.; Rigot, J.M.; Roussel, P. & Lafitte, J.J. (1996). Hypofertility with thick cervical mucus: another mild form of cystic fibrosis? *JAMA*, Vol.276, No.20, pp. 1638.

Gillen, A.E.; Gosalia, N.; Leir, S.H. & Harris, A. (2011). microRNA regulation of expression of the cystic fibrosis transmembrane conductance regulator gene. *Biochem.J.*, Vol.438, No.1, pp. 25-32.

Girodon, E.; Cazeneuve, C.; Lebargy, F.; Chinet, T.; Costes, B.; Ghanem, N.; Martin, J.; Lemay, S.; Scheid, P.; Housset, B.; Bignon, J. & Goossens, M. (1997). CFTR gene mutations in adults with disseminated bronchiectasis. *Eur.J.Hum.Genet.*, Vol.5, No.3, pp. 149-155.

Girodon, E.; Sternberg, D.; Chazouilleres, O.; Cazeneuve, C.; Huot, D.; Calmus, Y.; Poupon, R.; Goossens, M. & Housset, C. (2002). Cystic fibrosis transmembrane conductance regulator (CFTR) gene defects in patients with primary sclerosing cholangitis. *J.Hepatol.*, Vol.37, No.2, pp. 192-197.

Gomez Lira, M.; Benetazzo, M.G.; Marzari, M.G.; Bombieri, C.; Belpinati, F.; Castellani, C.; Cavallini, G.C.; Mastella, G. & Pignatti, P.F. (2000). High frequency of cystic fibrosis transmembrane regulator mutation L997F in patients with recurrent idiopathic pancreatitis and in newborns with hypertrypsinemia. *Am.J.Hum.Genet.*, Vol.66, No.6, pp. 2013-2014.

Green, A. & Kirk, J. (2007). Guidelines for the performance of the sweat test for the diagnosis of cystic fibrosis. *Ann.Clin.Biochem.*, Vol.44, No.Pt 1, pp. 25-34.

Griesenbach, U. & Alton, E.W. (2011). Current status and future directions of gene and cell therapy for cystic fibrosis. *BioDrugs.*, Vol.25, No.2, pp. 77-88.

Groman, J.D.; Meyer, M.E.; Wilmott, R.W.; Zeitlin, P.L. & Cutting, G.R. (2002). Variant cystic fibrosis phenotypes in the absence of CFTR mutations. *N.Engl.J.Med.*, Vol.347, No.6, pp. 401-407.

Gruenert, D.C.; Bruscia, E.; Novelli, G.; Colosimo, A.; Dallapiccola, B.; Sangiuolo, F. & Goncz, K.K. (2003). Sequence-specific modification of genomic DNA by small DNA fragments. *J.Clin.Invest*, Vol.112, No.5, pp. 637-641.

Hallows, K.R.; Raghuram, V.; Kemp, B.E.; Witters, L.A. & Foskett, J.K. (2000). Inhibition of cystic fibrosis transmembrane conductance regulator by novel interaction with the metabolic sensor AMP-activated protein kinase. *J.Clin.Invest*, Vol.105, No.12, pp. 1711-1721.

Hanukoglu, A.; Bistritzer, T.; Rakover, Y. & Mandelberg, A. (1994). Pseudohypoaldosteronism with increased sweat and saliva electrolyte values and frequent lower respiratory tract infections mimicking cystic fibrosis. *J.Pediatr.*, Vol.125, No.5 Pt 1, pp. 752-755.

Hayslip, C.C.; Hao, E. & Usala, S.J. (1997). The cystic fibrosis transmembrane regulator gene is expressed in the human endocervix throughout the menstrual cycle. *Fertil.Steril.*, Vol.67, No.4, pp. 636-640.

Hojo, S.; Fujita, J.; Miyawaki, H.; Obayashi, Y.; Takahara, J. & Bartholomew, D.W. (1998). Severe cystic fibrosis associated with a deltaF508/R347H + D979A compound heterozygous genotype. *Clin.Genet.,* Vol.53, No.1, pp. 50-53.

Huber, R.; Krueger, B.; Diakov, A.; Korbmacher, J.; Haerteis, S.; Einsiedel, J.; Gmeiner, P.; Azad, A.K.; Cuppens, H.; Cassiman, J.J.; Korbmacher, C. & Rauh, R. (2010). Functional characterization of a partial loss-of-function mutation of the epithelial sodium channel (ENaC) associated with atypical cystic fibrosis. *Cell Physiol Biochem.,* Vol.25, No.1, pp. 145-158.

Hummler, E.; Barker, P.; Gatzy, J.; Beermann, F.; Verdumo, C.; Schmidt, A.; Boucher, R. & Rossier, B.C. (1996). Early death due to defective neonatal lung liquid clearance in alpha-ENaC-deficient mice. *Nat.Genet.,* Vol.12, No.3, pp. 325-328.

Jakubiczka, S.; Bettecken, T.; Stumm, M.; Nickel, I.; Musebeck, J.; Krebs, P.; Fischer, C.; Kleinstein, J. & Wieacker, P. (1999). Frequency of CFTR gene mutations in males participating in an ICSI programme. *Hum.Reprod.,* Vol.14, No.7, pp. 1833-1834.

Jarvi, K.; McCallum, S.; Zielenski, J.; Durie, P.; Tullis, E.; Wilchanski, M.; Margolis, M.; Asch, M.; Ginzburg, B.; Martin, S.; Buckspan, M.B. & Tsui, L.C. (1998). Heterogeneity of reproductive tract abnormalities in men with absence of the vas deferens: role of cystic fibrosis transmembrane conductance regulator gene mutations. *Fertil.Steril.,* Vol.70, No.4, pp. 724-728.

Johnson, L.G.; Olsen, J.C.; Sarkadi, B.; Moore, K.L.; Swanstrom, R. & Boucher, R.C. (1992). Efficiency of gene transfer for restoration of normal airway epithelial function in cystic fibrosis. *Nat.Genet.,* Vol.2, No.1, pp. 21-25.

Joo N.S.; Irokawa T.; Robbins R.C. & Wine J.J. (2006). Hyposecretion, not hyperabsorption, is the basic defect of cystic fibrosis airway glands. *J. Biol. Chem.,* Vol.281, No.11, pp. 7392-7398.

Kalin, N.; Dork, T. & Tummler, B. (1992). A cystic fibrosis allele encoding missense mutations in both nucleotide binding folds of the cystic fibrosis transmembrane conductance regulator. *Hum.Mutat.,* Vol.1, No.3, pp. 204-210.

Karijolich, J. & Yu, Y.T. (2011). Converting nonsense codons into sense codons by targeted pseudouridylation. *Nature,* Vol.474, No.7351, pp. 395-398.

Kerem, B.; Rommens, J.M.; Buchanan, J.A.; Markiewicz, D.; Cox, T.K.; Chakravarti, A.; Buchwald, M. & Tsui, L.C. (1989). Identification of the cystic fibrosis gene: genetic analysis. *Science,* Vol.245, No.4922, pp. 1073-1080.

Kerem, E. (2005). Pharmacological induction of CFTR function in patients with cystic fibrosis: mutation-specific therapy. *Pediatr.Pulmonol.,* Vol.40, No.3, pp. 183-196.

Kerem, E. (2006). Atypical CF and CF related diseases. *Paediatr.Respir.Rev.,* Vol.7 Suppl 1, pp. S144-S146.

Kiesewetter, S.; Macek, M., Jr.; Davis, C.; Curristin, S.M.; Chu, C.S.; Graham, C.; Shrimpton, A.E.; Cashman, S.M.; Tsui, L.C.; Mickle, J. & . (1993). A mutation in CFTR produces different phenotypes depending on chromosomal background. *Nat.Genet.,* Vol.5, No.3, pp. 274-278.

Kim, D. & Steward, M.C. (2009). The role of CFTR in bicarbonate secretion by pancreatic duct and airway epithelia. *J.Med.Invest,* Vol.56 Suppl, pp. 336-342.

Lai, H.J.; Cheng, Y. & Farrell, P.M. (2005). The survival advantage of patients with cystic fibrosis diagnosed through neonatal screening: evidence from the United States Cystic Fibrosis Foundation registry data. *J.Pediatr.,* Vol.147, No.3 Suppl, pp. S57-S63.

Laroche, D. & Travert, G. (1991). Abnormal frequency of delta F508 mutation in neonatal transitory hypertrypsinaemia. *Lancet,* Vol.337, No.8732, pp. 55.

Le Marechal, C.; Audrezet, M.P.; Quere, I.; Raguenes, O.; Langonne, S. & Ferec, C. (2001). Complete and rapid scanning of the cystic fibrosis transmembrane conductance regulator (CFTR) gene by denaturing high-performance liquid chromatography (D-HPLC): major implications for genetic counselling. *Hum.Genet.,* Vol.108, No.4, pp. 290-298.

Legrys, V.A.; Yankaskas, J.R.; Quittell, L.M.; Marshall, B.C. & Mogayzel, P.J., Jr. (2007). Diagnostic sweat testing: the Cystic Fibrosis Foundation guidelines. *J.Pediatr.,* Vol.151, No.1, pp. 85-89.

Leoni, G.B.; Pitzalis, S.; Podda, R.; Zanda, M.; Silvetti, M.; Caocci, L.; Cao, A. & Rosatelli, M.C. (1995). A specific cystic fibrosis mutation (T3381) associated with the phenotype of isolated hypotonic dehydration. *J.Pediatr.,* Vol.127, No.2, pp. 281-283.

Lucarelli, M.; Grandoni, F.; Rossi, T.; Mazzilli, F.; Antonelli, M. & Strom, R. (2002). Simultaneous cycle sequencing assessment of (TG)m and Tn tract length in CFTR gene. *Biotechniques,* Vol.32, No.3, pp. 540-547.

Lucarelli, M.; Narzi, L.; Pierandrei, S.; Bruno, S.M.; Stamato, A.; d'Avanzo, M.; Strom, R. & Quattrucci, S. (2010). A new complex allele of the CFTR gene partially explains the variable phenotype of the L997F mutation. *Genet.Med.,* Vol.12, No.9, pp. 548-555.

Lucarelli, M.; Narzi, L.; Piergentili, R.; Ferraguti, G.; Grandoni, F.; Quattrucci, S. & Strom, R. (2006). A 96-well formatted method for exon and exon/intron boundary full sequencing of the CFTR gene. *Anal.Biochem.,* Vol.353, No.2, pp. 226-235.

Ludwig, M.; Bolkenius, U.; Wickert, L.; Marynen, P. & Bidlingmaier, F. (1998). Structural organisation of the gene encoding the alpha-subunit of the human amiloride-sensitive epithelial sodium channel. *Hum.Genet.,* Vol.102, No.5, pp. 576-581.

Maire, F.; Bienvenu, T.; Ngukam, A.; Hammel, P.; Ruszniewski, P. & Levy, P. (2003). [Frequency of CFTR gene mutations in idiopathic pancreatitis]. *Gastroenterol.Clin.Biol.,* Vol.27, No.4, pp. 398-402.

Mak, V.; Zielenski, J.; Tsui, L.C.; Durie, P.; Zini, A.; Martin, S.; Longley, T.B. & Jarvi, K.A. (2000). Cystic fibrosis gene mutations and infertile men with primary testicular failure. *Hum.Reprod.,* Vol.15, No.2, pp. 436-439.

Mall, M.; Bleich, M.; Greger, R.; Schreiber, R. & Kunzelmann, K. (1998). The amiloride-inhibitable Na^+ conductance is reduced by the cystic fibrosis transmembrane conductance regulator in normal but not in cystic fibrosis airways. *J.Clin.Invest,* Vol.102, No.1, pp. 15-21.

Massie, R.J.; Poplawski, N.; Wilcken, B.; Goldblatt, J.; Byrnes, C. & Robertson, C. (2001). Intron-8 polythymidine sequence in Australasian individuals with CF mutations R117H and R117C. *Eur.Respir.J.,* Vol.17, No.6, pp. 1195-1200.

Massie, R.J.; Wilcken, B.; Van, A.P.; Dorney, S.; Gruca, M.; Wiley, V. & Gaskin, K. (2000). Pancreatic function and extended mutation analysis in DeltaF508 heterozygous infants with an elevated immunoreactive trypsinogen but normal sweat electrolyte levels. *J.Pediatr.,* Vol.137, No.2, pp. 214-220.

Matsui, H.; Grubb, B.R.; Tarran, R.; Randell, S.H.; Gatzy, J.T.; Davis, C.W. & Boucher, R.C. (1998). Evidence for periciliary liquid layer depletion, not abnormal ion composition, in the pathogenesis of cystic fibrosis airways disease. *Cell,* Vol.95, No.7, pp. 1005-1015.

Mattoscio, D.; Evangelista, V.; De, C.R.; Recchiuti, A.; Pandolfi, A.; Di, S.S.; Manarini, S.; Martelli, N.; Rocca, B.; Petrucci, G.; Angelini, D.F.; Battistini, L.; Robuffo, I.; Pensabene, T.; Pieroni, L.; Furnari, M.L.; Pardo, F.; Quattrucci, S.; Lancellotti, S.; Davi, G. & Romano, M. (2010). Cystic fibrosis transmembrane conductance regulator (CFTR) expression in human platelets: impact on mediators and mechanisms of the inflammatory response. *FASEB J.*, Vol.24, No.10, pp. 3970-3980.

Mayell, S.J.; Munck, A.; Craig, J.V.; Sermet, I.; Brownlee, K.G.; Schwarz, M.J.; Castellani, C. & Southern, K.W. (2009). A European consensus for the evaluation and management of infants with an equivocal diagnosis following newborn screening for cystic fibrosis. *J.Cyst.Fibros.*, Vol.8, No.1, pp. 71-78.

McGinniss, M.J.; Chen, C.; Redman, J.B.; Buller, A.; Quan, F.; Peng, M.; Giusti, R.; Hantash, F.M.; Huang, D.; Sun, W. & Strom, C.M. (2005). Extensive sequencing of the CFTR gene: lessons learned from the first 157 patient samples. *Hum.Genet.*, Vol.118, No.3-4, pp. 331-338.

Mekus, F.; Ballmann, M.; Bronsveld, I.; Dork, T.; Bijman, J.; Tummler, B. & Veeze, H.J. (1998). Cystic-fibrosis-like disease unrelated to the cystic fibrosis transmembrane conductance regulator. *Hum.Genet.*, Vol.102, No.5, pp. 582-586.

Mercier, B.; Verlingue, C.; Lissens, W.; Silber, S.J.; Novelli, G.; Bonduelle, M.; Audrezet, M.P. & Ferec, C. (1995). Is congenital bilateral absence of vas deferens a primary form of cystic fibrosis? Analyses of the CFTR gene in 67 patients. *Am.J.Hum.Genet.*, Vol.56, No.1, pp. 272-277.

Merlo, C.A. & Boyle, M.P. (2003). Modifier genes in cystic fibrosis lung disease. *J.Lab Clin.Med.*, Vol.141, No.4, pp. 237-241.

Mutesa, L.; Azad, A.K.; Verhaeghe, C.; Segers, K.; Vanbellinghen, J.F.; Ngendahayo, L.; Rusingiza, E.K.; Mutwa, P.R.; Rulisa, S.; Koulischer, L.; Cassiman, J.J.; Cuppens, H. & Bours, V. (2008). Genetic Analysis of Rwandan Patients With Cystic Fibrosis-Like Symptoms: Identification of Novel Cystic Fibrosis Transmembrane Conductance Regulator and Epithelial Sodium Channel Gene Variants. *Chest*,

Nagel G.; Barbry P.; Chabot H.; Brochiero E.; Hartung K. & Grygorczyk R. (2005). CFTR fails to inhibit the epithelial sodium channel ENaC expressed in Xenopus laevis oocytes. *J. Physiol.*, Vol.564, No.3, pp. 671-682.

Narzi, L.; Ferraguti, G.; Stamato, A.; Narzi, F.; Valentini, S.B.; Lelli, A.; Delaroche, I.; Lucarelli, M.; Strom, R. & Quattrucci, S. (2007). Does cystic fibrosis neonatal screening detect atypical CF forms? Extended genetic characterization and 4-year clinical follow-up. *Clin.Genet.*, Vol.72, No.1, pp. 39-46.

Narzi, L.; Lucarelli, M.; Lelli, A.; Grandoni, F.; Lo, C.S.; Ferraro, A.; Matarazzo, P.; Delaroche, I.; Quattrucci, S.; Strom, R. & Antonelli, M. (2002). Comparison of two different protocols of neonatal screening for cystic fibrosis. *Clin.Genet.*, Vol.62, No.3, pp. 245-249.

Niel, F.; Legendre, M.; Bienvenu, T.; Bieth, E.; Lalau, G.; Sermet, I.; Bondeux, D.; Boukari, R.; Derelle, J.; Levy, P.; Ruszniewski, P.; Martin, J.; Costa, C.; Goossens, M. & Girodon, E. (2006). A new large CFTR rearrangement illustrates the importance of searching for complex alleles. *Hum.Mutat.*, Vol.27, No.7, pp. 716-717.

Noone, P.G. & Knowles, M.R. (2001). 'CFTR-opathies': disease phenotypes associated with cystic fibrosis transmembrane regulator gene mutations. *Respir.Res.*, Vol.2, No.6, pp. 328-332.

O'Sullivan, B.P. & Freedman, S.D. (2009). Cystic fibrosis. *Lancet,* Vol.373, No.9678, pp. 1891-1904.

Padoan, R.; Bassotti, A.; Seia, M. & Corbetta, C. (2002). Negative sweat test in hypertrypsinaemic infants with cystic fibrosis carrying rare CFTR mutations. *Eur.J.Pediatr.,* Vol.161, No.4, pp. 212-215.

Pallares-Ruiz, N.; Carles, S.; Des, G.M.; Guittard, C.; Arnal, F.; Humeau, C. & Claustres, M. (1999). Complete mutational screening of the cystic fibrosis transmembrane conductance regulator gene: cystic fibrosis mutations are not involved in healthy men with reduced sperm quality. *Hum.Reprod.,* Vol.14, No.12, pp. 3035-3040.

Pallares-Ruiz, N.; Carles, S.; Des, G.M.; Guittard, C.; Claustres, M.; Larrey, D. & Pageaux, G. (2000). Is isolated idiopathic pancreatitis associated with CFTR mutations? *Gut,* Vol.46, No.1, pp. 141.

Parad, R.B. & Comeau, A.M. (2005). Diagnostic dilemmas resulting from the immunoreactive trypsinogen/DNA cystic fibrosis newborn screening algorithm. *J.Pediatr.,* Vol.147, No.3 Suppl, pp. S78-S82.

Patrizio, P. & Salameh, W.A. (1998). Expression of the cystic fibrosis transmembrane conductance regulator (CFTR) mRNA in normal and pathological adult human epididymis. *J.Reprod.Fertil.Suppl,* Vol.53, pp. 261-270.

Pawankar, R. (2003). Nasal polyposis: an update: editorial review. *Curr.Opin.Allergy Clin.Immunol.,* Vol.3, No.1, pp. 1-6.

Peckham, D.; Conway, S.P.; Morton, A.; Jones, A. & Webb, K. (2006). Delayed diagnosis of cystic fibrosis associated with R117H on a background of 7T polythymidine tract at intron 8. *J.Cyst.Fibros.,* Vol.5, No.1, pp. 63-65.

Peters, K.W.; Qi, J.; Johnson, J.P.; Watkins, S.C. & Frizzell, R.A. (2001). Role of snare proteins in CFTR and ENaC trafficking. *Pflugers Arch.,* Vol.443 Suppl 1, pp. S65-S69.

Pier, G.B.; Grout, M. & Zaidi, T.S. (1997). Cystic fibrosis transmembrane conductance regulator is an epithelial cell receptor for clearance of Pseudomonas aeruginosa from the lung. *Proc.Natl.Acad.Sci.U.S.A,* Vol.94, No.22, pp. 12088-12093.

Pignatti, P.F.; Bombieri, C.; Marigo, C.; Benetazzo, M. & Luisetti, M. (1995). Increased incidence of cystic fibrosis gene mutations in adults with disseminated bronchiectasis. *Hum.Mol.Genet.,* Vol.4, No.4, pp. 635-639.

Prince, L.S.; Peter, K.; Hatton, S.R.; Zaliauskiene, L.; Cotlin, L.F.; Clancy, J.P.; Marchase, R.B. & Collawn, J.F. (1999). Efficient endocytosis of the cystic fibrosis transmembrane conductance regulator requires a tyrosine-based signal. *J.Biol.Chem.,* Vol.274, No.6, pp. 3602-3609.

Priou-Guesdon, M.; Malinge, M.C.; Augusto, J.F.; Rodien, P.; Subra, J.F.; Bonneau, D. & Rohmer, V. (2010). Hypochloremia and hyponatremia as the initial presentation of cystic fibrosis in three adults. *Ann.Endocrinol.(Paris),* Vol.71, No.1, pp. 46-50.

Raman, V.; Clary, R.; Siegrist, K.L.; Zehnbauer, B. & Chatila, T.A. (2002). Increased prevalence of mutations in the cystic fibrosis transmembrane conductance regulator in children with chronic rhinosinusitis. *Pediatrics,* Vol.109, No.1, pp. E13.

Ratjen, F. & Doring, G. (2003). Cystic fibrosis. *Lancet,* Vol.361, No.9358, pp. 681-689.

Ravnik-Glavac, M.; Atkinson, A.; Glavac, D. & Dean, M. (2002). DHPLC screening of cystic fibrosis gene mutations. *Hum.Mutat.,* Vol.19, No.4, pp. 374-383.

Ravnik-Glavac, M.; Glavac, D.; Chernick, M.; di, S.P. & Dean, M. (1994). Screening for CF mutations in adult cystic fibrosis patients with a directed and optimized SSCP strategy. *Hum.Mutat.,* Vol.3, No.3, pp. 231-238.

Riordan, J.R. (2008). CFTR function and prospects for therapy. *Annu.Rev.Biochem.*, Vol.77, pp. 701-726.

Rogan, M.P.; Stoltz, D.A. & Hornick, D.B. (2011). Cystic fibrosis transmembrane conductance regulator intracellular processing, trafficking, and opportunities for mutation-specific treatment. *Chest*, Vol.139, No.6, pp. 1480-1490.

Rohlfs, E.M.; Zhou, Z.; Sugarman, E.A.; Heim, R.A.; Pace, R.G.; Knowles, M.R.; Silverman, L.M. & Allitto, B.A. (2002). The I148T CFTR allele occurs on multiple haplotypes: a complex allele is associated with cystic fibrosis. *Genet.Med.*, Vol.4, No.5, pp. 319-323.

Romey, M.C.; Guittard, C.; Chazalette, J.P.; Frossard, P.; Dawson, K.P.; Patton, M.A.; Casals, T.; Bazarbachi, T.; Girodon, E.; Rault, G.; Bozon, D.; Seguret, F.; Demaille, J. & Claustres, M. (1999). Complex allele [-102T>A+S549R(T>G)] is associated with milder forms of cystic fibrosis than allele S549R(T>G) alone. *Hum.Genet.*, Vol.105, No.1-2, pp. 145-150.

Rommens, J.M.; Iannuzzi, M.C.; Kerem, B.; Drumm, M.L.; Melmer, G.; Dean, M.; Rozmahel, R.; Cole, J.L.; Kennedy, D.; Hidaka, N. & . (1989). Identification of the cystic fibrosis gene: chromosome walking and jumping. *Science*, Vol.245, No.4922, pp. 1059-1065.

Rossi, T.; Grandoni, F.; Mazzilli, F.; Quattrucci, S.; Antonelli, M.; Strom, R. & Lucarelli, M. (2004). High frequency of (TG)mTn variant tracts in the cystic fibrosis transmembrane conductance regulator gene in men with high semen viscosity. *Fertil.Steril.*, Vol.82, No.5, pp. 1316-1322.

Rubenstein, R.C.; Lockwood, S.R.; Lide, E.; Bauer, R.; Suaud, L. & Grumbach, Y. (2011). Regulation of endogenous ENaC functional expression by CFTR and DeltaF508-CFTR in airway epithelial cells. *Am.J.Physiol Lung Cell Mol.Physiol*, Vol.300, No.1, pp. L88-L101.

Salvatore, D.; Buzzetti, R.; Baldo, E.; Forneris, M.P.; Lucidi, V.; Manunza, D.; Marinelli, I.; Messore, B.; Neri, A.S.; Raia, V.; Furnari, M.L. & Mastella, G. (2011). An overview of international literature from cystic fibrosis registries. Part 3. Disease incidence, genotype/phenotype correlation, microbiology, pregnancy, clinical complications, lung transplantation, and miscellanea. *J.Cyst.Fibros.*, Vol.10, No.2, pp. 71-85.

Salvatore, D.; Tomaiuolo, R.; Abate, R.; Vanacore, B.; Manieri, S.; Mirauda, M.P.; Scavone, A.; Schiavo, M.V.; Castaldo, G. & Salvatore, F. (2004). Cystic fibrosis presenting as metabolic alkalosis in a boy with the rare D579G mutation. *J.Cyst.Fibros.*, Vol.3, No.2, pp. 135-136.

Salvatore, F.; Scudiero, O. & Castaldo, G. (2002). Genotype-phenotype correlation in cystic fibrosis: the role of modifier genes. *Am.J.Med.Genet.*, Vol.111, No.1, pp. 88-95.

Sangiuolo, F.; Bruscia, E.; Serafino, A.; Nardone, A.M.; Bonifazi, E.; Lais, M.; Gruenert, D.C. & Novelli, G. (2002). In vitro correction of cystic fibrosis epithelial cell lines by small fragment homologous replacement (SFHR) technique. *BMC.Med.Genet.*, Vol.3, pp. 8.

Sangiuolo, F.; Scaldaferri, M.L.; Filareto, A.; Spitalieri, P.; Guerra, L.; Favia, M.; Caroppo, R.; Mango, R.; Bruscia, E.; Gruenert, D.C.; Casavola, V.; De, F.M. & Novelli, G. (2008). Cftr gene targeting in mouse embryonic stem cells mediated by Small Fragment Homologous Replacement (SFHR). *Front Biosci.*, Vol.13, pp. 2989-2999.

Savov, A.; Angelicheva, D.; Balassopoulou, A.; Jordanova, A.; Noussia-Arvanitakis, S. & Kalaydjieva, L. (1995). Double mutant alleles: are they rare? *Hum.Mol.Genet.*, Vol.4, No.7, pp. 1169-1171.

Schroeder, T.H.; Lee, M.M.; Yacono, P.W.; Cannon, C.L.; Gerceker, A.A.; Golan, D.E. & Pier, G.B. (2002). CFTR is a pattern recognition molecule that extracts Pseudomonas aeruginosa LPS from the outer membrane into epithelial cells and activates NF-kappa B translocation. *Proc.Natl.Acad.Sci.U.S.A,* Vol.99, No.10, pp. 6907-6912.

Scotet, V.; De Braekeleer, M.; Audrezet, M.P.; Lode, L.; Verlingue, C.; Quere, I.; Mercier, B.; Dugueperoux, I.; Codet, J.P.; Moineau, M.P.; Parent, P. & Ferec, C. (2001). Prevalence of CFTR mutations in hypertrypsinaemia detected through neonatal screening for cystic fibrosis. *Clin.Genet.,* Vol.59, No.1, pp. 42-47.

Seidler, U.; Singh, A.K.; Cinar, A.; Chen, M.; Hillesheim, J.; Hogema, B. & Riederer, B. (2009). The role of the NHERF family of PDZ scaffolding proteins in the regulation of salt and water transport. *Ann.N.Y.Acad.Sci.,* Vol.1165, pp. 249-260.

Sermet-Gaudelus, I.; Mayell, S.J. & Southern, K.W. (2010). Guidelines on the early management of infants diagnosed with cystic fibrosis following newborn screening. *J.Cyst.Fibros.,* Vol.9, No.5, pp. 323-329.

Sharma, M.; Benharouga, M.; Hu, W. & Lukacs, G.L. (2001). Conformational and temperature-sensitive stability defects of the delta F508 cystic fibrosis transmembrane conductance regulator in post-endoplasmic reticulum compartments. *J.Biol.Chem.,* Vol.276, No.12, pp. 8942-8950.

Sheridan, M.B.; Fong, P.; Groman, J.D.; Conrad, C.; Flume, P.; Diaz, R.; Harris, C.; Knowles, M. & Cutting, G.R. (2005). Mutations in the beta-subunit of the epithelial Na^+ channel in patients with a cystic fibrosis-like syndrome. *Hum.Mol.Genet.,* Vol.14, No.22, pp. 3493-3498.

Sheth, S.; Shea, J.C.; Bishop, M.D.; Chopra, S.; Regan, M.M.; Malmberg, E.; Walker, C.; Ricci, R.; Tsui, L.C.; Durie, P.R.; Zielenski, J. & Freedman, S.D. (2003). Increased prevalence of CFTR mutations and variants and decreased chloride secretion in primary sclerosing cholangitis. *Hum.Genet.,* Vol.113, No.3, pp. 286-292.

Shimkets, R.A.; Warnock, D.G.; Bositis, C.M.; Nelson-Williams, C.; Hansson, J.H.; Schambelan, M.; Gill, J.R., Jr.; Ulick, S.; Milora, R.V.; Findling, J.W. & . (1994). Liddle's syndrome: heritable human hypertension caused by mutations in the beta subunit of the epithelial sodium channel. *Cell,* Vol.79, No.3, pp. 407-414.

Slieker, M.G.; Sanders, E.A.; Rijkers, G.T.; Ruven, H.J. & van der Ent, C.K. (2005). Disease modifying genes in cystic fibrosis. *J.Cyst.Fibros.,* Vol.4 Suppl 2, pp. 7-13.

Southern, K.W. (2007). Cystic fibrosis and formes frustes of CFTR-related disease. *Respiration,* Vol.74, No.3, pp. 241-251.

Southern, K.W.; Munck, A.; Pollitt, R.; Travert, G.; Zanolla, L.; nkert-Roelse, J. & Castellani, C. (2007). A survey of newborn screening for cystic fibrosis in Europe. *J.Cyst.Fibros.,* Vol.6, No.1, pp. 57-65.

Steiner, B.; Rosendahl, J.; Witt, H.; Teich, N.; Keim, V.; Schulz, H.U.; Pfutzer, R.; Luhr, M.; Gress, T.M.; Nickel, R.; Landt, O.; Koudova, M.; Macek, M., Jr.; Farre, A.; Casals, T.; Desax, M.C.; Gallati, S.; Gomez-Lira, M.; Audrezet, M.P.; Ferec, C.; Des, G.M.; Claustres, M. & Truninger, K. (2011). Common CFTR haplotypes and susceptibility to chronic pancreatitis and congenital bilateral absence of the vas deferens. *Hum.Mutat.,* Vol.32, No.8, pp. 912-920.

Steiner, B.; Truninger, K.; Sanz, J.; Schaller, A. & Gallati, S. (2004). The role of common single-nucleotide polymorphisms on exon 9 and exon 12 skipping in nonmutated CFTR alleles. *Hum.Mutat.,* Vol.24, No.2, pp. 120-129.

Stuhrmann, M. & Dork, T. (2000). CFTR gene mutations and male infertility. *Andrologia,* Vol.32, No.2, pp. 71-83.

Stutts, M.J.; Canessa, C.M.; Olsen, J.C.; Hamrick, M.; Cohn, J.A.; Rossier, B.C. & Boucher, R.C. (1995). CFTR as a cAMP-dependent regulator of sodium channels. *Science,* Vol.269, No.5225, pp. 847-850.

Su, Z.; Ning, B.; Fang, H.; Hong, H.; Perkins, R.; Tong, W. & Shi, L. (2011). Next-generation sequencing and its applications in molecular diagnostics. *Expert.Rev.Mol.Diagn.,* Vol.11, No.3, pp. 333-343.

Tang, B.L.; Gee, H.Y. & Lee, M.G. (2011). The cystic fibrosis transmembrane conductance regulator's expanding SNARE interactome. *Traffic.,* Vol.12, No.4, pp. 364-371.

Teem, J.L.; Berger, H.A.; Ostedgaard, L.S.; Rich, D.P.; Tsui, L.C. & Welsh, M.J. (1993). Identification of revertants for the cystic fibrosis delta F508 mutation using STE6-CFTR chimeras in yeast. *Cell,* Vol.73, No.2, pp. 335-346.

Thomas, C.P.; Loftus, R.W.; Liu, K.Z. & Itani, O.A. (2002). Genomic organization of the 5' end of human beta-ENaC and preliminary characterization of its promoter. *Am.J.Physiol Renal Physiol,* Vol.282, No.5, pp. F898-F909.

Tomaiuolo, A.C.; Alghisi, F.; Petrocchi, S.; Surace, C.; Roberti, M.C.; Bella, S.; Lucidi, V. & Angioni, A. (2010). Clinical hallmarks and genetic polymorphisms in the CFTR gene contribute to the disclosure of the A1006E mutation. *Clin.Invest Med.,* Vol.33, No.4, pp. E234-E239.

Tomaiuolo, R.; Spina, M. & Castaldo, G. (2003). Molecular diagnosis of cystic fibrosis: comparison of four analytical procedures. *Clin.Chem.Lab Med.,* Vol.41, No.1, pp. 26-32.

Trezise, A.E.; Chambers, J.A.; Wardle, C.J.; Gould, S. & Harris, A. (1993a). Expression of the cystic fibrosis gene in human foetal tissues. *Hum.Mol.Genet.,* Vol.2, No.3, pp. 213-218.

Trezise, A.E.; Linder, C.C.; Grieger, D.; Thompson, E.W.; Meunier, H.; Griswold, M.D. & Buchwald, M. (1993b). CFTR expression is regulated during both the cycle of the seminiferous epithelium and the oestrous cycle of rodents. *Nat.Genet.,* Vol.3, No.2, pp. 157-164.

van der Ven, K.; Messer, L.; van, d., V; Jeyendran, R.S. & Ober, C. (1996). Cystic fibrosis mutation screening in healthy men with reduced sperm quality. *Hum.Reprod.,* Vol.11, No.3, pp. 513-517.

Vankeerberghen, A.; Cuppens, H. & Cassiman, J.J. (2002). The cystic fibrosis transmembrane conductance regulator: an intriguing protein with pleiotropic functions. *J.Cyst.Fibros.,* Vol.1, No.1, pp. 13-29.

Voilley, N.; Bassilana, F.; Mignon, C.; Merscher, S.; Mattei, M.G.; Carle, G.F.; Lazdunski, M. & Barbry, P. (1995). Cloning, chromosomal localization, and physical linkage of the beta and gamma subunits (SCNN1B and SCNN1G) of the human epithelial amiloride-sensitive sodium channel. *Genomics,* Vol.28, No.3, pp. 560-565.

Voilley, N.; Lingueglia, E.; Champigny, G.; Mattei, M.G.; Waldmann, R.; Lazdunski, M. & Barbry, P. (1994). The lung amiloride-sensitive Na^+ channel: biophysical properties, pharmacology, ontogenesis, and molecular cloning. *Proc.Natl.Acad.Sci.U.S.A,* Vol.91, No.1, pp. 247-251.

Wagner, K.; Greil, I.; Schneditz, P.; Pommer, M. & Rosenkranz, W. (1994). A cystic fibrosis patient with delta F508, G542X and a deletion at the D7S8 locus. *Hum.Mutat.,* Vol.3, No.3, pp. 327-329.

Wang, S.; Yue, H.; Derin, R.B.; Guggino, W.B. & Li, M. (2000a). Accessory protein facilitated CFTR-CFTR interaction, a molecular mechanism to potentiate the chloride channel activity. *Cell,* Vol.103, No.1, pp. 169-179.

Wang, X.; Moylan, B.; Leopold, D.A.; Kim, J.; Rubenstein, R.C.; Togias, A.; Proud, D.; Zeitlin, P.L. & Cutting, G.R. (2000b). Mutation in the gene responsible for cystic fibrosis and predisposition to chronic rhinosinusitis in the general population. *JAMA,* Vol.284, No.14, pp. 1814-1819.

Wang, X.; Venable, J.; LaPointe, P.; Hutt, D.M.; Koulov, A.V.; Coppinger, J.; Gurkan, C.; Kellner, W.; Matteson, J.; Plutner, H.; Riordan, J.R.; Kelly, J.W.; Yates, J.R., III & Balch, W.E. (2006). Hsp90 cochaperone Aha1 downregulation rescues misfolding of CFTR in cystic fibrosis. *Cell,* Vol.127, No.4, pp. 803-815.

Wei, L.; Vankeerberghen, A.; Jaspers, M.; Cassiman, J.; Nilius, B. & Cuppens, H. (2000). Suppressive interactions between mutations located in the two nucleotide binding domains of CFTR. *FEBS Lett.,* Vol.473, No.2, pp. 149-153.

Weixel, K.M. & Bradbury, N.A. (2000). The carboxyl terminus of the cystic fibrosis transmembrane conductance regulator binds to AP-2 clathrin adaptors. *J.Biol.Chem.,* Vol.275, No.5, pp. 3655-3660.

Xu, W.; Hui, C.; Yu, S.S.; Jing, C. & Chan, H.C. (2011a). MicroRNAs and cystic fibrosis--an epigenetic perspective. *Cell Biol.Int.,* Vol.35, No.5, pp. 463-466.

Xu, W.M.; Chen, J.; Chen, H.; Diao, R.Y.; Fok, K.L.; Dong, J.D.; Sun, T.T.; Chen, W.Y.; Yu, M.K.; Zhang, X.H.; Tsang, L.L.; Lau, A.; Shi, Q.X.; Shi, Q.H.; Huang, P.B. & Chan, H.C. (2011b). Defective CFTR-dependent CREB activation results in impaired spermatogenesis and azoospermia. *PLoS.ONE.,* Vol.6, No.5, pp. e19120.

Xu, W.M.; Shi, Q.X.; Chen, W.Y.; Zhou, C.X.; Ni, Y.; Rowlands, D.K.; Yi, L.G.; Zhu, H.; Ma, Z.G.; Wang, X.F.; Chen, Z.H.; Zhou, S.C.; Dong, H.S.; Zhang, X.H.; Chung, Y.W.; Yuan, Y.Y.; Yang, W.X. & Chan, H.C. (2007). Cystic fibrosis transmembrane conductance regulator is vital to sperm fertilizing capacity and male fertility. *Proc.Natl.Acad.Sci.U.S.A,* Vol.104, No.23, pp. 9816-9821.

Yoshimura, K.; Nakamura, H.; Trapnell, B.C.; Chu, C.S.; Dalemans, W.; Pavirani, A.; Lecocq, J.P. & Crystal, R.G. (1991a). Expression of the cystic fibrosis transmembrane conductance regulator gene in cells of non-epithelial origin. *Nucleic Acids Res.,* Vol.19, No.19, pp. 5417-5423.

Yoshimura, K.; Nakamura, H.; Trapnell, B.C.; Dalemans, W.; Pavirani, A.; Lecocq, J.P. & Crystal, R.G. (1991b). The cystic fibrosis gene has a "housekeeping"-type promoter and is expressed at low levels in cells of epithelial origin. *J.Biol.Chem.,* Vol.266, No.14, pp. 9140-9144.

Yueksekdag, G.; Drechsel, M.; Rossner, M.; Schmidt, C.; Kormann, M.; Illenyi, M.C.; Rudolph, C. & Rosenecker, J. (2010). Repeated siRNA application is a precondition for successful mRNA gammaENaC knockdown in the murine airways. *Eur.J.Pharm.Biopharm.,* Vol.75, No.3, pp. 305-310.

Zhang, L.; Button, B.; Gabriel, S.E.; Burkett, S.; Yan, Y.; Skiadopoulos, M.H.; Dang, Y.L.; Vogel, L.N.; McKay, T.; Mengos, A.; Boucher, R.C.; Collins, P.L. & Pickles, R.J. (2009). CFTR delivery to 25% of surface epithelial cells restores normal rates of mucus transport to human cystic fibrosis airway epithelium. *PLoS.Biol.,* Vol.7, No.7, pp. e1000155.

Zhang, L.N.; Karp, P.; Gerard, C.J.; Pastor, E.; Laux, D.; Munson, K.; Yan, Z.; Liu, X.; Godwin, S.; Thomas, C.P.; Zabner, J.; Shi, H.; Caldwell, C.W.; Peluso, R.; Carter, B.

& Engelhardt, J.F. (2004). Dual therapeutic utility of proteasome modulating agents for pharmaco-gene therapy of the cystic fibrosis airway. *Mol.Ther.,* Vol.10, No.6, pp. 990-1002.

Zhou, Z.; Treis, D.; Schubert, S.C.; Harm, M.; Schatterny, J.; Hirtz, S.; Duerr, J.; Boucher, R.C. & Mall, M.A. (2008). Preventive but not late amiloride therapy reduces morbidity and mortality of lung disease in betaENaC-overexpressing mice. *Am.J.Respir.Crit Care Med.,* Vol.178, No.12, pp. 1245-1256.

Zielenski, J.; Rozmahel, R.; Bozon, D.; Kerem, B.; Grzelczak, Z.; Riordan, J.R.; Rommens, J. & Tsui, L.C. (1991). Genomic DNA sequence of the cystic fibrosis transmembrane conductance regulator (CFTR) gene. *Genomics,* Vol.10, No.1, pp. 214-228.

Websites

Consortium for CF genetic analysis database
http://www.genet.sickkids.on.ca/cftr/Home.html

Ensembl
http://www.ensembl.org/Homo_sapiens/Gene/Summary?db=core;g=ENSG00000001626;r=7:117105838-117308719

European CF thematic network
http://cf.eqascheme.org/info/public/index.xhtml

European CF society
http://www.ecfs.eu/

Human gene mutation database (HGMD)
http://www.hgmd.org/

OMIM
http://omim.org/entry/602421

U.S. CF Foundation drug development pipeline
http://www.cff.org/treatments/Pipeline/

U.S. National Institutes of Health Clinical Trials registry and database
http://www.clinicaltrials.gov/ct2/results?term=Cystic+Fibrosis

6

Biochemical and Molecular Genetic Testing Used in the Diagnosis and Assessment of Cystic Fibrosis

Donovan McGrowder
Department of Pathology, Faculty of Medical Sciences, University of the West Indies, Mona Campus, Kingston, Jamaica

1. Introduction

1.1 Mutations in the CFTR gene

Cystic fibrosis (CF) is the most common life-threatening autosomal recessive genetic disease among the Caucasian population, with an estimated incidence throughout the world of between 0.25 - 5 per 10,000 live births (Lewis et al., 1995). It is caused by mutations on both CF transmembrane conductance regulator (CFTR) alleles, resulting in pancreatic exocrine insufficiency in 95% of patients, abnormal sweat electrolytes, sino-pulmonary disease and male infertility (MacCready, 1963). In its classic form, this multi-system disease is characterized by one or more of several features varying in severity, including a progressive decline of pulmonary function secondary to chronic lung infections, pancreatic exocrine insufficiency leading to malnutrition and growth impairment, liver disease, and decreased reabsorption of chloride ions from sweat (Zielenski et al., 2000). The disease is easily diagnosed early in life, through a combination of clinical evaluation and laboratory testing including sweat testing and CFTR mutation analysis (Ross, 2008). However, 7% of CF patients are not diagnosed until age 10 years, with a proportion not diagnosed until after age 15 years. Because the phenotype in these patients may vary widely some of these patients present a considerable challenge in establishing a diagnosis of CF (Wilcken et al., 1995; Hammond et al., 1991).

The heterogeneity of CF disease is partially explained by the identification of 1890 mutations in the CFTR gene (Cystic Fibrosis Mutation Database). The delta F508 (ΔF508) mutation, the most common CF allele is a 3-base pair deletion in exon 10 causing a loss of phenylalanine at the amino acid position 508 of the protein product (Kerem et al., 1989). The ΔF508 mutation reaches frequencies of 70% or more in northern European populations, with lower frequencies in southern European populations. In the United States of America (USA), two-thirds of patients carry at least one copy of the ΔF508 mutation, with approximately 50% of CF patients being homozygous for this mutation (Crossley et al., 1979). Other common mutations existing in most populations include G542X, G551D, R553X, W1282X and N1303K. These mutations have population frequencies of approximately 1 - 2% (De Boeck, 2006).

The CFTR gene consists of a TATA-less promoter and 27 exons spanning about 215 kb of genomic sequence (Zielenski et al., 1991). It encodes a transmembrane protein with a symmetrical, multi-domain structure, consisting of two nucleotide-binding domains (NBD1, NBD2), two membrane-spanning domains (MSD1, MSD2), and a central, highly charged regulatory domain (R) with multiple phosphorylation consensus sites (Riordan et al., 1989). The principal function of CFTR is that of cyclic adenosine-5'-monophosphate (cAMP)-regulated chloride transport at the apical membranes of epithelial cells. It has also been implicated in many other processes such as membrane trafficking regulation of other ion channels and pH, and apoptosis (Quinton, 1999; Sheppard & Welsh, 1999).

Mutations in CFTR may result in: (1) defective processing of CFTR, such as ΔF508 or G480C, where the mutant protein is not processed to its mature glycosylated form and is not correctly localised to the apical membrane, but is retained in the endoplasmic reticulum and degraded, (2) defective CFTR production, such as R553X, due to unstable messenger ribonucleic acid (mRNA) and/or premature protein truncation and/or (3) defective ion channel function, such as G551D or R117H, in which case some of the mutant protein becomes correctly localised but results in either very little residual function (in the case of G551D) or a substantially reduced level of ion transport (in the case of R117H). In each class of mutation the level of functional CFTR at the apical membrane of epithelial cells in CF patients falls below a critical level, resulting in the characteristic clinical abnormalities observed in the organs in which CFTR is expressed (Comeau et al., 2004).

Mutations in CFTR result in abnormalities in epithelial ion and water transport, which are associated with derangements in airway mucociliary clearance and other cellular functions related to normal cell biology (Sontag et al., 2005). Furthermore, mutations in the CFTR gene can alter the structure, function, or production of a cAMP-dependent trans-membrane chloride channel protein that is critical for normal functioning of multiple organs. The organs and systems that are affected in CF include: pancreas, liver, sweat glands, genitourinary and gastrointestinal tracts, the lungs and upper respiratory tract (Welsh et al., 2001). It is the involvement of the latter which leads to most morbidity and is the most common cause of death. A large retrospective cohort study of approximately 17,000 patients from the USA CF Foundation National Registry, confirmed that the CFTR genotype affects mortality (McKone et al., 2003).

Extensive genetic studies have produced both greater awareness of the spectrum of mutations in specific population groups (Alper et al., 2004) and increased the understanding of genotype-phenotype relationships (Groman et al., 2005; Mickle, 2000), illuminating distinctions between CFTR mutations with limited or no functional effects and those known or predicted to cause CF disease. Most classically diagnosed patients with CF carry severe loss-of-function mutations on both alleles and have evidence of pancreatic insufficiency (Kerem et al., 1999). Those with non-classic CF carry a mild CFTR gene mutation on at least one allele, and usually retain sufficient residual pancreatic function to confer pancreatic sufficiency (Cystic Fibrosis Genotype-Phenotype Consortium, 1993; Zielenski, 2000). Both pancreatic insufficiency and sufficiency are associated with specific CFTR mutations.

The CFTR gene mutations have been placed into five classes depending on their effect on the CFTR protein (Welsh et al., 2001). Classes I – III are associated with complete loss of cAMP-regulated chloride channel function and are identified as "severe" mutations. Class I mutations lead to defective protein production, class II to defective protein maturation and processing, and class III to defective channel regulation/gating. Mutations in classes IV - V might allow for residual CFTR function, and lead to altered channel conductance in class IV and altered protein stability in class V. They are usually associated with milder phenotypes and pancreatic sufficiency (Welsh et al., 2001; Ahmed et al., 2003). Persons who have two mutations from within classes I, II, or III almost invariably experience pancreatic insufficiency, and those with < 2 mutations from classes IV or V usually maintain pancreatic insufficiency. The common ΔF508 mutation is a class II mutation that is associated with pancreatic insufficiency (Ahmed et al., 2003).

The sensitivity of a given DNA mutation panel for detecting persons with CF varies by race and ethnicity as different populations have different mutation frequencies. The inclusion of mutations specific to racial and ethnic minority populations can improve detection of CF among those populations (Bobadilla et al., 2002). Data from US newborn screening programs showed that birth prevalence is 1/2,500 - 3,500 births among non-Hispanic whites, 1/4,000 - 10,000 births among Hispanics, and 1/15,000 - 20,000 births among non-Hispanic Blacks (Comeau et al., 2004; Parad & Comeau, 2003). Non-Hispanic Whites constituted >90% of USA patients who received a diagnosis of CF (Cystic Fibrosis Foundation, 2001).

The spectrum of CFTR mutation frequencies varies in populations of each ethnicity, and a large proportion of CFTR mutations is still unidentified in Hispanic and Black people. Heim and colleagues in their study used a 70- and 86-DNA mutation panel, and reported a detection rate of 62% in Black infants, 58% in Hispanic infants, 38% in Asian infants, and 81% in Native American infants in the USA compared with 85% in White infants and 95% in Ashkenazi Jewish infants (Heim et al., 2001). Identification of infants with CF can be enhanced by choosing an appropriate mutation panel. A 75% detection rate can be achieved in Black populations by screening for 16 "common white" mutations and 8 "common African" mutations (Macek et al., 1997).

This review will examine the advances in adult and newborn screening for CF that are reported in the literature such as the use of genetic testing techniques to identify CFTR gene mutations. It will also critically examine the use of biochemical tests capable of diagnosis, detecting and monitoring the end-organ disease processes in patients with CF. These tests include sweat test, immunoreactive trypsinogen (IRT), nasal potential difference (NPD), pancreatic associated protein (PAP) and intestinal current measurement (ICM).

2. Analysis of CFTR gene mutations for diagnostic purposes

2.1 Mutations within the CFTR gene

According to The Cystic Fibrosis Genetic Analysis Consortium (1994), the ΔF508 mutation, the most common CFTR defect identified among Caucasians accounted for 66% of 43,849 tested CF chromosomes (The Cystic Fibrosis Genetic Analysis Consortium, 1994). However its occurrence varies considerably between geographical locations and different populations with the lowest reported incidence in Tunisia (17.9%) and highest in Denmark (90%) (Messaoud et al., 1996; Schwartz et al., 1990). The spectrum of remaining CFTR mutations is highly variable and is represented by a large number of rare alleles. All types of mutations are represented (missense, frameshift, nonsense, splice, small and large in-frame deletions or insertions), and are distributed throughout the entire gene (The Cystic Fibrosis Genetic Analysis Consortium, 1994).

A mutation detection rate of 90% in a specific population signifies that a mutation will be identified on both CFTR genes in 81% of the typical CF patients; a mutation will be found on only one CFTR gene in 18%; and no mutation will be found on either CFTR gene in 1% (De Boeck et al., 2006). Although currently available mutation screening panels can identify 90% of CFTR mutations, 9.7% of genotyped individuals in the Cystic Fibrosis Foundation Patient Registry have at least 1 un-identified mutation (Cystic Fibrosis Foundation Patient Registry, 2005).

2.2 Techniques used to analyze and detect CFTR gene mutations

The analysis and interpretation of CF genotype information requires the use of appropriate testing techniques to identify CFTR mutations, standardized criteria for defining a CF-causing mutation, and an understanding of the contribution of the genetic background to the phenotypic variability of CF. Rapid accurate identification of CFTR gene mutations is important for confirming the clinical diagnosis, for cascade screening in families at risk for CF, for understanding the correlation between genotype and phenotype, and moreover it is also the only means for prenatal diagnosis (Kolesár et al., 2008). The scanning of the whole coding region of the CFTR gene permits to identify about 90% of alleles from patients bearing CF and a lower percentage in patients bearing atypical CF. Several techniques such as allele specific oligonucleotide (ASO) dot-blot, reverse dot-blot, amplification refractory mutation (ARMS), and an oligo-ligation assay, are available to detect the most common mutations (Eshaque & Dixon, 2006). The ARMS is routinely used for the identification of specific mutations within genomes. This polymerase chain reaction (PCR)-based assay, although simple, is performed at a low-throughput scale, usually requiring gel-electrophoresis for the identification of specific mutations (Eaker et al., 2005). An extensive mutation screening of both CFTR genes may be required with assays such as single strand conformation polymorphism (SSCP) assay, sequencing, denaturing gradient gel electrophoresis (DGGE) and denaturing high pressure liquid chromatography (DHPLC) (Cuppens et al., 1993; Le Mare´chal et al., 2001). Sequencing approaches 100% sensitivity while the other techniques are indirect mutation scanning assays with sensitivities varying from close to 100% to as low as 90%. Other available commercial assays for CFTR mutation screening include the INNO-LiPA CFTR Assay (Innogenetics NV, Technologiepark, Gent, Belgium), oligonucleotide ligation assay (OLA) Cystic Fibrosis Assay (Abbott Laboratories, Abbott Park, Illinois, USA), and the Elucigene CF Assay (Tepnel Diagnostics Ltd, Oxon, UK). Most of these tests only screen for about 30 mutations, the majority of which are associated with classic CF (Dequeker et al., 2000).

A number of methods have been proposed for the detection of ΔF508. The multiplex ARMS analysis identified the ΔF508 mutation at an allele frequency of 24.0% in Indian CF cases (Ashavaid et al., 2005). Another study has reported that quantitative real-time PCR with melting curve analysis is a reliable and fast method for the detection of ΔF508 mutation. By using this method, the results are ready in 1 h following the DNA isolation. The applied primer-probe set with melting curve analysis gives additional information for the presence of other mutations in the ΔF508del region (Nagy et al., 2007). Furthermore, the ΔF508 mutation has been identified by PCR-SSCP. The appropriate 98 bp region of the CFTR gene was amplified by PCR and the reaction products were analysed by SSCP-electrophoresis using silver staining for band visualization. Single-strand DNA fragments gave a reproducible pattern of bands, characteristic for the ΔF508 mutation (Kakavas et al., 2006). However, detecting compound heterozygotes between ΔF508 and other mutations which are rare is difficult as some mutations are common only to particular ethnic groups. Therefore, diagnostic tests such as restriction enzyme assays and SSCP have been designed to recognize rare and population-specific mutations (Eshaque & Dixon, 2006).

2.3 Analysis, spectrum and frequency of CFTR mutations in different populations

One challenging aspect of genetic analysis as it relates to CF is the identification of CF mutations in some populations. There are a number of studies that have examined the spectrum and frequency of mutations in different countries. In a study conducted in Minas Gerais State, Brazil, the frequency of 8 mutations (ΔF508, G542X, R1162X, N1303K, W1282X, G85E, 3120+1G>A, and 711+1G>T) was analyzed using by ASO-PCR with specially designed primers in 111 newborn patients. An allele frequency of 48.2% was observed for the ΔF508 mutation, and allele frequencies of 5.41%, 4.50%, 4.05%, and 3.60% were found for the R1162X, G542X, 3120+1G>A, and G85E mutations, respectively (Perone et al., 2010). Mutational analysis of the CFTR gene was performed in 49 Lithuanian CF patients through a combined approach of ASO-PCR and DGGE analysis. A CFTR mutation was characterized in 62.2% of CF chromosomes and ΔF508 (52.0%) was the most frequent Lithuanian CF mutation. Seven CFTR mutations, N1303K (2.0%), R75Q (1.0%), G314R (1.0%), R553X (4.2%), W1282X (1.0%), and 3944delGT (1.0%), accounted for 10.1% of Lithuanian CF chromosomes (Giannattasio et al., 2006).

There is a reported high incidence of the CFTR mutations 3272-26A-->G and L927P in Belgian CF patients. The technique DGGE was used to extensively analyse the CFTR gene in those patients with at least one unknown mutation after preliminary screening. There was also the identification of three new CFTR mutations (186-2A-->G, E588V, and 1671insTATCA). The mutation, 3272-26A-->G has a frequency of 3.8%, while L927P, 2.4% (Storm et al., 2007). In another study, different methods, such as ARMS-PCR, SSCP analysis, restriction enzyme digestion analysis, direct sequencing, and MLPA (Multiplex Ligation-mediated Probe Amplification) were used to analyse mutations in the complete coding region, and its exon/intron junctions, of the CFTR gene in 69 Iranian CF patients. CFTR mutation analysis revealed the identification of 37 mutations with a CFTR mutation detection rate of 81.9% (Alibakhsh et al., 2007). The most common mutations were ΔF508 (18.1%), 2183AA>G (6.5%), S466X (5.8%), N1303K (4.3%), 2789+5G>A (4.3%), G542X (3.6%), 3120+1G>A (3.6%), R334W (2.9%) and 3130delA (2.9%). These 9 types of mutant CFTR genes accounted for 52.0% of all CFTR genes derived from the Iranian CF patients (Alibakhsh et al., 2007).

Extensive CFTR gene sequencing can detect rare mutations which are not found with other screening and diagnostic tests, and can thus establish a definitive diagnosis in symptomatic patients with previously negative results. This enables carrier detection and prenatal diagnosis in additional family members (McGinniss et al., 2005). Prenatal diagnosis and carrier screening of relatives can be performed by segregation analysis of polymorphisms within or linked to the CFTR gene. Most commercial tests screen for the T5 allele, a splicing error in intron 8 that is considered to be a mild mutation with an incomplete penetrance (Rave-Harel et al., 1997). The T5 polymorphism is found on about 5% of the CFTR genes in the general White ethnic population, but on about 21% of the CFTR genes derived from patients with congenital bilateral absence of the vas deferens (CBAVD) (Chillo'n et al., 1995) and it may even confer non-classic CF (Cuppens et al., 1998; Noone et al., 2000). In most cases the partial penetrance is explained by the polymorphic TGm locus (11, 12 or 13 TG repeats) in front of the T5 allele. Analysis of the TGm locus can be accurately determined by sequencing (De Boeck et al., 2006). A higher number of TG repeats also results in less efficient splicing of CFTR transcripts (Cuppens et al., 1998). In patients with CBAVD and non-classic CF, the milder TG11-T5 allele is infrequent while the TG12-T5 allele is most frequently found (Cuppens et al., 1998). The TG13-T5 is rarer but also more frequently found in patients with CBAVD and non-classic CF (Cuppens et al., 1998; Groman et al., 2004).

Mutation analysis of the CFTR gene in Slovak CF patients by DHPLC and subsequent sequencing resulted in the identified four novel mutations (G437D, H954P, H1375N, and 3120+33G>T). This was done by the gene scanning approach using DHPLC system for analysing specifically all CFTR exons. There was the identification of a total of 28 different mutations in Slovak CF patients, and 17 different polymorphisms (Kolesár et al., 2008). Elce et al. (2009) reported three novel CFTR polymorphic repeats (IVS3polyA, IVS4polyA, and IVS10CA repeats) which improve segregation analysis for CF. They also developed and validated a procedure based on PCR followed by capillary electrophoresis (CE) for large-scale analysis of these polymorphisms. The allelic distribution and heterozygosity results suggest that the 3 novel intragenic polymorphic repeats strongly contribute to carrier and prenatal diagnosis of CF in families in which 1 or both causal mutations have not been identified (Elce et al., 2009). A universal array-based multiplexed test for CF carrier screening using the Tag-It multiplex mutation platform and the Cystic Fibrosis Mutation Detection Kit have been introduced. The Tag-It CF assay is a multiplexed genotyping assay that detects a panel of 40 CFTR mutations including the 23 mutations recommended by the American College of Medical Genetics (ACMG) and American College of Obstetricians and Gynecologists (ACOG) for population screening. A total of 16 additional mutations detected by the Tag-It CF assay may also be common (Amos et al., 2006).

Methods that include genetic testing can be done using a single sample. The controversy is the appropriate number of mutations to include in the genetic test. The answer depends in part on the heterogeneity of the population. The ΔF508 mutation is found in 72% of the US Non-Hispanic Caucasian CF population, but in much lower percentages of patients with CF from other ethnicities (Hispanic Caucasian, 54%; African American, 44%; Asian American, 39%; Ashekenazi Jewish, 31%) (Watson et al., 2004). In 2001, the ACMG Cystic Fibrosis Carrier Screening Working Group recommended a panel of 25 mutations which would account for > 80% of CF alleles in the pan-ethnic US population with CF (Grody et al., 2001). This panel was updated in 2004 based on a larger more pan-ethnic CF data-base that finds six additional mutations with a frequency > 0.10% and another 14 that occurred at slightly lower frequency but would be useful for specific ethnic minority communities (Watson et al., 2004).

2.4 Detection of rearrangements in CFTR gene

Large rearrangements (deletions, duplications, or insertion/deletion mutations) have recently been reported to constitute 1-2% of CFTR mutations (Svensson et al., 2010). The developments in quantitative PCR technologies have greatly improved our ability to detect large genome rearrangements. In particular oligonucleotide-based array comparative genomic hybridisation has become a useful tool for appropriate and rapid detection of breakpoints (Ramos et al., 2010). Using quantitative PCR analysis of all coding regions, the occurrence of CFTR rearrangements in 130 alleles from classic CF patients bearing unidentified mutations after the scanning of CFTR were assessed in the Italian population. Seven rearrangements (i.e. dele1, dele2, dele23, dele 14b17b, dele17a18, dele2223, and dele2224) were identified in 26.0% of CF alleles bearing undetected mutations (Tomaiuolo et al., 2008).

Ramos et al. (2010) analysed 80 samples (42 unknown CF alleles) applying three quantitative technologies (MLPA, quantitative PCR and array-comparative genomic hybridization) to detect recurrent as well as novel large rearrangements in the Spanish CF population. They identified three deletions and one duplication in five alleles. The new duplication in this cohort, CFTRdupProm-3 mutation spans 35.7 kb involving the 5'-end of the CFTR gene. Additionally, RNA analysis revealed a cryptic sequence with a premature termination codon leading to a disrupted protein (Ramos et al. 2010). In another study, de Becdelièvre et al. determined the contribution of large CFTR gene rearrangements in fetuses with bowel anomalies using a semi-quantitative fluorescent multiplex PCR (QFM-PCR) assay. Deletions were found in 5/70 cases in which QFM-PCR was applied, dele19, dele22_23, dele2_6b, dele14b_15 and dele6a_6b, of which the last three remain un-described (de Becdelièvre et al. 2010).

Schneider et al. (2007) used the CFTR MLPA Kit (MRC-Holland, Amsterdam, Netherlands) that allows the exact detection of copy numbers from all 27 exons in the CFTR gene, to screen 50 patients with only one identified mutation for large deletions in the CFTR gene. Detected deletion in the CFTR gene was confirmed using real-time PCR assay and deletion-specific PCR reactions using junction fragment primers. Large deletions were detected in eight CF alleles belonging to four different deletion types (CFTRindel2, CFTRdele14b-17b, CFTRdele17a-17b and CFTRdele 2-9) (Schneider et al., 2006). The LightCycler assay allows reliable and rapid screening for large deletions in the CFTR gene and detects the copy number of all 27 exons (Schneider et al., 2007).

3. Diagnosis of CF using sweat test

3.1 Methods used for assessing sweat chloride

The report of the Consensus Conference initiated by the CF Foundation in the USA stated that the criteria for the diagnosis of CF should include the following: (1) one or more characteristic phenotypic features, or a history of CF in a sibling, or positive newborn screening test results; and (2) an elevated sweat chloride concentration by pilocarpine iontophoresis (>60 mmol/L) on two or more occasions, or identification of two CF mutations (Rosen & Cutting, 1998), or 3) *in vivo* demonstration of characteristic abnormalities in ion transport across the nasal epithelium (Welsh et al., 2001; Rosenstein & Cutting, 1998).

The chloride ion is most directly related to CFTR dysfunction. Chloride concentration measurement is the analysis of choice because the chloride ion concentration shows the greatest discrimination between normal individuals and CF subjects. Concurrent measurement of sodium acts as a quality control. The sweat test is based on the observation in 1953 by Darting et al. (1953) that stimulated sweat of CF patients contains elevated levels of sodium and chloride ions. The development of the quantitative pilocarpine iontophoresis by Gibson and Cooke dates from 1959 and is preferred method of sweat stimulation (Gibson & Cooke, 1959). The sweat test involves transdermal administration of pilocarpine by iontophoresis to stimulate sweat gland secretion, followed by collection and quantitation of sweat onto gauze or filter paper or into a Macroduct coil (Wescor Inc, Logan, Utah) and analysis of chloride concentration as described by Clinical Laboratory Standards Institute (2000). If carried out properly and with considerable care, this method is still the most specific biochemical test for CF (Shwachman, 1979). There is documentation in the literature of a semi-quantitative test, based on die production of a white silver chloride precipitate ring on a brown silver chromate background that was originally proposed by Shwachman and Gahm (1956) and adapted to die so-called paper patch test (Yeung et al., 1984). Although intended for the non-specialist centre, die method is very subjective and liable to misinterpretation and has not gained popularity.

One of the major consequences of mutations in the CFTR gene is a dysfunction of ion channels resulting in elevated sweat chloride concentrations, progressive lung disease and pancreatic insufficiency (Pilewski & Frizzell, 1999; Bals et al., 1999). In CF subjects the sweat chloride is usually higher than the sweat sodium, but the converse is true in normal persons. Normal sweat contains less than 60 mmol/L chloride and sodium (Association of Clinical Biochemistry, 2002). The 60 mmol/L value of sweat chloride concentrations has been used for a long time to discriminate between the populations of patients with CF and without CF (LeGrys, 1996). An elevated sweat chloride level has been the "gold standard" for diagnosis of CF (Gibson & Cooke, 1959). All patients with a sweat chloride level above 60 mmol/L and a clinical phenotype compatible with CF have a diagnosis of classic CF. However patients have been reported with characteristic manifestations of CF, and chloride levels, below 60 mmol/L (Highsmith et al., 1994; Cystic Fibrosis Genotype-Phenotype Consortium, 1993). Most of the studies exploring these patients with equivocal sweat tests have focused on the chloride range 40 - 60 mmol/L (Desmarquest et al., 2000). In the UK guidelines on sweat testing (Association of Clinical Biochemistry, 2000), 40 mmol/L is considered as the lower limit for equivocal sweat tests because this value represents the mean +2SD in carriers.

3.2 Intermediate sweat test results

The evidence that a proportion of CF patients with chloride concentrations of 30 - 60 mmol/L with two CFTR mutations following testing is documented in the literature (Lebecque et al., 2002). Sweat chloride concentrations of 30 - 60 mmol/L are seen in about 4% of sweat tests; 23% of these patients will subsequently be found to have two CFTR mutations. CF affected patients occur with similar frequency in the 30 - 40 mmol/L range as in the 40 - 60 mmol/L range (Lebecque et al., 2002). Furthermore, in the 2005 Cystic Fibrosis Foundation Patient Registry, only 3.5% of patients with a diagnosis of CF had a sweat chloride value <60 mmol/L, and only 1.2% had a value <40 mmol/L (Cystic Fibrosis Foundation Patient Registry, 2005). A Canadian study reported that sweat chloride values <60 mmol/L were observed in 21% with pancreatic-sufficient CF (Wilschanski et al., 2006).

Increasing recognition of the wide range of CF phenotypic variability (Nick & Rodman, 2005; Bishop et al., 2005) should lead to increasing diagnosis of CF in individuals with intermediate sweat chloride values. Farrell et al. (2008) recommends that sweat chloride values ≥40 mmol/L in individuals over age 6 months should be considered beyond the normal range and merit further evaluation, to include repeat sweat chloride testing and DNA analysis for CFTR mutations. A sweat chloride level above 60 mmol/L in the absence of CF is rare, although it has been reported in a number of unusual clinical conditions that can usually be readily distinguished from CF (Rosenstein, 2000). In patients with a sweat chloride level below 30 mmol/L the diagnosis of CF becomes very unlikely.

3.3 Sweat tests in infants

New born screening (NBS) of CF identifies only newborns at risk for CF. A positive screening result, indicating persistent hypertrypsinogenemia, should be followed by referral for direct diagnostic testing (i.e. sweat chloride test) to confirm a diagnosis of CF. With sufficient experience, sweat testing can be performed adequately in infants, but interpreting the results can be problematic. Studies of sweat chloride testing in infants have demonstrated most infants identified by NBS will undergo sweat testing after 2 weeks of age. Earlier testing could lead to misleading results, because sweat chloride concentrations in healthy newborns gradually decrease over the first weeks of life (Parad et al., 2005). A study in 103 infants without CF found a mean sweat chloride value of 23.3 ± 5.7 mmol/L at age 3 to 7 days, decreasing to 17.6 ± 5.6 mmol/L by age 8 to 14 days and then to 13.1 ± 7.4 mmol/L after age 6 weeks (Eng et al., 2005). This gradual early decline in sweat chloride values suggests that sweat test results are less likely to be difficult to interpret after age 2 weeks (Eng et al., 2005).

The Consensus Committee recommends based on the available data on sweat chloride test results in healthy and CF-affected infants, the following sweat chloride reference ranges for infants up to age 6 months: ≤29 mmol/L, CF unlikely; 30 to 59 mmol/L, intermediate; ≥60 mmol/L, indicative of CF (Farrell et al., 2008). A study of 725 infants identified as being at risk through NBS or based on clinical presentation who carried 0, 1, or 2 copies of the common CFTR gene mutation ΔF508, showed that all of the ΔF508 homozygous infants had sweat chloride concentrations >60 mmol/L. The findings from this study are in accordance with other studies from Australia (Massie et al., 2000; Parad et al., 2005). Although sweat chloride values are generally ≥60 mmol/L in infants with CF, lower values also can occur (Taceetti et al., 2004; Rock et al., 2005). In a 4-year cohort of infants in the Massachusetts NBS program in the USA who had clinician-diagnosed CF, 8.2% had a sweat chloride concentration of 30 to 59 mmol/L and 2.7% had a concentration <30 mmol/L (Parad & Comeau, 2005).

There are studies which support the recommendation that a sweat chloride value ≥ 30 mmol/L in infants <age 6 months should be considered abnormal and trigger further patient evaluation (Eng et al., 2005; Barben et al., 2005). A sweat chloride value ≤39 mmol/L after age 6 months generally is not consistent with a diagnosis of CF, although CF can occur in this group in rare cases (Lebecque et al., 2002; O'Sullivan et al., 2006). Some infants have been particularly difficult to classify, such as those with 2 CF mutations and a sweat chloride value <40 mmol/L and those with only 1 CF mutation and a slightly elevated sweat chloride value. Although such infants represent only a small fraction of patients, they may be at risk for developing complications of CF and thus should be identified and followed (Farrell et al., 2008). Sweat testing can be performed accurately on the majority of infants at age 2-3 weeks; however, not all infants have sufficient quantities of sweat for reliable testing (Boyle, 2003).

3.4 Limitations, advantages and disadvantages of sweat test

The sweat test is cheap and, in nearly all populations, will result in a greater diagnostic yield than a standard CFTR deoxyribonucleic acid (DNA) screening test. Sweat should be collected for 30 minutes onto pre-weighed gauze or filter paper low in sodium chloride. A minimum sweat rate of 1 g/m^2 body surface area/min is required; thus a sweat volume of 50 -100 mL is adequate. Testing can be carried out after the first 2 weeks of life in infants weighing more than 3 kg who are normally hydrated and without significant illness. Testing should be delayed in infants who are acutely ill or dehydrated, who have eczema or oedema, or who are receiving supplemental oxygen. Raised sweat electrolyte concentrations can be found in infants who are underweight or dehydrated.

Sweat electrolyte concentrations can be lowered by systemic steroids and oedema. Sweat electrolytes are not affected by administration of intravenous fluids, diuretics or intake of flucloxacillin (Association of Clinical Biochemistry, 2002; National Committee for Clinical Laboratory Standards, 2000). False negative results have been reported (LeGrys & Wood, 1988) as well as consistently borderline values (Canciam et al., 1988). False positive results can also occur (Smalley et al., 1979) often due to lack of care during sweat collection, resulting in evaporation of collected sweat prior to analysis. Consequently the test which is time-consuming should be done only by properly trained personnel. An additional problem is that in the very young and those with dry skin, sweat collection volumes may be too small for analysis.

As the appropriate performance of the sweat test is crucial for the accurate diagnosis of CF, the Cystic Fibrosis Foundation (2007) requires that sweat testing conducted at accredited CF care centers adheres to the standards recommended by a Cystic Fibrosis Foundation Committee comprising CF center directors (LeGrys et al., 2007). Laboratories accredited by the College of American Pathologists must follow the protocols and procedures outlined in the College's Laboratory Accreditation Program Inspection Checklist (College of American Pathologists, 2007). Because of the additional technical challenges involved in obtaining sweat from newborns, it is often recommended that NBS-positive newborns undergo sweat testing only at a Cystic Fibrosis Foundation certified laboratory.

4. Immunoreactive trypsinogen (IRT) in CF neonatal screening

4.1 The sensitivity and specificity of IRT

The purpose of CF newborn screening is identification of CF-affected infants. Strategies used by CF newborn screening programs have included measuring for elevated levels of IRT which is relatively inexpensive and adaptable to large numbers (Crossley et al., 1981). The IRT is an indirect measure of pancreatic injury that is present at birth in most newborns who have CF on serial dried blood spot specimens (Hammond et al., 1991) or measuring for elevated IRT followed by assaying for ΔF508 on the same dried blood spot (2-tier algorithm)

(Gregg et al., 1993). Increased IRT concentrations at birth are characteristic of newborns affected by CF, but can also be found in healthy infants. In 1979, Crossley et al. reported a two to threefold increase in IRT in blood from CF neonates, compared with normal (non-CF) infants. The test was based on a radioimmunoassay for serum trypsin, and was adapted for use on dried blood-spots.

The IRT levels tend to remain elevated for several months in newborns with CF, because pancreatic trypsinogen leaks back through interstitial fluid due to partial obstruction of pancreatic ducts (Crossley et al., 1979). The lack of specificity of IRT means, however, that they may also be false positives (Wilcken et al., 1983). The 'falsely' elevated IRT levels usually return to normal within the first weeks of life of the child's birth. This presents a diagnostic dilemma. CF should be confirmed or ruled out as quickly as possible in these situations to alleviate parental distress and allow earlier therapeutic intervention and genetic counseling. In most older CF children IRT levels are subnormal and there is considerable child to child variation (Chatfield et al., 1991). To improve the specificity of neonatal screening, a second blood sample is obtained in neonates with raised levels of IRT at birth, and only infants with persistently raised IRT values progress to a sweat test. Furthermore, standard diagnostic strategy calls for extensive analysis of the CFTR gene and repetition of the sweat Cl^- measurement (De Boeck et al., 2006; Rosenstein & Cutting, 1998).

Prospective studies have shown false positive incidence of 0.5% (from first blood spots) but the false negative incidence was very low if infants presenting with meconium ileus were excluded (Crossley et al., 1981; Heeley et al., 1982). The false positive incidence could be significantly reduced by repeating the test on a second blood spot (Travert, 1988). The results of routine screening from 16 centres around the world were correlated and it was found that false positive rate ranged from 0.2 - 0.5% although this was higher in those laboratories where a lower cut-off point was taken (Travert, 1988). There have been reports concerning improvement in sensitivity and specificity for the IRT test, by including the use of complementary tests (Pederzini et al., 1990) have suggested a combination of meconium screening by measurement of lactase, on those infants who are IRT positive. Sweat tests are done on those patients who test positive, either by the lactase test or where blood spots are above a certain value by IRT test. This approach achieved a marked drop in false negative incidence but it seems likely that the extra work and expense will be unacceptable (Pederzini et al., 1990).

In most neonatal screening protocols, IRT retesting in infants with an initially raised value has been replaced by analysis of a panel of CF causing mutations in the neonatal blood sample (Ranieri, 1994). Comeau et al. (2004) implemented statewide CF newborn screening in Massachusetts, USA using a 2-tier algorithm in which all specimens were assayed for IRT. Those with elevated IRT then had multiple- CFTR-mutation testing. Infants who screened positive by detection of 1 or 2 mutations or extremely elevated IRT (>99.8%; failsafe protocol) were then referred for definitive diagnosis by sweat testing. The authors reported that by using the multiple-CFTR-mutation panel, a screening result with a genetic "diagnosis" of CF was made in 75% of screened-positive CF-affected infants, compared with 50% had they used ΔF508 alone, thus facilitating more rapid referral and intervention (Comeau et al., 2004).

4.2 The use of the IRT/IRT method in neonatal screening

Multiple protocols and algorithms are used to screen newborns for CF. All protocols begin with a first-tier phenotypic test that measures IRT in dried blood spots. Different laboratory kits for IRT produce varying distributions of IRT measures, and screening programs set cut-offs on the basis of evaluations of specimens from their own populations and the screening protocols and algorithms used. Screening programs in five states in the USA (Colorado, Connecticut, Montana, New Jersey, and Wyoming) have set absolute cut-offs for a normal IRT value on the first newborn blood spot (range: 90 - 105 ng/mL) (Wilfond et al., 2003).

The IRT-IRT algorithm involves measurement of IRT during the first week on the Guthrie blood spot and repeating the measurement at 3 - 4 weeks in those with initial high levels. The sensitivity of a raised 3 - 5 day IRT is high, but the positive predictive value is low. Because blood levels of IRT decay slowly in CF infants, a second IRT at 3 - 4 weeks increases the specificity, but about 1 in 200 newborn infants progress to the second blood test (Price, 2006).

In the USA, because normal IRT reference values vary slightly, the individual NBS program in the state in which the newborn is being tested sets the specific cut-off value that defines an elevated IRT. After an abnormal IRT value is identified, most NBS programs perform DNA testing to identify known CFTR gene mutations (IRT/DNA strategy), while other programs repeat the IRT measurement in a second blood sample obtained from the infant at age approximately 2 weeks (IRT/IRT strategy) (Comeau et al., 2007). These strategies have been reported to provide approximately 90% to 95% sensitivity (Wilcken et al., 1995) and have identified newborns at risk for a wide spectrum of disease severity (Farrell et al., 1997). However, there are studies which have shown that IRT/DNA screening suggested better sensitivity than IRT/IRT (Gregg et al., 1997; Padoan et al., 2002), but relatively small populations were previously studied.

In the IRT/IRT algorithm, both the first and the second IRT values must be above the fixed cut-offs to recommend a sweat test; therefore, the initial IRT is the more crucial step. In the USA, a first IRT value of 100 or 105 ng/mL, and a second value of 70 ng/mL are used. These values have been set in an attempt to maximize sensitivity and positive predictive value. Although the initial cut-off for IRT/IRT algorithm decreased over time from 140 ng/mL (Hammond et al., 1991) to 100 or 105 ng/mL (Sontag et al., 2005) in attempts to decrease false negative results in the IRT/IRT, there are concerns regarding sub-optimal sensitivity and observations which have revealed that the second specimens of some patients with CF showed precipitous decreases which have led Wisconsin in the USA (Rock et al., 1990) and Australia (Gregg et al., 1993) to develop the 2-tier IRT/DNA (ΔF508) method.

4.3 IRT/DNA and IRT/DNA/IRT protocols in neonatal screening

According to Price (2006), IRT/DNA employs DNA analysis instead of a second IRT at 3 - 4 weeks. Infants with very high IRT in the first week undergo DNA analysis and those with at least one mutation have a sweat test. The advantage of the IRT/DNA protocol is that both tests can be done on the initial blood spot sample (Price, 2006). However, the sensitivity of the IRT/DNA protocol is, however, dependent on the gene frequency of common CFTR mutations in the population. Many programs that use an IRT/DNA methodology also recommend sweat testing on children with a very high IRT level without mutations in an attempt to capture children who have rare mutations. This safeguard will reduce the number of false negatives (Benhardtet et al., 1987).

If an IRT/DNA method is used, the number of carriers detected will depend on the number of mutations included in the screening test. The more mutations included, the more children will be identified with one common mutation. The screening panel should include more rather than less mutations to avoid disproportionate number of missed screened cases (false negatives) in USA ethnic minorities. In order to capture a high percentage of cases involving ethnic minorities, full sequencing of the CFTR gene is required (Ross, 2008). Kammesheidt et al. (2006) have shown the feasibility of temporal temperature gradient electrophoresis-based full sequence analysis and targeted sequencing from DNA in newborn blood specimens which can increase the identification of mutations in ethnic minorities. This method allowed a more comprehensive diagnosis on one blood sample because only children with two mutations and/or variants would need to undergo sweat testing. It should reduce the overall number of cases referred for sweat tests, unless questionable variants are more common than previously anticipated (Kammesheidt et al., 2006).

The IRT/DNA/IRT protocol use 2 IRT measurements and DNA testing. This method, applies a mutation panel to primary samples with an elevated IRT. Children whose sample has at least one mutation or whose sample has a very high initial IRT measurement are asked to provide a second sample for a second IRT measurement. Only those with an elevated IRT levels on the second sample undergo sweat testing (Ross, 2008). Corbetta et al. (2002) assessed the performance of IRT/DNA/IRT based on IRT followed by direct CFTR gene analysis (based on a panel of up to 31 mutations) in hypertrypsinaemic newborn infants in Italy. The screening strategy consisted of an IRT assay from dried blood spots, a PCR followed by an OLA (PCR-OLA), and a sequence code separation. The researchers reported that the IRT/DNA/IRT protocol with an OLA showed the identification of 94% of infants with CF. They concluded that PCR-OLA assay was a reliable, robust method to apply to the neonatal screening programme (Corbetta et al., 2002).

In the UK approximately 4% of children diagnosed with CF are non-Caucasian in origin. A DNA panel comprising the most common 31 CF mutations will detect 97% of mutations in a Caucasian population, but only just over 65% of mutations in a non-Caucasian population. The gene frequency of ΔF508 in the UK Indian sub-continent CF population is less than half that in the UK Caucasian CF population (McCormick et al., 2002). A three stage IRT/DNA/IRT protocol is reported to likely increase the chances of detecting CF in non-Caucasian infants (McCormick et al., 2002).

The main benefits of the IRT/DNA/IRT protocol over a single IRT/DNA methodology is that they reduce the number of children who need to undergo sweat testing, and the number of parents who are informed of their child's carrier status and need genetic counselling (Ross, 2008). However, the main disadvantage of the IRT/DNA/IRT protocol is its complexity and the anxiety generated for families who have to wait for the result of a second IRT (McCormick et al., 2002). Both the IRT/DNA/IRT and IRT/DNA protocols involve DNA testing, and may fail to detect ethnic minorities with rare mutations. Some ethnic minority children with rare mutations may still be detected to the extent that the IRT/DNA/IRT method employs the safeguard of recommending sweat testing of children with a very high IRT measurement even if no mutations are detected. Modeling in different ethnic communities using different DNA panels would be necessary to determine whether the costs of the extra laboratory testing are outweighed by the benefits achieved by reducing the number of children who need to undergo sweat testing and genetic counselling (Ross, 2008).

5. The use of the nasal potential difference (NPD) in aiding the diagnosis of CF

Genetic studies sometimes take several weeks and may find no useful information, neither confirming nor ruling out CF, such as when one or both mutant alleles remain unidentified or when the CF-causing nature of the mutations cannot be proven (Castellani et al., 2001). In addition, there are ancillary tests currently used by clinicians to clarify the diagnostic status of individuals with less CF-specific gastrointestinal or pulmonary symptomatology. The NPD test, which has been used in CF research for decades, has been introduced to clinical practice to aid diagnosis (Knowles et al., 1995). It may be particularly helpful in individuals with inconclusive sweat chloride values (Wilson et al., 1998). In *vivo* demonstration of abnormal CFTR-related ion transport across nasal epithelium could serve as an important diagnostic tool in these difficult situations.

Measurements of trans-epithelial NPD in adults accurately characterize CFTR-related ion transport. Nasal PD is determined by standard criteria as described by Knowles et al (1995). The PD is measured between a fluid filled exploring bridge on the nasal mucosa and a reference bridge on the skin of the forearm. The reference bridge may be applied to the skin by a thin needle inserted subcutaneously or placed directly on the skin after performing a small abrasion (Gelrud et al., 2004). After consistent baseline PD measurements have been obtained, the effect of amiloride superfusion through a second tube overriding the exploring catheter is evaluated. To study nasal chloride permeability and cAMP activation of chloride permeability, a large chloride chemical gradient is generated across the apical membrane by superfusion of the nasal mucosa for 3 minutes with a chloride free solution containing 10^{-4} M amiloride in Ringer's solution with gluconate substituted for chloride at a rate of 5 ml/min. Sodium (Na^+) transport and CFTR-related Cl^- transport is measured electrically by recording the changes in the nasal transepithelial PD (Knowles et al., 1995).

The nasal PD of a patient with classic CF is remarkably different from controls. The profile of classic CF patients is characterized by hyperpolarization of basal PD, increased Na^+ channel activity, an amiloride response that is exaggerated, and there is very little or no response to chloride free and isoproterenol solutions. In non-classic CF the nasal PD may be borderline and there is not yet a total consensus as to what exactly constitutes an abnormal result, but a formula which takes into account both sodium and chloride transport has been proposed by Wilschanski and colleagues (Wilschanski et al., 2001).

There have been several reports on the usefulness of NPD measurements for diagnosing CF (Hubert et al., 2004; Schüler et al., 2004). Nasal PD measurement has been widely validated in adults (Knowles et al., 1995) and provides an easy, quick and painless tool to discriminate between adults with atypical CF and those presenting some CF symptoms without CF (Delmarco et al., 1997; Wilschanski et al., 2001). Therefore a NPD test showing a significant response to zero-chloride perfusate containing isoproterenol may be useful in ruling out a diagnosis of CF. But the quantitative aspects of NPD results that are clearly indicative of CF are not defined consistently across all CF-testing centers. Moreover, some overlap likely occurs between CF and non-CF values for both the basal PD and response to zero-chloride and isoproterenol, analogous to the overlap in sweat chloride values. The NPD test's predictive capability improves somewhat when analyses of sodium and chloride channel abnormalities are combined (Standaert et al., 1997).

The NPD measurements in infants reported so far come mostly from case reports (Barker et al., 1997; Southern et al., 2001). These few studies used either the equipment already validated in adults, or specially designed one-of-a-kind devices. In a study, Sermet-Gaudelus et al. (2006) sought to validate NPD testing as a diagnostic tool for children with borderline results in neonatal screening. They adapted the standard NPD protocol for young children, designed a special catheter for them, used a slower perfusion rate, and shortened the protocol to include only measurement of basal PD, transepithelial sodium (Na^+) transport in response to amiloride, and CFTR-mediated Cl^- secretion in response to isoproterenol. The authors reported that the new protocol was well tolerated and produced NPD measurements that did not differ significantly from those obtained with the standard protocol. They conclude that this preliminary study will provide a basis for interpreting NPD measurements in patients with suspected CF after neonatal screening (Sermet-Gaudelus et al., 2005).

It is important however to standardize the protocol and to verify that the reference data and patterns in infants are similar to the values previously validated in adults. It is not yet known, for example, whether airway epithelium undergoes maturation during the first months of life, as renal and sweat gland epithelia do (Wilken and Travert, 1999). Therefore, before this test is implemented as a diagnostic tool for cases with borderline observations in neonatal screening, there is an urgent need to obtain and validate reference data for NPD measurements in infants and very young children with CF, and in healthy controls of the same age (Wilken and Travert, 1999). Properly conducted NPD testing at a research center can provide valuable information for diagnosis when clinical evidence is not clear-cut; however, access to the test is limited. Because there are no clear reference values, validation studies, or standardized technical protocols for NPD testing for diagnostic purposes, the test should be used only to provide contributory evidence in a diagnostic evaluation (Standaert et al., 2004).

6. The value of pancreatic associated protein (PAP) as a screening test for CF

Genetic analysis has certain drawbacks, the most important of which being the management of heterozygotes, and in France the requirement by law of previous informed consent (Barthellemy et al., 2001). In cases of CF, pancreatic alterations are already present in utero. Previous studies have demonstrated the value of PAP as a screening test for CF, and has indicated that a feasible two-stage strategy could involve the selection of infants with elevated PAP levels, and in this group of infants, subsequent detection of those with elevated IRT levels for direct CF diagnosis by the sweat test thereby avoiding the use of genetic analysis (Sarles et al., 1999; Sarles et al., 2005).

The IRT/PAP protocol can be done on one sample and preliminary data show comparable sensitivity and specificity with the other methods using the Guthrie cards (Sarles et al.,

2005). Barthellemy et al. (2001) evaluated PAP levels in a prospective study involving 47, 213 infants in the Provence region of France. In infants with a PAP > 7.5 ng/mL, 1.28% had an elevated IRT level > 700 ng/mL (0.37%). In this limited population sample (0.37% of the total), the sweat test diagnosed five cases of CF. The authors concluded that the PAP/IRT technique for CF detection seems to be suitable for mass screening, without the drawbacks of genetic testing (Barthellemy et al., 2001).

A recent study Sommerburg et al. (2010) used a prospective and sequential IRT/PAP strategy, and validated this biochemical approach against the widely used IRT/DNA protocol in a population-based NBS study in southwest Germany. The study involved the prospective quantitation of PAP and genetic analysis for the presence of four mutations in the CFTR gene most prevalent in southwest Germany (ΔF508, R553X, G551D, G542X) on all newborns with IRT >99.0th percentile. New born screening was rated positive when either PAP was ≥1.0 ng/mL and/or at least one CFTR mutation was detected. The results showed that out of 73,759 newborns tested, 0.13% were positive with IRT/PAP and 0.08% with IRT/DNA. In addition, after sweat testing of 135 CF NBS-positive infants, 13 were diagnosed with CF. The authors reported that the detection rates were similar for both IRT/PAP and IRT/DNA protocols (Sommerburg et al., 2010).

Sequential measurement of IRT/PAP provides good sensitivity and specificity and allows reliable and cost-effective CF NBS which circumvents the necessity of genetic testing with its inherent ethical problems. However, to-date it has not been tested outside of Europe and its benefits and harms in a pan-ethnic community have not been clarified.

7. Intestinal current measurement (ICM) as a diagnostic tool for CF

As many intestinal ion transport processes are electrogenic, measuring the electrical current that they generate (ICM) can be used to monitor their activity. Intestinal current measurements on rectal suction biopsies are a tool for the *ex vivo* diagnosis of classical and atypical CF. The ICM technique allows the registration of CF-induced changes in electrogenic transepithelial ion transport (Cl^-, HCO_3^-, K^+) in a Cl^- secretory epithelium, and on the basis of pharmacological criteria, is able to discriminate between CFTR-mediated Cl^- secretion, and secretion through alternative anion channels. In CF, intestinal chloride secretion is impaired while absorptive processes remain unchanged and may even be enhanced. Furthermore, ICM is particularly useful for the classification of individuals with CF-like clinical features with equivocal sweat test values (De Jonge et al., 2004).

There is a clear difference between ICM measurement in classic CF and in normal individuals. There is information in the literature about the use of ICM as a clinical diagnostic tool (De Jonge et al., 2004; Hug et al., 2004). Derichs et al. (2010) described reference values and validated ICM for the diagnostic classification of questionable CF at all patient ages. The ICM method was performed in 309 rectal biopsies from 130 infants, children and adults including patients with known pancreatic-insufficient, pancreatic-sufficient, patients with an unclear diagnosis with mild CF symptoms, intermediate sweat test and/or *CFTR* mutation screening and healthy controls. The researchers found that the cumulative chloride secretory response of $\Delta I_{sc,carbachol}$, $\Delta I_{sc,cAMP/forskolin}$ and $\Delta I_{sc,histamine}$ was the best diagnostic ICM parameter, differentiating patients with questionable CF into pancreatic-sufficient-CF and 'CF unlikely' groups. The study underlines the diagnostic value of ICM, especially for confirmation of CF in the absence of two disease-causing *CFTR* mutations, exclusion of CF despite intermediate sweat test and age groups unsuitable for NPD measurements (Derichs et al., 2010). They conclude that ICM is an important tool for functional assessment in *CFTR* mutations of unknown clinical relevance (Derichs et al., 2010). However at present the technique has remained mainly in the research setting, so it is not yet included in the diagnostic algorithms.

8. Conclusion

Cystic fibrosis, a recessively inherited condition caused by mutation of the CFTR gene is a disease with the complex, multi-faceted clinical phenotype and is one of the most investigated monogenic disorders. More than 1800 different disease-causing mutations within the CFTR gene have been described. Mutations affect CFTR through a variety of molecular mechanisms, which can produce little or no functional gene product at the apical membrane. This results in abnormal viscous mucoid secretions in multiple organs and the main clinical features are chronic infection and progressive obstruction of the respiratory tract, pancreatic insufficiency and intestinal disease. Disease severity, to some extent, correlates with organ sensitivity to CFTR dysfunction and to the amount of functional protein, which is influenced by the type of mutation.

CFTR gene studies are now one of the most frequent activities in clinical molecular genetics laboratories and with advances in DNA analysis there is an increased knowledge of the mutational spectrum for cystic fibrosis. Genetic testing can confirm a clinical diagnosis of CF and can be used for infants with meconium ileus, for carrier detection in individuals with positive family history and partners of proven CF carriers, and for prenatal diagnostic testing if both parents are carriers. A growing number of tests capable of simultaneously detecting several frequent CF mutations are being developed, and commercial kits are now available.

The sweat chloride test remains the gold standard for CF diagnosis but does not always give a clear answer. For patients in whom sweat chloride concentrations are normal or borderline and in whom two CF mutations are not identified, an abnormal NPD measurement recorded on 2 separate days can be used as evidence of CFTR dysfunction. Newborn infants with CF have raised levels of IRT in their serum. Measurement of IRT in the first week of life has enabled CF to be incorporated into existing NBS blood spot protocols. The IRT detection test is practical, adaptable to large scale screening of dried neonatal blood spots, relatively inexpensive, and promising for the detection of newborns with CF who have pancreatic insufficiency. However, IRT is not a specific test for CF and NBS therefore requires a further tier of tests to avoid unnecessary referral for diagnostic testing. DNA analysis for common CF-associated mutations has been increasingly used as a second tier test. The sequential measurement of IRT/PAP provides good sensitivity and specificity and allows reliable and cost-effective CF newborn screening which circumvents the necessity of genetic testing. ICM is particularly useful for the classification of individuals with CF-like clinical features with equivocal sweat test values However, standardization of international programs for newborns has not yet been achieved. The significant advances in our understanding of CF and the development of new technologies now allow prenatal diagnosis. However, despite steady improvements in prenatal diagnosis, NBS and adult, CF remains a serious disease which places a heavy burden on affected families.

9. References

Ahmed, N., Corey, M., Forstner, G., Zielenski, J., Tsui, L.C., Ellis, L., Tullis, E. & Durie P. (2003). Molecular consequences of Cystic Fibrosis Transmembrane Regulator (CFTR) gene mutations in the exocrine pancreas. *Gut*, Vol. 52, pp. 1159-1164.

Alibakhshi, R., Kianishirazi, R., Cassiman, J.J., Zamani, M. & Cuppens H. (2008). Analysis of the CFTR gene in Iranian cystic fibrosis patients: identification of eight novel mutations. J Cyst Fibros Vol. 7, pp. 102-109.

Alper, O.M., Wong, L.J., Young, S., Pearl, M., Graham, S., Sherwin, J., Nussbaum, E., Nielson, D., Platzker, A., Davies, Z., Lieberthal, A., Chin, T., Shay, G., Hardy, K. & Kharrazi, M. (2004). Identification of novel and rare mutations in California Hispanic and African-American cystic fibrosis patients. *Hum Mutat* Vol. 24, pp. 353.

Amos, J.A., Bridge-Cook, P., Ponek, V. & Jarvis M.R. (2006). A universal array-based multiplexed test for cystic fibrosis carrier screening. Expert Rev Mol Diagn Vol. 6, pp. 15-22.

Ashavaid, T.F., Kondkar, A.A., Dherai, A.J., Raghavan, R., Udani, S.V., Udwadia, Z.F. & Desai, D. (2005). Application of multiplex ARMS and SSCP/HD analysis in molecular diagnosis of cystic fibrosis in Indian patients. Mol Diagn Vol. 9, pp. 59-66.

Association of Clinical Biochemistry. Guidelines for the performance of the sweat test for the investigation of cystic fibrosis in the UK, Report from the Multidisciplinary Working Group, 2002. Available at http://www.acb.org.uk.

Bals, R., Weiner, D. & Wilson J. (1999). The innate immune system in cystic fibrosis lung disease. *J Clin Invest* Vol. 103, pp.303-307.

Barben, J., Ammann, R.A., Metlagel, A. & Schoeni, M.H. (2005). Conductivity determined by a new sweat analyzer compared to chloride concentrations for the diagnosis of cystic fibrosis. *J Pediatr* Vol. 146, pp. 183-188.

Barker, P.M., Gowen, C.W., Lawson, E.E. & Knowles, M.R. (1997). Decreased sodium ion absorption across nasal epithelium of very premature infants with respiratory distress syndrome. *J Pediatr* Vol. 130, pp. 373-377.

Barthellemy, S., Maurin, N., Roussey, M., Férec, C., Murolo, S., Berthézène, P., Iovanna, J.L., Dagorn, J.C. & Sarles J. (2001). Evaluation of 47,213 infants in neonatal screening for cystic fibrosis, using pancreatitis-associated protein and immunoreactive trypsinogen assays. *Arch Pediatr* Vol. 8, pp.275-281.

Bernhardt, B.A., Weiner, J., Foster, E.C., Tumpson, J.E. & Pyeritz RE. (1987). The economics of clinical genetics services. II. A time analysis of a medical genetics clinic. *American Journal of Human Genetics* Vol. 41, pp. 559-565.

Bishop, M.D., Freedman, S.D., Zielenski, J., Ahmed, N., Dupuis, A., Martin, S., Ellis, L., Shea, J., Hopper, I., Corey, M., Kortan, P., Haber, G., Ross, C., Tzountzouris, J., Steele, L. Ray, P.N., Tsui, L.C. & Durie, P.R. (2005). The cystic fibrosis transmembrane conductance regulator gene and ion channel function in patients with idiopathic pancreatitis. *Hum Genet* Vol. 118, pp.372-381.

Bobadilla, J.L., Macek, M. Jr., Fine, J.P. & Farrell, P.M. (2002). Cystic fibrosis: a worldwide analysis of CFTR mutations-correlation with incidence data and application to screening. *Hum Mutat* Vol. 19, pp. 575-606.

Boyle, M.P. (2003). Nonclassic cystic fibrosis and CFTR-related diseases. *Curr Opin Pulm Med* Vol. 9, pp. 498-503.

Canciam, M., Fomo, S. & Mastella, G. (1988). Borderline sweat test Criteria for cystic fibrosis diagnosis. *Scand J Gastroenterol* Vol. 143, pp. 19-27.

Castellani, C., Benetazzo, M.G., Tamanini, A., Begnini, A., Mastella, G. & Pignatti, P. (2001). Analysis of the entire coding region of the cystic fibrosis transmembrane regulator gene in neonatal. hypertrypsinaemia with normal sweat test. *J Med Genet* Vol. 38, pp. 202-205.

Castellani, C., Tamanini, A. & Mastella, G. (2000). Protracted neonatal hypertrypsinogenaemia, normal sweat chloride, and cystic fibrosis. *Arch Dis Child* Vol. 82, pp. 481-482.

Chatfield, S., Owen, G., Ryley, H.C., *Williams, J., Alfaham, M., Weller, P.H., Goodchild, M.C., Carter, R.A., Bradley, D. & Dodge, J.A. (1991).* Neonatal Screening for cystic fibrosis in Wales and the West Midlands Clinical assessment after five years of screening. *Arch Dis Child* Vol. 66, pp. 29-33.

Cheillan, D., Vercherat, M., Cheavlier-Porst, F., Charcosset, M., Rolland, M.O. & Dorche, C. (2005). False positive results in neonatal screening for cystic fibrosis based on a three-stage protocol (IRT/DNA/IRT): Should we adjust IRT cut-off to ethnic origin? *Journal of Inherited Metabolic Disease* Vol. 28, pp. 813-818.

Chillo´n, M., Casals, T., Mercier, B., Bassas, L., Lissens, W., Silber, S., Romey, M.C., Ruiz-Romero, J., Verlingue, C., Claustres, M., Nunes, D.V., Férec, C. & Estivill, X. (1995). Mutations in the cystic fibrosis gene in patients with congenital absence of the vas deferens. *N Engl J Med* Vol. 332, pp. 1475-1480.

Clinical Laboratory Standards Institute (formerly National Committee for Clinical Laboratory Standards) Approved guideline. National Committee for Clinical Laboratory Standards; 2000. Sweat testing: sample collection and quantitative analysis. Document, pp. C34-A2.

College of American Pathologists. Chemistry checklist, laboratory accreditation program. [Accessed August 10, 2011]. Available from:

http://www.cap.org/apps/docs/laboratory_accreditation/checklists/chemistry_and_toxicology_april2006.pdf

Comeau, A.M., Accurso, F.J., White, T.B., Campbell, P.W., III, Hoffman, G., Parad, R.B., Wilfond, B.S., Rosenfeld, M., Sontag, M.K., Massie, J., Farrell, P.M. & O'Sullivan, B.P. (2007). Cystic Fibrosis Foundation. Guidelines for implementation of cystic fibrosis newborn screening programs: Cystic Fibrosis Foundation workshop report. *Pediatrics* Vol. 119, pp. 495-518.

Comeau, A.M., Parad, R.B., Dorkin, H.L., Dovey, M., Gerstle, R., Haver, K., Lapey, A., O'Sullivan, B.P., Waltz, D.A., Zwerdling, R.G. & Eaton, R.B. (2004). Population-based newborn screening for genetic disorders when multiple mutation DNA testing is incorporated: a cystic fibrosis newborn screening model demonstrating increased sensitivity but more carrier detections. *Pediatrics* Vol. 113:1573-1581.

Corbetta, C., Seia, M., Bassotti, A., Ambrosioni, A., Giunta, A. & Padoan, R. (2002). Screening for cystic fibrosis in newborn infants: results of a pilot programme based on a two tier protocol (IRT/DNA/IRT) in the Italian population. *J Med Screen* Vol. 9, pp. 60-63.

Crossley, J.R., Smith, P.A., Edgar, B.W., Gluckman, P.D. & Elliott, R.B. (1981). Neonatal screening for cystic fibrosis using Immunoreactive trypsin assay in dried blood spots. *Clin Chim Acta* Vol. 113, pp. 111-121.

Crossley, J.R., Elliott, R.B. & Smith, P.A. (1979). Dried blood spot screening for cystic fibrosis in the newborn *Lancet* Vol. 1, pp. 472-474.

Crossley, J.R., Smith P.A., Edgar, B.W., Gluckman, P.D. & Elliott, R.B. (1981). Neonatal screening for cystic fibrosis, using immunoreactive trypsin assay dried blood spots. *Clin Chim Acta* Vol. 113, pp. 111-121.

Cuppens, H., Lin, W., Jaspers, M., Costes, B., Teng, H., Vankeerberghen, A., Jorissen, M., Droogmans, G., Reynaert, I., Goossens, M., Nilius, B. & Cassiman, J.J. (1998). Polyvariant mutant cystic fibrosis transmembrane conductance regulator genes: the polymorphic (TG)m locus explains the partial penetrance of the T5 polymorphism as a disease mutation. *J Clin Invest* Vol. 101, pp. 487-496.

Cuppens, H., Marynen, P., De Boeck, K. & Cassiman, J.J. (1993). Detection of 98.5% of the mutations in 200 Belgian cystic fibrosis alleles by reverse dot blot and sequencing of the complete coding regin and exon/intron junctions of the CFTR gene. *Genomics* Vol. 18, pp.693-697.

Cystic Fibrosis Foundation. Patient registry 2001 annual report. Bethesda, MD: Cystic Fibrosis Foundation, 2002.

Cystic Fibrosis Foundation Patient Registry. Annual Data Report to the Center Directors. Bethesda, MD: Cystic Fibrosis Foundation, 2005.

Cystic Fibrosis Genotype-Phenotype Consortium. (1993). Correlation between genotype and phenotype in patients with cystic fibrosis. *N Engl J Med* Vol. 329, pp. 1308-1313.

Cystic Fibrosis Mutation Database. [www.genet.sickkids.on.ca/cftr]. Accessed 10 August 2011.

Darting, R.C., di Sant'Agnese, P.A., Perera, G.A. & Anderson, D.H. (1953). Electrolyte abnormalities of sweat in fibrocysic disease of the pancreas. *Am J Med Sci* Vol. 225, pp. 67-70.

De Boeck, K., Wilschanski, M., Castellani, C., Taylor, C., Cuppens, H., Dodge, J. & Sinaasappel, M. (2006). Cystic fibrosis: terminology and diagnostic algorithms. *Thorax* Vol. 61, pp. 627-635.

de Becdelièvre, A., Costa, C., LeFloch, A., Legendre, M., Jouannic, J.M., Vigneron, J., Bresson, J.L., Gobin, S., Martin, J., Goossens, M. & Girodon, E. (2010). Notable contribution of large CFTR gene rearrangements to the diagnosis of cystic fibrosis in fetuses with bowel anomalies. *Eur J Hum Genet* Vol. 18, pp. 1166-1169.

De Jonge, H.R., Ballmann, M., Veeze, H., Bronsveld, I., Stanke, F., Tümmler, B. & Sinaasappel, M. (2004). Ex vivo CF diagnosis by intestinal current measurements (ICM) in small aperture, circulating Ussing chambers. *J Cyst Fibros* Vol. 3, pp. 159-163.

Delmarco, A., Pradal, U., Cabrini, G., Bonizzato, A. & Mastella G. (1997). Nasal potential difference in cystic fibrosis patients presenting borderline sweat test. *Eur Respir J* Vol. 10, pp. 1145-1149.

Dequeker, E., Cuppens, H., Dodge, J., Estivill, X., Goossens, M., Pignatti, P.F., Scheffer, H., Schwartz, M., Schwarz, M., Tümmler, B. & Cassiman, J.J. (2000). Recommendations for quality improvement in genetic testing for cystic fibrosis. European Concerted Action on Cystic Fibrosis. *Eur J Hum Genet* Vol. 8, pp. S1-S24.

Derichs, N., Sanz, J., Von Kanel, T., Stolpe, C., Zapf, A., Tümmler, B., Gallati, S. & Ballmann, M. (2010). Intestinal current measurement for diagnostic classification of patients with questionable cystic fibrosis: validation and reference data. *Thorax* Vol. 65, pp. 594-599.

Desmarquest, P., Feldman, D., Tamalat, A., Estivill, X., Goossens, M., Pignatti, P.F., Scheffer, H., Schwartz, M., Schwarz, M., Tümmler, B. & Cassiman, J.J. (2000). Genotype analysis and phenotypic manifestation of children with intermediate sweat chloride test results. *Chest* Vol. 118, pp. 1591-1597.

Eaker, S., Johnson, M., Jenkins, J., Bauer, M. & Little, S. (2005). Detection of CFTR mutations using ARMS and low-density microarrays. Biosens Bioelectron Vol. 21, pp. 933-939.

Elce, A., Boccia, A., Cardillo, G., Giordano, S., Tomaiuolo, R., Paolella, G. & Castaldo, G. (2009). Three novel CFTR polymorphic repeats improve segregation analysis for cystic fibrosis. *Clin Chem* Vol. 55, pp. 1372-1379.

Eng, W., LeGrys, V.A., Schechter, M.S., Laughon, M.M. & Barker, P.M. (2005). Sweat-testing in preterm and full-term infants less than 6 weeks of age. *Pediatr Pulmonol* Vol. 40, pp. 64-67.

Eshaque, B. & Dixon, B. (2006). Technology platforms for molecular diagnosis of cystic fibrosis. Biotechnol Adv Vol. 24, pp. 86-93.

Farrell, P.M., Kosorok, M.R., Laxova, A., Shen, G., Koscik, R.E., Bruns, W.T., Splaingard, M. & Mischler, E.H. (1997). Nutritional benefits of neonatal screening for cystic fibrosis. Wisconsin Cystic Fibrosis Neonatal Screening Study Group. *N Engl J Med* Vol. 337, pp. 963-969.

Farrell, P.M., Rosenstein, B.J., White, T.B., Accurso, F.J., Castellani, C., Cutting, G.R., Durie, P.R., Legrys, V.A., Massie, J., Parad, R.B., Rock, M.J. & Campbell, P.W. (2008). 3rd; Cystic Fibrosis Foundation. Guidelines for diagnosis of cystic fibrosis in newborns through older adults: Cystic Fibrosis Foundation consensus report. J Pediatr Vol. 153, pp. S4-S14.

Gelrud, A., Sheth, S., Banerjee, S., Weed, D., Shea,, J., Chuttani, R., Howell, D.A., Telford, J.J., Carr-Locke, D.L., Regan, M.M., Ellis, L., Durie, P.R. & Freedman, S.D. (2004). Analysis of CFTR function in patients with pancreas divisum and recurrent acute pancreatitis. *Am J Gastroenterol* Vol. 99, pp. 1557-1562.

Giannattasio, S., Bobba, A., Jurgelevicius, V., Vacca, R.A., Lattanzio, P., Merafina, R.S., Utkus, A., Kucinskas, V. & Marra, E. (2006). Molecular basis of cystic fibrosis in Lithuania: incomplete CFTR mutation detection by PCR-based screening protocols. Genet Test Vol. 10, pp. 169-173.

Gibson, L.E. & Cooke, R.E. (1959). A test for concentration of electrolytes in sweat in cystic fibrosis of the pancreas utilizing pilocarpine by iontophoresis. *Pediatrics* Vol. 23, pp. 545-549.

Gregg, R.G., Simantel, A., Farrell, P.M., Koscik, R., Kosorok, M.R., Laxova, A., Laessig, R., Hoffman, G., Hassemer, D., Mischler, E.H. & Splaingard M. (1997). Newborn screening for cystic fibrosis in Wisconsin: comparison of biochemical and molecular methods. *Pediatrics* Vol. 99, pp. 819-824.

Gregg, R.G., Wilfond, B.S., Farrell, P.M., Laxova, A., Hassemer, D. & Mischler EH. (1993). Application of DNA analysis in a population screening program for neonatal diagnosis of cystic fibrosis: comparison of screening protocols. *Am J Hum Genet* Vol. 52, pp. 616-626.

Grody, W.W., Cutting, G.R., Klinger, K.W., Richards, C.S., Watson, M.S. & Desnick, R.J. (2001). Laboratory standards and guidelines for population-based cystic fibrosis carrier screening. *Genetics in Medicine* Vol. 3, pp. 149-154.

Groman, J.D., Hefferon, T.W., Casals, T., Bassas, L., Estivill, X., Des Georges, M., Guittard, C., Koudova, M., Fallin, M.D., Nemeth, K., Fekete, G., Kadasi, L., Friedman, K., Schwarz, M., Bombieri, C., Pignatti, P.F., Kanavakis, E., Tzetis, M., Schwartz, M., Novelli, G., D'Apice, M.R., Sobczynska-Tomaszewska, A., Bal, J., Stuhrmann, M., Macek, M. Jr., Claustres, M. & Cutting, G.R. (2004). Variation in a repeat sequence determines whether a common variant of the cystic fibrosis transmembrane conductance regulator gene is pathogenic or benign. *Am J Hum Genet* Vol. 74, pp. 176-179.

Groman, J.D., Karczeski, B., Sheridan, M., Robinson, T.E., Fallin, M.D. & Cutting, G.R. (2005). Phenotypic and genetic characterization of patients with features of "nonclassic" forms of cystic fibrosis. *J Pediatr* Vol. 146, pp. 675-680.

Hammond, K.B., Abman, S.H., Sokol, R.J. & Accurso, F.J. (1991). Efficacy of statewide neonatal screening for cystic fibrosis by assay of trypsinogen concentrations. *New Engl J Med* Vol. 325, pp. 769-774.

Heim, R., Sugarman, E. & Allitto B. (2001). Improved detection of cystic fibrosis mutations in the heterogeneous U.S. population using an expanded, pan-ethnic mutation panel. *Genet Med* Vol. 3, pp. 168-176.

Highsmith, W.E., Burch, L.H., Zhou, Z., Olsen, J.C., Boat, T.E., Spock, A., Gorvoy, J.D., Quittel, L., Friedman, K.J. & Silverman, L.M. (1994). A novel mutation in the cystic fibrosis gene in patients with pulmonary disease but normal sweat chloride concentrations. *N Engl J Med* Vol. 331, pp. 97-80.

Heeley, A.F., Heeley, M.E., King, D.N., Kuzemko, J.A. & Walsh, M.P. (1982). Screening for cystic fibrosis by dried blood spot trypsin assay. *Arch Dis Child* Vol. 57, pp. 18-21.

Hubert, D., Jajac, I., Bienvenu, T., Desmazes-Dufeu, N., Ellaffi, M., Dall'ava-Santucci, J. & Dusser, D. (2004). Diagnosis of cystic fibrosis in adults with diffuse bronchiectasis. *J Cyst Fibros* Vol. 3, pp. 15-22.

Hug, M.J. & Tummler, B. (2004). Ex vivo CF diagnosis by intestinal current measurement (ICM) in small aperture, circulating Ussing chambers. *J Cyst Fibros* Vol. 3(Suppl 2), pp. 157-158.

Kakavas, K.V., Noulas, A.V., Kanakis, I., Bonanou, S. & Karamanos, N.K. (2006). Identification of the commonest cystic fibrosis transmembrane regulator gene DeltaF508 mutation: evaluation of PCR-single-strand conformational polymorphism and polyacrylamide gel electrophoresis. Biomed Chromatogr Vol. 20, pp. 1120-1125.

Kammesheidt, A., Kharrazi, M., Graham, S., Young, S., Pearl, M., Dunlop, C. & Keiles S. (2006). Comprehensive genetic analysis of the cystic fibrosis transmembrane conductance regulator from dried blood specimens - Implications for newborn screening. *Genetics in Medicine* Vol. 8, pp. 557-562.

Kerem, B., Rommens, J.M., Buchanan, J.A., Markiewicz, D., Cox, T.K., Chakravarti, A., Buchwald, M. & Tsui, L.C. (1989). Identification of the cystic fibrosis gene: Genetic analysis. *Science* Vol. 245, pp. 1073-1080.

Kerem, E., Corey, M., Kerem, B.S., Rommens, J., Markiewicz, D., Levison, H., Tsui, L.C. & Durie, P. (1990). The relation between genotype and phenotype in cystic fibrosis: analysis of the most common mutation (delta F508). *N Engl J Med* Vol. 323, pp. 1517-1522.

Knowles, M.R., Paradiso, A.M. & Boucher, R.C. (1995). In vivo nasal potential difference: techniques and protocols for assessing efficacy of gene transfer in cystic fibrosis. *Hum Gene Ther* Vol. 6, pp. 445-455.

Kolesár, P., Minárik, G., Baldovic, M., Ficek, A., Kovács, L. & Kádasi L. (2008). Mutation analysis of the CFTR gene in Slovak cystic fibrosis patients by DHPLC and subsequent sequencing: identification of four novel mutations. Gen Physiol Biophys Vol. 27, pp. 299-305.

Kristidis, P., Bozon, D., Corey, M., Markiewicz, D., Rommens, J., Tsui, L.C. & Durie P. (1992). Genetic determination of exocrine pancreatic function in cystic fibrosis. *Am J Hum Genet* Vol. 50, pp. 1178-1184.

Lebecque, P., Leal, T., De Boeck, C., Jaspers, M., Cuppens, H. & Cassiman, J.J. (2002). Mutations of the cystic fibrosis gene and intermediate sweat chloride levels in children. *Am J Respir Crit Care Med* Vol. 165, pp. 757-761.

LeGrys, V.A. & Wood, R.E. (1988). Incidence and implications of false negative sweat test reports in patients with cystic fibrosis. *Pediatr Pulmonol* Vol. 4, pp. 169-172.

LeGrys, V. (1996). Sweat testing for the diagnosis of cystic fibrosis: practical considerations. *J Pediatr* Vol. 129, pp. 892-897.

LeGrys, V.A., Yankaskas, J.R., Quittell, L.M., Marshall, B.C. & Mogayzel, P.J. Jr. (2007). Diagnostic sweat testing: the Cystic Fibrosis Foundation guidelines. *J Pediatr* Vol. 151, pp. 85-89.

Le Mare´chal, C., Audrezet, M.P., Quere, I., Quéré, I., Raguénès, O., Langonné, S. & Férec, C. (2001). Complete and rapid scanning of the cystic fibrosis conductance regulator (CFTR) gene by denaturing high performance liquid chromatography (D-HPLC): major implications for genetic counselling. *Hum Genet* Vol. 108, pp.290-298.

Lewis, P.A. (1995). The epidemiology of cystic fibrosis. In: Hodson ME, Geddes DM, editor(s). Cystic Fibrosis. London: Chapman & Hall Medical, pp. 1-5.

MacCready, R. (1963). Phenylketonuria screening program. *N Engl J Med* Vol. 269, pp. 52-56.

Macek, M. Jr., Mackova, A., Hamosh, A., Hilman, B.C., Selden, R.F., Lucotte, G., Friedman, K.J., Knowles, M.R., Rosenstein, B.J. & Cutting, G.R. (1997). Identification of common cystic fibrosis mutations in African-Americans with cystic fibrosis increases the detection rate to 75%. *Am J Hum Genet* Vol. 60, pp. 1122-1127.

Massie, J., Gaskin, K., Van Asperen, P. & Wilcken, B. (2000). Sweat testing following newborn screening for cystic fibrosis. *Pediatr Pulmonol* Vol. 29, pp. 452-456.

Messaoud, T., Verlingue, C., Denamur, E., Pascaud, O., Quere, I., Fattoum, S., Elion, J. & Ferec, C. (1996). Distribution of CFTR mutations in cystic fibrosis patients of Tunisian origin: Identification of two novel mutations. *Eur J Hum Genet* Vol. 4, pp. 20-24.

McCormick, J., Green, M., Mehta, G., Culross, F. & Mehta, A. (2002). Demographics of the UK cystic fibrosis population: implications for neonatal screening. *Eur J Hum Genet* Vol. 10, pp. 583-590.

McGinniss, M.J., Chen, C., Redman, J.B., Buller, A., Quan, F., Peng, M., Giusti, R., Hantash, F.M., Huang, D., Sun, W. & Strom, C.M. (2005). Extensive sequencing of the CFTR gene: lessons learned from the first 157 patient samples. Hum Genet Vol. 118, pp. 331-338.

McKone, E.F., Emerson, S.S., Edwards, K.L. & Aitken, M.L. (2003). Effect of genotype on phenotype and mortality in cystic fibrosis: a retrospective cohort study. *Lancet* Vol. 361, pp. 1671-1676.

Mickle, J.E. & Cutting, G.R. (2000). Genotype-phenotype relationships in cystic fibrosis. *Med Clin North Am* Vol. 84, pp. 597-607.

Nagy, B., Nagy, G.R., Lázár, L., Bán, Z. & Papp, Z. (2007). Detection of DeltaF508del using quantitative real-time PCR, comparison of the results obtained by fluorescent PCR. Fetal Diagn Ther Vol. 22, pp. 63-67.

National Committee for Clinical Laboratory Standards (NCCLS). (2000). Sweat testing: sample collection and quantitative analysis, Approved guideline C34-A2. Wayne, PA: NCCLS.

Nick, J.A. & Rodman, D.M. (2005). Manifestations of cystic fibrosis diagnosed in adulthood. *Curr Opin Pulm Med* Vol. 11, pp. 513-518.

Noone, P.G., Pue, C.A., Zhou, Z., Friedman, K.J., Wakeling, E.L., Ganeshananthan, M., Simon, R.H., Silverman, L.M. & Knowles, M.R. (2000). Lung disease associated with the IVS8 5T allele of the CFTR gene. *Am J Respir Crit Care Med* Vol. 162, pp. 1919-1924.

O'Sullivan, B.P., Zwerdling, R.G., Dorkin, H.L., Comeau, A.M. & Parad R. (2006). Early pulmonary manifestation of cystic fibrosis in children with the deltaF508/R117H-7T genotype. *Pediatrics* Vol. 118, pp. 1260-1265.

Padoan, R., Genoni, S., Moretti, E., Seia, M., Giunta, A. & Corbetta, C. (2002). Genetic and clinical features of false-negative infants in a neonatal screening programme for cystic fibrosis. *Acta Paediatr* Vol. 91, pp. 82-87.

Parad, R.B. & Comeau, A.M. (2003). Newborn screening for cystic fibrosis. *Pediatr Ann* Vol. 32, pp. 528-535.

Parad, R.B. & Comeau, A.M. (2005). Diagnostic dilemmas resulting from the immunoreactive trypsinogen/DNA cystic fibrosis newborn screening algorithm. *J Pediatr* Vol. 147(Suppl), pp. S78-S82.

Parad, R.B., Comeau, A.M., Dorkin, H.L., Dovey, M., Gerstle, R., Martin, T. & O'Sullivan, B.P. (2005). Sweat testing newborn infants detected by cystic fibrosis newborn screening. *J Pediatr* Vol. 147(Suppl), pp. S69-S72.

Pederziru, F., Faraguna, D., Giglio, L., Pedrotti, D., Perobelh, L. & Mastella, G. (1990). Development of a screening system for cystic fibrosis meconium or blood spot trypsin assay or both? *Acta Paediatr* Scand Vol. 79, pp. 935-942.

Perone, C., Medeiros, G.S., del Castillo, D.M., de Aguiar, M.J., Januário, J.N. (2010). Frequency of 8 CFTR gene mutations in cystic fibrosis patients in Minas Gerais, Brazil, diagnosed by neonatal screening. *Braz J Med Biol Res* Vol. 43, pp. 134-138.

Pilewski, J. & Frizzell, R. (1999). Role of CFTR in airway disease. *Physiol Rev* Vol. 79(1 Suppl), pp. S215-S255.

Price, J.F. (2006). Newborn screening for cystic fibrosis: do we need a second IRT? *Arch Dis Child* Vol. 91, pp. 209-210.

Quinton, P.M. (1999). Physiological basis of cystic fibrosis: A historical perspective. *Physiol Rev* Vol. 79, pp. S3-S22.

Ramos, M.D., Masvidal, L., Giménez, J., Bieth, E., Seia, M., des Georges, M., Armengol, L. Casals, T. (2010). CFTR rearrangements in Spanish cystic fibrosis patients: first new duplication (35kb) characterised in the Mediterranean countries. *Ann Hum Genet* Vol. 74, pp. 463-469.

Ranieri, E., Lewis, B.D., Gerase, R.L., Ryall, R.G., Morris, C.P., Nelson, P.V., Carey, W.F. & Robertson, E.F. (1994). Neonatal screening for cystic fibrosis using immunoreactive trypsinogen and direct gene analysis: four years' experience. *BMJ* Vol. 308, pp. 1469-1472.

Rave-Harel, N., Kerem, E., Nissim-Rafinia, M., Madjar, I., Goshen, R., Augarten, A., Rahat, A., Hurwitz, A., Darvasi, A. & Kerem. (1997). The molecular basis of partial penetrance of splicing mutations in cystic fibrosis. *Am J Hum Genet* Vol. 60, pp. 87-94.

Riordan, J.R., Rommens, J.M., Kerem, B., Alon, N., Rozmahel, R., Grzelczak, Z., Zielenski, J., Lok, S., Plavsic, N. & Chou, J.L. (1989). Identification of the cystic fibrosis gene: Cloning and characterization of complementary DNA. *Science* Vol. 245, pp. 1066-1073.

Rock, M.J., Mischler, E.H., Farrell, P.M., Wei, L.J., Bruns, W.T., Hassemer, D.J. Laessig, R.H. (1990). Newborn screening for cystic fibrosis is complicated by age-related decline in immunoreactive trypsinogen levels. *Pediatrics* Vol. 85, pp. 1001-1007.

Rock, M.J., Hoffman, G., Laessig, R.H., Kopish, G.J., Litsheim, T.J. & Farrell, P.M. (2005). Newborn screening for cystic fibrosis in Wisconsin: nine years experience with routine trypsinogen/DNA testing. *J Pediatr* Vol. 147(Suppl), pp. S73-S77.

Rock, M.J., Mischler, E.H., Farrell, P.M., Bruns, W.T., Hassemer, D.J. & Laessig R.H. (1989). Immunoreactive Trypsinogen Screening for Cystic Fibrosis: Characterization of Infants with a False-Positive Screening Test. *Pediatric Pulmonology* Vol. 6, pp. 42-48.

Ross, L.F. (2008). Newborn screening for cystic fibrosis: a lesson in public health disparities. *Pediatr* Vol. 153, pp. 308-313.

Rosenstein, B.J. (2000). Diagnostic methods. In: Hodson M, Geddes D, eds. Cystic fibrosis. 2nd ed. Arnold Publishers, pp. 177-188.

Rosenstein, B.J. & Cutting, G.R. (1998) for the Cystic Fibrosis Foundation Consensus Panel. The diagnosis of cystic fibrosis: a consensus statement. *J Pediatr* Vol. 132, pp. 589-595.

Sarles, J., Berthezene. P,, Le Louarn, C., Somma, C., Perini, J.M., Catheline, M., Mirallie, S., Luzet, K., Roussey, M., Farriaux, J.P., Berthelot, J. & Dagorn, J.C. (2005). Combining immunoreactive trypsinogen and pancreatitisassociated protein assays, a method of newborn screening for cystic fibrosis that avoids DNA analysis. *Journal of Pediatrics* Vol. 147, pp. 302-305.

Sarles, J., Barthellemy, S., Ferec, C., Iovanna, J., Roussey, M., Farriaux, J.P., Toutain, A., Berthelot, J., Maurin, N., Codet, J.P., Berthezene, P. & Dagorn, J.C. (1999). Blood concentrations of pancreatitis associated protein in neonates: relevance to neonatal screening for cystic fibrosis. *Archives of Disease in Childhood Fetal & Neonatal Edition* Vol. 80, pp. F118-F122.

Schneider, M., Joncourt, F., Sanz, J., von Känel, T. & Gallati, S. (2006). Detection of exon deletions within an entire gene (CFTR) by relative quantification on the Light Cycler. Clin Chem Vol. 52, pp. 2005-2012.

Schneider, M., Hirt, C., Casaulta, C., Barben, J., Spinas, R., Bühlmann, U., Spalinger, J., Schwizer, B., Chevalier-Porst, F., Gallati, S. (2007). Large deletions in the CFTR gene: clinics and genetics in Swiss patients with CF. Clin Genet Vol. 72, pp. 30-38.

Schüler, D., Sermet-Gaudelus, I., Wilschanski, M., Ballmann, M., Dechaux, M., Edelman, A., Hug, M., Leal, T., Lebacq, J., Lebecque, P., Lenoir, G., Stanke, F., Wallemacq, P., Tümmler, B. & Knowles, M.R. (2004). Basic protocol for transepithelial potential difference measurements. *J Cyst Fibros* Vol. 3, pp. 151-156.

Schwartz, M., Johansen, H.K., Koch, C. & Brandt, N.J. (1990). Frequency of the delta F508 mutation on cystic fibrosis chromosomes in Denmark. *Hum Genet* Vol. 85, pp. 427-428.

Sermet-Gaudelus, I., Roussel, D., Bui, S., Deneuville, E., Huet, F., Reix, P., Bellon, G., Lenoir, G. & Edelman, A. (2006). The CF-CIRC study: a French collaborative study to assess the accuracy of cystic fibrosis diagnosis in neonatal screening. *BMC Pediatr* Vol. 6:25.

Sermet-Gaudelus, I., Dechaux, M., Vallee, B., Fajac, A., Girodon, E., Nguyen-Khoa, T., Marianovski, R., Hurbain, I., Bresson, J.L., Lenoir, G. & Edelman, A. (2005). Chloride transport in nasal ciliated cells of cystic fibrosis heterozygotes. *Am J Respir Crit Care Med* Vol. 171, pp. 1026-1031.

Sheppard, D.N. & Welsh, M.J. (1999). Structure and function of the CFTR chloride channel. *Physiol Rev* Vol. 79, pp. S23-S45.

Shwachman, H. & Gahm, N. (1956). Studies in cystic fibrosis of the pancreas. A simple test for the detection of excess chloride on the skin. *N Eng J Med* Vol. 255, pp. 999-1001.

Smalley, C.A., Addy, D.P. & Anderson, C.M. (1978). Does that child really have cystic fibrosis? *Lancet* Vol. n, pp. 415-416.

Sommerburg, O., Lindner, M., Muckenthaler, M., Kohlmueller, D., Leible, S., Feneberg, R., Kulozik, A.E., Mall, M.A. & Hoffmann, G.F. (2010). Initial evaluation of a biochemical cystic fibrosis newborn screening by sequential analysis of immunoreactive trypsinogen and pancreatitis-associated protein (IRT/PAP) as a strategy that does not involve DNA testing in a Northern European population. *J Inherit Metab Dis* Vol. 33(Suppl 2), pp. S263-S271.

Sontag, M.K., Hammond, K.B., Zielenski, J., Wagener, J.S. & Accurso, F.J. (2005). Two-tiered immunoreactive trypsinogen-based newborn screening for cystic fibrosis in Colorado: screening efficacy and diagnostic outcomes. *J Pediatr* Vol. 147(3 Suppl), pp. S83-S88.

Southern, K.W., Noone, P.G., Bosworth, D.G., Legrys, V.A., Knowles, M.R. & Barker PM. (2001). A modified technique for measurement of nasal transepithelial potential difference in infants. J *Pediatr* Vol. 139, pp. 353-358.

Standaert, T.A., Boitano, L., Emerson, J., Milgram, L.J., Konstan, M.W., Hunter, J., Hunter, J., Berclaz, P.Y., Brass, L., Zeitlin, P.L., Hammond, K., Davies, Z., Foy, C., Noone, P.G., Knowles, M.R. (2004). Standardized procedure for measurement of nasal potential difference: an outcome measure in multi-center cystic fibrosis clinical trials. *Pediatr Pulmonol* Vol. 37, pp. 385-392.

Stewart, B., Zabner, J., Shuber, A., Welsh, M.J. & McCray, P.B. (1995). Normal sweat chloride values do not exclude the diagnosis of cystic fibrosis. *Am J Respir Crit Care Med* Vol. 151, pp. 899-903.

Storm, K., Moens, E., Vits, L., De Vlieger, H., Delaere, G., D'Hollander, M., Wuyts, W., Biervliet, M., Van Schil, L., Desager, K. & Nöthen, M.M. (2007). High incidence of the CFTR mutations 3272-26A-->G and L927P in Belgian cystic fibrosis patients, and identification of three new CFTR mutations (186-2A-->G, E588V, and 1671insTATCA). J Cyst Fibros Vol. 6, pp. 371-375.

Svensson, A.M., Chou, L.S., Miller, C.E., Robles, J.A., Swensen, J.J., Voelkerding, K.V., Mao, R. & Lyon, E. (2010). Detection of large rearrangements in the cystic fibrosis transmembrane conductance regulator gene by multiplex ligation-dependent probe amplification assay when sequencing fails to detect two disease-causing mutations. *Genet Test Mol Biomarkers* Vol. 14, pp. 171-174.

Taccetti, G., Festini, F., Braccini, G., Campana, S. & deMartino, M. (2004). Sweat testing in newborns positive to neonatal screening for cystic fibrosis. *Arch Dis Child Fetal Neonatal Ed* Vol. 89, pp. F463-F464.

The Cystic Fibrosis Genetic Analysis Consortium: Population variation of common cystic fibrosis mutations. (1994). The Cystic Fibrosis Genetic Analysis Consortium. *Hum Mutat* Vol. 4, pp. 167-177.

Tomaiuolo, R., Sangiuolo, F., Bombieri, C., Bonizzato, A., Cardillo, G., Raia, V., D'Apice, M.R., Bettin, M.D., Pignatti, P.F., Castaldo, G. & Novelli, G. (2008). Epidemiology and a novel procedure for large scale analysis of CFTR rearrangements in classic and atypical CF patients: a multicentric Italian study. J Cyst Fibros Vol. 7, pp. 347-351.

Travert G. (1988). Analyse de l'expenence mondiale de depistage neonatal de la mucoviscidose par dosage de la trypsirje immunoreactive (Conference Internationale Mucoviscidose- Deistage neonatal et pnse en charge precore). *Caen*, pp. 1-23.

Watson, M.S., Cutting, G.R., Desnick, R.J., Driscoll, D.A., Klinger, K., Mennuti, M., Palomaki, G.E., Popovich, B.W., Pratt, V.M., Rohlfs, E.M., Strom, C.M., Richards, C.S., Witt, D.R. & Grody, W.W. (2004). Cystic fibrosis population carrier screening: 2004 revision of American College of Medical Genetics mutation panel. *Genetics in Medicine* Vol. 6, pp. 387-391.

Welsh, M.J., Ramsey, B.W., Accurso, F. & Cutting, G.R. (2001). Cystic fibrosis. In: Scriver AB, Sly WS, Valle D, eds. The Molecular and Metabolic Basis of Inherited Disease. New York: McGraw-Hill, pp. 5121-5188.

Wilcken, B. & Travert, G. (1999). Neonatal screening for cystic fibrosis: present and future. *Acta Paediatr Suppl* Vol. 88, pp. 33-35.

Wilcken, B., Wiley, V., Sherry, G. & Bayliss, U. (1995). Neonatal screening for cystic fibrosis: a comparison of two strategies for case detection in 1.2 million babies. *J Pediatr* Vol. 127, pp. 965-970.

Wilcken, B., Brown, A.R., Urwin, R. & Brown, D.A. (1983). Cystic fibrosis screening by dried blood spot trypsin assay: results in 75,000 newborn infants. *J Pediatr* Vol. 102, pp. 383-387.

Wilfond, B.S. & Gollust, S.E. (2003). Policy issues for expanding newborn screening programs: a look "behind the curtain" at cystic fibrosis newborn screening programs in the United States [presentation]. Newborn Screening for Cystic Fibrosis Meeting; November 21, 2003; Atlanta, GA.

Wilschanski, M., Dupuis, A., Ellis, L., Jarvi, K., Zielenski, J., Tullis, E., Martin, S., Corey, M., Tsui, L.C. & Durie P. (2006). Mutations in the cystic fibrosis transmembrane regulator gene and in vivo transepithelial potentials. *Am J Respir Crit Care Med* Vol. 174, pp. 787-794.

Wilschanski, M., Famini, H., Strauss-Liviatan, N., Rivlin, J., Blau, H., Bibi, H., Bentur, L., Yahav, Y., Springer, H., Kramer, M.R., Klar, A., Ilani, A., Kerem, B. & Kerem E. (2001). Nasal potential difference measurements in patients with atypical cystic fibrosis. *Eur Respir J* Vol. 17, pp. 1208-1215.

Wilson, D.C., Ellis, L., Zielenski, J., Corey, M., Ip, W.F., Tsui, L.C., Tullis, E., Knowles, M.R. & Durie, P.R. (1998). Uncertainty in the diagnosis of cystic fibrosis: possible role of *in vivo* nasal potential difference measurements. *J Pediatr* Vol. 132, pp. 596-599.

Yeung, W.H., Palmer, J., Schidlow, D., Bye, M.R. & Huang, N.N. (1984). Evaluation of a paper patch test for sweat chloride determination *Clin Pediatr* Vol. 23, pp. 603-607.

Zielenski, J. (2000). Genotype and phenotype in cystic fibrosis. *Respiration* Vol. 67, pp. 117-133.

Zielenski, J., Rozmahel, R., Bozon, D., Kerem, B., Grzelczak, Z., Riordan, J.R., Rommens, J. & Tsui, L.C. (1991). Genomic DNA sequence of the cystic fibrosis transmembrane conductance regulator (CFTR) gene. *Genomics* Vol. 10, pp. 214-228.

Part 3

Microbiology and Immunology

7

Pseudomonas aeruginosa Biofilm Formation in the CF Lung and Its Implications for Therapy

Gregory G. Anderson
Indiana University Purdue University Indianapolis
USA

1. Introduction

Numerous microorganisms colonize or are associated with the airways of individuals with Cystic Fibrosis (CF). Impairment of the mucociliary clearance in CF lungs leads to a greater number of microbes present for the simple fact that they are not physically removed (Gibson, Burns et al. 2003; Boucher 2004). Microbes thrive in the large mucus plugs in CF airways, probably due to optimal growth temperatures and the abundance of nutrients. Additionally, CF patients display defective antimicrobial peptide activity in their lungs, which can further enhance microbial colonization (Gibson, Burns et al. 2003; Boucher 2004). As a result of these abnormalities, CF lungs are extraordinarily susceptible to infection with a number of bacteria, fungi, and viruses, including *Pseudomonas aeruginosa*, *Staphylococcus aureus*, *Burkholderia cepacia* complex, *Stenotrophomonas maltophilia*, *Haemophilus influenzae*, *Aspergillus fumigatus*, *Candida albicans*, Respiratory Syncytial virus, and Influenza Virus (Govan and Deretic 1996; Lyczak, Cannon et al. 2002; Saiman and Siegel 2004; Lipuma 2010). The relative abundance and rate of isolation of these various microorganisms varies over time. For instance, early in life, *S. aureus* is the most often isolated microbe, but by adolescence to young adulthood, *P. aeruginosa* becomes the predominate microorganism isolated from the airways (Gibson, Burns et al. 2003; Pressler, Bohmova et al. 2011).

P. aeruginosa is a Gram-negative bacterium that causes opportunistic infections. With a large number of genes involved in metabolism of many different substrates, as well as numerous regulatory genes, this bacterium has the genetic flexibility to colonize a wide range of different habitats (Stover, Pham et al. 2000; Yoon and Hassett 2004; Gomez and Prince 2007). Though typically considered an obligate aerobe, *P. aeruginosa* had been shown to undergo anaerobic respiration, in particular by denitrification processes utilizing nitrate, nitrite, or nitric oxide as terminal electron acceptors (Davies, Lloyd et al. 1989; Yoon and Hassett 2004). Furthermore, *P. aeruginosa* produces an arsenal of virulence factors, including pili, flagella, exopolysaccharides, proteases, elastase, lipases, iron chelators (pyoverdine and pyochelin), and a number of different toxins, including pyocyanin, hydrogen cyanide, exotoxin A, and the Type III Secretion System (T3SS) toxins ExoS, ExoT, ExoU, and ExoY (Lyczak, Cannon et al. 2000; Ran, Hassett et al. 2003; Shaver and Hauser 2004; Sadikot, Blackwell et al. 2005; Yahr and Wolfgang 2006; Gomez and Prince 2007). Utilizing these pathogenic tools, *P. aeruginosa* can infect a wide range of hosts, including animals (Rahme, Stevens et al. 1995), plants (Rahme, Stevens et al. 1995), insects (Miyata, Casey et al. 2003), nematodes (Gallagher and Manoil 2001), and fungi (Hogan and Kolter 2002). In humans, in addition to CF lung infections, *P. aeruginosa* can cause acute pneumonia (especially in the context of ventilator-associated pneumonia), burn wound infections, ulcerative keratitis, otitis media, otitis externa, bacteremia, urinary tract infections, and meningitis (Lyczak, Cannon et al. 2000; Sadikot, Blackwell et al. 2005; Moore and Flaws 2011).

The unique pathogenic characteristics of *P. aeruginosa* also promote efficient infection in the CF lung. Studies suggest that 20%-25% of CF infants have had a positive *P. aeruginosa* culture in the United States, and infection rates steadily increase with increasing age, such that 80% of adults 25 years old and older are chronically infected with *P. aeruginosa* (Gibson, Burns et al. 2003; Stuart, Lin et al. 2010; Woodward, Brown et al. 2010). Initially, individuals with CF experience intermittent infection, wherein transient colonization is followed by *P. aeruginosa*-free periods (Hoiby, Frederiksen et al. 2005; Stuart, Lin et al. 2010). Clinically, intermittent infection has been defined as either 1) "at least 1 isolate of [*P. aeruginosa*] with normal [*P. aeruginosa*] antibody levels," or 2) "[*P. aeruginosa*] cultures were positive in 50% or less of the 12 months" (Stuart, Lin et al. 2010). Other definitions are possible. These initial, intermittent strains are thought to originate from the environment, but there have also been cases of epidemic strains, demonstrating the potential for direct or indirect person-to-person spread (Salunkhe, Smart et al. 2005; Lipuma 2010; Mowat, Paterson et al. 2011; Saiman 2011). Following the intermittent colonization period, *P. aeruginosa* eventually establishes chronic infection (Gibson, Burns et al. 2003; Pressler, Bohmova et al. 2011). One of the hallmark characteristics of chronic *P. aeruginosa* infection in the CF lung is a switch in the colony morphology of *P. aeruginosa* isolates from a non-mucoid to a mucoid phenotype (Gibson, Burns et al. 2003; Yoon and Hassett 2004). It has been estimated that this conversion to mucoidy takes approximately 1.8 years to occur (Stuart, Lin et al. 2010). Because of mucoidy and other changes (as described below), the bacteria in the chronic state survive the intense immune reaction that occurs in the CF lung as well as the high-dose antibiotic treatment given to CF patients to kill infecting microbes (Lyczak, Cannon et al. 2002; Gomez and Prince 2007). Because of their location within the mucus airway plugs, these mucoid bacteria are further protected from immune clearance (Worlitzsch, Tarran et al. 2002; Bjarnsholt, Jensen et al. 2009). Thus, once the chronic infection is established, *P. aeruginosa* persists for the life of the individual. This chronic colonization is the cause of much of the morbidity and mortality associated with CF (Gibson, Burns et al. 2003).

Chronic *P. aeruginosa* infection also contributes significantly to the economic burden associated with treatment and care for individuals with CF. Recent studies have calculated an average of $48,098 (US) in overall medical costs per CF patient per year in the United States, with similar estimates for some European countries (Ouyang, Grosse et al. 2009). Thus, with approximately 30,000 CF individuals in the United States (Gibson, Burns et al. 2003), CF accounts for over $1.4 billion (US) in medical expenditures in the United States alone. This calculation is a gross underestimate because it omits increased costs for transplantation, malnutrition, CF-associated diabetes, and other complications (Ouyang, Grosse et al. 2009). Additional analysis has estimated that the costs of treatment with the anti-Pseudomonal antibiotic tobramycin can reach $22,481 per person per year in the United States, which is nearly half of the aforementioned per person total expenditures ($48,098) (Woodward, Brown et al. 2010). It is evident, then, that development of more effective anti-Pseudomonal therapies might lead to decreased *P. aeruginosa* infection rates and decreased economic burden. Development of new drugs will come through a better understanding of the mechanisms used by *P. aeruginosa* to establish chronic infection.

2. Transition to the chronic infection phenotype

2.1 Biofilm formation

It is generally well accepted that the chronic nature of *P. aeruginosa* in the CF lung results from the association of the bacteria into organized structures called biofilms (Gibson, Burns et al. 2003; Gomez and Prince 2007). Biofilms are communities of microorganisms bound to a surface, or to each other. During biofilm formation, bacteria undergo phenotypic, and often genotypic, changes that lead to self-aggregation and transition to a lifestyle distinct from their free-swimming (planktonic) counterparts (Costerton, Lewandowski et al. 1995). Numerous infectious states involve a biofilm component, including *P. aeruginosa* infection in the CF lung, infectious kidney stones, bacterial endocarditis, otitis media, chronic prostatitis, urinary tract infections, periodontitis, and medical device-related infections (Costerton 2001; Donlan and Costerton 2002; Parsek and Singh 2003). Often, these biofilm infections are chronic and/or recurrent.

While the characteristics of biofilms vary depending upon microbial species and growth conditions, there are several general properties that can be used to describe and define biofilms (Figure 1). Focusing specifically on *P. aeruginosa*, biofilm formation is initiated as planktonic bacteria bind to a surface via their polar flagella (O'Toole and Kolter 1998; Sauer, Camper et al. 2002), although pili have also been shown to mediate attachment to cells and other surfaces (Woods, Straus et al. 1980; Chiang and Burrows 2003). At this point, the bacterium can spin in place as the flagellum continues to rotate (Sauer, Camper et al. 2002; Hinsa, Espinosa-Urgel et al. 2003; Caiazza and O'Toole 2004). However, this initial attachment is reversible because polarly-bound bacteria can detach and swim away from the site of initial attachment (Sauer, Camper et al. 2002; Hinsa, Espinosa-Urgel et al. 2003; Caiazza and O'Toole 2004; Monds, Newell et al. 2007). This initial reversible attachment stage has been referred to as a "sampling" of the surface before full commitment to biofilm formation has been made (Caiazza and O'Toole 2004). Full commitment to the biofilm mode of growth is signaled as the initially-bound *P. aeruginosa* rods lay down on the surface along their long axis (Sauer, Camper et al. 2002; Caiazza and O'Toole 2004). The bacteria become irreversibly bound at this point and remain on the surface (Stoodley, Sauer et al. 2002)(Figure 1: Inset). Next, through type IV pilus-mediated twitching motility, the individual bacteria begin to associate into structures called microcolonies (O'Toole, Kaplan et al. 2000; Sauer, Camper et al. 2002). Through the efforts of specific signaling molecules called quorum sensing signals (described below), and the resultant change in gene expression, these microcolonies mature into large structures, which can reach a thickness of 100 μM, depending upon the growth conditions (Sauer, Camper et al. 2002). During the maturation process, the constituent bacteria begin to excrete polysaccharides, such that the bacteria in the mature biofilm are encased in a matrix of exopolysaccharides that they produced (Costerton, Lewandowski et al. 1995; Ryder, Byrd et al. 2007). DNA and protein have also been shown to be components of *P. aeruginosa* biofilms (Parsek and Singh 2003; Bjarnsholt, Tolker-Nielsen et al. 2010). Finally, as the biofilm ages, a sub-population of the bacteria break away from the biofilm bulk, revert to the planktonic state (become motile), and disperse from the biofilm (O'Toole, Kaplan et al. 2000; Sauer, Camper et al. 2002; Kirov, Webb et al. 2007; Harmsen, Yang et al. 2010). Dispersion events appear to be influenced by the production of virulent bacteriophage from dormant prophage (Rice, Tan et al. 2009). While very few studies investigating *P. aeruginosa* biofilm formation on living tissue have been performed, it is thought that these steps are conserved during infection (Hoffmann, Rasmussen et al. 2005; Anderson, Moreau-Marquis et al. 2008; Moreau-Marquis, Bomberger et al. 2008; Woodworth, Tamashiro et al. 2008; Moreau-Marquis, Redelman et al. 2010)(Figure 1).

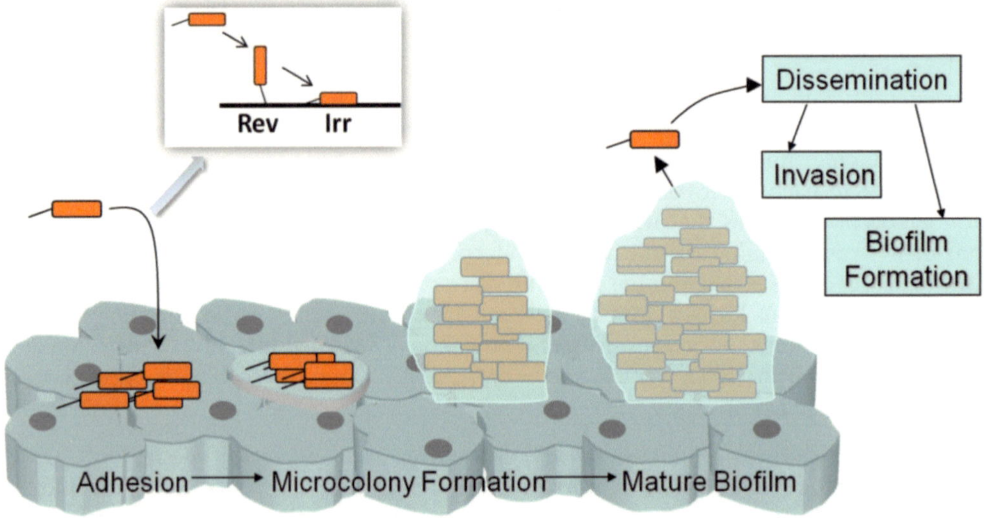

Fig. 1. Proposed biofilm formation cascade on living tissue. It is thought that many of the steps involved in bacterial biofilm formation on non-living surfaces also occur as bacteria form biofilms on human cells. Inset: Initially *P. aeruginosa* bind reversibly (Rev) by their flagellum. Irreversible binding (Irr) begins when the bacteria lay down on the surface along their long axis. See text for details.

2.2 Quorum sensing

As mentioned above, the production of quorum sensing (QS) molecules greatly influences biofilm maturation. QS is a method of self-recognition and cell density-dependent gene regulation (Cooley, Chhabra et al. 2008; Galloway, Hodgkinson et al. 2011). As a population of bacteria grows, small molecules (the QS signal) are produced and secreted. Once the density of the population is sufficiently high, the QS signal binds to an intracellular receptor that activates (or represses) a sub-set of genes (Galloway, Hodgkinson et al. 2011). Recognition of the QS signal is a stochastic process and the probability of a QS molecule binding to a receptor is low until the culture reaches a threshold density (Galloway, Hodgkinson et al. 2011). Hence, QS molecules allow bacteria to "sense the quorum", or the relative density of the population, and in this manner, they can coordinate their behaviors (Cooley, Chhabra et al. 2008). Because of the high bacterial density achieved in biofilms, QS plays a large role in regulating gene expression during biofilm development (Bjarnsholt, Tolker-Nielsen et al. 2010). *P. aeruginosa* contains 3 overlapping QS systems: Las, Rhl, and PQS (Wagner, Bushnell et al. 2003; Harmsen, Yang et al. 2010; Heeb, Fletcher et al. 2011). These systems regulate expression of virulence factors, exopolysaccharides, and other factors important for biofilm formation (Sauer, Camper et al. 2002; Wagner, Bushnell et al. 2003; Bjarnsholt, Tolker-Nielsen et al. 2010; Heeb, Fletcher et al. 2011). It has been found that QS systems are activated during biofilm maturation, and that mutation of QS genes leads to aberrations in overall biofilm architecture and sensitivity of the biofilm to stresses (Sauer, Camper et al. 2002; Bjarnsholt, Tolker-Nielsen et al. 2010; Harmsen, Yang et al. 2010; Heeb, Fletcher et al. 2011). As detailed below, much research is being devoted to the development of QS inhibitors for the disruption of biofilms.

2.3 The acute/chronic infection regulatory switch

There are numerous phenotypic changes that occur as planktonic *P. aeruginosa* transitions to the biofilm state, including a general decrease in expression of toxins and other tissue damaging virulence factors important for acute infections (Furukawa, Kuchma et al. 2006; Gooderham and Hancock 2009; Bjarnsholt, Tolker-Nielsen et al. 2010; Diaz, King et al. 2011). This suggests that *P. aeruginosa* displays 2 different infection phenotypes: an acute infection phenotype characterized by production of toxins, and a chronic infection phenotype characterized by biofilm formation and secretion of exopolysaccharides. In fact, recent evidence has revealed an inverse regulation of biofilm formation and virulence attributes associated with acute infections (Goodman, Kulasekara et al. 2004; Furukawa, Kuchma et al. 2006; Harmsen, Yang et al. 2010). For instance, expression of the AlgU alternative sigma factor leads to decreased expression of T3SS and increased production of the biofilm exopolysaccharide alginate (Wu, Badrane et al. 2004; Diaz, King et al. 2011). Similarly, the SadARS (also known as RocARS) three component regulatory system positively regulates biofilm maturation but inhibits the transcription of genes encoding components of the T3SS (Kuchma, Connolly et al. 2005; Kulasekara, Ventre et al. 2005). The LadS and GacS sensor proteins also enhance biofilm formation and exopolysaccharide production, but repress T3SS (Ventre, Goodman et al. 2006; Gooderham and Hancock 2009; Harmsen, Yang et al. 2010; Diaz, King et al. 2011). These sensors activate GacA, which, in addition to modulation of T3SS and exopolysaccharide production, can alter levels of pyocyanin, hydrogen cyanide, elastase, and lipase (Burrowes, Baysse et al. 2006; Gooderham and Hancock 2009). On the other hand, the regulatory protein RetS (also known as RtsM) inhibits the actions of GacA, and expression of RetS negatively influences exopolysaccharide production and biofilm formation but positively regulates T3SS gene expression and production of the toxins ToxA and LipA (Goodman, Kulasekara et al. 2004; Laskowski, Osborn et al. 2004). This alternate regulation of genes involved in acute toxicity and genes involved in biofilm formation suggests that during an infection, local environmental conditions might influence the infection phenotype of *P. aeruginosa*, producing an acute, toxic infection or a chronic, biofilm infection. Indeed, taking the human lung as an example, *P. aeruginosa* infection can lead to either acute pneumonia or, in the case of the CF lung, chronic colonization (Chastre and Fagon 2002; Furukawa, Kuchma et al. 2006). Depending upon the activity levels of the various acute and chronic regulators, a variety of intermediate bacterial phenotypes could occur on the acute to chronic spectrum. Investigation into this Acute/Chronic regulatory switch, and how it impacts human infections, is ongoing.

2.4 Evidence for biofilm formation in the CF lung

Numerous lines of evidence have confirmed that *P. aeruginosa* persists in CF lungs as biofilms. Perhaps most importantly, microscopic examinations of sputum samples and lung tissue sections have revealed the presence of microcolonies and large biofilm-like structures in the airways (Lam, Chan et al. 1980; Singh, Schaefer et al. 2000; Worlitzsch, Tarran et al. 2002; Bjarnsholt, Jensen et al. 2009; Hoiby, Ciofu et al. 2010; Hoiby, Ciofu et al. 2011). These biofilms can grow to larger than 100 μM in diameter (Worlitzsch, Tarran et al. 2002), and the bacteria within these biofilms have been identified as *P. aeruginosa* by fluorescent *in situ* hybridization (FISH) (Bjarnsholt, Jensen et al. 2009). Studies have suggested that in those individuals without sufficient antimicrobial therapy, these biofilms exist throughout the lungs, whereas in those patients that have had aggressive antibiotic therapy, biofilms are confined to the conductive zone and are absent from the lower airways (Bjarnsholt, Jensen et al. 2009).

As further confirmation of biofilm formation in the CF lung, *P. aeruginosa* QS signaling molecules have been identified and characterized in CF patient sputum samples (Singh, Schaefer et al. 2000). Importantly, the ratios and relative proportion of the different QS molecules was similar to that of *P. aeruginosa* biofilms grown on abiotic surfaces. These data suggest that the bacteria within CF airways receive signals that induce them toward a chronic biofilm infection phenotype.

Indeed, *P. aeruginosa* isolates from CF airways display a number of characteristics indicative of biofilm formation. The conversion to mucoidy seen with chronically-infecting strains results from an overproduction of the biofilm exopolysaccharide alginate (Gibson, Burns et al. 2003; Ramsey and Wozniak 2005). Initially, steep hypoxic gradients in the mucus plugs of the CF airways stimulate the production of alginate (Worlitzsch, Tarran et al. 2002; Yoon and Hassett 2004). Over time, mutations in the gene *mucA*, encoding the membrane-localized anti-sigma factor MucA, result in constitutive expression of the alginate biosynthesis genes, through activation of the alternative sigma factor AlgU (Ohman and Chakrabarty 1981; Hughes and Mathee 1998; Hentzer, Teitzel et al. 2001; Ramsey and Wozniak 2005; Hoiby, Ciofu et al. 2010). It is thought that the constant oxidative stress encountered in the CF lung environment induces these mutations (Yoon and Hassett 2004; Hoiby, Ciofu et al. 2010).

CF lung isolates also accumulate mutations in T3SS genes (Dacheux, Attree et al. 2001; Jain, Ramirez et al. 2004; Smith, Buckley et al. 2006). Studies have shown an increasing number of T3SS defective isolates with increasing length of *P. aeruginosa* colonization (Jain, Ramirez et al. 2004). However, T3SS-competent bacteria have also been isolated from the lungs of CF patients (Dacheux, Toussaint et al. 2000; Jain, Ramirez et al. 2004; Jain, Bar-Meir et al. 2008), and it is possible that hyperactivation of AlgU might inhibit T3SS in these strains (Wu, Badrane et al. 2004; Diaz, King et al. 2011). Thus, both mutation and regulation appear to inhibit T3SS production in the CF lung during chronic infection, and this decrease in T3SS further supports the hypothesis that *P. aeruginosa* forms biofilms in the CF lung.

Intriguingly, many other mutations appear in genes involved in acute toxicity, including genes for lipopolysaccharide (LPS) biosynthesis, twitching motility, regulation of exotoxin A, pyoverdine synthesis, and QS factors (Smith, Buckley et al. 2006). A particular subset of chronic CF isolates, called small-colony variants (SCVs) due to their small colony morphology on agar plates, contains mutations in intracellular signaling proteins that lead to altered expression of polysaccharides, flagella, and type VI secretion (Starkey, Hickman et al. 2009). Thus, chronic CF *P. aeruginosa* isolates generally display a decrease in acute virulence. It is interesting to note that several studies have shown decreased virulence of chronic *P. aeruginosa* strains in mouse models of acute infection (Smith, Buckley et al. 2006; Bragonzi, Paroni et al. 2009). This adapted virulence of SCVs and other chronic CF isolates is thought to promote bacterial survival in the CF lung environment. T3SS toxins and other secreted factors are highly immunogenic, and mutation might protect the infecting bacteria from immune clearance. Furthermore, decreased bacterial toxicity would potentially inhibit the destruction of the biofilm habitat.

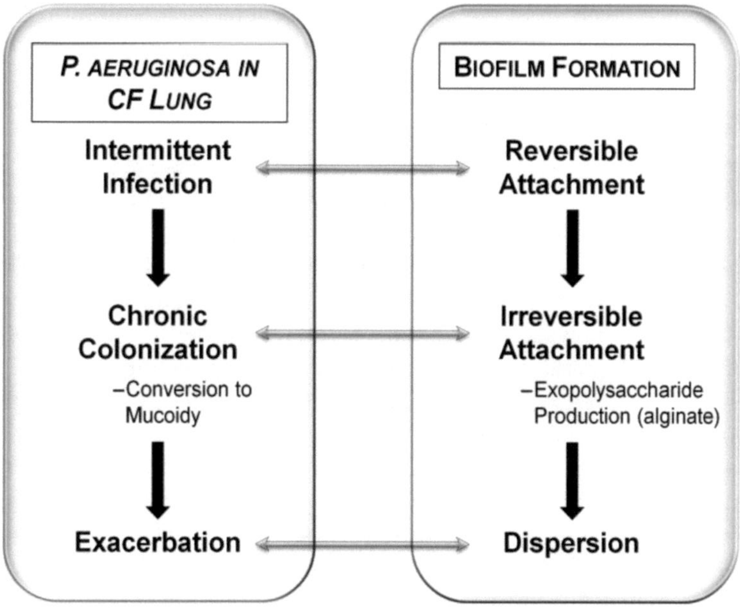

Fig. 2. Similarities between *P. aeruginosa* colonization of the CF lung and *in vitro P. aeruginosa* biofilm formation. The transition from reversible to irreversible attachment is mirrored in the transition from intermittent to chronic colonization. Similarly, just as bacteria in mature biofilms secrete exopolysaccharides, the conversion to mucoidy observed with CF isolates signals the overproduction of the exopolysaccharide alginate. Finally, it is possible that bacteria present during an exacerbation could represent bacteria that have dispersed from the biofilm and reverted to the planktonic phenotype expressing acute virulence factors.

Taken together, the presence of biofilm-like microcolonies and QS molecules, the increase in alginate production, and the decrease in T3SS and other acute infection phenotype factors strongly indicate that *P. aeruginosa* persists in the CF lung as biofilms. When comparing the biofilm formation cascade to the history of *P. aeruginosa* in an individual with CF, several intriguing parallels become apparent (Figure 2). Thus, the progression of intermittent infection, followed by chronic infection and conversion to mucoidy, is analogous to reversible binding, followed by irreversible binding and maturation of the *in vitro* biofilms, albeit chronic infection occurs on a much longer time scale than biofilms grown in the laboratory.

3. Consequences of biofilm formation in the CF lung

The formation of *P. aeruginosa* biofilms promotes chronic infection in the CF airways. As discussed in the following sections, several unique properties of biofilms contribute to this bacterial persistence, including antibiotic resistance, resistance to the activities of the immune system, and the high-frequency generation of bacterial mutants. Additionally, it has been found that *P. aeruginosa* contact with airway fluid leads to reduced flagella production (Wolfgang, Jyot et al. 2004), which potentially limits spread of the microorganism. Indeed, bacterial colonizers of the CF lung generally remain localized to the airways, and systemic spread rarely occurs (Govan and Deretic 1996). The biofilms that result from the growth and accumulation of infecting bacteria confer several survival advantages.

3.1 Antibiotic resistance

Biofilm bacteria are more resistant to many stresses than their planktonic counterparts (Costerton, Stewart et al. 1999; Stewart and Costerton 2001; Donlan and Costerton 2002; Dunne 2002; Patel 2005). In fact, biofilm bacteria can display up to 1,000 fold greater antibiotic resistance than planktonic bacteria (Mah and O'Toole 2001). This increased antibiotic resistance is due to several factors, including reduced antibiotic diffusion through the biofilm exopolysaccharide matrix, reduced growth rates of biofilm bacteria, the development of dormant persister cells, and the production of specific antibiotic-resistance factors (Donlan and Costerton 2002; Mah, Pitts et al. 2003; Lewis 2005; del Pozo and Patel 2007; Anderson 2008). All of these factors appear to influence the antibiotic-resistant nature of *P. aeruginosa* biofilms. In particular, alginate has been shown to retard the movement of cationic antimicrobial peptides, quaternary ammonium compounds, and aminoglycosides (including tobramycin) through *P. aeruginosa* biofilms (Nichols, Dorrington et al. 1988; Campanac, Pineau et al. 2002; Chan, Burrows et al. 2005). Additionally, *P. aeruginosa* produces biofilm-specific antimicrobial inhibitors (Mah, Pitts et al. 2003). Antibiotic treatment of *P. aeruginosa* biofilms also stimulates increased production of resistance factors, such as β-lactamases and antibiotic efflux pumps (Whiteley, Bangera et al. 2001; Bagge, Schuster et al. 2004). Further compounding the problem of biofilm antibiotic resistance, chronic *P. aeruginosa* CF isolates can accumulate mutations in antibiotic resistance genes, resulting in increased expression and activity of the resistance factors. These mutations confer increased survival in the presence of particular antibiotics (Smith, Buckley et al. 2006). The combination of these activities enables *P. aeruginosa* biofilms to survive the intense, often daily, antibiotic treatment regime taken by individuals with CF.

3.2 Immune resistance

P. aeruginosa biofilms also persist despite the high level inflammatory reaction that occurs in the CF lung (Gibson, Burns et al. 2003; Boucher 2004). The biofilm matrix acts as a shield preventing opsonophagocytosis of biofilm bacteria (Worlitzsch, Tarran et al. 2002; Gibson, Burns et al. 2003; Parsek and Singh 2003). In sputum and lung samples, neutrophils have been seen surrounding *P. aeruginosa* biofilms, but they have rarely been observed within the biofilms (Bjarnsholt, Jensen et al. 2009; Hoiby, Ciofu et al. 2010). *P. aeruginosa* can also counteract the effects of harmful chemical species produced by immune cells. Alginate has been shown to protect biofilm bacteria from reactive oxygen species (Cochran, Suh et al. 2000; Battan, Barnes et al. 2004; Gomez and Prince 2007; Hoiby, Ciofu et al. 2010), and denitrification pathways expressed in *P. aeruginosa* can metabolize reactive nitrogen intermediates, such as nitric oxide (Davies, Lloyd et al. 1989; Yoon and Hassett 2004). Thus, neutrophils appear to be recruited to CF lung biofilms, but the bacteria are protected from attack. Of greatest concern, lysis of spent neutrophils has been shown to add to biofilm viscosity and volume due to the release of DNA and protein (Walker, Tomlin et al. 2005; Parks, Young et al. 2009).

Chronic biofilm growth might also inhibit immune recognition of *P. aeruginosa*. Reduced production of flagella, T3SS, and acute phase virulence factors in biofilms can lead to reduced antibody detection of these antigens (Adamo, Sokol et al. 2004; Jain, Ramirez et al. 2004; Wolfgang, Jyot et al. 2004; Smith, Buckley et al. 2006; Starkey, Hickman et al. 2009). Furthermore, some chronic *P. aeruginosa* isolates display a modified LPS, which can further contribute to immune evasion (Ernst, Yi et al. 1999).

3.3 The insurance hypothesis

Biofilm formation can also result in genetic diversity. In addition to mutations in virulence factors and antibiotic resistance factors, a host of other *P. aeruginosa* genes are mutated within biofilms (Boles, Thoendel et al. 2004; Smith, Buckley et al. 2006; Starkey, Hickman et al. 2009). It is thought that the constant stress encountered in the CF lung environment leads to DNA damage, and hence mutations. Several studies have found mutations in DNA mismatch repair genes in chronic CF *P. aeruginosa* isolates, which enhances the mutation rate (Smith, Buckley et al. 2006; Doring, Parameswaran et al. 2011). It has been suggested that this genetic diversification with *P. aeruginosa* biofilms supports the "Insurance Hypothesis", which states that diversity within a population provides protection for the community as a whole against a wide range of adverse or changing conditions (Boles, Thoendel et al. 2004). In other words, in the CF lung, mutation of individual *P. aeruginosa* cells within a biofilm will give rise to subpopulations with resistance to a wide range of different stresses and the ability to grow in a variety of different environments. In fact, it has been shown that genetic diversity within *P. aeruginosa* biofilms confers protection from oxidative stress (Boles, Thoendel et al. 2004). In this manner, genotypic changes, along with antibiotic resistance and immune evasion, promote *P. aeruginosa* survival and chronic infection in the CF lung.

3.4 Seed for recurring exacerbations?

Considering the presence of a large persistent population of *P. aeruginosa* in the lungs of individuals with CF, it is possible that biofilms serve as a reservoir of bacterial pathogens that emerge during a pulmonary exacerbation (VanDevanter and Van Dalfsen 2005). Indeed, during an exacerbation, lung function decreases while the symptoms of bacterial infection increase (VanDevanter, O'Riordan et al. 2010). Clinically, exacerbations have been defined as a sudden worsening of symptoms requiring physician intervention and the need for altered antibiotic treatment (Rogers, Hoffman et al. 2011), although some clinicians and researchers argue for more objective criteria (Bilton, Canny et al. 2011). This definition implies that bacterial activity is a large part of an exacerbation. However, the role of bacteria during an exacerbation remains a mystery. Some studies have shown that bacterial densities increase during an exacerbation (Mowat, Paterson et al. 2011), while others report similar bacterial levels before and during an exacerbation (Stressmann, Rogers et al. 2011). It has also been suggested that a virulent sub-population of bacteria emerge during an exacerbation, thus leading to symptoms of acute infection (Jaffar-Bandjee, Lazdunski et al. 1995; Stressmann, Rogers et al. 2011). In support of this hypothesis, researchers have found increased levels of *P. aeruginosa* exoenzyme S, exotoxin A, elastase, and alkaline protease in sputum samples during exacerbations (Grimwood, Semple et al. 1993; Jaffar-Bandjee, Lazdunski et al. 1995).

Moreover, it has been shown that high-dose antibiotic intervention for exacerbations decreases bacterial density and results in improved pulmonary symptoms, indication that bacterial activity plays a large role in initiation and progression of an exacerbation (Jaffar-Bandjee, Lazdunski et al. 1995; VanDevanter, O'Riordan et al. 2010; Tunney, Klem et al. 2011). Thus, during an exacerbation, it is possible that some fraction of the biofilm bacteria disperses from the biofilm and reverts to the acute planktonic phenotype, which will cause more tissue damage and lead to greater immune stimulation (Figure 2).

4. Treatment of *P. aeruginosa* infections of the CF lung: Triumphs and challenges

Treatment of *P. aeruginosa* lung infections remains challenging. The best course of action might be prevention of infection through aggressive infection control procedures. These procedures are meant to prevent person-to-person transmission as well as transmission from contaminated surfaces. It has been found that sputum-encased *P. aeruginosa* can survive on inanimate surfaces for up to 8 days (Saiman and Siegel 2004). Thus, thorough cleaning and sterilization of clinical rooms, apparatuses, and home respirators is recommended (Saiman and Siegel 2004; Saiman 2011). Furthermore, healthcare workers should practice good hand and respiratory hygiene (Saiman and Siegel 2004; Hoiby, Ciofu et al. 2011; Saiman 2011). Isolation and separation of individuals infected with particular pathogens, such as *P. aeruginosa* and multi-drug resistant bacteria, has also been suggested to reduce patient-to-patient spread. Many clinics also encourage re-gowning and re-gloving with each new patient contact. However, despite the best infection control protocols, most CF individuals still acquire *P. aeruginosa*, either from environmental sources or from other CF patients. As discussed below, there are a number of antimicrobial therapies implemented to control lung infection with *P. aeruginosa*.

4.1 Antibiotic treatments

Numerous antibiotics have been used to treat CF lung infection with *P. aeruginosa*, although the aminoglycoside antibiotic tobramycin has most often been used and has been studied the most (Gibson, Burns et al. 2003; Ryan, Singh et al. 2011). In order to achieve high concentration in the airways, tobramycin and other antibiotics are often inhaled in a nebulized form (Ryan, Singh et al. 2011). Studies have investigated the efficacy of a number of inhaled antibiotics, including tobramycin, colistin, gentamicin, ceftazidime, cephaloridine, aztreonam lysine, taurolidine, and a gentamicin/carbenicillin combination (Ryan, Singh et al. 2011). The use of inhaled antibiotics, can lead to increased lung function and decreased exacerbation frequency over placebo (Ryan, Singh et al. 2011). During stable periods, inhaled antibiotics such as tobramycin or colistin can be given as chronic suppressive therapies to maintain low bacterial levels within the airways (Hoiby, Ciofu et al. 2011). An economics study estimated that increased usage of inhaled tobramycin would lead to increased cost for medication but decreased physician and hospital visits. This would have a net decrease in healthcare costs (Woodward, Brown et al. 2010). It has also been suggested that this maintenance therapy be supplemented with 2-week courses of intravenous (IV) antibiotic combinations every 3 months for added anti-Pseudomonal pressure (Hoiby, Ciofu et al. 2011). In addition to antimicrobial therapies, other medications such as DNase and hypertonic saline are widely used to increase airway clearance (Fuchs, Borowitz et al. 1994; Donaldson, Bennett et al. 2006; Elkins, Robinson et al. 2006; Parks, Young et al. 2009).

However, despite suppressive therapies, pulmonary exacerbations still occur. The types of antibiotics, dosing, and treatment schedules for exacerbation therapy vary greatly country-to-country and site-to-site. Synergy and a reduction in antibiotic resistance have been shown with thrice daily IV infusions of an aminoglycoside antibiotic and a β-lactam antibiotic (Bals, Hubert et al. 2011; Plummer and Wildman 2011). A recent study has found that twice daily treatments of tobramycin and ceftazidime are just as effective as thrice daily infusions, and this reduced treatment regimen can be safer and more convenient than a three times a day schedule. Studies have demonstrated that the bacterial response to antibiotic treatment is completed within 14 days (Adeboyeku, Jones et al. 2011), although in some cases, patients respond better to shorter or longer treatments (VanDevanter, O'Riordan et al. 2010; Plummer and Wildman 2011). Many more antibiotic treatment regimens are used in clinics and hospitals, and optimization of therapy for an individual exacerbation event often relies on symptoms and pulmonary function testing. Home-based IV antibiotic therapy of exacerbation has also been explored as an alternative to inpatient treatment. At-home therapy, while requiring specialized training for family members and friends, can reduce costs to families and hospitals, reduce incidence of hospital-acquired infections, improve disease manifestations, and can be more convenient for the affected individual (Balaguer and Gonzalez de Dios 2008).

4.2 Early colonization eradication

The period of intermittent infection, before the establishment of chronic *P. aeruginosa* biofilms, presents a unique opportunity for therapeutic intervention. Many studies have shown the efficacy of early aggressive antibiotic therapy to eradicate *P. aeruginosa* during this early colonization period. In the Copenhagen Model, which has been in place for over 20 years in the Copenhagen CF center, infected CF patients are given inhaled colistin and IV ciprofloxacin for 3 months (Hoiby, Frederiksen et al. 2005; Hansen, Pressler et al. 2008). 80% of patients treated with this regimen were free of chronic *P. aeruginosa* infection for up to 15 years, and the bacterial isolates recovered exhibited little resistance to colistin and ciprofloxacin (Hansen, Pressler et al. 2008). In a different study of other European CF centers, treatment with inhaled colistin and IV ciprofloxacin for 3 months was found to be 81% effective (Taccetti, Campana et al. 2005). In this study, treated patients were completely free from *P. aeruginosa* infection for an average of 18 months, and 73% of subsequent *P. aeruginosa* infections were found to involve a genotypically distinct strain, suggesting that the original isolate had been eradicated (Taccetti, Campana et al. 2005). This treatment was also associated with reduced overall treatment costs and little development of antibiotic resistance (Taccetti, Campana et al. 2005).

There are numerous variations on eradication therapies, and many studies evaluating the efficacy of these treatments (Stuart, Lin et al. 2010; Hayes, Feola et al. 2011). In an effort to develop standardized treatment guidelines for early eradication therapies, there have been 2 large, multicenter studies: the Early Inhaled Tobramycin for Eradication (ELITE) study in Europe, and the Early *Pseudomonas* Infection Control (EPIC) program in the United States. The

EPIC program, the results of which have yet to be published, is comparing standard culture-based therapy with twice daily inhaled tobramycin (300 mg) for 28 days every yearly quarter (Stuart, Lin et al. 2010; Hayes, Feola et al. 2011). The tobramycin-treatment group is further split into groups that additionally receive 14 days of either oral ciprofloxacin or oral placebo. The ELITE study treated participants for 28 days with twice daily inhaled tobramycin (300mg/5mL), and found that 93% of those treated were *P. aeruginosa*-free after 1 month (Ratjen, Munck et al. 2010). 66% of participants were free of *P. aeruginosa* infection for 2 years (Ratjen, Munck et al. 2010). Similar results were obtained with individuals treated for 56 days.

The early promise of eradication therapy studies demonstrates that these treatments will likely enhance overall patient health and reduce healthcare costs related to *P. aeruginosa* infection. Indeed, such early eradication protocols have dramatically increased the age at which chronic *P. aeruginosa* infection is established (Hoiby, Frederiksen et al. 2005; Hansen, Pressler et al. 2008). Furthermore, eradication can be achieved regardless of the age of the patient, provided there has been no evidence of prior *P. aeruginosa* infection (Hayes, Feola et al. 2011). However, even with constant monitoring and treatment, intermittent *P. aeruginosa* infection will eventually give way to chronic biofilm formation. It is well established that once chronic infection is initiated, eradication of *P. aeruginosa* from the CF lung is essentially impossible (Hoiby, Frederiksen et al. 2005; Hansen, Pressler et al. 2008).

4.3 Antibiotic resistance

Perhaps not surprisingly, treatment of CF lung infections with large doses of antibiotics leads to high levels of antibiotic resistance. Resistance of a CF lung isolate to a particular antibiotic is generally associated with treatment with that antibiotic (Emerson, McNamara et al. 2010). Greater resistance leads to longer therapies, which consequently induces more resistance (Plummer and Wildman 2011). The formation of *P. aeruginosa* biofilms plays a large role in the emergence of antibiotic resistance. In addition to the general resistance of biofilms and other stresses (Costerton, Stewart et al. 1999; Stewart and Costerton 2001; Donlan and Costerton 2002; Dunne 2002; Patel 2005), the high mutation rate and generation of diversity that occurs in *P. aeruginosa* biofilms results in variant strains that display increased resistance to antibiotics, through mutation of antibiotic targets and increased production and activity of multidrug efflux pumps (Smith, Buckley et al. 2006; Bals, Hubert et al. 2011; Mowat, Paterson et al. 2011). Moreover, the SCVs that develop in biofilms, and appear with increasing prevalence in CF patient sputum samples over time, are more innately resistant to a multitude of antibiotics (Starkey, Hickman et al. 2009; Bals, Hubert et al. 2011). The appearance of multidrug-resistant *P. aeruginosa* clones, which are associated with more severe lung disease and declining lung function (Plummer and Wildman 2011), has lead to an antibiotic dilemma. Novel antimicrobial strategies must be developed to combat these multidrug-resistant *P. aeruginosa* infections in the CF lung.

5. Hope for the future: Novel therapies and model systems

Recent investigations into anti-Pseudomonal treatments, with an eye toward inhibiting *P. aeruginosa* biofilm formation, have led to new drugs and novel implementation strategies of existing antimicrobials (Table 1). Likewise, advances in CF lung infection model systems are leading to new insights into the nature of chronic *P. aeruginosa* infection in the CF lung.

Strategy	References
Anti-biofilm Testing	
MBEC testing of current antibiotics	(Ceri, Olson et al. 1999; Keays, Ferris et al. 2009; Moskowitz, Emerson et al. 2011)
Quorum Sensing Inhibitors	
Furanones	(Steinberg, Schneider et al. 1997; Hentzer, Riedel et al. 2002)
Garlic extract	(Rasmussen and Givskov 2006; Harmsen, Yang et al. 2010)
Patulin	(Rasmussen, Skindersoe et al. 2005)
Penicillin acid	(Rasmussen, Skindersoe et al. 2005)
cis-2 decanoic acid	(Bjarnsholt, Tolker-Nielsen et al. 2010)
Salicylic acid	(Bjarnsholt, Tolker-Nielsen et al. 2010)
4-NPO	(Rasmussen and Givskov 2006; Bjarnsholt, Tolker-Nielsen et al. 2010)
Solenopsin A	(Bjarnsholt, Tolker-Nielsen et al. 2010)
Azithromycin	(Skindersoe, Alhede et al. 2008; Bjarnsholt, Tolker-Nielsen et al. 2010)
Clarithromycin	(Wozniak and Keyser 2004)
Ceftazidime	(Skindersoe, Alhede et al. 2008)
Ciprofloxacin	(Skindersoe, Alhede et al. 2008)
Inhaled Antibiotics	
Aztreonam lysine	(McCoy, Quittner et al. 2008; Retsch-Bogart, Burns et al. 2008; Parkins and Elborn 2010)
Levofloxacin	(Anderson 2010; Bals, Hubert et al. 2011)
Fosfomycin/Tobramycin	(Anderson 2010)
Tobramycin, inhalable powder	(Bals, Hubert et al. 2011)
Ciprofloxacin, inhalable powder	(Anderson 2010; Bals, Hubert et al. 2011)
Liposomally-encased Antibiotics	
Amikacin	(Anderson 2010; Bals, Hubert et al. 2011)
Tobramycin	(Bals, Hubert et al. 2011)
Polymyxin B	(Bals, Hubert et al. 2011)
New Antibiotics	
Tigecycline	(Parkins and Elborn 2010)
Doripenem	(Parkins and Elborn 2010)
Ceftibiprole	(Parkins and Elborn 2010)
Tomopenem	(Parkins and Elborn 2010)
CXA-101	(Parkins and Elborn 2010; Bals, Hubert et al. 2011)
NXL104/Ceftazidime	(Parkins and Elborn 2010)
ACHN-490	(Parkins and Elborn 2010)
CB182,804	(Parkins and Elborn 2010)
BLI-489/Pipericillin	(Parkins and Elborn 2010)
Disruption of Iron Metabolism	
Gallium	(Kaneko, Thoendel et al. 2007)
Desferasirox	(Moreau-Marquis, O'Toole et al. 2009)
Desferoxamine	(Moreau-Marquis, O'Toole et al. 2009)
Virulence Factor Modulation	
T3SS Inhibitors	(Aiello, Williams et al. 2010)
Vaccination	(Doring and Pier 2008)

Table 1. Novel and Emerging Therapies for *P. aeruginosa* Infection of CF Lungs

5.1 Novel therapies

5.1.1 Anti-biofilm strategies

Because biofilm formation plays an integral role in the persistence and antibiotic resistance of *P. aeruginosa* in the CF lung, many researchers have begun searching out ways to specifically destroy biofilms. The most obvious place to start in the development of anti-biofilm therapies is testing the efficacy of our current antibiotics against *P. aeruginosa* biofilms (Moskowitz, Emerson et al. 2011)(Table 1). In one retrospective analysis, the reported planktonic antibiotic susceptibilities of *P. aeruginosa* CF isolates were compared to the antibiotic susceptibilities of these strains grown as biofilms (Keays, Ferris et al. 2009). Those patients that were treated with antibiotics that could kill biofilm-state bacteria experienced lower treatment failure, decreased exacerbation risk, and decreased hospital stays (Keays, Ferris et al. 2009). Other studies have also shown that treatment tailored to biofilm susceptibility patterns can be effective (Moskowitz, Emerson et al. 2011). The recent development of the Minimum Biofilm Eradication Concentration (MBEC) Assay (also known as the Calgary Biofilm Device, distributed through Innovotech, Edmonton, CA), has permitted high throughput analysis of biofilm formation and biofilm susceptibilities of *P. aeruginosa* and other CF pathogens (Ceri, Olson et al. 1999; Tomlin, Malott et al. 2005; Davies, Harrison et al. 2007; Alfa and Howie 2009). Anti-biofilm therapies developed using the MBEC or other biofilm assays can thus be of great clinical benefit.

Another promising avenue of anti-biofilm research is the identification of molecules that interrupt QS signaling (Geske, Wezeman et al. 2005; Rasmussen and Givskov 2006; Galloway, Hodgkinson et al. 2011)(Table 1). By interfering with inter-bacterial communication and gene regulation, these compounds can lead to the dispersion of biofilm bacteria as well as alter virulence factor production. Generally, QS inhibitors fall into one of three categories: 1) those that block production of the QS signaling molecule, 2) those that degrade the QS molecule, and 3) those that prevent bacterial recognition of the QS signal (Rasmussen and Givskov 2006). Many large screens of natural compounds have been completed or are taking place to identify novel QS inhibitors, and several active compounds have emerged from these studies. For instance, halogenated furanones from the alga *Delisea pulchra* and synthetic furanones have been shown to block *P. aeruginosa* QS and biofilm formation, and they lead to increased *P. aeruginosa* killing when used in combination with traditional antibiotics (Steinberg, Schneider et al. 1997; Hentzer, Riedel et al. 2002; Bjarnsholt, Tolker-Nielsen et al. 2010). Likewise, garlic extract, patulin and penicillic acid from *Penicillium* species, *cis*-2-decanoic acid from *P. aeruginosa,* salicylic acid, 4-nitro-pyridine-N-oxide (4-NPO), and solenopsin A from fire ant venom have all demonstrated inhibition of *P. aeruginosa* QS, and some have shown direct biofilm disruption activity (Rasmussen, Skindersoe et al. 2005; Rasmussen and Givskov 2006; Bjarnsholt, Tolker-Nielsen et al. 2010; Harmsen, Yang et al. 2010). Some of these QS inhibitors, such as garlic extract, patulin, 4-NPO, and furanones, have also displayed a therapeutic effect in models of *P. aeruginosa* infection (Rasmussen and Givskov 2006). Importantly, it is thought that resistance to QS inhibitors will not develop because these compounds do not directly affect bacterial growth, and thus exert little selective pressure (Bjarnsholt, Tolker-Nielsen et al. 2010).

Intriguingly, it has been found that some traditional antibiotics can affect biofilm formation and virulence factor production through QS inhibition or other mechanisms. For instance, azithromycin, ceftazidime, and ciprofloxacin were all shown to affect *P. aeruginosa* QS and virulence factor production (Skindersoe, Alhede et al. 2008; Bjarnsholt, Tolker-Nielsen et al. 2010). Sub-inhibitory concentrations of clarithromycin can also alter biofilm morphology (Wozniak and Keyser 2004). Thus, treatment with these antibiotics has yielded unexpected consequences for *P. aeruginosa* infection.

5.1.2 Newer antimicrobial strategies

Development of traditional antibiotics, and novel delivery methods for antibiotics, has also yielded some successes (Table 1). Several new antibiotics have recently hit the markets in various countries, including tigecycline, doripenem, and the 5th generation cephalosporin ceftibiprole (Parkins and Elborn 2010). Many more antibiotics with potential efficacy against Gram-negative CF pathogens are in development, such as tomopenem, CXA-101, NXL104/ceftazidime, ACHN-490, CB182,804, and BLI-489/pipericillin (Parkins and Elborn 2010; Bals, Hubert et al. 2011). However, because many of these compounds are derivatives of existing antibiotics, resistance and toxicity might hinder further research on these novel therapies (Parkins and Elborn 2010).

On the other hand, the development of inhaled versions of existing antibiotics has been shown to improve delivery times and concentrate the antibiotic at the site of infection (Anderson 2010; Bals, Hubert et al. 2011; Ryan, Singh et al. 2011). Nebulized tobramycin has been used for years as an effective anti-Pseudomonal therapy, and many other inhaled antibiotic formulation have been studied (Ryan, Singh et al. 2011). Recently, Aztreonam Lysine for Inhalation has been approved in many countries for treatment of chronic CF lung infections, and studies have shown that use of this drug can improve quality of life and pulmonary function of CF patients, while decreasing *P. aeruginosa* burden and lower exacerbation severity (McCoy, Quittner et al. 2008; Retsch-Bogart, Burns et al. 2008; Anderson 2010; Parkins and Elborn 2010; Bals, Hubert et al. 2011). Work continues on other inhaled antibiotics, including aerosolized levofloxacin, fosfomycin/tobramycin, and inhalable dry powers of tobramycin and ciprofloxacin (Anderson 2010; Bals, Hubert et al. 2011). Inhalation of liposomally-encased antibiotics shows great promise for therapy of biofilm infections, as liposome delivery is thought to increase the penetration of biofilms (Smith 2005; Bals, Hubert et al. 2011). Patients treated with liposomally-encased amikacin showed improved lung function and reduction in sputum *P. aeruginosa* levels (Anderson 2010; Bals, Hubert et al. 2011). Similarly, liposomal encasement of tobramycin and polymyxin B might hold great promise as alternative treatments for chronic CF infections (Bals, Hubert et al. 2011).

Looking toward the future, there is great interest in identifying and developing novel chemical agents that disrupt bacterial metabolism, adhesins, virulence factor production, efflux pump activity, and bacterial intracellular signaling (Parkins and Elborn 2010; Bals, Hubert et al. 2011)(Table 1). Indeed, treatment with iron chelators (desferasirox and desferoxamine) or gallium, which is a non-reducible mimic for iron, can interfere with *P. aeruginosa* metabolism, resulting in biofilm disruption and protection against *P. aeruginosa* infection in animal models (Kaneko, Thoendel et al. 2007; DeLeon, Balldin et al. 2009; Moreau-Marquis, O'Toole et al. 2009). Inhibitors of *P. aeruginosa* T3SS have also been found

(Aiello, Williams et al. 2010). Further screening of chemical compound libraries will likely reveal many additional molecules with anti-Pseudomonal activity.

5.1.3 Vaccination

Vaccines against *P. aeruginosa* have also been proposed as a potential therapy for preventing chronic CF infections (Table 1). Researchers have explored vaccines against *P. aeruginosa* LPS, alginate, flagella, outer membrane proteins, pili, T3SS components, DNA, and killed whole bacteria (Doring and Pier 2008). Many of these vaccines have been tested in clinical trials, with moderate efficacy. It is thought that clearance and prevention of *P. aeruginosa* infection by aggressive early eradication programs masks the true effectiveness of these vaccines, and none of them have reached the market (Doring and Pier 2008). Passive immunotherapy with monoclonal antibodies or pooled immune serum has also been investigated for anti-Pseudomonal therapy (Doring and Pier 2008).

5.2 Novel model systems

5.2.1 Animal models

Researchers have tried for decades to develop an animal CF model that can maintain a chronic *P. aeruginosa* infection. Mice with various *CFTR* alleles and/or overexpression of βENaC have been tested as infection models, but *P. aeruginosa* is generally cleared from the lungs of these animals (Grubb and Boucher 1999; Mall, Grubb et al. 2004; Wilke, Buijs-Offerman et al. 2011; Zhou, Duerr et al. 2011). Mice and humans have very different lung physiologies, which most likely account for the inability to establish chronic infection in "CF" mice (Wilke, Buijs-Offerman et al. 2011). The recently developed pig and ferret CF animal models have been reported to develop spontaneous bacterial infections, and it is possible that chronic *P. aeruginosa* infection could be reproduced in these animals (Fisher, Zhang et al. 2011). However, these CF animals generally require surgery to correct the meconium ileus that develops in the young (Fisher, Zhang et al. 2011). Thus, the cost of these model systems is high.

5.2.2 Artificial sputum

In order to model the CF lung environment *in vitro*, several groups have created artificial sputum media. These media replicate the experimentally-determined composition of CF sputum samples, and they can support similar *P. aeruginosa* growth rates, gene expression patterns, nutritional preferences, and QS patterns as found in CF sputum (Sriramulu, Lunsdorf et al. 2005; Palmer, Aye et al. 2007). These media have also been useful for investigations of *P. aeruginosa* biofilm formation (Sriramulu, Lunsdorf et al. 2005; Garbe, Wesche et al. 2010). These models could lead to a better understanding of metabolic flux in *P. aeruginosa* biofilms in the context of CF lung infection.

5.2.3 Biofilms co-cultured with airway cells

Recently, several investigators have developed *P. aeruginosa* biofilms on cultured airway cells *in vitro* (Figure 3). These co-culture biofilm models were developed to more closely mimic the CF lung environment and potential signals that the bacteria receive from mammalian cells during infection. In one model, *P. aeruginosa* bind to a monolayer or air-liquid interface differentiated layer of immortalized CF-derived (*CFTR* ΔF508 homozygous) bronchial epithelial cells (Moreau-Marquis, Bomberger et al. 2008; Moreau-Marquis, Redelman et al. 2010). Fresh culture medium then flows across the system and large bacterial aggregates form on the epithelial cells. The aggregates appear morphologically similar to biofilms formed on abiotic surfaces (Moreau-Marquis, Bomberger et al. 2008; Moreau-Marquis, Redelman et al. 2010). Furthermore, formation of these co-culture biofilms requires factors necessary for abiotic biofilm formation, and bacteria within co-culture biofilms display a pattern of gene expression consistent with that found in abiotic biofilms. In a different study, similar co-culture biofilms were formed by static incubation of *P. aeruginosa* and CF airway cells in the presence of arginine (Anderson, Moreau-Marquis et al. 2008; Moreau-Marquis, Redelman et al. 2010). Importantly, in both systems, the antibiotic resistance of the co-culture biofilms was greatly increased compared to both planktonic bacteria and abiotic biofilms (Anderson, Moreau-Marquis et al. 2008; Moreau-Marquis, Bomberger et al. 2008; Moreau-Marquis, O'Toole et al. 2009). It was also discovered that the co-culture biofilms displayed a different genetic response to tobramycin treatment than biofilms formed on plastic (Anderson, Moreau-Marquis et al. 2008). These data suggest that the surface upon which a biofilm forms can affect the properties of that biofilm, and they also offer clues into the high antibiotic resistance of *P. aeruginosa* biofilms that form in the CF lung. *P. aeruginosa* biofilms have also been shown to form on cultured mouse nasal septal epithelial cells (Woodworth, Tamashiro et al. 2008).

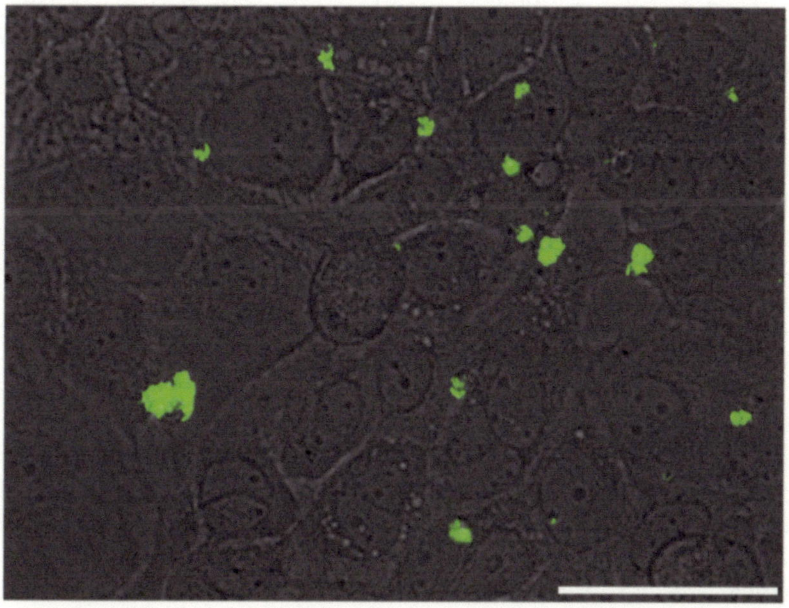

Fig. 3. *P. aeruginosa* biofilm microcolonies on cultured human CF-derived airway cells. Immortalized human bronchial epithelial cells, originally isolated from an individual with CF, were inoculated with *P. aeruginosa* constitutively expressing green fluorescent protein. Biofilm microcolonies (green) are attached to the surface of the cells. Bar = 50μm.

6. Conclusion

There have been a number of great advances in recent years in anti-Pseudomonal therapy of CF lung infections. In particular, early eradication treatments appear to show much promise in delaying the onset of chronic *P. aeruginosa* biofilm formation. The increasing arsenal against *P. aeruginosa,* including inhaled aztreonam and liposomal amikacin, will likely prove a benefit for *P. aeruginosa* treatment. Eradication of chronic *P. aeruginosa* may be possible, but it will take creative thinking. It is clear that new anti-biofilm treatments need to be discovered and implemented. The development of clinically-relevant models will further aid this process by providing appropriate systems for testing novel molecules. With renewed focus on the biofilm nature of the infection, much progress can be made toward eliminating chronic *P. aeruginosa* from the CF lung.

7. Acknowledgements

Many thanks are given to C. Redelman, C. McCaslin, and M. Howenstine for helpful comments and technical support. This work was supported by RSFG from IUPUI and PRF from Purdue University to GGA.

8. References

Adamo, R., S. Sokol, G. Soong, M. I. Gomez and A. Prince (2004). Pseudomonas aeruginosa flagella activate airway epithelial cells through asialoGM1 and toll-like receptor 2 as well as toll-like receptor 5. *Am J Respir Cell Mol Biol* 30(5): 627-34.

Adeboyeku, D., A. L. Jones and M. E. Hodson (2011). Twice vs three-times daily antibiotics in the treatment of pulmonary exacerbations of cystic fibrosis. *J Cyst Fibros* 10(1): 25-30.

Aiello, D., J. D. Williams, H. Majgier-Baranowska, I. Patel, N. P. Peet, J. Huang, S. Lory, T. L. Bowlin and D. T. Moir (2010). Discovery and characterization of inhibitors of Pseudomonas aeruginosa type III secretion. *Antimicrob Agents Chemother* 54(5): 1988-99.

Alfa, M. J. and R. Howie (2009). Modeling microbial survival in buildup biofilm for complex medical devices. *BMC Infect Dis* 9: 56.

Anderson, G. G., S. Moreau-Marquis, B. A. Stanton and G. A. O'Toole (2008). In vitro analysis of tobramycin-treated Pseudomonas aeruginosa biofilms on cystic fibrosis-derived airway epithelial cells. *Infect Immun* 76(4): 1423-33.

Anderson, G. G., O'Toole. G. A. (2008). Innate and Induced Resistance Mechanisms of Bacterial Biofilms. *Bacterial Biofilms*. T. Romeo. Berlin, Springer-Verlag. 322: 85-105.

Anderson, P. (2010). Emerging therapies in cystic fibrosis. *Ther Adv Respir Dis* 4(3): 177-85.

Bagge, N., M. Schuster, M. Hentzer, O. Ciofu, M. Givskov, E. P. Greenberg and N. Hoiby (2004). Pseudomonas aeruginosa biofilms exposed to imipenem exhibit changes in global gene expression and beta-lactamase and alginate production. *Antimicrob Agents Chemother* 48(4): 1175-87.

Balaguer, A. and J. Gonzalez de Dios (2008). Home intravenous antibiotics for cystic fibrosis. *Cochrane Database Syst Rev*(3): CD001917.

Bals, R., D. Hubert and B. Tummler (2011). Antibiotic treatment of CF lung disease: from bench to bedside. *J Cyst Fibros* 10 Suppl 2: S146-51.

Battan, P. C., A. I. Barnes and I. Albesa (2004). Resistance to oxidative stress caused by ceftazidime and piperacillin in a biofilm of Pseudomonas. *Luminescence* 19(5): 265-70.

Bilton, D., G. Canny, S. Conway, S. Dumcius, L. Hjelte, M. Proesmans, B. Tummler, V. Vavrova and K. De Boeck (2011). Pulmonary exacerbation: towards a definition for use in clinical trials. Report from the EuroCareCF Working Group on outcome parameters in clinical trials. *J Cyst Fibros* 10 Suppl 2: S79-81.

Bjarnsholt, T., P. O. Jensen, M. J. Fiandaca, J. Pedersen, C. R. Hansen, C. B. Andersen, T. Pressler, M. Givskov and N. Hoiby (2009). Pseudomonas aeruginosa biofilms in the respiratory tract of cystic fibrosis patients. *Pediatr Pulmonol* 44(6): 547-58.

Bjarnsholt, T., T. Tolker-Nielsen, N. Hoiby and M. Givskov (2010). Interference of Pseudomonas aeruginosa signalling and biofilm formation for infection control. *Expert Rev Mol Med* 12: e11.

Boles, B. R., M. Thoendel and P. K. Singh (2004). Self-generated diversity produces "insurance effects" in biofilm communities. *Proc Natl Acad Sci U S A* 101(47): 16630-5.

Boucher, R. C. (2004). New concepts of the pathogenesis of cystic fibrosis lung disease. *Eur Respir J* 23(1): 146-58.

Bragonzi, A., M. Paroni, A. Nonis, N. Cramer, S. Montanari, J. Rejman, C. Di Serio, G. Doring and B. Tummler (2009). Pseudomonas aeruginosa microevolution during cystic fibrosis lung infection establishes clones with adapted virulence. *Am J Respir Crit Care Med* 180(2): 138-45.

Burrowes, E., C. Baysse, C. Adams and F. O'Gara (2006). Influence of the regulatory protein RsmA on cellular functions in Pseudomonas aeruginosa PAO1, as revealed by transcriptome analysis. *Microbiology* 152(Pt 2): 405-18.

Caiazza, N. C. and G. A. O'Toole (2004). SadB is required for the transition from reversible to irreversible attachment during biofilm formation by Pseudomonas aeruginosa PA14. *J Bacteriol* 186(14): 4476-85.

Campanac, C., L. Pineau, A. Payard, G. Baziard-Mouysset and C. Roques (2002). Interactions between biocide cationic agents and bacterial biofilms. *Antimicrob Agents Chemother* 46(5): 1469-74.

Ceri, H., M. E. Olson, C. Stremick, R. R. Read, D. Morck and A. Buret (1999). The Calgary Biofilm Device: new technology for rapid determination of antibiotic susceptibilities of bacterial biofilms. *J Clin Microbiol* 37(6): 1771-6.

Chan, C., L. L. Burrows and C. M. Deber (2005). Alginate as an auxiliary bacterial membrane: binding of membrane-active peptides by polysaccharides. *J Pept Res* 65(3): 343-51.

Chastre, J. and J. Y. Fagon (2002). Ventilator-associated pneumonia. *Am J Respir Crit Care Med* 165(7): 867-903.

Chiang, P. and L. L. Burrows (2003). Biofilm formation by hyperpiliated mutants of Pseudomonas aeruginosa. *J Bacteriol* 185(7): 2374-8.

Cochran, W. L., S. J. Suh, G. A. McFeters and P. S. Stewart (2000). Role of RpoS and AlgT in Pseudomonas aeruginosa biofilm resistance to hydrogen peroxide and monochloramine. *J Appl Microbiol* 88(3): 546-53.

Cooley, M., S. R. Chhabra and P. Williams (2008). N-Acylhomoserine lactone-mediated quorum sensing: a twist in the tail and a blow for host immunity. *Chem Biol* 15(11): 1141-7.

Costerton, J. W. (2001). Cystic fibrosis pathogenesis and the role of biofilms in persistent infection. *Trends Microbiol* 9(2): 50-2.

Costerton, J. W., Z. Lewandowski, D. E. Caldwell, D. R. Korber and H. M. Lappin-Scott (1995). Microbial biofilms. *Annu Rev Microbiol* 49: 711-45.

Costerton, J. W., P. S. Stewart and E. P. Greenberg (1999). Bacterial biofilms: a common cause of persistent infections. *Science* 284(5418): 1318-22.

Dacheux, D., I. Attree and B. Toussaint (2001). Expression of ExsA in trans confers type III secretion system-dependent cytotoxicity on noncytotoxic Pseudomonas aeruginosa cystic fibrosis isolates. *Infect Immun* 69(1): 538-42.

Dacheux, D., B. Toussaint, M. Richard, G. Brochier, J. Croize and I. Attree (2000). Pseudomonas aeruginosa cystic fibrosis isolates induce rapid, type III secretion-dependent, but ExoU-independent, oncosis of macrophages and polymorphonuclear neutrophils. *Infect Immun* 68(5): 2916-24.

Davies, J. A., J. J. Harrison, L. L. Marques, G. R. Foglia, C. A. Stremick, D. G. Storey, R. J. Turner, M. E. Olson and H. Ceri (2007). The GacS sensor kinase controls phenotypic reversion of small colony variants isolated from biofilms of Pseudomonas aeruginosa PA14. *FEMS Microbiol Ecol* 59(1): 32-46.

Davies, K. J., D. Lloyd and L. Boddy (1989). The effect of oxygen on denitrification in Paracoccus denitrificans and Pseudomonas aeruginosa. *J Gen Microbiol* 135(9): 2445-51.

del Pozo, J. L. and R. Patel (2007). The challenge of treating biofilm-associated bacterial infections. *Clin Pharmacol Ther* 82(2): 204-9.

DeLeon, K., F. Balldin, C. Watters, A. Hamood, J. Griswold, S. Sreedharan and K. P. Rumbaugh (2009). Gallium maltolate treatment eradicates Pseudomonas aeruginosa infection in thermally injured mice. *Antimicrob Agents Chemother* 53(4): 1331-7.

Diaz, M. R., J. M. King and T. L. Yahr (2011). Intrinsic and extrinsic regulation of type III secretion gene expression in Pseudomonas aeruginosa. *Frontiers in Microbiology* 2.

Donaldson, S. H., W. D. Bennett, K. L. Zeman, M. R. Knowles, R. Tarran and R. C. Boucher (2006). Mucus clearance and lung function in cystic fibrosis with hypertonic saline. *N Engl J Med* 354(3): 241-50.

Donlan, R. M. and J. W. Costerton (2002). Biofilms: survival mechanisms of clinically relevant microorganisms. *Clin Microbiol Rev* 15(2): 167-93.

Doring, G., I. G. Parameswaran and T. F. Murphy (2011). Differential adaptation of microbial pathogens to airways of patients with cystic fibrosis and chronic obstructive pulmonary disease. *FEMS Microbiol Rev* 35(1): 124-46.

Doring, G. and G. B. Pier (2008). Vaccines and immunotherapy against Pseudomonas aeruginosa. *Vaccine* 26(8): 1011-24.

Dunne, W. M., Jr. (2002). Bacterial adhesion: seen any good biofilms lately? *Clin Microbiol Rev* 15(2): 155-66.

Elkins, M. R., M. Robinson, B. R. Rose, C. Harbour, C. P. Moriarty, G. B. Marks, E. G. Belousova, W. Xuan and P. T. Bye (2006). A controlled trial of long-term inhaled hypertonic saline in patients with cystic fibrosis. *N Engl J Med* 354(3): 229-40.

Emerson, J., S. McNamara, A. M. Buccat, K. Worrell and J. L. Burns (2010). Changes in cystic fibrosis sputum microbiology in the United States between 1995 and 2008. *Pediatr Pulmonol* 45(4): 363-70.

Ernst, R. K., E. C. Yi, L. Guo, K. B. Lim, J. L. Burns, M. Hackett and S. I. Miller (1999). Specific lipopolysaccharide found in cystic fibrosis airway Pseudomonas aeruginosa. *Science* 286(5444): 1561-5.

Fisher, J. T., Y. Zhang and J. F. Engelhardt (2011). Comparative biology of cystic fibrosis animal models. *Methods Mol Biol* 742: 311-34.

Fuchs, H. J., D. S. Borowitz, D. H. Christiansen, E. M. Morris, M. L. Nash, B. W. Ramsey, B. J. Rosenstein, A. L. Smith and M. E. Wohl (1994). Effect of aerosolized recombinant human DNase on exacerbations of respiratory symptoms and on pulmonary function in patients with cystic fibrosis. The Pulmozyme Study Group. *N Engl J Med* 331(10): 637-42.

Furukawa, S., S. L. Kuchma and G. A. O'Toole (2006). Keeping their options open: acute versus persistent infections. *J Bacteriol* 188(4): 1211-7.

Gallagher, L. A. and C. Manoil (2001). Pseudomonas aeruginosa PAO1 kills Caenorhabditis elegans by cyanide poisoning. *J Bacteriol* 183(21): 6207-14.

Galloway, W. R., J. T. Hodgkinson, S. D. Bowden, M. Welch and D. R. Spring (2011). Quorum sensing in Gram-negative bacteria: small-molecule modulation of AHL and AI-2 quorum sensing pathways. *Chem Rev* 111(1): 28-67.

Garbe, J., A. Wesche, B. Bunk, M. Kazmierczak, K. Selezska, C. Rohde, J. Sikorski, M. Rohde, D. Jahn and M. Schobert (2010). Characterization of JG024, a pseudomonas aeruginosa PB1-like broad host range phage under simulated infection conditions. *BMC Microbiol* 10: 301.

Geske, G. D., R. J. Wezeman, A. P. Siegel and H. E. Blackwell (2005). Small molecule inhibitors of bacterial quorum sensing and biofilm formation. *J Am Chem Soc* 127(37): 12762-3.

Gibson, R. L., J. L. Burns and B. W. Ramsey (2003). Pathophysiology and management of pulmonary infections in cystic fibrosis. *Am J Respir Crit Care Med* 168(8): 918-51.

Gomez, M. I. and A. Prince (2007). Opportunistic infections in lung disease: Pseudomonas infections in cystic fibrosis. *Curr Opin Pharmacol* 7(3): 244-51.

Gooderham, W. J. and R. E. Hancock (2009). Regulation of virulence and antibiotic resistance by two-component regulatory systems in Pseudomonas aeruginosa. *FEMS Microbiol Rev* 33(2): 279-94.

Goodman, A. L., B. Kulasekara, A. Rietsch, D. Boyd, R. S. Smith and S. Lory (2004). A signaling network reciprocally regulates genes associated with acute infection and chronic persistence in Pseudomonas aeruginosa. *Dev Cell* 7(5): 745-54.

Govan, J. R. and V. Deretic (1996). Microbial pathogenesis in cystic fibrosis: mucoid Pseudomonas aeruginosa and Burkholderia cepacia. *Microbiol Rev* 60(3): 539-74.

Grimwood, K., R. A. Semple, H. R. Rabin, P. A. Sokol and D. E. Woods (1993). Elevated exoenzyme expression by Pseudomonas aeruginosa is correlated with exacerbations of lung disease in cystic fibrosis. *Pediatr Pulmonol* 15(3): 135-9.

Grubb, B. R. and R. C. Boucher (1999). Pathophysiology of gene-targeted mouse models for cystic fibrosis. *Physiol Rev* 79(1 Suppl): S193-214.

Hansen, C. R., T. Pressler and N. Hoiby (2008). Early aggressive eradication therapy for intermittent Pseudomonas aeruginosa airway colonization in cystic fibrosis patients: 15 years experience. *J Cyst Fibros* 7(6): 523-30.

Harmsen, M., L. Yang, S. J. Pamp and T. Tolker-Nielsen (2010). An update on Pseudomonas aeruginosa biofilm formation, tolerance, and dispersal. *FEMS Immunol Med Microbiol* 59(3): 253-68.

Hayes, D., Jr., D. J. Feola, B. S. Murphy, R. J. Kuhn and G. A. Davis (2011). Eradication of Pseudomonas aeruginosa in an adult patient with cystic fibrosis. *Am J Health Syst Pharm* 68(4): 319-22.

Heeb, S., M. P. Fletcher, S. R. Chhabra, S. P. Diggle, P. Williams and M. Camara (2011). Quinolones: from antibiotics to autoinducers. *FEMS Microbiol Rev* 35(2): 247-74.

Hentzer, M., K. Riedel, T. B. Rasmussen, A. Heydorn, J. B. Andersen, M. R. Parsek, S. A. Rice, L. Eberl, S. Molin, N. Hoiby, S. Kjelleberg and M. Givskov (2002). Inhibition of quorum sensing in Pseudomonas aeruginosa biofilm bacteria by a halogenated furanone compound. *Microbiology* 148(Pt 1): 87-102.

Hentzer, M., G. M. Teitzel, G. J. Balzer, A. Heydorn, S. Molin, M. Givskov and M. R. Parsek (2001). Alginate overproduction affects Pseudomonas aeruginosa biofilm structure and function. *J Bacteriol* 183(18): 5395-401.

Hinsa, S. M., M. Espinosa-Urgel, J. L. Ramos and G. A. O'Toole (2003). Transition from reversible to irreversible attachment during biofilm formation by Pseudomonas fluorescens WCS365 requires an ABC transporter and a large secreted protein. *Mol Microbiol* 49(4): 905-18.

Hoffmann, N., T. B. Rasmussen, P. O. Jensen, C. Stub, M. Hentzer, S. Molin, O. Ciofu, M. Givskov, H. K. Johansen and N. Hoiby (2005). Novel mouse model of chronic Pseudomonas aeruginosa lung infection mimicking cystic fibrosis. *Infect Immun* 73(4): 2504-14.

Hogan, D. A. and R. Kolter (2002). Pseudomonas-Candida interactions: an ecological role for virulence factors. *Science* 296(5576): 2229-32.

Hoiby, N., O. Ciofu and T. Bjarnsholt (2010). Pseudomonas aeruginosa biofilms in cystic fibrosis. *Future Microbiol* 5(11): 1663-74.

Hoiby, N., O. Ciofu, H. K. Johansen, Z. J. Song, C. Moser, P. O. Jensen, S. Molin, M. Givskov, T. Tolker-Nielsen and T. Bjarnsholt (2011). The clinical impact of bacterial biofilms. *Int J Oral Sci* 3(2): 55-65.

Hoiby, N., B. Frederiksen and T. Pressler (2005). Eradication of early Pseudomonas aeruginosa infection. *J Cyst Fibros* 4 Suppl 2: 49-54.

Hughes, K. T. and K. Mathee (1998). The anti-sigma factors. *Annu Rev Microbiol* 52: 231-86.

Jaffar-Bandjee, M. C., A. Lazdunski, M. Bally, J. Carrere, J. P. Chazalette and C. Galabert (1995). Production of elastase, exotoxin A, and alkaline protease in sputa during pulmonary exacerbation of cystic fibrosis in patients chronically infected by Pseudomonas aeruginosa. *J Clin Microbiol* 33(4): 924-9.

Jain, M., M. Bar-Meir, S. McColley, J. Cullina, E. Potter, C. Powers, M. Prickett, R. Seshadri, B. Jovanovic, A. Petrocheilou, J. D. King and A. R. Hauser (2008). Evolution of Pseudomonas aeruginosa type III secretion in cystic fibrosis: a paradigm of chronic infection. *Transl Res* 152(6): 257-64.

Jain, M., D. Ramirez, R. Seshadri, J. F. Cullina, C. A. Powers, G. S. Schulert, M. Bar-Meir, C. L. Sullivan, S. A. McColley and A. R. Hauser (2004). Type III secretion phenotypes of Pseudomonas aeruginosa strains change during infection of individuals with cystic fibrosis. *J Clin Microbiol* 42(11): 5229-37.

Kaneko, Y., M. Thoendel, O. Olakanmi, B. E. Britigan and P. K. Singh (2007). The transition metal gallium disrupts Pseudomonas aeruginosa iron metabolism and has antimicrobial and antibiofilm activity. *J Clin Invest* 117(4): 877-88.

Keays, T., W. Ferris, K. L. Vandemheen, F. Chan, S. W. Yeung, T. F. Mah, K. Ramotar, R. Saginur and S. D. Aaron (2009). A retrospective analysis of biofilm antibiotic susceptibility testing: a better predictor of clinical response in cystic fibrosis exacerbations. *J Cyst Fibros* 8(2): 122-7.

Kirov, S. M., J. S. Webb, Y. O'May C, D. W. Reid, J. K. Woo, S. A. Rice and S. Kjelleberg (2007). Biofilm differentiation and dispersal in mucoid Pseudomonas aeruginosa isolates from patients with cystic fibrosis. *Microbiology* 153(Pt 10): 3264-74.

Kuchma, S. L., J. P. Connolly and G. A. O'Toole (2005). A three-component regulatory system regulates biofilm maturation and type III secretion in Pseudomonas aeruginosa. *J Bacteriol* 187(4): 1441-54.

Kulasekara, H. D., I. Ventre, B. R. Kulasekara, A. Lazdunski, A. Filloux and S. Lory (2005). A novel two-component system controls the expression of Pseudomonas aeruginosa fimbrial cup genes. *Mol Microbiol* 55(2): 368-80.

Lam, J., R. Chan, K. Lam and J. W. Costerton (1980). Production of mucoid microcolonies by Pseudomonas aeruginosa within infected lungs in cystic fibrosis. *Infect Immun* 28(2): 546-56.

Laskowski, M. A., E. Osborn and B. I. Kazmierczak (2004). A novel sensor kinase-response regulator hybrid regulates type III secretion and is required for virulence in Pseudomonas aeruginosa. *Mol Microbiol* 54(4): 1090-103.

Lewis, K. (2005). Persister cells and the riddle of biofilm survival. *Biochemistry (Mosc)* 70(2): 267-74.

Lipuma, J. J. (2010). The changing microbial epidemiology in cystic fibrosis. *Clin Microbiol Rev* 23(2): 299-323.

Lyczak, J. B., C. L. Cannon and G. B. Pier (2000). Establishment of Pseudomonas aeruginosa infection: lessons from a versatile opportunist. *Microbes Infect* 2(9): 1051-60.

Lyczak, J. B., C. L. Cannon and G. B. Pier (2002). Lung infections associated with cystic fibrosis. *Clin Microbiol Rev* 15(2): 194-222.

Mah, T. F. and G. A. O'Toole (2001). Mechanisms of biofilm resistance to antimicrobial agents. *Trends Microbiol* 9(1): 34-9.

Mah, T. F., B. Pitts, B. Pellock, G. C. Walker, P. S. Stewart and G. A. O'Toole (2003). A genetic basis for Pseudomonas aeruginosa biofilm antibiotic resistance. *Nature* 426(6964): 306-10.

Mall, M., B. R. Grubb, J. R. Harkema, W. K. O'Neal and R. C. Boucher (2004). Increased airway epithelial Na+ absorption produces cystic fibrosis-like lung disease in mice. *Nat Med* 10(5): 487-93.

McCoy, K. S., A. L. Quittner, C. M. Oermann, R. L. Gibson, G. Z. Retsch-Bogart and A. B. Montgomery (2008). Inhaled aztreonam lysine for chronic airway Pseudomonas aeruginosa in cystic fibrosis. *Am J Respir Crit Care Med* 178(9): 921-8.

Miyata, S., M. Casey, D. W. Frank, F. M. Ausubel and E. Drenkard (2003). Use of the Galleria mellonella caterpillar as a model host to study the role of the type III secretion system in Pseudomonas aeruginosa pathogenesis. *Infect Immun* 71(5): 2404-13.

Monds, R. D., P. D. Newell, R. H. Gross and G. A. O'Toole (2007). Phosphate-dependent modulation of c-di-GMP levels regulates Pseudomonas fluorescens Pf0-1 biofilm formation by controlling secretion of the adhesin LapA. *Mol Microbiol* 63(3): 656-79.

Moore, N. M. and M. L. Flaws (2011). Epidemiology and pathogenesis of Pseudomonas aeruginosa infections. *Clin Lab Sci* 24(1): 43-6.

Moreau-Marquis, S., J. M. Bomberger, G. G. Anderson, A. Swiatecka-Urban, S. Ye, G. A. O'Toole and B. A. Stanton (2008). The {Delta}F508-CFTR mutation results in increased biofilm formation by Pseudomonas aeruginosa by increasing iron availability. *Am J Physiol Lung Cell Mol Physiol* 295(1): L25-37.

Moreau-Marquis, S., G. A. O'Toole and B. A. Stanton (2009). Tobramycin and FDA-approved iron chelators eliminate Pseudomonas aeruginosa biofilms on cystic fibrosis cells. *Am J Respir Cell Mol Biol* 41(3): 305-13.

Moreau-Marquis, S., C. V. Redelman, B. A. Stanton and G. G. Anderson (2010). Co-culture Models of Pseudomonas aeruginosa Biofilms Grown on Live Human Airway Cells. *J Vis Exp*(44): e2186.

Moskowitz, S. M., J. C. Emerson, S. McNamara, R. D. Shell, D. M. Orenstein, D. Rosenbluth, M. F. Katz, R. Ahrens, D. Hornick, P. M. Joseph, R. L. Gibson, M. L. Aitken, W. W. Benton and J. L. Burns (2011). Randomized trial of biofilm testing to select antibiotics for cystic fibrosis airway infection. *Pediatr Pulmonol* 46(2): 184-92.

Mowat, E., S. Paterson, J. L. Fothergill, E. A. Wright, M. J. Ledson, M. J. Walshaw, M. A. Brockhurst and C. Winstanley (2011). Pseudomonas aeruginosa Population Diversity and Turnover in Cystic Fibrosis Chronic Infections. *Am J Respir Crit Care Med* 183(12): 1674-9.

Nichols, W. W., S. M. Dorrington, M. P. Slack and H. L. Walmsley (1988). Inhibition of tobramycin diffusion by binding to alginate. *Antimicrob Agents Chemother* 32(4): 518-23.

O'Toole, G., H. B. Kaplan and R. Kolter (2000). Biofilm formation as microbial development. *Annu Rev Microbiol* 54: 49-79.

O'Toole, G. A. and R. Kolter (1998). Flagellar and twitching motility are necessary for Pseudomonas aeruginosa biofilm development. *Mol Microbiol* 30(2): 295-304.

Ohman, D. E. and A. M. Chakrabarty (1981). Genetic mapping of chromosomal determinants for the production of the exopolysaccharide alginate in a Pseudomonas aeruginosa cystic fibrosis isolate. *Infect Immun* 33(1): 142-8.

Ouyang, L., S. D. Grosse, D. D. Amendah and M. S. Schechter (2009). Healthcare expenditures for privately insured people with cystic fibrosis. *Pediatr Pulmonol* 44(10): 989-96.

Palmer, K. L., L. M. Aye and M. Whiteley (2007). Nutritional cues control Pseudomonas aeruginosa multicellular behavior in cystic fibrosis sputum. *J Bacteriol* 189(22): 8079-87.

Parkins, M. D. and J. S. Elborn (2010). Aztreonam lysine: a novel inhalational antibiotic for cystic fibrosis. *Expert Rev Respir Med* 4(4): 435-44.

Parkins, M. D. and J. S. Elborn (2010). Newer antibacterial agents and their potential role in cystic fibrosis pulmonary exacerbation management. *J Antimicrob Chemother* 65(9): 1853-61.

Parks, Q. M., R. L. Young, K. R. Poch, K. C. Malcolm, M. L. Vasil and J. A. Nick (2009). Neutrophil enhancement of Pseudomonas aeruginosa biofilm development: human F-actin and DNA as targets for therapy. *J Med Microbiol* 58(Pt 4): 492-502.

Parsek, M. R. and P. K. Singh (2003). Bacterial biofilms: an emerging link to disease pathogenesis. *Annu Rev Microbiol* 57: 677-701.

Patel, R. (2005). Biofilms and antimicrobial resistance. *Clin Orthop Relat Res* 437: 41-7.

Plummer, A. and M. Wildman (2011). Duration of intravenous antibiotic therapy in people with cystic fibrosis. *Cochrane Database Syst Rev*(1): CD006682.

Pressler, T., C. Bohmova, S. Conway, S. Dumcius, L. Hjelte, N. Hoiby, H. Kollberg, B. Tummler and V. Vavrova (2011). Chronic Pseudomonas aeruginosa infection definition: EuroCareCF Working Group report. *J Cyst Fibros* 10 Suppl 2: S75-8.

Rahme, L. G., E. J. Stevens, S. F. Wolfort, J. Shao, R. G. Tompkins and F. M. Ausubel (1995). Common virulence factors for bacterial pathogenicity in plants and animals. *Science* 268(5219): 1899-902.

Ramsey, D. M. and D. J. Wozniak (2005). Understanding the control of Pseudomonas aeruginosa alginate synthesis and the prospects for management of chronic infections in cystic fibrosis. *Mol Microbiol* 56(2): 309-22.

Ran, H., D. J. Hassett and G. W. Lau (2003). Human targets of Pseudomonas aeruginosa pyocyanin. *Proc Natl Acad Sci U S A* 100(24): 14315-20.

Rasmussen, T. B. and M. Givskov (2006). Quorum-sensing inhibitors as anti-pathogenic drugs. *Int J Med Microbiol* 296(2-3): 149-61.

Rasmussen, T. B., M. E. Skindersoe, T. Bjarnsholt, R. K. Phipps, K. B. Christensen, P. O. Jensen, J. B. Andersen, B. Koch, T. O. Larsen, M. Hentzer, L. Eberl, N. Hoiby and M. Givskov (2005). Identity and effects of quorum-sensing inhibitors produced by Penicillium species. *Microbiology* 151(Pt 5): 1325-40.

Ratjen, F., A. Munck, P. Kho and G. Angyalosi (2010). Treatment of early Pseudomonas aeruginosa infection in patients with cystic fibrosis: the ELITE trial. *Thorax* 65(4): 286-91.

Retsch-Bogart, G. Z., J. L. Burns, K. L. Otto, T. G. Liou, K. McCoy, C. Oermann and R. L. Gibson (2008). A phase 2 study of aztreonam lysine for inhalation to treat patients with cystic fibrosis and Pseudomonas aeruginosa infection. *Pediatr Pulmonol* 43(1): 47-58.

Rice, S. A., C. H. Tan, P. J. Mikkelsen, V. Kung, J. Woo, M. Tay, A. Hauser, D. McDougald, J. S. Webb and S. Kjelleberg (2009). The biofilm life cycle and virulence of Pseudomonas aeruginosa are dependent on a filamentous prophage. *ISME J* 3(3): 271-82.

Rogers, G. B., L. R. Hoffman, M. W. Johnson, N. Mayer-Hamblett, J. Schwarze, M. P. Carroll and K. D. Bruce (2011). Using bacterial biomarkers to identify early indicators of cystic fibrosis pulmonary exacerbation onset. *Expert Rev Mol Diagn* 11(2): 197-206.

Ryan, G., M. Singh and K. Dwan (2011). Inhaled antibiotics for long-term therapy in cystic fibrosis. *Cochrane Database Syst Rev*(3): CD001021.

Ryder, C., M. Byrd and D. J. Wozniak (2007). Role of polysaccharides in Pseudomonas aeruginosa biofilm development. *Curr Opin Microbiol* 10(6): 644-8.

Sadikot, R. T., T. S. Blackwell, J. W. Christman and A. S. Prince (2005). Pathogen-host interactions in Pseudomonas aeruginosa pneumonia. *Am J Respir Crit Care Med* 171(11): 1209-23.

Saiman, L. (2011). Infection prevention and control in cystic fibrosis. *Curr Opin Infect Dis* 24(4): 390-5.

Saiman, L. and J. Siegel (2004). Infection control in cystic fibrosis. *Clin Microbiol Rev* 17(1): 57-71.

Salunkhe, P., C. H. Smart, J. A. Morgan, S. Panagea, M. J. Walshaw, C. A. Hart, R. Geffers, B. Tummler and C. Winstanley (2005). A cystic fibrosis epidemic strain of Pseudomonas aeruginosa displays enhanced virulence and antimicrobial resistance. *J Bacteriol* 187(14): 4908-20.

Sauer, K., A. K. Camper, G. D. Ehrlich, J. W. Costerton and D. G. Davies (2002). Pseudomonas aeruginosa displays multiple phenotypes during development as a biofilm. *J Bacteriol* 184(4): 1140-54.

Shaver, C. M. and A. R. Hauser (2004). Relative contributions of Pseudomonas aeruginosa ExoU, ExoS, and ExoT to virulence in the lung. *Infect Immun* 72(12): 6969-77.

Singh, P. K., A. L. Schaefer, M. R. Parsek, T. O. Moninger, M. J. Welsh and E. P. Greenberg (2000). Quorum-sensing signals indicate that cystic fibrosis lungs are infected with bacterial biofilms. *Nature* 407(6805): 762-4.

Skindersoe, M. E., M. Alhede, R. Phipps, L. Yang, P. O. Jensen, T. B. Rasmussen, T. Bjarnsholt, T. Tolker-Nielsen, N. Hoiby and M. Givskov (2008). Effects of antibiotics on quorum sensing in Pseudomonas aeruginosa. *Antimicrob Agents Chemother* 52(10): 3648-63.

Smith, A. W. (2005). Biofilms and antibiotic therapy: is there a role for combating bacterial resistance by the use of novel drug delivery systems? *Adv Drug Deliv Rev* 57(10): 1539-50.

Smith, E. E., D. G. Buckley, Z. Wu, C. Saenphimmachak, L. R. Hoffman, D. A. D'Argenio, S. I. Miller, B. W. Ramsey, D. P. Speert, S. M. Moskowitz, J. L. Burns, R. Kaul and M. V. Olson (2006). Genetic adaptation by Pseudomonas aeruginosa to the airways of cystic fibrosis patients. *Proc Natl Acad Sci U S A* 103(22): 8487-92.

Sriramulu, D. D., H. Lunsdorf, J. S. Lam and U. Romling (2005). Microcolony formation: a novel biofilm model of Pseudomonas aeruginosa for the cystic fibrosis lung. *J Med Microbiol* 54(Pt 7): 667-76.

Starkey, M., J. H. Hickman, L. Ma, N. Zhang, S. De Long, A. Hinz, S. Palacios, C. Manoil, M. J. Kirisits, T. D. Starner, D. J. Wozniak, C. S. Harwood and M. R. Parsek (2009). Pseudomonas aeruginosa rugose small-colony variants have adaptations that likely promote persistence in the cystic fibrosis lung. *J Bacteriol* 191(11): 3492-503.

Steinberg, P. D., R. Schneider and S. Kjelleberg (1997). Chemical defenses of seaweeds against microbial colonization. *Biodegradation* 8(3): 211-220.

Stewart, P. S. and J. W. Costerton (2001). Antibiotic resistance of bacteria in biofilms. *Lancet* 358(9276): 135-8.

Stoodley, P., K. Sauer, D. G. Davies and J. W. Costerton (2002). Biofilms as complex differentiated communities. *Annu Rev Microbiol* 56: 187-209.

Stover, C. K., X. Q. Pham, A. L. Erwin, S. D. Mizoguchi, P. Warrener, M. J. Hickey, F. S. Brinkman, W. O. Hufnagle, D. J. Kowalik, M. Lagrou, R. L. Garber, L. Goltry, E. Tolentino, S. Westbrock-Wadman, Y. Yuan, L. L. Brody, S. N. Coulter, K. R. Folger, A. Kas, K. Larbig, R. Lim, K. Smith, D. Spencer, G. K. Wong, Z. Wu, I. T. Paulsen, J. Reizer, M. H. Saier, R. E. Hancock, S. Lory and M. V. Olson (2000). Complete genome sequence of Pseudomonas aeruginosa PA01, an opportunistic pathogen. *Nature* 406(6799): 959-64.

Stressmann, F. A., G. B. Rogers, P. Marsh, A. K. Lilley, T. W. Daniels, M. P. Carroll, L. R. Hoffman, G. Jones, C. E. Allen, N. Patel, B. Forbes, A. Tuck and K. D. Bruce (2011). Does bacterial density in cystic fibrosis sputum increase prior to pulmonary exacerbation? *J Cyst Fibros*.

Stuart, B., J. H. Lin and P. J. Mogayzel, Jr. (2010). Early eradication of Pseudomonas aeruginosa in patients with cystic fibrosis. *Paediatr Respir Rev* 11(3): 177-84.

Taccetti, G., S. Campana, F. Festini, M. Mascherini and G. Doring (2005). Early eradication therapy against Pseudomonas aeruginosa in cystic fibrosis patients. *Eur Respir J* 26(3): 458-61.

Tomlin, K. L., R. J. Malott, G. Ramage, D. G. Storey, P. A. Sokol and H. Ceri (2005). Quorum-sensing mutations affect attachment and stability of Burkholderia cenocepacia biofilms. *Appl Environ Microbiol* 71(9): 5208-18.

Tunney, M. M., E. R. Klem, A. A. Fodor, D. F. Gilpin, T. F. Moriarty, S. J. McGrath, M. S. Muhlebach, R. C. Boucher, C. Cardwell, G. Doering, J. S. Elborn and M. C. Wolfgang (2011). Use of culture and molecular analysis to determine the effect of antibiotic treatment on microbial community diversity and abundance during exacerbation in patients with cystic fibrosis. *Thorax* 66(7): 579-84.

VanDevanter, D. R., M. A. O'Riordan, J. L. Blumer and M. W. Konstan (2010). Assessing time to pulmonary function benefit following antibiotic treatment of acute cystic fibrosis exacerbations. *Respir Res* 11: 137.

VanDevanter, D. R. and J. M. Van Dalfsen (2005). How much do Pseudomonas biofilms contribute to symptoms of pulmonary exacerbation in cystic fibrosis? *Pediatr Pulmonol* 39(6): 504-6.

Ventre, I., A. L. Goodman, I. Vallet-Gely, P. Vasseur, C. Soscia, S. Molin, S. Bleves, A. Lazdunski, S. Lory and A. Filloux (2006). Multiple sensors control reciprocal expression of Pseudomonas aeruginosa regulatory RNA and virulence genes. *Proc Natl Acad Sci U S A* 103(1): 171-6.

Wagner, V. E., D. Bushnell, L. Passador, A. I. Brooks and B. H. Iglewski (2003). Microarray analysis of Pseudomonas aeruginosa quorum-sensing regulons: effects of growth phase and environment. *J Bacteriol* 185(7): 2080-95.

Walker, T. S., K. L. Tomlin, G. S. Worthen, K. R. Poch, J. G. Lieber, M. T. Saavedra, M. B. Fessler, K. C. Malcolm, M. L. Vasil and J. A. Nick (2005). Enhanced Pseudomonas aeruginosa biofilm development mediated by human neutrophils. *Infect Immun* 73(6): 3693-701.

Whiteley, M., M. G. Bangera, R. E. Bumgarner, M. R. Parsek, G. M. Teitzel, S. Lory and E. P. Greenberg (2001). Gene expression in Pseudomonas aeruginosa biofilms. *Nature* 413(6858): 860-4.

Wilke, M., R. M. Buijs-Offerman, J. Aarbiou, W. H. Colledge, D. N. Sheppard, L. Touqui, A. Bot, H. Jorna, H. R. de Jonge and B. J. Scholte (2011). Mouse models of cystic fibrosis: phenotypic analysis and research applications. *J Cyst Fibros* 10 Suppl 2: S152-71.

Wolfgang, M. C., J. Jyot, A. L. Goodman, R. Ramphal and S. Lory (2004). Pseudomonas aeruginosa regulates flagellin expression as part of a global response to airway fluid from cystic fibrosis patients. *Proc Natl Acad Sci U S A* 101(17): 6664-8.

Woods, D. E., D. C. Straus, W. G. Johanson, Jr., V. K. Berry and J. A. Bass (1980). Role of pili in adherence of Pseudomonas aeruginosa to mammalian buccal epithelial cells. *Infect. Immun.* 29(3): 1146-1151.

Woodward, T. C., R. Brown, P. Sacco and J. Zhang (2010). Budget impact model of tobramycin inhalation solution for treatment of Pseudomonas aeruginosa in cystic fibrosis patients. *J Med Econ* 13(3): 492-9.

Woodworth, B. A., E. Tamashiro, G. Bhargave, N. A. Cohen and J. N. Palmer (2008). An in vitro model of Pseudomonas aeruginosa biofilms on viable airway epithelial cell monolayers. *Am J Rhinol* 22(3): 235-8.

Worlitzsch, D., R. Tarran, M. Ulrich, U. Schwab, A. Cekici, K. C. Meyer, P. Birrer, G. Bellon, J. Berger, T. Weiss, K. Botzenhart, J. R. Yankaskas, S. Randell, R. C. Boucher and G. Doring (2002). Effects of reduced mucus oxygen concentration in airway Pseudomonas infections of cystic fibrosis patients. *J Clin Invest* 109(3): 317-25.

Wozniak, D. J. and R. Keyser (2004). Effects of subinhibitory concentrations of macrolide antibiotics on Pseudomonas aeruginosa. *Chest* 125(2 Suppl): 62S-69S; quiz 69S.

Wu, W., H. Badrane, S. Arora, H. V. Baker and S. Jin (2004). MucA-mediated coordination of type III secretion and alginate synthesis in Pseudomonas aeruginosa. *J Bacteriol* 186(22): 7575-85.

Yahr, T. L. and M. C. Wolfgang (2006). Transcriptional regulation of the Pseudomonas aeruginosa type III secretion system. *Mol Microbiol* 62(3): 631-40.

Yoon, S. S. and D. J. Hassett (2004). Chronic Pseudomonas aeruginosa infection in cystic fibrosis airway disease: metabolic changes that unravel novel drug targets. *Expert Rev Anti Infect Ther* 2(4): 611-23.

Zhou, Z., J. Duerr, B. Johannesson, S. C. Schubert, D. Treis, M. Harm, S. Y. Graeber, A. Dalpke, C. Schultz and M. A. Mall (2011). The ENaC-overexpressing mouse as a model of cystic fibrosis lung disease. *J Cyst Fibros* 10 Suppl 2: S172-82.

8

Outcome and Prevention of *Pseudomonas aeruginosa-Staphylococcus aureus* Interactions During Pulmonary Infections in Cystic Fibrosis

Gabriel Mitchell and François Malouin
Université de Sherbrooke
Canada

1. Introduction

Several microorganisms take advantages of the most common single gene disorder afflicting Caucasians and colonize the airways of cystic fibrosis (CF) patients. Although CF is a multi-system disorder, the associated mortality is mostly due to respiratory problems subsequent to chronic bacterial infections. CF is the result of mutations in the cystic fibrosis transmembrane conductance regulator (CFTR) which is a cAMP-regulated chloride channel and a regulator of the activity of other channels. Consequently, there is a significant dehydration of the airway mucus when CFTR is dysfunctional. However, the exact reason why CF predisposes the lungs to microbial infections is not completely understood. It is thought that the obstruction of the airways by mucus and the proinflammatory status associated with this disease may be part of the explanation (Lyczak *et al.*, 2002; Riordan, 2008).

The recalcitrance of CF pathogens to antibiotic therapies is a major problem and is responsible for most of the morbidity and the mortality associated with CF (Chmiel & Davis, 2003; Lyczak *et al.*, 2002). The ever-growing and overwhelming problems caused by antibiotic-resistant bacteria in human medicine have not spared CF patients. Antibiotic-resistant bacteria are frequently recovered from CF samples (George *et al.*, 2009; Parkins & Elborn, 2010). The evolution of drug resistance has been accelerated by the extensive use of an antibiotic arsenal which has become limited due to insufficient innovation in the development of antimicrobials (Shah, 2005; Talbot *et al.*, 2006). Indeed, the development of new classes of antibiotics has been almost abandoned for the last four decades and antibiotics that were introduced during this period usually consisted of new-generation molecules derived from existing antibiotics (Wenzel *et al.*, 2005). Furthermore, long-term infections of the CF airways not only allow pathogens to adapt and circumvent the host immune system, but also allow them time to adapt to antibiotic therapies (Goerke & Wolz, 2010; Hogardt & Heesemann, 2010). Several mechanisms that decrease the susceptibility to antimicrobials are known to be at play in the CF airways. Conventional resistance mechanisms include the upregulation of bacterial efflux pumps and mutations of antibiotic target molecules (Høiby *et al.*, 2010). In addition, the formation of persister cells (Mulcahy *et al.*, 2010) and of small-colony variants (Goerke & Wolz, 2010; Proctor *et al.*, 2006; Schneider *et al.*, 2008) as well as bacterial growth in biofilms (Høiby *et al.*, 2010; Mitchell *et al.*, 2010a,

2010b; Wagner & Iglewski, 2008) are mechanisms that are well known for their involvement in difficult-to-treat infections (Galli *et al.*, 2007; Stewart, 2002).

The formation of bacterial biofilms may explain, at least in part, the failure of many antimicrobial therapies. Biofilm-growing bacteria are highly persistent in CF because they appear to be physically protected from the host immune system and are inherently resistant to antimicrobials (Costerton *et al.*, 1999; Davies & Bilton, 2009; Høiby *et al.*, 2010; Stewart, 2002). These bacteria are thought to be as much as 1000 times more resistant to antimicrobials than their planktonic counterparts (George *et al.*, 2009). Biofilms also represent complex integrated polymicrobial communities that are strongly influenced by cell-to-cell intraspecies and interspecies communications (Costerton *et al.*, 1999; Hall-Stoodley *et al.*, 2004; Stoodley *et al.*, 2002). The different species of microbes found in polymicrobial infections such as in CF most probably respond to each other's chemical signals in order to survive and this is likely to influence the course of any particular infection (Brogden *et al.*, 2005; Ryan & Dow, 2008).

In the surge to develop new therapies against CF pathogens, multiple aspects should be considered. Indeed, several diverse phenotypic adaptations confer a selective advantage in the host environment or toward antibiotic therapies. Also to consider are the various bacterial signals used for cell-to-cell communication that are involved in the establishment and the development of an infection. These mechanisms enable pathogens from polymicrobial communities to adjust their behavior in response to other neighboring bacteria and they deserve particular attention. This chapter aims to describe some of the mechanisms used by *Pseudomonas aeruginosa* and *Staphylococcus aureus* for their mutual coexistence and persistence in the host environment, and to emphasize those that are potential targets for the development of anti-pathogenesis therapies.

2. Microbiology of CF

Colonization of the CF airways by bacteria usually occurs in infancy and results in the establishment of chronic infections which eventually lead to respiratory failure and death (Harrison, 2007; Lyczak *et al.*, 2002). Recent investigations have shown that the CF airways are colonized by complex polymicrobial communities constituted by numerous bacterial species and not only by the relatively few predominant species originally described that include *P. aeruginosa, S. aureus, Heamophilus influenzae,* bacteria from the *Burkholderia cepacia* complex and *Stenotrophomonas maltophilia* (Sibley & Surette, 2011). Notwithstanding this polymicrobial mixture, *P. aeruginosa* and *S. aureus* are still among the most prevalent and dominant bacterial species encountered in CF (Canadian Cystic Fibrosis Foundation, 2009; Cystic Fibrosis Foundation, 2009; European Cystic Fibrosis Society, 2007). It is also important to note that the prevalence of the different pathogens varies as a function of the age of patients, with *S. aureus* and *H. influenzae* being more frequent in early childhood and *P. aeruginosa* being more important as patients become older. Several other microorganisms such as *Mycobacterium* spp., pathogenic viruses, fungal pathogens (*e.g. Aspergillus fulmigatus*) and yeasts (*e.g. Candida albicans*) have also been recovered from the CF airways and may also contribute to disease (Harrison, 2007; Lyczak *et al.*, 2002; Moskowitz *et al.*, 2005). It should be kept in mind that the chronically infected CF airways represent a complex and diverse ecosystem and that the precise contribution of the different microbes to the morbidity of the disease remains undetermined, even for the less frequently encountered microorganisms (Harrison, 2007).

2.1 Pathogenesis of *P. aeruginosa* in CF

P. aeruginosa is a Gram-negative bacterium that has the ability to survive in several different natural environments. However, it is better known as an opportunistic antibiotic-resistant human pathogen often encountered in hospital settings (Bodey *et al.*, 1983). This bacterium is also known as the major cause of lung function decline and mortality in CF (Lyczak *et al.*, 2002). *P. aeruginosa* establishes infections using several virulence factors. The production of these virulence factors varies as a function of the cell density of the bacterial population and is controlled by cell-to-cell chemical communication, *i.e.* quorum-sensing or QS (R. S. Smith & Iglewski, 2003). QS systems are used by many bacteria to promote collective behaviors and depend on the action of diffusible signal molecules. QS systems are typically composed of a signal synthase that produces the signal molecule and a signal receptor that modulates the expression of target genes subsequent to the binding of the signal molecule.

QS in *P. aeruginosa* is controlled by the *las* and *rhl* *N*-acylhomoserine lactone (AHL) regulatory circuits and by the 2-alkyl-4-quinolone (AQ) system (Dubern & Diggle, 2008). In the *las* and *rhl* system, the *las*I and *rhl*I gene products direct the synthesis of the homoserine lactones (HSL) 3-oxo-C12-HSL and C4-HSL, which interact with the transcription regulators LasR and RhlR, respectively, and activate target promoters. The *las* and *rhl* systems are hierarchically connected and interact together to regulate the production of several virulence determinants such as pyocyanin biosynthesis and biofilm formation (Dubern & Diggle, 2008; R. S. Smith & Iglewski, 2003). The AQ system is also interconnected with *las* and *rhl* and leads to the production of 2-heptyl-4-quinolone (HHQ) and the *Pseudomonas* quinolone signal (PQS). Both HHQ and PQS also have a role in cell-to-cell communication. However, PQS has a number of other biologically important functions (Dubern & Diggle, 2008). *P. aeruginosa* produces several other quinolone compounds, some of which, such as 4-hydroxy-2-heptylquinoline-*N*-oxide (HQNO), have antibiotic activity (Leisinger & Margraff, 1979; Lépine *et al.*, 2004; Machan *et al.*, 1992). It should also be kept in mind that the control of virulence factors by these systems is growth and environment dependent. This complex mixture of factors allows *P. aeruginosa* to modulate its behavior only when necessary (Williams & Camara, 2009). Interestingly, *P. aeruginosa* QS signals not only serve for intraspecies communications, but are also known to affect other microorganisms and the host (Williams & Camara, 2009). The association between the environment, *P. aeruginosa* QS systems and virulence is schematized in Fig. 1.

Substantial adaptive and genetic changes occur in the genome of *P. aeruginosa* during chronic infections of the CF airways (Foweraker *et al.*, 2005; E. E. Smith *et al.*, 2006; Sriramulu *et al.*, 2005). These changes cause bacteria to diversify and to exhibit characteristics differing from isolates found in the environment outside the body. The adaptation of *P. aeruginosa* during persistent infection of CF lungs can often lead to antimicrobial resistance, alginate overproduction and improved metabolic fitness. Overall, *P. aeruginosa* seems able to adopt a less aggressive profile by repressing its virulence factors and its immunostimulatory products, by growing in biofilms and by metabolically adapting to the microaerobic environment created by airway mucus plugs (Hogardt & Heesemann, 2010). Of these characteristics it appears that the formation of drug-resistant biofilms is strongly associated with the persistence of this bacterium in the CF airways (Høiby *et al.*, 2010; Wagner &

Iglewski, 2008). Also, non-mucoid strains that colonize CF patients can, with time, switch to the mucoid phenotype, show resistance to various antibiotics and become more difficult to eradicate from the airways (George *et al.*, 2009). Other phenotypic variants associated with chronic infections and antibiotic tolerance have also been recovered from the CF airways such as persister cells (Mulcahy *et al.*, 2010) and small-colony variants (Häußler *et al.*, 1999; Schneider *et al.*, 2008). The hypermutability of *P. aeruginosa* CF strains is thought to accelerate the development of antibiotic resistances and the adaptation required for long-term persistence in the host (Maciá *et al.*, 2005).

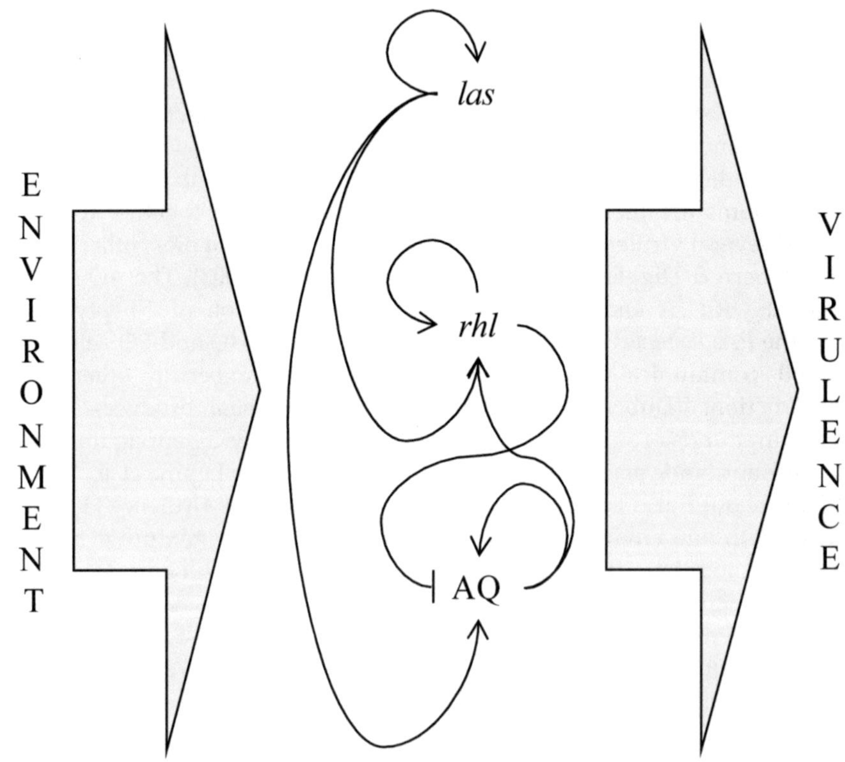

Fig. 1. The virulence of *P. aeruginosa* is controlled by interconnected quorum-sensing (QS) systems that integrate environmental cues and influence virulence gene expression. The two *N*-acylhomoserine lactone systems *las* and *rhl* and the 2-alkyl-4-quinolone (AQ) system are hierarchically interconnected. The *las* system is usually activated first. These QS systems regulate the production of several virulence factors as a function of growth and in response to the environment not only to influence *P. aeruginosa* behavior but also other bacteria of the microbial community as well as host-pathogen interactions.

2.2 Pathogenesis of *S. aureus* in CF

S. aureus can live as a human commensal but also can be an opportunistic Gram-positive pathogen associated with significant mortality in hospitals (Talbot *et al.*, 2006). This bacterium demonstrates an impressive versatility being able to infect several hosts, organs and body sites and cause both life-threatening and chronic infections (Archer, 1998; Goerke & Wolz, 2010). The treatment of *S. aureus* is seriously impeded by antibiotic resistance that has spread among staphylococci and is now being considered as a serious threat to the general population (Witte *et al.*, 2008).

The presence of numerous virulence genes in the genome of *S. aureus* is thought to explain the ability of this bacterium to cause a broad spectrum of diseases (Archer, 1998). The genes involved in pathogenesis are tightly controlled by complex regulatory networks that allow the bacteria to express its virulence factors as a function of the bacterial population density and of its environment (Novick, 2003). One of the most characterized regulatory systems influencing the virulence of *S. aureus* is *agr*, the quorum-sensing accessory gene regulator, that upregulates the production of several extracellular proteins while downregulating many cell-surface proteins (Novick & Geisinger, 2008). Other regulatory networks that govern the expression of accessory genes in *S. aureus* include several two-component regulatory systems and transcription factors such as the alternative sigma factor SigB (Bronner *et al.*, 2004; Novick, 2003). The activity of particular virulence regulators is thought to allow the expression of different sets of factors likely to be required at specific steps during infection or needed for different types of infections.

The contribution of *S. aureus* to the progression of disease in CF is less obvious than that of *P. aeruginosa*. Although the presence of this bacterium in the lower respiratory tract is considered as representative of a pathologic situation, there are still questions concerning the impact of *S. aureus* on the progression of the disease (Lyczak *et al.*, 2002). However, recent data indicate that while the prevalence of *P. aeruginosa* has declined among CF patients over the past few years, the incidence of methicillin-suceptible and methicillin-resistant *S. aureus* (MSSA and MRSA, respectively) has increased in the USA (Razvi *et al.*, 2009). Importantly, detection of persistent MRSA in the respiratory tract of CF patients has been associated with a decrease in survival and with a more rapid decline in lung function (Dasenbrook *et al.*, 2008; Dasenbrook *et al.*, 2010). Furthermore, MRSA bacteria often present a phenotype of mutiresistance to antibiotics (Chambers & Deleo, 2009; Pruneau *et al.*, 2011) and are proficient in biofilm production (Molina *et al.*, 2008).

Notwithstanding these findings, *S. aureus* often persists in the CF lungs for many months or even years and is the cause of recurrent and relapsing infections despite antibiotic treatments (Goerke & Wolz, 2010; B. C. Kahl, 2010). Long-term adaptation of *S. aureus* to the CF environment may occur through mutations (such as those causing the small-colony variant [SCV] phenotype) or through regulatory mechanisms that are still not well understood and that may result in the repression of the *agr* system and establishment of biofilms (Goerke & Wolz, 2010).

SCVs of *S. aureus* are often isolated from chronic infections such as those of the CF airways (Kahl *et al.*, 1998; Moisan *et al.*, 2006; Proctor *et al.*, 2006). The SCV phenotype is frequently caused by either mutations in genes required for electron transport (*e.g.* genes involved in the biosynthesis of hemin or menadione) or by mutations in genes enabling thymidine biosynthesis. Almost all the phenotypic characteristics of SCVs such as the slow growth (*i.e.*, the formation of pin-point colonies when grown on solid media), the altered susceptibility to aminoglycoside antibiotics and the decreased production of exotoxins can be explained by their dysfunctional electron transport (Proctor *et al.*, 2006). Several studies have reported that SCVs are less virulent than prototypical strains *in vivo* yet they can persist as well as the normal strains (Proctor *et al.*, 2006). Our group and others have demonstrated that SCVs are relatively more persistent than their normal counterparts under antibiotic pressure (Bates *et al.*, 2003; Brouillette *et al.*, 2004). A recent study supports the theory that bacterial switching between wild-type and SCV phenotypes is required to sustain chronic infections (Tuchscherr *et al.*, 2011).

The hypothesis that SCVs play a role in the development of chronic infections is well supported by *in vitro* experiments demonstrating that these variants have an increased ability to adhere to host tissue components (Mitchell *et al.*, 2008; Vaudaux *et al.*, 2002), to form biofilms (Mitchell *et al.*, 2010a, 2010b; Singh *et al.*, 2009, 2010) and to infect and persist within non-professional phagocytes (Mitchell *et al.*, 2011b; Sendi & Proctor, 2009). These *in vitro* characteristics can be explained by the impact of the defective electron transport chain on the expression of virulence factors which seem to be mostly controlled by the activity of SigB rather than by the *agr* system in SCVs (Moisan *et al.*, 2006; Senn *et al.*, 2005). This altered activation of virulence regulators triggers a sustained expression of several genes encoding cell-surface proteins (*e.g.* the fibronectin-binding protein A *fnbA* gene) and the down-regulation of several exoprotein genes (*e.g.* the hemolysin-α *hla* gene) (Mitchell *et al.*, 2008; Moisan *et al.*, 2006). The sustained expression of *fnbA* has been associated with efficient binding of SCVs to fibronectin (Mitchell *et al.*, 2008). In turn, the formation of a fibronectin bridge between *S. aureus* fibronectin-binding proteins and the $\alpha_5\beta_1$-integrin of eukaryotic cells (Sinha *et al.*, 1999) probably explains the proficient cellular internalization of SCVs (Sendi & Proctor, 2009). Additionally, the low production of exoproteins and toxins by SCVs is likely to account for their increased persistence within host cells (Sendi & Proctor, 2009). Moreover, the increased production of biofilm by SCVs in comparison with wild-type strains may possibly be explained by the relative influence and the interconnection of the *agr* system and SigB that manipulate the maturation of protein-dependent biofilms (Lauderdale *et al.*, 2009). Furthermore, SCVs have been shown to activate the innate immune response to a lesser extent than that observed with wild-type strains (Tuchscherr *et al.*, 2010). This reduced ability of SCVs to induce an inflammatory response may also be attributable to the repression of the *agr* system (Grundmeier *et al.*, 2010) and supports the idea that the SCV phenotype confers on *S. aureus* the ability to remain hidden from the host immune system inside non-professional phagocytes. However, to date, the *in vitro* observations that suggest that the formation of biofilms and the infection of host cells by SCVs allow *S. aureus* to establish long-term infections in CF patients have not been supported by *in vivo* experiments. Further work is required, especially in CF models of pulmonary infections, in order to fully understand the role of SCVs in the pathogenesis of *S. aureus*. Some of the characteristics of the normal and SCV strains are compared in Fig. 2.

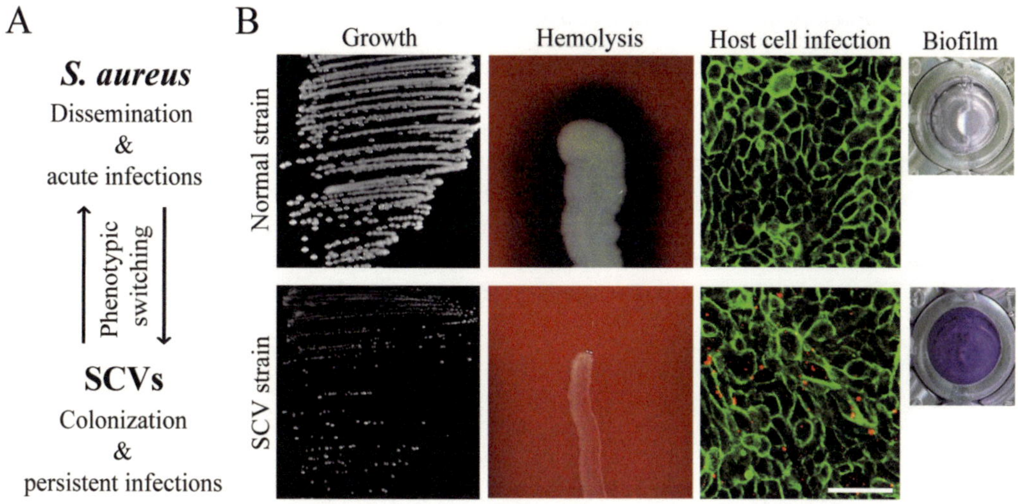

Fig. 2. The ability to switch from the normal to the small-colony variant (SCV) phenotype may have an impact on the virulence of *S. aureus*. (A) *S. aureus* can switch from a normal to a SCV phenotype. The normal and SCV phenotypes are associated with the dissemination of bacteria and acute infections, and with host tissue colonization and persistent infections, respectively. In comparison to normal strains, SCVs form pinpoint colonies, are less or non-hemolytic on blood agar plates and have an increased ability to infect non-professional phagocytes and to form biofilms (B). The host-cell infection pictures were prepared as previously described (Mitchell *et al.*, 2011a, 2011b) and show Calu-3 cells with actin colored in green and internalized *S. aureus* bacteria in red. Scale bar is 50 µm. Biofilm formation was evaluated by crystal violet staining as previously decribed (Mitchell *et al.*, 2010a, 2010b).

3. Interspecies interactions between CF pathogens

It is now accepted that bacteria can sense signal molecules across species' boundaries and that this signaling influences the development of microbial communities and the virulence and persistence of pathogens during infections (Ryan & Dow, 2008). The clinical impact of polymicrobial infections is receiving more and more recognition from the medical community. There are indeed several examples of polymicrobial infections where at least two different microorganisms influence the course of the disease by synergistic, additive or antagonistic effects. Also, biofilms are thought to be of major importance for the pathogenesis of bacteria in the context of CF lung infections (Davies & Bilton, 2009) and can be considered as integrated and complex polymicrobial communities whose development is controlled by interspecies communications (Stoodley *et al.*, 2002). Accordingly, and as previously underlined, infections of the CF airways is highly polymicrobic and there is growing evidence that many of these microorganisms interact (Sibley & Surette, 2011) as observed between *P. aeruginosa* and *S. aureus* (Biswas *et al.*, 2009; Hoffman *et al.*, 2006; Mashburn *et al.*, 2005; Mitchell *et al.*, 2010b; Qazi *et al.*, 2006; Yang *et al.*, 2011), *P. aeruginosa* and *Burkholderia* spp. (Bakkal *et al.*, 2010; Chattoraj *et al.*, 2010; Riedel *et al.*, 2001; Weaver & Kolter, 2004), *P. aeruginosa* and *S. maltophilia* (Ryan *et al.*, 2008), *P. aeruginosa* and *C. albicans* (McAlester *et al.*, 2008), and more generally with a large proportion of the organisms found in the CF airways (Duan *et al.*, 2003; Sibley *et al.*, 2008).

3.1 Interactions between *P. aeruginosa* and *S. aureus*

Given that *P. aeruginosa* and *S. aureus* are highly prevalent and commonly co-isolated from the CF airways (Harrison, 2007; Hoffman *et al.*, 2006), a great deal of effort has been directed toward the characterization of the interaction between them. Historically, synergistic interactions between these two species have been proposed and it was thought that *S. aureus* could sensitize the lungs for subsequent infections by *P. aeruginosa* (Lyczak *et al.*, 2002). However, it is now clear that antagonistic interactions also exist between these bacteria as *P. aeruginosa* has the ability to provoke lysis of *S. aureus* cells (Mashburn *et al.*, 2005; Palmer *et al.*, 2005). The structures of some *P. aeruginosa* exoproducts that are known to impact on *S. aureus* are shown in Fig. 3.

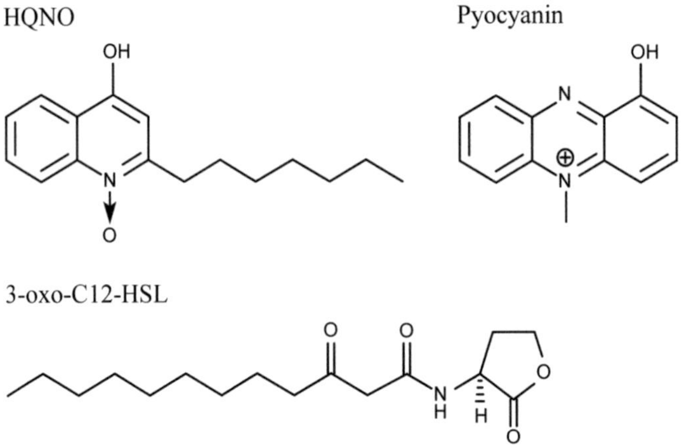

Fig. 3. Structure of *P. aeruginosa* molecules influencing *S. aureus* viability and pathogenesis.

The antistaphylococcal activities of pseudomonal HQNO (see Fig. 3) and other 4-hydroxy-2-alkylquinolines (HAQs) have been known for many years and are molecules that can generally suppress the growth of many Gram-positive bacteria (Lightbown & Jackson, 1954; Machan *et al.*, 1992). Mashburn *et al.* (2005) suggested that *P. aeruginosa* could exploit this property to lyse *S. aureus* cells in order to use the released iron for growth in low-iron environments. Interestingly, HQNO also allows some Gram-positive to grow slowly in presence of aminoglycoside antibiotics (Lightbown, 1954) and the reason for this has remained a mystery for several years. The protection provided by HQNO against the inhibitory activity of aminoglycosides was finally found to be related to the ability of this molecule to inhibit the Gram-positive electron transport chain (Hoffman *et al.*, 2006), which is required for aminoglycoside uptake (Bryan & Van Den Elzen, 1977). It was further shown that prolonged exposure of *S. aureus* to HQNO (or to *P. aeruginosa)* selects for SCVs (Hoffman *et al.*, 2006). We subsequently demonstrated that HQNO produced by *P. aeruginosa* not only stimulates the formation of *S. aureus* biofilms but also modulates the activity of virulence regulators. More particularly, while increasing the activity of SigB and the expression of *sarA*, HQNO downregulates the expression of the effector of the *agr* system (RNAIII). This modulation of regulator activities is likely to influence the expression of several virulence factors as was shown for *fnbA* and *hla* (Mitchell *et al.*, 2010b). The interaction of PQS with the cell envelope of *P. aeruginosa* is also known to trigger the release of membrane vesicles (MVs) which contain toxins, DNA, antimicrobials as well as HHQ, PQS and HQNO. It is thought that MVs are important for the trafficking of PQS within the *P aeruginosa* population as PQS is poorly soluble in water. However, since MVs contain AQs including HQNO, they could also inhibit staphylococcal growth (Mashburn & Whiteley, 2005). Furthermore, *P. aeruginosa* produces other small-molecule respiratory inhibitors such as pyocyanin (see Fig. 3) and hydrogen cyanide which can affect the respiration of *S. aureus* (Voggu *et al.*, 2006) and potentially select for the SCV phenotype (Biswas *et al.*, 2009). Whether and how these other respiratory inhibitors influence the virulence of *S. aureus* remains to be determined. Fig. 4 shows the effect of *P. aeruginosa* on the growth of *S. aureus*, the HQNO-mediated emergence of SCVs and the stimulation of *S. aureus* biofilm production by HQNO.

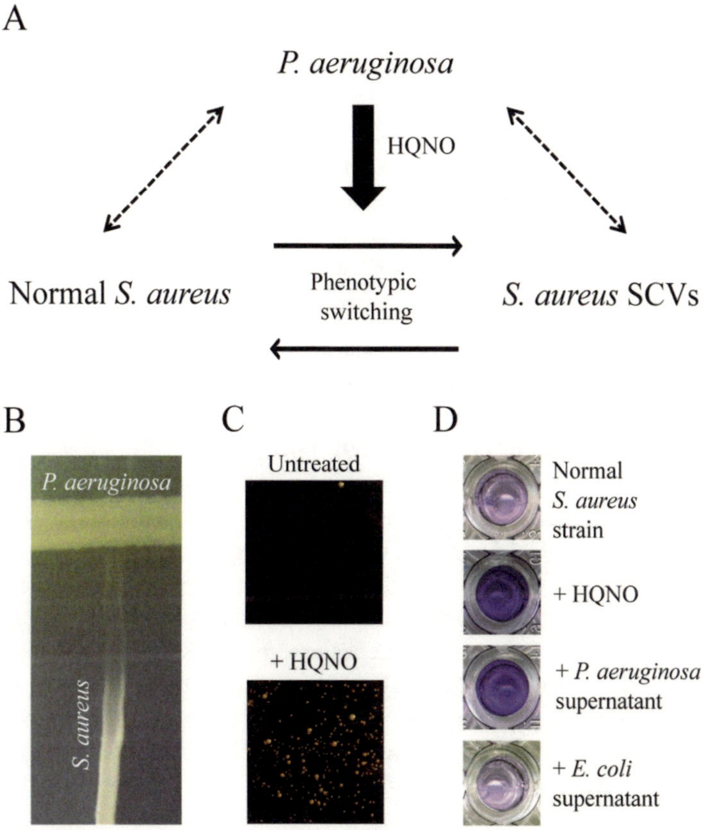

Fig. 4. *P. aeruginosa* influences the phenotypic switching of *S. aureus* and may have an impact on its virulence. (A) *P. aeruginosa* promotes the emergence of SCVs from normal *S. aureus* strains through the production of respiratory inhibitors such as HQNO and pyocyanin. Dotted arrows indicate other potential interactions between these bacterial species. (B) *P. aeruginosa* inhibits the growth of *S. aureus*. (C) HQNO stimulates the emergence of SCVs in *S. aureus*. Bacteria were treated or not with 10 µg/ml of HQNO for 18 h and plated on agar containing gentamicin at 4 µg/ml to reveal the presence of SCVs. (D) HQNO and *P. aeruginosa* culture supernatants enhance biofilm production by a normal *S. aureus* strain. *S. aureus* biofilms were produced in the presence of 10 µg/ml of HQNO or in the presence of culture supernatants from *P. aeruginosa* or *Escherichia coli* (acting as a negative control) and were revealed by crystal violet staining as previously described (Mitchell *et al.*, 2010a, 2010b).

It also appears that factors other than pseudomonal respiratory inhibitors are involved in the microbial interactions occurring between *P. aeruginosa* and *S. aureus*. Importantly, most of the antistaphylococcal activity found in *P. aeruginosa* culture supernatant is attributed to the staphylolytic endopeptidase LasA (Kessler *et al.*, 1993). Qazi *et al.* (2006) demonstrated that some long-chain 3-oxo-substituted *N*-acylhomoserine lactones (AHL) such as 3-oxo-C12-homoserine lactone (see Fig. 3) can inhibit the growth of *S. aureus* as a function of their concentrations. The 3-oxo-C12-HSL also modulates the production of *S. aureus* exotoxins and cell-surface proteins through the repression of *sarA* and *agr* by interaction with a specific and saturable receptor(s) at the cytoplasmic membrane. Furthermore, the 3-oxo-C12-HSL is capable of undergoing internal re-arrangement to form the 3-oxo-C12-tetrameric acid, which also has an inhibitory activity against Gram-positive bacteria (Kaufmann *et al.*, 2005). A recent study investigated the formation of biofilms by *P. aeruginosa-S. aureus* co-cultures using a flow chamber system and confocal microscopy (Yang *et al.*, 2011). This study demonstrated that wild-type *P. aeruginosa* facilitates *S. aureus* microcolony formation, but that *mucA* and *rpoN* mutants do not have this property and tend to outcompete *S. aureus*. A role for type IV pili in this phenomenon was proposed to occur through binding of extracellular DNA, and it was demonstrated that *P. aeruginosa* protects *S. aureus* against *Dictyostelium discoideum* phagocytosis when in co-culture biofilms.

Some studies have been carried out to substantiate the interactions between *P. aeruginosa* and *Staphylococcus epidermidis,* a bacterium closely related to *S. aureus*. It was shown that some *P. aeruginosa* extracellular products (possibly polysaccharides) provide a competitive advantage over *S. epidermidis* (Qin *et al.*, 2009). Furthermore, Pihl *et al.* (Pihl *et al.*, 2010a, 2010b) demonstrated that some *S. epidermidis* strains were better fitted than others to coexist in biofilms with *P. aeruginosa* whereas the ability of *P. aeruginosa* to inhibit *S. epidermidis* biofilms varied between clinical isolates. These authors suggested that specific *P. aeruginosa* strains might be selected during infections to counteract chronic colonization by *S. epidermidis* in order to allow the persistence and dominance of *P. aeruginosa.* Whether the genetic background of each strain also influences interspecies interactions between *S. aureus* and *P. aeruginosa* and whether the outcome of these interactions varies in each CF patient remains to be determined. Recent studies, which demontrate that *P. aeruginosa lasR* mutants are frequently found in CF, indicate that some of the abilities of this bacterium to influence the virulence of *S. aureus* may indeed be lost during CF lung infections (D'Argenio *et al.*, 2007; Hoffman *et al.*, 2009).

Other questions remain open. For example, the real impact of *S. aureus-P. aeruginosa* co-infections in CF is not known and convincing clinical data as well as co-infection in adequate experimental models are clearly missing. Whether *S. aureus* and *P. aeruginosa* have a synergistic or antagonistic effect on the progression of the disease is not known and may potentially be influenced by the nature of each clinical isolate. Furthermore, whereas the effect of *P. aeruginosa* on *S. aureus* has been studied widely, almost no investigations address the potential effect of *S. aureus* on the virulence of *P. aeruginosa*. Interestingly, Korgaonkar and Whiteley (2011) proposed a model in which *P. aeruginosa* senses surrounding bacteria by monitoring the presence of exogenous peptidoglycan and responds to it by increasing the production of the virulence factor pyocyanin.

4. New therapeutic approaches in CF

Humanity is now facing a post-antibiotic era defined by its limited capability to combat microbial infections caused by antibiotic resistant pathogens. The increased number of nosocomial and community-acquired infections caused by microorganisms resistant to at least two classes of conventional antibiotics is becoming an important public health problem. The global rise of antimicrobial resistance combined with the slow discovery and approval processes for classical antibiotics has resulted in the present urgent need for new and innovative therapeutic approaches. One of the reasons for multidrug resistance is that current antibiotics were designed around a limited number of chemical scaffolds with few major modifications since the 1980s. This has left plenty of opportunities for antibiotic resistance mechanisms to develop and spread worldwide (Shah, 2005; Talbot *et al.*, 2006). The identification of new antimicrobial targets and the development of novel therapeutic approaches may be facilitated by a better understanding of bacterial pathogenesis both at the single species and bacterial community levels. Antibiotic resistant bacteria are often recovered from CF patients but recalcitrance to antibiotic therapies is not only caused by bacterial genes that encode conventional mechanisms of antibiotic resistance. Indeed, the ever changing epidemiology of the CF airways (Razvi *et al.*, 2009) and the acquisition of bacterial phenotypes inherently resistant to antimicrobials contribute to treatment failures. Although some antibiotics have recently been approved or are close to being approved for clinical use and are promising in the context of CF (Parkins & Elborn, 2010), this section will talk about some novel therapeutic approaches that take into account the pathogenesis and the adaptation of CF pathogens in the context of polymicrobial infections. However, in order to appreciate the entirety of the efforts directed toward the cure of CF, it should be kept in mind that a number of strategies other than those using antibiotherapies are also being considered (George *et al.*, 2009).

4.1 Modulation of biofilm-forming microbial communities

The formation of biofilms by CF pathogens is thought to be a major virulence asset that promotes resistance both to antimicrobials and the host immune system (Costerton *et al.*, 1999; Davies & Bilton, 2009; Høiby *et al.*, 2010; Stewart, 2002). This fully justifies current research aimed at the development of therapeutic strategies that target biofilm formation and dispersal (Simões, 2011). Current management practices for *P. aeruginosa* infections include hygienic measures (Høiby & Pedersen, 1989), early aggressive eradication by antimicrobial therapy (Döring & Høiby, 2004), the use of nebulized DNAse (Frederiksen *et al.*, 2006) and chronic suppressive antibiotic therapy (Bjarnsholt *et al.*, 2009; Döring *et al.*, 2000). However, even if these methods are undeniably successful to a certain extent, chronic infection ultimately occurs and a gradual increase in the level of resistance is observed (Ciofu *et al.*, 1994). New therapeutic approaches specifically targeting biofilms should thus be useful in the context of CF lung infections and should decrease the occurrence or development of antibiotic resistance.

Most natural biofilms are polymicrobial (Stoodley *et al.*, 2002) and the polymicrobial nature of CF lung infections needs to be considered in novel therapeutic approaches (Sibley *et al.*, 2009; Sibley & Surette, 2011). Whereas some microbes may predispose the tissue toward the colonization by others, there may also be competition among bacterial populations and the removal of one pathogen could create an opportunity for another to expand (Harrison,

2007). On the other hand, tampering with the CF airway microbial community may lead to more effective treatment of chronic infections (Moore *et al.*, 2005). Some data even suggest that a healthy gut microflora protects against some respiratory pathogens (Alvarez *et al.*, 2001; Villena *et al.*, 2005) and that care should be taken not to deplete the gut microflora when oral or intravenous routes of antibiotic administration are used. It is also conceivable that monitoring the population dynamics of polymicrobial infections can be used to predict the efficacy of antimicrobial therapy and to optimize treatments (Rogers *et al.*, 2010). As such, the impact of antimicrobial chemotherapies on microbial communities should be assessed to detect unwanted effects. As an example, aminoglycosides, which are indicated for the management of acute exacerbations, the control of chronic infections and the eradication of recently acquired *P. aeruginosa*, have also been shown to induce bacterial biofilms in both *P. aeruginosa* (Hoffman *et al.*, 2005) and *S. aureus* (Mitchell *et al.*, 2010a).

The next sections provide examples of methods by which biofilm infections may be potentially overcome using different strategies that include targeting specific microbial phenotypes, influencing the pathogenesis of bacteria through the manipulation of cell-to-cell signaling and the enhancement of preexisting antimicrobial therapies against persistent forms of bacteria.

4.2 Targeting the persistent microbial phenotype

Bacteria often encounter unfavorable conditions during infection that limit bacterial growth and oblige the microorganisms to enter a quiescent state in order to persist within the host (Kolter *et al.*, 1993; Nataro *et al.*, 2000). Dormant bacteria are well-known for their tolerance to antibiotics normally active against rapidly dividing cells and often require prolonged periods of treatment (Coates *et al.*, 2002; Neu, 1992). The highly refractory nature of biofilms to eradication by chemotherapy is thought to be at least partly attributable to the presence of metabolically inactive cells (Fux *et al.*, 2005). The inefficacy of antibiotics against non-multiplying bacteria thus results in slow or partial death, prolonges the duration of therapy and increases the emergence of genotypic resistances. Accordingly, targeting slow-growing or non-dividing bacteria should provide substancial therapeutic benefits.

Membrane-acting agents are usually active against bacteria in all their phases of growth and are thus good candidates for the development of antimicrobials that target slow-growing and non-dividing bacteria. As an example, the novel porphyrin antibacterial agents XF-70 and XF-73 were shown to remain highly active against this type of bacteria (Ooi *et al.*, 2010). Hu *et al.* (2010) found that the small quinolone-derived compound HT61 was active against non-multiplying MSSA and MRSA by causing depolarization of the cell membrane and destruction of the cell wall. Antimicrobial peptides also interact and permeabilize the bacterial membrane and there is a good probability that they act on slow-growing bacteria that form biofilms (Batoni *et al.*, 2011). Bioactive peptides may even have additional benefits for CF therapeutic applications due to their anti-inflammatory and immunomodulating activities (Scott *et al.*, 2007; Zhang *et al.*, 2005).

The resistance of biofilms to killing by most antimicrobial agents is thought to be more specifically attributable to the presence of non-dividing persister cells (Lewis, 2007). Persisters are dormant bacteria that present a global slowdown in metabolic processes, do not divide and are tolerant to antibiotics. In other words, they have the ability to survive the effects of antibiotics without the use of drug-specific resistance mechanisms. Persisters have been described for *S. aureus* (Allison *et al.*, 2011; Singh *et al.*, 2009) and *P. aeruginosa*, with a recent study that shows the emergence of strains producing high levels of persister cells in CF patients (Mulcahy *et al.*, 2010). Currently, there are only a few therapeutic strategies that are considered for targeting persister cells. One such is the combination of conventional antibiotics with an inhibitor of an essential persister protein (Lewis, 2007). Also, repeated- or pulse-dosing of antibiotics could allow persister cells to resuscitate in order to be killed by subsequent antibiotic administration. The development of specific pro-antibiotics which could irreversibly bind to bacterial targets is also being considered (Lewis, 2007). An outstanding recent study shows that the use of specific metabolic stimuli enables the killing of persister cells with aminoglycoside antibiotics by modulating the proton-motive force required for the uptake of these drugs. The proof of concept for the latter approach has been demonstrated against biofilms and also in a model of chronic infection (Allison *et al.*, 2011).

As we have previously mentioned, SCVs are often associated with relapsing and persistent infections. In addition to the increased ability of these variants to form biofilms (Al Laham *et al.*, 2007; Häußler *et al.*, 2003; Mitchell *et al.*, 2010a, 2010b; Singh *et al.*, 2009, 2010; von Götz *et al.*, 2004), SCVs are well-known for their ability to infect and persist within non-professional phagocytes (Sendi & Proctor, 2009) and there is a limited choice of antibiotics able to act against intracellular bacteria. Nguyen *et al.* (Nguyen *et al.*, 2009a) reported a considerable decrease in the efficacy of most antibiotics against intracellular SCVs in comparison to that seen against extracellular bacteria, but, most importantly, in comparison to their efficacy against the normal-phenotype bacteria. Nevertheless, the authors noted that four antibiotics (quinupristin-dalfopristin, moxifloxacin, oritavancin and rifampicin) were more effective in killing intracellular SCVs. In addition, we recently described the first known molecule to specifically target the SCV phenotype of *S. aureus* (Mitchell *et al.*, 2011a). Tomatidine (TO) is the aglycone form of the plant secondary metabolite tomatine. The structure and the main biological activities of TO against *S. aureus* are presented in Fig. 5A. We found that TO has a bacteriostatic activity against SCVs, but not against normal strains. More importantly, we showed that TO has the ability to inhibit the replication of SCVs internalized in CF-like human airway epithelial cells (Mitchell *et al.*, 2011a). The specificity of the action of TO against SCVs was linked to the dysfunctional electron transport chain of these variants. Acordingly, HQNO sensitized normal *S. aureus* strains to TO (see Fig. 5B), which suggests that TO may be especially effective in the context where *P. aeruginosa* and *S. aureus* co-infect a CF patient. Although TO causes a marked inhibition of protein synthesis in bacteria showing a dysfunctional electron transport chain, the exact mechanism of action of TO on SCVs remains to be elucidated. Other biological activities for TO are discussed below.

4.3 Targeting virulence

Another emerging concept in the development of novel therapeutic approaches is the possibility to modulate the expression of virulence factors that are thought to be of major importance in the establishment of a particular infection. Modulators or blockers of pathogenesis are particularly interesting because it is speculated that, since they do not inhibit growth or kill bacteria, their use will not yield a strong selective pressure for resistance development. In this context, most attention has been directed toward the interference of bacterial QS and cell-to-cell signaling to inhibit virulence or biofilm

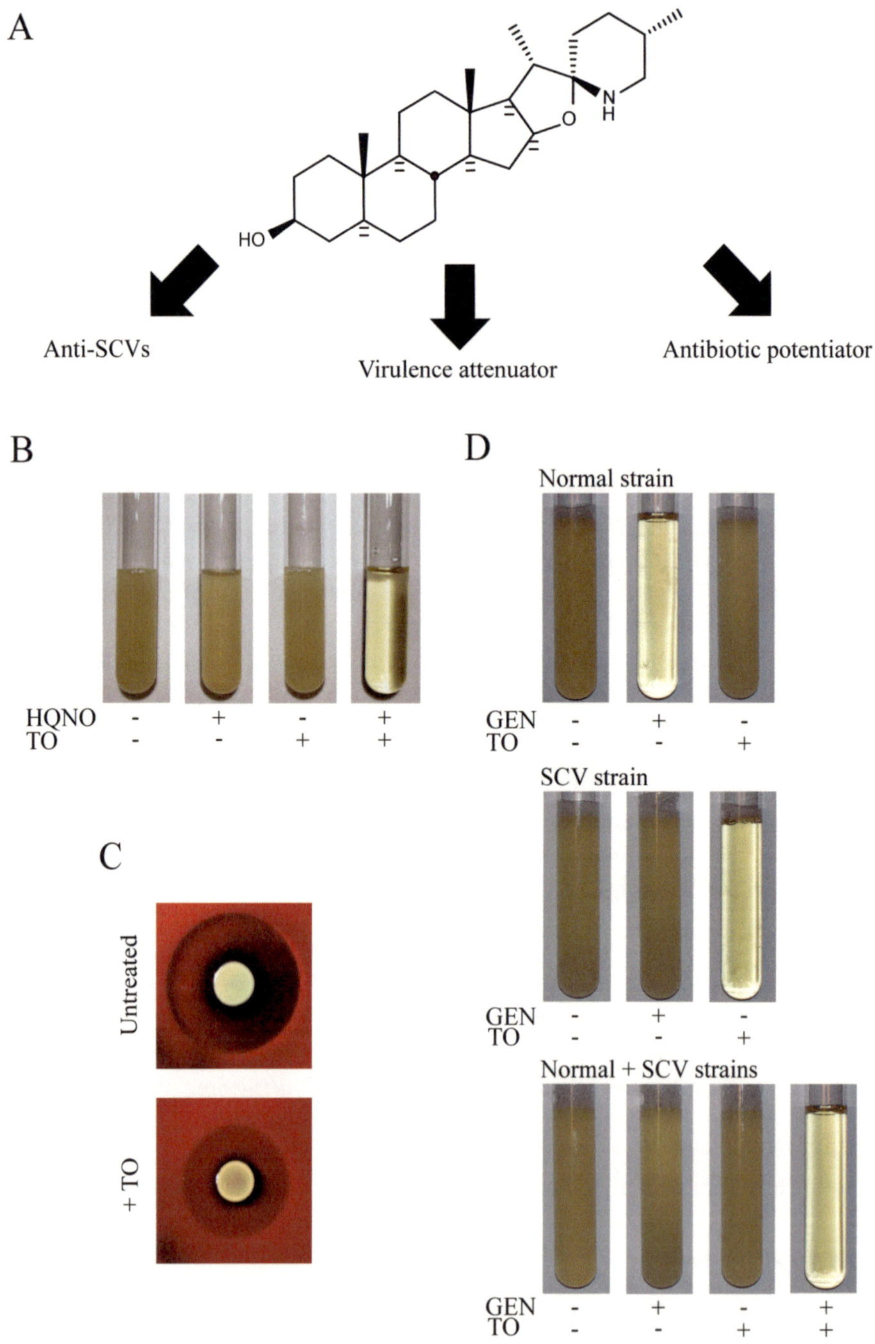

Fig. 5. Biological activities of tomatidine against *S. aureus*. (A) Tomatidine (TO) is a steroidal alkaloid molecule that inhibits both the extracellular and intracellular replication of SCVs, represses the expression of several *agr*-regulated exoproducts and potentiates the bactericidal activity of aminoglycoside antibiotics against prototypical *S. aureus*. (B) TO (8 µg/ml) inhibits the growth of a normal *S. aureus* strain in presence of HQNO (20 µg/ml).

Bacteria were inoculated at 10^5-10^6 CFU/ml and incubated 24 h at 35°C with shaking. (C) TO (8µg/ml) inhibits the hemolytic ability of a normal-growing *S. aureus* strain. (D) TO may be used in combination with aminoglycosides (*e.g.*, gentamicin [GEN]) to eradicate a population of *S. aureus* composed of normal and SCV bacteria. Bacteria were inoculated at 10^5-10^6 CFU/ml and incubated 24 h at 35°C with shaking in presence of 4 µg/ml of GEN and/or 0.12 µg/ml of TO. The clear test tubes show no bacterial growth.

formation (Njoroge & Sperandio, 2009; Rasko & Sperandio, 2010). However, although targeting the QS systems of *P. aeruginosa* in CF infections may increase the susceptibility of biofilms to clearance by antibiotics (Hentzer *et al.*, 2003), interference with the QS *agr* system of *S. aureus* may not be a good strategy since it could increase the formation of biofilms and increase bacterial persistence (Novick & Geisinger, 2008; Otto, 2004). The discovery of compounds that attenuate or abolish the cross talk between the QS systems of different bacterial species may be more promising. It remains to be determined whether interference with interspecies communications has the potential to decrease the overall virulence or the cohesion of polymicrobial communities and more particularly of those found in CF.

Several plant products have been shown to act as "virulence attenuators" of human pathogens (González-Lamothe *et al.*, 2009). Virulence attenuators modulate the virulence or the ability of the bacterium to adapt to the host environment. This gives a competitive advantage to the host immune system. As an example, a garlic extract was shown to interfere with the QS of *P. aeruginosa,* to sensitize its biofilm to tobramycin treatments and to improve clearance of bacteria in a pulmonary mouse model (Bjarnsholt *et al.*, 2005; Rasmussen *et al.*, 2005). Ginseng extract was also shown to alter the virulence of *P. aeruginosa* by interfering with QS, destroying biofilms, promoting phagocytosis by airway phagocytes and by protecting animals from the development of chronic lung infections (Song *et al.*, 1997a, 1997b, 2010; Wu *et al.*, 2011). Some of our own transcriptional analyses of bacteria exposed to plant products have shed light on the effect of TO on the expression of virulence factors by normal *S. aureus* strains (Bouarab *et al.*, 2007). We demonstrated that TO causes a repression in the expression of many extracellular toxins and of RNAIII, the effector molecule of the *agr* system, and thus it inhibits the hemolytic activity of *S. aureus*. We further showed that TO inhibits biofilm formation by *S. aureus* SCVs, probably through the induction of bacteriostasis (Mitchell *et al.*, 2009). We suggest that the overall negative effects of TO on the virulence and the growth of both normal and SCV *S. aureus* strains could be used in the management of both acute and chronic lung infections in CF patients. Fig. 5C shows the inhibitory effect of TO on the hemolytic ability of a normal *S. aureus* strain.

Other studies have also promoted the use of virulence factor-based therapies against *S. aureus.* For example, QS autoinducing peptide variants were shown to inhibit heterologous *agr* activation and were proposed as therapeutic agents (Novick & Geisinger, 2008). Also, a blocker of the synthesis of staphyloxanthin, the golden-carotenoid pigment of *S. aureus* that promotes resistance to reactive oxygen species and host neutrophil-based killing, increased the susceptibility of *S. aureus* to killing by human blood and the innate immune clearance in a mouse infection model (Liu *et al.*, 2008). Other researchers have attempted to achieve virulence attenuation by manipulation of bacterial metabolism (Lan *et al.*, 2010; Zhu *et al.*, 2009). Another possible approach is to target the bacterial pathways for programmed cell death which have been identified in several species (Engelberg-Kulka *et al.*, 2004).

4.4 Enhancing preexisting antimicrobial therapies

The use of synergistic combinations of antimicrobial compounds is an old strategy that continues to be tantalizing especially against the polymicrobial populations found in the CF airways. Accordingly, Høiby (2011) suggests that the effectiveness of combination therapies should be tested in the context of CF lung infections. Several combinations of old antibiotics indeed showed promising synergistic effects *in vitro* and/or *in vivo* such as fosfomycin-tobramycin, tobramycin-colistin and ciprofloxacin-colistin combinations, with the ciprofloxacin-colistin combination thought to be efficient even against *P. aeruginosa* biofilms (Høiby, 2011). A large screen of double and triple antibiotic combinations was tested on biofilm-grown *B. cepacia* and *P. aeruginosa* in order to identify effective antibiotic combinations for the treatment of CF patients (Dales *et al.*, 2009). Combinations of antibiotics may also be useful in order to improve the efficiency of antimicrobial treatments against intracellular SCVs. As an example, some drug combinations that included rifampicin were most effective against intracellular *S. aureus* of both normal and SCV phenotypes. (Baltch *et al.*, 2008). Nguyen *et al.* (2009b) also showed additive or synergistic effects between oritavancin, moxifloxacin and rifampicin against intracellular SCVs.

The combination of antimicrobial agents with non-antibiotic compounds is also an attractive approach (George *et al.*, 2009). Several plant products are "antibiotic potentiators" that can act as bacterial efflux pump inhibitors, cell wall-acting agents or membrane destabilizing agents to provide synergy with conventional antibiotics (González-Lamothe *et al.*, 2009). Interestingly, we have recently demonstrated that TO potentiates the bactericidal activity of aminoglycoside antibiotics against normal *S. aureus* strains of diverse clinical origins and antibiotic susceptibility patterns (unpublished results). Although the mechanism(s) by which this effect occurs is yet unknown, TO may prove useful in combination therapy with aminoglycoside antibiotics in the treatment of CF lung infections as exemplified in Fig. 5D. According to Mohtar *et al.* (Mohtar *et al.*, 2009), a vast number of other plant products with antimicrobial activity await discovery.

5. Conclusion

Complex polymicrobial communities colonize the CF airways and interspecies interactions are likely to play a role in the course of respiratory infections. *P. aeruginosa* and *S. aureus* are prevalent pathogens often simultaneously found in CF patients and for which microbial interactions that modulate virulence are already well documented. In communities and by using intraspecies and interspecies cell-to-cell communication, these pathogens have the ability to form biofilms and to adopt persistent phenotypes such as persister cells and SCVs. These phenotypes confer non-specific resistance to antimicrobials and to the host immune system. The development of novel therapeutic approaches that take into account polymicrobial communities and the various strategies that bacteria have elaborated to adapt and persist within the CF airways should help to eradicate chronic and life-threatening infections in CF.

6. Acknowledgment

François Malouin (FM) is supported by Cystic Fibrosis Canada and by a team grant from the Fonds Québécois de la Recherche sur la Nature et les Technologies (FQRNT) with Kamal Bouarab and Éric Marsault. Gabriel Mitchell was the recipient of an Alexander-Graham-Bell

Graduate Scholarship from the Natural Sciences and Engineering Research Council of Canada and received a research scholarship from FQRNT during the course of his doctoral program. The authors would like to thank Brian Talbot for critical review of this chapter, Gilles Grondin for technical assistance as well as Alexandre Fugère, David Lalonde Séguin, Éric Brouillette, Isabelle Guay, Karine Pépin Gaudreau and Simon Boulanger for their involvement in the CF research program taking place in the FM laboratory. We thank Josée Lessard and André Cantin from the CF clinic and Eric Frost and the personnel from the clinical microbiology laboratory of the Centre Hospitalier Universitaire de Sherbrooke, and of course, we gratefully thank all CF patients for their willingness and enthusiasm in participating to this research.

7. References

Al Laham, N., Rohde, H., Sander, G., Fischer, A., Hussain, M., Heilmann, C., Mack, D., Proctor, R., Peters, G., Becker, K. & von Eiff, C. (2007). Augmented expression of polysaccharide intercellular adhesin in a defined *Staphylococcus epidermidis* mutant with the small-colony-variant phenotype. *J Bacteriol*, Vol. 189, No. 12, pp. 4494-4501.

Allison, K.R., Brynildsen, M.P. & Collins, J.J. (2011). Metabolite-enabled eradication of bacterial persisters by aminoglycosides. *Nature*, Vol. 473, No. 7346, pp. 216-220.

Alvarez, S., Herrero, C., Bru, E. & Perdigon, G. (2001). Effect of *Lactobacillus casei* and yogurt administration on prevention of *Pseudomonas aeruginosa* infection in young mice. *J Food Prot*, Vol. 64, No. 11, pp. 1768-1774.

Archer, G.L. (1998). *Staphylococcus aureus*: a well-armed pathogen. *Clin Infect Dis*, Vol. 26, No. 5, pp. 1179-1181.

Bakkal, S., Robinson, S.M., Ordonez, C.L., Waltz, D.A. & Riley, M.A. (2010). Role of bacteriocins in mediating interactions of bacterial isolates taken from cystic fibrosis patients. *Microbiology*, Vol. 156, No. Pt 7, pp. 2058-2067.

Baltch, A.L., Ritz, W.J., Bopp, L.H., Michelsen, P. & Smith, R.P. (2008). Activities of daptomycin and comparative antimicrobials, singly and in combination, against extracellular and intracellular *Staphylococcus aureus* and its stable small-colony variant in human monocyte-derived macrophages and in broth. *Antimicrob Agents Chemother*, Vol. 52, No. 5, pp. 1829-1833.

Bates, D.M., von Eiff, C., McNamara, P.J., Peters, G., Yeaman, M.R., Bayer, A.S. & Proctor, R.A. (2003). *Staphylococcus aureus menD* and *hemB* mutants are as infective as the parent strains, but the menadione biosynthetic mutant persists within the kidney. *J Infect Dis*, Vol. 187, No. 10, pp. 1654-1661.

Batoni, G., Maisetta, G., Brancatisano, F.L., Esin, S. & Campa, M. (2011). Use of antimicrobial peptides against microbial biofilms: advantages and limits. *Curr Med Chem*, Vol. 18, No. 2, pp. 256-279.

Biswas, L., Biswas, R., Schlag, M., Bertram, R. & Götz, F. (2009). Small-colony variant selection as a survival strategy for *Staphylococcus aureus* in the presence of *Pseudomonas aeruginosa*. *Appl Environ Microbiol*, Vol. 75, No. 21, pp. 6910-6912.

Bjarnsholt, T., Jensen, P.Ø., Rasmussen, T.B., Christophersen, L., Calum, H., Hentzer, M., Hougen, H.P., Rygaard, J., Moser, C., Eberl, L., Høiby, N. & Givskov, M. (2005). Garlic blocks quorum sensing and promotes rapid clearing of pulmonary *Pseudomonas aeruginosa* infections. *Microbiology*, Vol. 151, No. Pt 12, pp. 3873-3880.

Bjarnsholt, T., Jensen, P.Ø., Fiandaca, M.J., Pedersen, J., Hansen, C.R., Andersen, C.B., Pressler, T., Givskov, M. & Høiby, N. (2009). *Pseudomonas aeruginosa* biofilms in the respiratory tract of cystic fibrosis patients. *Pediatr Pulmonol*, Vol. 44, No. 6, pp. 547-558.

Bodey, G.P., Bolivar, R., Fainstein, V. & Jadeja, L. (1983). Infections caused by *Pseudomonas aeruginosa*. *Rev Infect Dis*, Vol. 5, No. 2, pp. 279-313.

Bouarab, K., Ordi, M.E., Gattuso, M., Moisan, H. & Malouin, F. (2007). Plant stress response agents affect *Staphylococcus aureus* virulence genes. abstr. C1-1483, *Proceedings of 47th Intersci. Conf. Antimicrob. Agents Chemother*, Chicago, IL.

Brogden, K.A., Guthmiller, J.M. & Taylor, C.E. (2005). Human polymicrobial infections. *Lancet*, Vol. 365, No. 9455, pp. 253-255.

Bronner, S., Monteil, H. & Prévost, G. (2004). Regulation of virulence determinants in *Staphylococcus aureus*: complexity and applications. *FEMS Microbiol Rev*, Vol. 28, No. 2, pp. 183-200.

Brouillette, E., Martinez, A., Boyll, B.J., Allen, N.E. & Malouin, F. (2004). Persistence of a *Staphylococcus aureus* small-colony variant under antibiotic pressure *in vivo*. *FEMS Immunol Med Microbiol*, Vol. 41, No. 1, pp. 35-41.

Bryan, L.E. & Van Den Elzen, H.M. (1977). Effects of membrane-energy mutations and cations on streptomycin and gentamicin accumulation by bacteria: a model for entry of streptomycin and gentamicin in susceptible and resistant bacteria. *Antimicrob Agents Chemother*, Vol. 12, No. 2, pp. 163-177.

Canadian Cystic Fibrosis Foundation (2009) *Patient data registry report.* Toronton, ON, Canada.

Chambers, H.F. & Deleo, F.R. (2009). Waves of resistance: *Staphylococcus aureus* in the antibiotic era. *Nat Rev Microbiol*, Vol. 7, No. 9, pp. 629-641.

Chattoraj, S.S., Murthy, R., Ganesan, S., Goldberg, J.B., Zhao, Y., Hershenson, M.B. & Sajjan, U.S. (2010). *Pseudomonas aeruginosa* alginate promotes *Burkholderia cenocepacia* persistence in cystic fibrosis transmembrane conductance regulator knockout mice. *Infect Immun*, Vol. 78, No. 3, pp. 984-993.

Chmiel, J.F. & Davis, P.B. (2003). State of the art: why do the lungs of patients with cystic fibrosis become infected and why can't they clear the infection? *Respir Res*, Vol. 4, pp. 8.

Ciofu, O., Giwercman, B., Pedersen, S.S. & Høiby, N. (1994). Development of antibiotic resistance in *Pseudomonas aeruginosa* during two decades of antipseudomonal treatment at the Danish CF Center. *Apmis*, Vol. 102, No. 9, pp. 674-680.

Coates, A., Hu, Y., Bax, R. & Page, C. (2002). The future challenges facing the development of new antimicrobial drugs. *Nat Rev Drug Discov*, Vol. 1, No. 11, pp. 895-910.

Costerton, J.W., Stewart, P.S. & Greenberg, E.P. (1999). Bacterial biofilms: a common cause of persistent infections. *Science*, Vol. 284, No. 5418, pp. 1318-1322.

Cystic Fibrosis Foundation (2009). Patient registry annual report, Washington, D.C.

D'Argenio, D.A., Wu, M., Hoffman, L.R., Kulasekara, H.D., Déziel, E., Smith, E.E., Nguyen, H., Ernst, R.K., Larson Freeman, T.J., Spencer, D.H., Brittnacher, M., Hayden, H.S., Selgrade, S., Klausen, M., Goodlett, D.R., Burns, J.L., Ramsey, B.W. & Miller, S.I. (2007). Growth phenotypes of *Pseudomonas aeruginosa lasR* mutants adapted to the airways of cystic fibrosis patients. *Mol Microbiol*, Vol. 64, No. 2, pp. 512-533.

Dales, L., Ferris, W., Vandemheen, K. & Aaron, S.D. (2009). Combination antibiotic susceptibility of biofilm-grown *Burkholderia cepacia* and *Pseudomonas aeruginosa* isolated from patients with pulmonary exacerbations of cystic fibrosis. *Eur J Clin Microbiol Infect Dis*, Vol. 28, No. 10, pp. 1275-1279.

Dasenbrook, E.C., Merlo, C.A., Diener-West, M., Lechtzin, N. & Boyle, M.P. (2008). Persistent methicillin-resistant *Staphylococcus aureus* and rate of FEV1 decline in cystic fibrosis. *Am J Respir Crit Care Med*, Vol. 178, No. 8, pp. 814-821.

Dasenbrook, E.C., Checkley, W., Merlo, C.A., Konstan, M.W., Lechtzin, N. & Boyle, M.P. (2010). Association between respiratory tract methicillin-resistant *Staphylococcus aureus* and survival in cystic fibrosis. *JAMA*, Vol. 303, No. 23, pp. 2386-2392.

Davies, J.C. & Bilton, D. (2009). Bugs, biofilms, and resistance in cystic fibrosis. *Respir Care*, Vol. 54, No. 5, pp. 628-640.

Döring, G., Conway, S.P., Heijerman, H.G., Hodson, M.E., Høiby, N., Smyth, A. & Touw, D.J. (2000). Antibiotic therapy against *Pseudomonas aeruginosa* in cystic fibrosis: a European consensus. *Eur Respir J*, Vol. 16, No. 4, pp. 749-767.

Döring, G. & Høiby, N. (2004). Early intervention and prevention of lung disease in cystic fibrosis: a European consensus. *J Cyst Fibros*, Vol. 3, No. 2, pp. 67-91.

Duan, K., Dammel, C., Stein, J., Rabin, H. & Surette, M.G. (2003). Modulation of *Pseudomonas aeruginosa* gene expression by host microflora through interspecies communication. *Mol Microbiol*, Vol. 50, No. 5, pp. 1477-1491.

Dubern, J.F. & Diggle, S.P. (2008). Quorum sensing by 2-alkyl-4-quinolones in *Pseudomonas aeruginosa* and other bacterial species. *Mol Biosyst*, Vol. 4, No. 9, pp. 882-888.

Engelberg-Kulka, H., Sat, B., Reches, M., Amitai, S. & Hazan, R. (2004). Bacterial programmed cell death systems as targets for antibiotics. *Trends Microbiol*, Vol. 12, No. 2, pp. 66-71.

European Cystic Fibrosis Society (2007) *Patient Registry Report*.

Foweraker, J.E., Laughton, C.R., Brown, D.F. & Bilton, D. (2005). Phenotypic variability of *Pseudomonas aeruginosa* in sputa from patients with acute infective exacerbation of cystic fibrosis and its impact on the validity of antimicrobial susceptibility testing. *J Antimicrob Chemother*, Vol. 55, No. 6, pp. 921-927.

Frederiksen, B., Pressler, T., Hansen, A., Koch, C. & Høiby, N. (2006). Effect of aerosolized rhDNase (Pulmozyme) on pulmonary colonization in patients with cystic fibrosis. *Acta Paediatr*, Vol. 95, No. 9, pp. 1070-1074.

Fux, C.A., Costerton, J.W., Stewart, P.S. & Stoodley, P. (2005). Survival strategies of infectious biofilms. *Trends Microbiol*, Vol. 13, No. 1, pp. 34-40.

Galli, J., Ardito, F., Calo, L., Mancinelli, L., Imperiali, M., Parrilla, C., Picciotti, P.M. & Fadda, G. (2007). Recurrent upper airway infections and bacterial biofilms. *J Laryngol Otol*, Vol. 121, No. 4, pp. 341-344.

George, A.M., Jones, P.M. & Middleton, P.G. (2009). Cystic fibrosis infections: treatment strategies and prospects. *FEMS Microbiol Lett*, Vol. 300, No. 2, pp. 153-164.

Goerke, C. & Wolz, C. (2009). Adaptation of *Staphylococcus aureus* to the cystic fibrosis lung. *Int J Med Microbiol*, Vol. 300, No. 8, pp. 520-525.

González-Lamothe, R., Mitchell, G., Gattuso, M., Diarra, M.S., Malouin, F. & Bouarab, K. (2009). Plant antimicrobial agents and their effects on plant and human pathogens. *Int J Mol Sci*, Vol. 10, No. 8, pp. 3400-3419.

Grundmeier, M., Tuchscherr, L., Brück, M., Viemann, D., Roth, J., Willscher, E., Becker, K., Peters, G. & Löffler, B. (2010). Staphylococcal strains vary greatly in their ability to induce an inflammatory response in endothelial cells. *J Infect Dis*, Vol. 201, No. 6, pp. 871-880.

Hall-Stoodley, L., Costerton, J.W. & Stoodley, P. (2004). Bacterial biofilms: from the natural environment to infectious diseases. *Nat Rev Microbiol*, Vol. 2, No. 2, pp. 95-108.

Harrison, F. (2007). Microbial ecology of the cystic fibrosis lung. *Microbiology*, Vol. 153, No. Pt 4, pp. 917-923.

Häußler, S., Tümmler, B., Weißbrodt, H., Rohde, M. & Steinmetz, I. (1999). Small-colony variants of *Pseudomonas aeruginosa* in cystic fibrosis. *Clin Infect Dis*, Vol. 29, No. 3, pp. 621-625.

Häußler, S., Ziegler, I., Löttel, A., von Götz, F., Rohde, M., Wehmhöhner, D., Saravanamuthu, S., Tümmler, B. & Steinmetz, I. (2003). Highly adherent small-colony variants of *Pseudomonas aeruginosa* in cystic fibrosis lung infection. *J Med Microbiol*, Vol. 52, No. Pt 4, pp. 295-301.

Hentzer, M., Wu, H., Andersen, J.B., Riedel, K., Rasmussen, T.B., Bagge, N., Kumar, N., Schembri, M.A., Song, Z., Kristoffersen, P., Manefield, M., Costerton, J.W., Molin, S., Eberl, L., Steinberg, P., Kjelleberg, S., Høiby, N. & Givskov, M. (2003). Attenuation of *Pseudomonas aeruginosa* virulence by quorum sensing inhibitors. *Embo J*, Vol. 22, No. 15, pp. 3803-3815.

Hoffman, L.R., D'Argenio, D.A., MacCoss, M.J., Zhang, Z., Jones, R.A. & Miller, S.I. (2005). Aminoglycoside antibiotics induce bacterial biofilm formation. *Nature*, Vol. 436, No. 7054, pp. 1171-1175.

Hoffman, L.R., Déziel, E., D'Argenio, D.A., Lépine, F., Emerson, J., McNamara, S., Gibson, R.L., Ramsey, B.W. & Miller, S.I. (2006). Selection for *Staphylococcus aureus* small-colony variants due to growth in the presence of *Pseudomonas aeruginosa*. *Proc Natl Acad Sci U S A*, Vol. 103, No. 52, pp. 19890-19895.

Hoffman, L.R., Kulasekara, H.D., Emerson, J., Houston, L.S., Burns, J.L., Ramsey, B.W. & Miller, S.I. (2009). *Pseudomonas aeruginosa lasR* mutants are associated with cystic fibrosis lung disease progression. *J Cyst Fibros*, Vol. 8, No. 1, pp. 66-70.

Hogardt, M. & Heesemann, J. (2010). Adaptation of *Pseudomonas aeruginosa* during persistence in the cystic fibrosis lung. *Int J Med Microbiol*, Vol. 300, No. 8, pp. 557-562.

Høiby, N. & Pedersen, S.S. (1989). Estimated risk of cross-infection with *Pseudomonas aeruginosa* in Danish cystic fibrosis patients. *Acta Paediatr Scand*, Vol. 78, No. 3, pp. 395-404.

Høiby, N., Bjarnsholt, T., Givskov, M., Molin, S. & Ciofu, O. (2010). Antibiotic resistance of bacterial biofilms. *Int J Antimicrob Agents*, Vol. 35, No. 4, pp. 322-332.

Høiby, N. (2011). Recent advances in the treatment of *Pseudomonas aeruginosa* infections in cystic fibrosis. *BMC Med*, Vol. 9, pp. 32.

Hu, Y., Shamaei-Tousi, A., Liu, Y. & Coates, A. (2010). A new approach for the discovery of antibiotics by targeting non-multiplying bacteria: a novel topical antibiotic for staphylococcal infections. *PLoS One*, Vol. 5, No. 7, pp. e11818.

Kahl, B., Herrmann, M., Everding, A.S., Koch, H.G., Becker, K., Harms, E., Proctor, R.A. & Peters, G. (1998). Persistent infection with small colony variant strains of *Staphylococcus aureus* in patients with cystic fibrosis. *J Infect Dis*, Vol. 177, No. 4, pp. 1023-1029.

Kahl, B.C. (2010). Impact of *Staphylococcus aureus* on the pathogenesis of chronic cystic fibrosis lung disease. *Int J Med Microbiol*, Vol. 300, No. 8, pp. 514-519.

Kaufmann, G.F., Sartorio, R., Lee, S.H., Rogers, C.J., Meijler, M.M., Moss, J.A., Clapham, B., Brogan, A.P., Dickerson, T.J. & Janda, K.D. (2005). Revisiting quorum sensing: Discovery of additional chemical and biological functions for 3-oxo-N-acylhomoserine lactones. *Proc Natl Acad Sci U S A*, Vol. 102, No. 2, pp. 309-314.

Kessler, E., Safrin, M., Olson, J.C. & Ohman, D.E. (1993). Secreted LasA of *Pseudomonas aeruginosa* is a staphylolytic protease. *J Biol Chem*, Vol. 268, No. 10, pp. 7503-7508.

Kolter, R., Siegele, D.A. & Tormo, A. (1993). The stationary phase of the bacterial life cycle. *Annu Rev Microbiol*, Vol. 47, pp. 855-874.

Korgaonkar, A.K. & Whiteley, M. (2011). *Pseudomonas aeruginosa* enhances production of an antimicrobial in response to N-acetylglucosamine and peptidoglycan. *J Bacteriol*, Vol. 193, No. 4, pp. 909-917.

Lan, L., Cheng, A., Dunman, P.M., Missiakas, D. & He, C. (2010). Golden pigment production and virulence gene expression are affected by metabolisms in *Staphylococcus aureus*. *J Bacteriol*, Vol. 192, No. 12, pp. 3068-3077.

Lauderdale, K.J., Boles, B.R., Cheung, A.L. & Horswill, A.R. (2009). Interconnections between Sigma B, *agr*, and proteolytic activity in *Staphylococcus aureus* biofilm maturation. *Infect Immun*, Vol. 77, No. 4, pp. 1623-1635.

Leisinger, T. & Margraff, R. (1979). Secondary metabolites of the fluorescent pseudomonads. *Microbiol Rev*, Vol. 43, No. 3, pp. 422-442.

Lépine, F., Milot, S., Déziel, E., He, J. & Rahme, L.G. (2004). Electrospray/mass spectrometric identification and analysis of 4-hydroxy-2-alkylquinolines (HAQs) produced by *Pseudomonas aeruginosa*. *J Am Soc Mass Spectrom*, Vol. 15, No. 6, pp. 862-869.

Lewis, K. (2007). Persister cells, dormancy and infectious disease. *Nat Rev Microbiol*, Vol. 5, No. 1, pp. 48-56.

Lightbown, J.W. (1954). An antagonist of streptomycin and dihydrostreptomycin produced by *Pseudomonas aeruginosa*. *J Gen Microbiol*, Vol. 11, No. 3, pp. 477-492.

Lightbown, J.W. & Jackson, F.L. (1954). Inhibition of cytochrome system of heart muscle and of *Staphylococcus aureus* by 2-heptyl-4-hydroxyquinoline-N-oxide, an antagonist of dihydrostreptomycin. *Biochem J*, Vol. 58, No. 4, pp. xlix.

Liu, C.I., Liu, G.Y., Song, Y., Yin, F., Hensler, M.E., Jeng, W.Y., Nizet, V., Wang, A.H. & Oldfield, E. (2008). A cholesterol biosynthesis inhibitor blocks *Staphylococcus aureus* virulence. *Science*, Vol. 319, No. 5868, pp. 1391-1394.

Lyczak, J.B., Cannon, C.L. & Pier, G.B. (2002). Lung infections associated with cystic fibrosis. *Clin Microbiol Rev*, Vol. 15, No. 2, pp. 194-222.

Machan, Z.A., Taylor, G.W., Pitt, T.L., Cole, P.J. & Wilson, R. (1992). 2-Heptyl-4-hydroxyquinoline N-oxide, an antistaphylococcal agent produced by *Pseudomonas aeruginosa*. *J Antimicrob Chemother*, Vol. 30, No. 5, pp. 615-623.

Maciá, M.D., Blanquer, D., Togores, B., Sauleda, J., Pérez, J.L. & Oliver, A. (2005). Hypermutation is a key factor in development of multiple-antimicrobial resistance in *Pseudomonas aeruginosa* strains causing chronic lung infections. *Antimicrob Agents Chemother*, Vol. 49, No. 8, pp. 3382-3386.

Mashburn, L.M., Jett, A.M., Akins, D.R. & Whiteley, M. (2005). *Staphylococcus aureus* serves as an iron source for *Pseudomonas aeruginosa* during *in vivo* coculture. *J Bacteriol*, Vol. 187, No. 2, pp. 554-566.

Mashburn, L.M. & Whiteley, M. (2005). Membrane vesicles traffic signals and facilitate group activities in a prokaryote. *Nature*, Vol. 437, No. 7057, pp. 422-425.

McAlester, G., O'Gara, F. & Morrissey, J.P. (2008). Signal-mediated interactions between *Pseudomonas aeruginosa* and *Candida albicans*. *J Med Microbiol*, Vol. 57, No. Pt 5, pp. 563-569.

Mitchell, G., Lamontagne, C.A., Brouillette, E., Grondin, G., Talbot, B.G., Grandbois, M. & Malouin, F. (2008). *Staphylococcus aureus* SigB activity promotes a strong fibronectin-bacterium interaction which may sustain host tissue colonization by small-colony variants isolated from cystic fibrosis patients. *Mol Microbiol*, Vol. 70, No. 6, pp. 1540-1555.

Mitchell, G., Gattuso, M., Bouarab, K. & Malouin, F. (2009). Tomatidine (TO) affects virulence regulators of prototypical *Staphylococcus aureus* (SA) and small-colony variants (SCV) of cystic fibrosis patients, abstr. C1-1341, *Proceedings of 49th Intersci. Conf. Antimicrob. Agents Chemother*, San Francisco, CA.

Mitchell, G., Brouillette, E., Séguin, D.L., Asselin, A.E., Jacob, C.L. & Malouin, F. (2010a). A role for sigma factor B in the emergence of *Staphylococcus aureus* small-colony variants and elevated biofilm production resulting from an exposure to aminoglycosides. *Microb Pathog*, Vol. 48, No. 1, pp. 18-27.

Mitchell, G., Séguin, D.L., Asselin, A.E., Déziel, E., Cantin, A.M., Frost, E.H., Michaud, S. & Malouin, F. (2010b). *Staphylococcus aureus* sigma B-dependent emergence of small-colony variants and biofilm production following exposure to *Pseudomonas aeruginosa* 4-hydroxy-2-heptylquinoline-N-oxide. *BMC Microbiol*, Vol. 10, pp. 33.

Mitchell, G., Gattuso, M., Grondin, G., Marsault, E., Bouarab, K. & Malouin, F. (2011a). Tomatidine inhibits replication of *Staphylococcus aureus* small-colony variants in cystic fibrosis airway epithelial cells. *Antimicrob Agents Chemother*, Vol. 55, No. 5, pp. 1937-1945.

Mitchell, G., Grondin, G., Bilodeau, G., Cantin, A.M. & Malouin, F. (2011b). Infection of Polarized Airway Epithelial Cells by Normal and Small-Colony Variant Strains of *Staphylococcus aureus* is Increased in Cells with Abnormal CFTR function and is influenced by NF-κB. *Infect Immun*. Vol. 79, No. 9, pp. 3541-3551.

Mohtar, M., Johari, S.A., Li, A.R., Isa, M.M., Mustafa, S., Ali, A.M. & Basri, D.F. (2009). Inhibitory and resistance-modifying potential of plant-based alkaloids against methicillin-resistant *Staphylococcus aureus* (MRSA). *Curr Microbiol*, Vol. 59, No. 2, pp. 181-186.

Moisan, H., Brouillette, E., Jacob, C.L., Langlois-Bégin, P., Michaud, S. & Malouin, F. (2006). Transcription of virulence factors in *Staphylococcus aureus* small-colony variants isolated from cystic fibrosis patients is influenced by SigB. *J Bacteriol*, Vol. 188, No. 1, pp. 64-76.

Molina, A., Del Campo, R., Máiz, L., Morosini, M.I., Lamas, A., Baquero, F. & Cantón, R. (2008). High prevalence in cystic fibrosis patients of multiresistant hospital-acquired methicillin-resistant *Staphylococcus aureus* ST228-SCC*mecI* capable of biofilm formation. *J Antimicrob Chemother*, Vol. 62, No. 5, pp. 961-967.

Moore, J.E., Shaw, A., Millar, B.C., Downey, D.G., Murphy, P.G. & Elborn, J.S. (2005). Microbial ecology of the cystic fibrosis lung: does microflora type influence microbial loading? *Br J Biomed Sci*, Vol. 62, No. 4, pp. 175-178.

Moskowitz, S.M., Gibson, R.L. & Effmann, E.L. (2005). Cystic fibrosis lung disease: genetic influences, microbial interactions, and radiological assessment. *Pediatr Radiol*, Vol. 35, No. 8, pp. 739-757.

Mulcahy, L.R., Burns, J.L., Lory, S. & Lewis, K. (2010). Emergence of *Pseudomonas aeruginosa* strains producing high levels of persister cells in patients with cystic fibrosis. *J Bacteriol*, Vol. 192, No. 23, pp. 6191-6199.

Nataro J.P., Blaser M.J. & Cunningham-Rundles S. (2000). Persistent bacterial infections: commensalism gone awry or adaptive niche?, In *Persistent Bacterial Infections*, Nataro J.P., Blaser M.J. and Cunningham-Rundles S., pp. 3-10, American Society for Microbiology Press, Washington, DC.

Neu, H.C. (1992). General therapeutic principles., In *Infectious Diseases*, Gorbach, S.L., Bartlett, J.G. and Blacklow, N.R., pp. 153-160, WB Saunders Company, Philadelphia, PA.

Nguyen, H.A., Denis, O., Vergison, A., Theunis, A., Tulkens, P.M., Struelens, M.J. & Van Bambeke, F. (2009a). Intracellular activity of antibiotics in a model of human THP-1 macrophages infected by a *Staphylococcus aureus* small-colony variant strain isolated from a cystic fibrosis patient: pharmacodynamic evaluation and comparison with isogenic normal-phenotype and revertant strains. *Antimicrob Agents Chemother*, Vol. 53, No. 4, pp. 1434-1442.

Nguyen, H.A., Denis, O., Vergison, A., Tulkens, P.M., Struelens, M.J. & Van Bambeke, F. (2009b). Intracellular activity of antibiotics in a model of human THP-1 macrophages infected by a *Staphylococcus aureus* small-colony variant strain isolated from a cystic fibrosis patient: study of antibiotic combinations. *Antimicrob Agents Chemother*, Vol. 53, No. 4, pp. 1443-1449.

Njoroge, J. & Sperandio, V. (2009). Jamming bacterial communication: new approaches for the treatment of infectious diseases. *EMBO Mol Med*, Vol. 1, No. 4, pp. 201-210.

Novick, R.P. (2003). Autoinduction and signal transduction in the regulation of staphylococcal virulence. *Mol Microbiol*, Vol. 48, No. 6, pp. 1429-1449.

Novick, R.P. & Geisinger, E. (2008). Quorum sensing in staphylococci. *Annu Rev Genet*, Vol. 42, pp. 541-564.

Ooi, N., Miller, K., Randall, C., Rhys-Williams, W., Love, W. & Chopra, I. (2010). XF-70 and XF-73, novel antibacterial agents active against slow-growing and non-dividing cultures of *Staphylococcus aureus* including biofilms. *J Antimicrob Chemother*, Vol. 65, No. 1, pp. 72-78.

Otto, M. (2004). Quorum-sensing control in Staphylococci -- a target for antimicrobial drug therapy? *FEMS Microbiol Lett*, Vol. 241, No. 2, pp. 135-141.

Palmer, K.L., Mashburn, L.M., Singh, P.K. & Whiteley, M. (2005). Cystic fibrosis sputum supports growth and cues key aspects of *Pseudomonas aeruginosa* physiology. *J Bacteriol*, Vol. 187, No. 15, pp. 5267-5277.

Parkins, M.D. & Elborn, J.S. (2010). Newer antibacterial agents and their potential role in cystic fibrosis pulmonary exacerbation management. *J Antimicrob Chemother*, Vol. 65, No. 9, pp. 1853-1861.

Pihl, M., Chávez de Paz, L.E., Schmidtchen, A., Svensäter, G. & Davies, J.R. (2010a). Effects of clinical isolates of *Pseudomonas aeruginosa* on *Staphylococcus epidermidis* biofilm formation. *FEMS Immunol Med Microbiol*, Vol. 59, No. 3, pp. 504-512.

Pihl, M., Davies, J.R., Chávez de Paz, L.E. & Svensäter, G. (2010b). Differential effects of *Pseudomonas aeruginosa* on biofilm formation by different strains of *Staphylococcus epidermidis*. *FEMS Immunol Med Microbiol*, Vol. 59, No. 3, pp. 439-446.

Proctor, R.A., von Eiff, C., Kahl, B.C., Becker, K., McNamara, P., Herrmann, M. & Peters, G. (2006). Small colony variants: a pathogenic form of bacteria that facilitates persistent and recurrent infections. *Nat Rev Microbiol*, Vol. 4, No. 4, pp. 295-305.

Pruneau, M., Mitchell, G., Moisan, H., Dumont-Blanchette, E., Jacob, C.L. & Malouin, F. (2011). Transcriptional analysis of antibiotic resistance and virulence genes in multiresistant hospital-acquired MRSA. *FEMS Immunol Med Microbiol*. Jun 10 [Epub ahead of print]

Qazi, S., Middleton, B., Muharram, S.H., Cockayne, A., Hill, P., O'Shea, P., Chhabra, S.R., Camara, M. & Williams, P. (2006). N-acylhomoserine lactones antagonize virulence gene expression and quorum sensing in *Staphylococcus aureus*. *Infect Immun*, Vol. 74, No. 2, pp. 910-919.

Qin, Z., Yang, L., Qu, D., Molin, S. & Tolker-Nielsen, T. (2009). *Pseudomonas aeruginosa* extracellular products inhibit staphylococcal growth, and disrupt established biofilms produced by *Staphylococcus epidermidis*. *Microbiology*, Vol. 155, No. Pt 7, pp. 2148-2156.

Rasko, D.A. & Sperandio, V. (2010). Anti-virulence strategies to combat bacteria-mediated disease. *Nat Rev Drug Discov*, Vol. 9, No. 2, pp. 117-128.

Rasmussen, T.B., Bjarnsholt, T., Skindersoe, M.E., Hentzer, M., Kristoffersen, P., Köte, M., Nielsen, J., Eberl, L. & Givskov, M. (2005). Screening for quorum-sensing inhibitors (QSI) by use of a novel genetic system, the QSI selector. *J Bacteriol*, Vol. 187, No. 5, pp. 1799-1814.

Razvi, S., Quittell, L., Sewall, A., Quinton, H., Marshall, B. & Saiman, L. (2009). Respiratory microbiology of patients with cystic fibrosis in the United States, 1995 to 2005. *Chest*, Vol. 136, No. 6, pp. 1554-1560.

Riedel, K., Hentzer, M., Geisenberger, O., Huber, B., Steidle, A., Wu, H., Høiby, N., Givskov, M., Molin, S. & Eberl, L. (2001). N-acylhomoserine-lactone-mediated communication between *Pseudomonas aeruginosa* and *Burkholderia cepacia* in mixed biofilms. *Microbiology*, Vol. 147, No. Pt 12, pp. 3249-3262.

Riordan, J.R. (2008). CFTR function and prospects for therapy. *Annu Rev Biochem*, Vol. 77, pp. 701-726.

Rogers, G.B., Hoffman, L.R., Whiteley, M., Daniels, T.W., Carroll, M.P. & Bruce, K.D. (2010). Revealing the dynamics of polymicrobial infections: implications for antibiotic therapy. *Trends Microbiol*, Vol. 18, No. 8, pp. 357-364.

Ryan, R.P. & Dow, J.M. (2008). Diffusible signals and interspecies communication in bacteria. *Microbiology*, Vol. 154, No. Pt 7, pp. 1845-1858.

Ryan, R.P., Fouhy, Y., Garcia, B.F., Watt, S.A., Niehaus, K., Yang, L., Tolker-Nielsen, T. & Dow, J.M. (2008). Interspecies signalling via the *Stenotrophomonas maltophilia* diffusible signal factor influences biofilm formation and polymyxin tolerance in *Pseudomonas aeruginosa*. *Mol Microbiol*, Vol. 68, No. 1, pp. 75-86.

Schneider, M., Mühlemann, K., Droz, S., Couzinet, S., Casaulta, C. & Zimmerli, S. (2008). Clinical characteristics associated with isolation of small-colony variants of *Staphylococcus aureus* and *Pseudomonas aeruginosa* from respiratory secretions of patients with cystic fibrosis. *J Clin Microbiol*, Vol. 46, No. 5, pp. 1832-1834.

Scott, M.G., Dullaghan, E., Mookherjee, N., Glavas, N., Waldbrook, M., Thompson, A., Wang, A., Lee, K., Doria, S., Hamill, P., Yu, J.J., Li, Y., Donini, O., Guarna, M.M., Finlay, B.B., North, J.R. & Hancock, R.E. (2007). An anti-infective peptide that selectively modulates the innate immune response. *Nat Biotechnol*, Vol. 25, No. 4, pp. 465-472.

Sendi, P. & Proctor, R.A. (2009). *Staphylococcus aureus* as an intracellular pathogen: the role of small colony variants. *Trends Microbiol*, Vol. 17, No. 2, pp. 54-58.

Senn, M.M., Bischoff, M., von Eiff, C. & Berger-Bächi, B. (2005). σ^B activity in a *Staphylococcus aureus hemB* mutant. *J Bacteriol*, Vol. 187, No. 21, pp. 7397-7406.

Shah, P.M. (2005). The need for new therapeutic agents: what is the pipeline? *Clin Microbiol Infect*, Vol. 11 Suppl 3, pp. 36-42.

Sibley, C.D., Duan, K., Fischer, C., Parkins, M.D., Storey, D.G., Rabin, H.R. & Surette, M.G. (2008). Discerning the complexity of community interactions using a *Drosophila* model of polymicrobial infections. *PLoS Pathog*, Vol. 4, No. 10, pp. e1000184.

Sibley, C.D., Parkins, M.D., Rabin, H.R. & Surette, M.G. (2009). The relevance of the polymicrobial nature of airway infection in the acute and chronic management of patients with cystic fibrosis. *Curr Opin Investig Drugs*, Vol. 10, No. 8, pp. 787-794.

Sibley, C.D. & Surette, M.G. (2011). The polymicrobial nature of airway infections in cystic fibrosis: Cangene Gold Medal Lecture. *Can J Microbiol*, Vol. 57, No. 2, pp. 69-77.

Simões, M. (2011). Antimicrobial strategies effective against infectious bacterial biofilms. *Curr Med Chem*, Vol. 18, No. 14, pp. 2129-2145.

Singh, R., Ray, P., Das, A. & Sharma, M. (2009). Role of persisters and small-colony variants in antibiotic resistance of planktonic and biofilm-associated *Staphylococcus aureus*: an *in vitro* study. *J Med Microbiol*, Vol. 58, No. Pt 8, pp. 1067-1073.

Singh, R., Ray, P., Das, A. & Sharma, M. (2010). Enhanced production of exopolysaccharide matrix and biofilm by a menadione-auxotrophic *Staphylococcus aureus* small-colony variant. *J Med Microbiol*, Vol. 59, No. Pt 5, pp. 521-527.

Sinha, B., Francois, P.P., Nuße, O., Foti, M., Hartford, O.M., Vaudaux, P., Foster, T.J., Lew, D.P., Herrmann, M. & Krause, K.H. (1999). Fibronectin-binding protein acts as *Staphylococcus aureus* invasin via fibronectin bridging to integrin α5β1. *Cell Microbiol*, Vol. 1, No. 2, pp. 101-117.

Smith, E.E., Buckley, D.G., Wu, Z., Saenphimmachak, C., Hoffman, L.R., D'Argenio, D.A., Miller, S.I., Ramsey, B.W., Speert, D.P., Moskowitz, S.M., Burns, J.L., Kaul, R. & Olson, M.V. (2006). Genetic adaptation by *Pseudomonas aeruginosa* to the airways of cystic fibrosis patients. *Proc Natl Acad Sci U S A*, Vol. 103, No. 22, pp. 8487-8492.

Smith, R.S. & Iglewski, B.H. (2003). *P. aeruginosa* quorum-sensing systems and virulence. *Curr Opin Microbiol*, Vol. 6, No. 1, pp. 56-60.

Song, Z., Johansen, H.K., Faber, V., Moser, C., Kharazmi, A., Rygaard, J. & Høiby, N. (1997a). Ginseng treatment reduces bacterial load and lung pathology in chronic *Pseudomonas aeruginosa* pneumonia in rats. *Antimicrob Agents Chemother*, Vol. 41, No. 5, pp. 961-964.

Song, Z., Kong, K.F., Wu, H., Maricic, N., Ramalingam, B., Priestap, H., Schneper, L., Quirke, J.M., Høiby, N. & Mathee, K. (2010). Panax ginseng has anti-infective activity against opportunistic pathogen *Pseudomonas aeruginosa* by inhibiting quorum sensing, a bacterial communication process critical for establishing infection. *Phytomedicine*, Vol. 17, No. 13, pp. 1040-1046.

Song, Z.J., Johansen, H.K., Faber, V. & Høiby, N. (1997b). Ginseng treatment enhances bacterial clearance and decreases lung pathology in athymic rats with chronic *P. aeruginosa* pneumonia. *APMIS*, Vol. 105, No. 6, pp. 438-444.

Sriramulu, D.D., Nimtz, M. & Romling, U. (2005). Proteome analysis reveals adaptation of *Pseudomonas aeruginosa* to the cystic fibrosis lung environment. *Proteomics*, Vol. 5, No. 14, pp. 3712-3721.

Stewart, P.S. (2002). Mechanisms of antibiotic resistance in bacterial biofilms. *Int J Med Microbiol*, Vol. 292, No. 2, pp. 107-113.

Stoodley, P., Sauer, K., Davies, D.G. & Costerton, J.W. (2002). Biofilms as complex differentiated communities. *Annu Rev Microbiol*, Vol. 56, pp. 187-209.

Talbot, G.H., Bradley, J., Edwards, J.E., Jr., Gilbert, D., Scheld, M. & Bartlett, J.G. (2006). Bad bugs need drugs: an update on the development pipeline from the Antimicrobial Availability Task Force of the Infectious Diseases Society of America. *Clin Infect Dis*, Vol. 42, No. 5, pp. 657-668.

Tuchscherr, L., Heitmann, V., Hussain, M., Viemann, D., Roth, J., von Eiff, C., Peters, G., Becker, K. & Löffler, B. (2010). *Staphylococcus aureus* small-colony variants are adapted phenotypes for intracellular persistence. *J Infect Dis*, Vol. 202, No. 7, pp. 1031-1040.

Tuchscherr, L., Medina, E., Hussain, M., Völker, W., Heitmann, V., Niemann, S., Holzinger, D., Roth, J., Proctor, R.A., Becker, K., Peters, G. & Löffler, B. (2011). *Staphylococcus aureus* phenotype switching: an effective bacterial strategy to escape host immune response and establish a chronic infection. *EMBO Mol Med*, Vol. 3, No. 3, pp. 129-141.

Vaudaux, P., Francois, P., Bisognano, C., Kelley, W.L., Lew, D.P., Schrenzel, J., Proctor, R.A., McNamara, P.J., Peters, G. & Von Eiff, C. (2002). Increased expression of clumping factor and fibronectin-binding proteins by *hemB* mutants of *Staphylococcus aureus* expressing small colony variant phenotypes. *Infect Immun*, Vol. 70, No. 10, pp. 5428-5437.

Villena, J., Racedo, S., Agüero, G., Bru, E., Medina, M. & Alvarez, S. (2005). *Lactobacillus casei* improves resistance to pneumococcal respiratory infection in malnourished mice. *J Nutr*, Vol. 135, No. 6, pp. 1462-1469.

Voggu, L., Schlag, S., Biswas, R., Rosenstein, R., Rausch, C. & Götz, F. (2006). Microevolution of cytochrome bd oxidase in Staphylococci and its implication in resistance to respiratory toxins released by *Pseudomonas*. *J Bacteriol*, Vol. 188, No. 23, pp. 8079-8086.

von Götz, F., Häussler, S., Jordan, D., Saravanamuthu, S.S., Wehmhöner, D., Strüßmann, A., Lauber, J., Attree, I., Buer, J., Tümmler, B. & Steinmetz, I. (2004). Expression analysis of a highly adherent and cytotoxic small colony variant of *Pseudomonas aeruginosa* isolated from a lung of a patient with cystic fibrosis. *J Bacteriol*, Vol. 186, No. 12, pp. 3837-3847.

Wagner, V.E. & Iglewski, B.H. (2008). *P. aeruginosa* Biofilms in CF Infection. *Clin Rev Allergy Immunol*, Vol. 35, No. 3, pp. 124-134.

Weaver, V.B. & Kolter, R. (2004). *Burkholderia* spp. alter *Pseudomonas aeruginosa* physiology through iron sequestration. *J Bacteriol*, Vol. 186, No. 8, pp. 2376-2384.

Wenzel, R., Bate, G. & Kirkpatrick, P. (2005). Tigecycline. *Nat Rev Drug Discov*, Vol. 4, No. 10, pp. 809-810.

Williams, P. & Camara, M. (2009). Quorum sensing and environmental adaptation in *Pseudomonas aeruginosa*: a tale of regulatory networks and multifunctional signal molecules. *Curr Opin Microbiol*, Vol. 12, No. 2, pp. 182-191.

Witte, W., Cuny, C., Klare, I., Nübel, U., Strommenger, B. & Werner, G. (2008). Emergence and spread of antibiotic-resistant Gram-positive bacterial pathogens. *Int J Med Microbiol*, Vol. 298, No. 5-6, pp. 365-377.

Wu, H., Lee, B., Yang, L., Wang, H., Givskov, M., Molin, S., Høiby, N. & Song, Z. (2011). Effects of ginseng on *Pseudomonas aeruginosa* motility and biofilm formation. *FEMS Immunol Med Microbiol*, Vol. 62, No. 1, pp. 49-56.

Yang, L., Liu, Y., Markussen, T., Høiby, N., Tolker-Nielsen, T. & Molin, S. (2011). Pattern differentiation in co-culture biofilms formed by *Staphylococcus aureus* and *Pseudomonas aeruginosa*. *FEMS Immunol Med Microbiol*.

Zhang, L., Parente, J., Harris, S.M., Woods, D.E., Hancock, R.E. & Falla, T.J. (2005). Antimicrobial peptide therapeutics for cystic fibrosis. *Antimicrob Agents Chemother*, Vol. 49, No. 7, pp. 2921-2927.

Zhu, Y., Xiong, Y.Q., Sadykov, M.R., Fey, P.D., Lei, M.G., Lee, C.Y., Bayer, A.S. & Somerville, G.A. (2009). Tricarboxylic acid cycle-dependent attenuation of *Staphylococcus aureus in vivo* virulence by selective inhibition of amino acid transport. *Infect Immun*, Vol. 77, No. 10, pp. 4256-4264.

9

Infection by Non Tuberculous Mycobacteria in Cystic Fibrosis

María Santos[1], Ana Gil-Brusola[1] and Pilar Morales[2]
[1]*Microbiology Department,*
[2]*Lung Transplant Unit, University Hospital La Fe, Valencia,*
Spain

1. Introduction

Cystic fibrosis (CF) is a common autosomal recessive genetic condition affecting white population with an approximate incidence of 1 per 2500 live births (Davis et al., 1996), nearly 30,000 people in the USA (Olivier et al., 2003). Patients with this life-shortening disease have abnormally thickened secretions that facilitate chronic infection of the airways, bronchiectasis and early death. The respiratory pathogens most frequently isolated in these patients are *Staphylococcus aureus* and *Pseudomonas aeruginosa.*

As the survival of this group of patients has been improved by better nutrition, intensive therapy to clear airway secretions and more aggressive use of antibiotics (FitzSimmons, 1993, Ramsey, 1996), new pathogens such as *Stenotrophomonas maltophilia, Burkholderia cepacia, Alkaligenes xylosoxidans, Nocardia* spp., fungi and non tuberculous mycobacteria (NTM) are evolving (Burns et al., 1998; Burns & Saiman, 1999; Olivier et al., 1996)

NTM have increasingly been reported in the world as pulmonary pathogens not only in immunosuppressed but also in non immunocompromised persons, mainly in patients with lung disease (bronchiectasis, hypersensitivity, pneumonitis, chest wall disorders, previous mycobacteriosis and CF) (Huang et al., 1999; Prince et al., 1989; Hjelte et al., 1990; Fauroux et al., 1997)

Two important issues to consider are: 1) the clinical significance of isolation of a NTM (contamination, colonization or disease) (Hayes, 2005); and 2) bacterial overgrowth, especially with *P. aeruginosa,* leading to difficulty in the isolation of the mycobacterium from sputum samples.

NTM produce insidious infections that require several months of combined antibiotic therapy, difficult eradication and frequent relapses with progressive lung function deterioration (Esther et al., 2010). They represent an important social and health problem (Olivier et al., 2003), with not well defined and unsolved aspects, such as mode of infection, pathogenic role, standardized treatment or prophylaxis.

In this chapter we will review the main epidemiological, clinical, diagnostic, therapeutic and prophylactic aspects of NTM infections in CF patients.

2. Epidemiology and pathogenesis

2.1 General aspects

The term NTM refers to *Mycobacterium* spp. different to *M. tuberculosis complex* and *M. leprae*. These microorganisms are widely distributed in the environment (water, soil, dust, animals and food). Almost all NTM are less virulent and contagious than *M. tuberculosis* (Runyon, 1959; Brown-Elliot et al., 2002). There are more than 100 described species, of which only 15-20 produce infections in humans.

NTM are resistant to chlorination and ozonation (Prim et al., 2004) and to multiple antiseptics and antibiotics. They are opportunistic microorganisms capable of causing disease in a different range of locations (skin and soft tissues, lymph nodes and lung) as well as disseminated diseases.

The extent and severity of infection depends on the anatomic and immune integrity of the host. These bacteria can adhere to biomedical materials (catheters, prosthesis, filters or membranes of inhalation systems) forming a biofilm that may complicate the pharmacological treatment of such infections (Williams et al., 2009).

Infection by NTM was first reported in a patient with CF in 1980 (Boxerbaum, 1980). Few infections were described before 1990, but in the last 20 years, NTM have emerged as new pathogens in CF (Griffith, 2003; Olivier et al., 1996). This increase may be due to several factors: greater survival of patients with CF, increasing their environmental exposure; more aggressive therapies, which facilitate susceptibility to infection; improved microbiological diagnostic methods; and better interaction between clinicians and microbiologists. In 1997, the American Thoracic Society (ATS) published a Consensus Statement that identified CF as a risk factor for NTM pulmonary disease in HIV-seronegative patients and provided recommendations for laboratory and clinical diagnosis of NTM infection (Official Statement ATS, 1997).

In summary, NTM are common in patients with CF but neither person to person nor nosocomial acquisition explain their high prevalence. Clinical significance of NTM is incompletely defined but patients with these organisms should be monitored with repeated sample cultures (Olivier et al., 2003).

2.2 Pathogenesis

Patients with CF have abnormally viscous and thickened airway and gastrointestinal secretions as a result of a defect or decrease in the transmembrane conductance regulator protein or gene product which regulates chloride and liquid secretions across epithelial surfaces and resorption of sodium and liquid. These thick respiratory secretions occlude the airways and ductal lumens leading to recurrent pulmonary infections, pancreatic insufficiency and intestinal obstruction (Welsh, 1990).

NTM, which enter mainly through the respiratory tract, are phagocytosed by macrophages and survive and reproduce within patients until symptomatic infection occurs. The disease manifestations depend on the immune cellular response and the possible granulome formation; hence, its difficult eradication and its tendency to persistence or recurrence (Morales et al., 2011).

2.3 Frequency and distribution

Prevalence rates of NTM infections in patients with CF are variable, due mainly to the few multicenter studies (Olivier et al., 2003; Roux et al., 2009; Mussaffi, et al., 2005; Levy et al., 2008) and their diversity in the methodology used, since some refer to patients who had at least one positive culture and others to those who met disease criteria following the ATS recommendations from 1997 (Official Statement ATS, 1997) or 2007 (Griffith et al., 2007), obtaining fewer cases.

Infection data vary between 2 and 30%, with an average of 13 to 15%. These differences are due to the number of cases reported in each study - the most numerous being Olivier et al, 1186 and Roux et al, 1582-, the geographical location - with differences between continents (America greater reports) and within countries (the highest prevalence values were those reported for coastal states) - and the age of the patients included. In general, more isolates may be found in teenagers (10-20%) and young adults with CF (American Academy of Paediatrics, 2006).

Regarding age, both multicenter studies and general observations, suggest that NTM infections occur as a complication in adolescents and young adults (10 to 25 years old) although with small differences between mycobacteria, since the rapidly growing can be acquired at almost any age and *M. avium complex* (MAC) in older patients (Roux et al., 2009). Some do not find significant differences among sex (Olivier et al., 2003), while as others describe more cases in women than men (Roux et al., 2009).

2.4 Isolated NTM

In relation to the isolated species of NTM, most authors agree that both, MAC and the rapidly growing mycobacteria (RGM), are the most frequent, accounting around 80% (Roux et al., 2009). Infection is usually caused by a single species and exceptionally by a mixture of two mycobacteria.

MAC is composed of a group of slow, fastidiously growing mycobacteria that includes *M. avium, M. intracellulare* and unnamed genetically related species. It ranks first in North America with 72% of the isolates, mainly *M. avium* (Olivier et al., 2003) but is second and third in frequency in other series. *M. abscessus*, a member of the RGM (culture growth in less than 7 days) seems to prevail in Western Europe (Roux et al., 2009; Jönsson et al., 2007; Sermet-Gaudelus et al., 2003) and Israel (Levy et al., 2008), where *M. simiae* is also frequent. (Figure 1).

M. abscessus may be confused due to its different classification in time, since it was first included within *M. chelonae* group, then as a different species by itself, and more recently as part of the *M. abscessus complex* (MABSC), together with *M. massiliense* (Adékambi et al., 2004) and *M. bolletii* (Adékambi et al., 2006).

The prevalence of these two groups - MAC and MABSC - varies with age. MABSC may appear at any age, but most frequently in teenagers age 11 to 15 years old, while as MAC is more common in young adults aged 20 to 25 (Pierre-Audigier et al., 2005; Rodman et al., 2005). In all series, there is a minority group of varied mycobacteria named "others", which includes *M. gordonae* (possible contaminant), *M. fortuitum, M. kansasii, M. simiae, M. peregrinum, M. malmoense*, all of them infrequent and poorly representative.

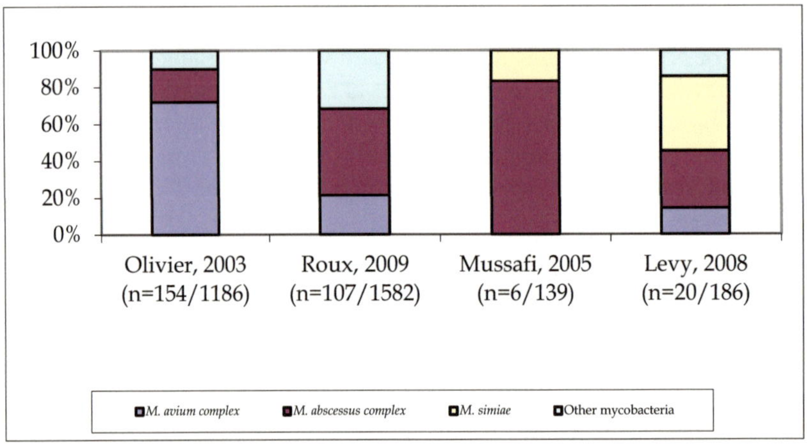

Fig. 1. Frequency of NTM species isolated in CF patients according to several studies (Olivier et al., 2003; Roux et al., 2009; Mussaffi et al., 2005; Levy et al., 2008).

2.5 Transmission

Given the ubiquitous nature of NTM, the port of entry for infection may be diverse: cutaneous, oropharyngeal mucosa, digestive or respiratory. NTM are frequently present in tap water and shower heads, where they remain viable in aerosols (Parker et al., 1983). Some, such as MAC, are resistant to chlorine and ozone, as already mentioned. Most infections remain near the port of entry but may also disseminate to other organs if the patient is immunocompromised. There is no evidence of person-to-person transmission of NTM infection. Therefore, no patient isolation but only universal precautions are necessary. Infections usually present as single cases, but outbreaks have also been reported, some of them by molecular techniques, secondary to a common focus neither identified nor corrected (Wallace et al., 1998; Kim et al., 2007; Viana-Niero et al, 2008).

2.6 Risk factors

In the last ten years, several authors have sought the relationship between NTM infection and different aspects of the patients, the disease or the microorganisms involved, describing some predisposing or risk factors (Table 1). (Olivier et al., 2003; Roux et al., 2009; Mussafi et al., 2005; Levy et al., 2008).

Age	Sweat chloride	*P. aeruginosa*
Race	Insulin-requiring diabetes	*S. aureus*
Sex	Pancreatic enzymes use	*Aspergillus spp.*
BMI	Steroids	Sputums cultured
Place of residence	Severe genotypes	FEV1

BMI, body mass index; FEV1, forced espiratory volume in the 1st second.

Table 1. Predictors of NTM infection in CF patients

Olivier et al, compared CF patients with and without positive culture for NTM. The culture-positive patients were significantly older (26 versus 22, $p<0,001$), had higher FEV1 (60% versus 54%), higher frequency of *S. aureus* (43% versus 31%) and lower frequency of *P. aeruginosa* co-infection (71% versus 82%). Another related factor was the body mass index (BMI). There were no significant differences between *M. abscessus* and *MAC*. When several risk factors are present (for example, age, FEV1 and *S. aureus* co-infection) the probability of having NTM is 50-fold higher.

Roux et al, found nuances in age between the two groups of mycobacteria, as previously mentioned, suggesting that this difference may be due to the different degree of virulence of these mycobacteria. Women were more frequently affected, a fact not previously referenced. Little is known about the clinical significance and the risk factors of the new species of RGM, apart from their tendency to produce cutaneous lesions. A recent study has also found clinical differences between *M. maxiliense* and *M. abscessus* infection (Zelazny et al., 2009).

Levy et al, found that the presence of *Aspergillus* spp. in sputum and the number of the sputum specimens processed for mycobacteria were the most significant predictors for isolation of NTM.

Mussafi et al, have found a relationship between pulmonary *M. abscessus* disease and allergic bronchopulmonary aspergillosis and corticosteroid therapy. Eradication of infection was more difficult in these circumstances.

In addition to the risk factors analyzed, we must not forget that, back in 1997, the ATS published a consensus document identifying CF as a risk factor itself for NTM infection, providing extensive information about it.

3. Clinical manifestations and radiology

Clinical manifestations, together with radiological findings and the microbiological cultures that will be commented further on, constitute the three basic pillars for the diagnosis of NTM disease (Table 2) (Griffith et al., 2007).

CATEGORY	REQUIREMENTS
Clinical findings	Pulmonary symptoms Exclusion of other diagnoses
Radiological findings	Chest X-ray: nodular or cavitary images; or HRCT: multifocal bronchiectasis with multiple small nodules.
Bacteriological findings	Sputum: 2 or more positive cultures or BAS or BAL: ≥ 1 positive culture or lung biopsy: granulomatous inflammation or positive staining for AFB together with one or more positive cultures (biopsy, sputum, BAS; BAL)

Table 2. ATS / IDSA criteria for the diagnosis of lung disease caused by NTM

Diagnosis requires: all the clinical criteria + 1 radiological criterion + 1 bacteriological criterion. ATS: American Thoracic Society; IDSA: Infectious Diseases Society of America; NTM: Non-tuberculous Mycobacteria; HRCT: high-resolution computerized tomography; BAS: bronchoalveolar secretions (aspirate); BAL: bronchoalveolar lavage; AFB: acid-alcohol resistant bacilli.

Lung infections in general tend to have non specific symptoms (cough, dyspnea, weight loss, increased expectoration, sometimes hemoptysis) and chest radiographic findings that vary from innocuous or no findings, to infiltrates or nodules, sometimes cavitated, (Morales et al., 2007) with HRCT scanning chest abnormalities - nodules and/or multifocal bronchiectasis (Hayes, 2005).

The chest radiography in NTM pulmonary disease caused by RGM is likely to show multilobular, patchy, reticulonodular or mixed interstitial and alveolar infiltrates with upper lobe predominance and cavitation in only 15% of cases (Griffith et al., 1993, Daley & Griffith, 2002) (Figure 2).

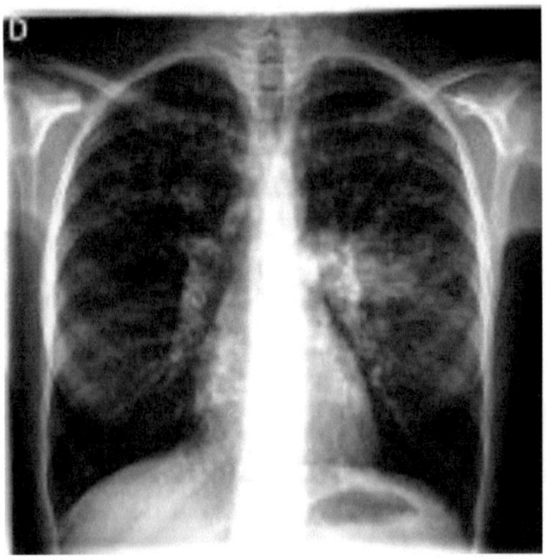

Fig. 2. Chest radiography of *M. abscessus* infection in CF patient.

The most common radiographic changes in MAC infection are cavitary disease and fibronodular bronchiectasis (Goo & Im, 2002). Cavities are finer and surrounded by less parenchymal opacification than in the case of tuberculosis (TB) (Erasmus et al., 1999). Bronchiectasis appear preferentially in the middle lobe and lingula (Lynch et al., 1995). Pleural effusion is not common. In HRCT scanning, the presence of bronchiectasis and multiple small nodules are predictive of MAC lung disease (Maycher et al., 2000).

Cutaneous manifestations may vary from small single nodes to ulcers, sometimes coincident with skin disruptions such as wounds, burns, surgical incisions, catheter implantation sites and so forth. These cutaneous lesions are very important in lung transplant recipients (LTx), since they can be the first sign of dissemination (Taylor & Palmer, 2006, Morales et al., 2007).

In isolated cases and, especially, in immunossuppressed patients, including transplant recipients, infection may diseminate to other organs, like from skin to lungs, intestine or other sites.

3.1 Clinical course and evolution

Clinical course is similar to that of TB, with insidious and slow progression that requires combined treatment for various months. This is difficult to comply due to its adverse effects and interactions with other drugs. Initial clinical and microbiological response is usually good but, even after complete compliance, with apparently successful therapy, there is a tendency to persistance and relapse (Mussaffi et al., 2005). NTM affects pulmonary function and chronic lung infection in CF patients is the main cause of morbidity and mortality (Esther et al., 2010). There is no data of mortality directly associated to mycobaterial infection, since these patients usually suffer simultaneous infections by different microorganisms (Figure 3).

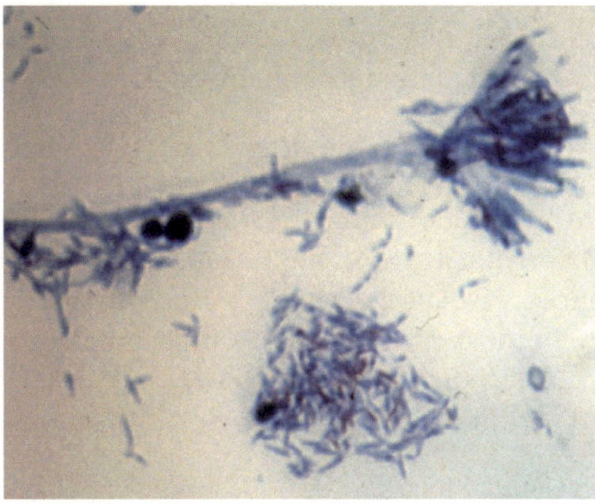

Fig. 3. Modified Ziehl-Neelsen stain showing co-infection of *Mycobacterium* spp. with *Aspergillus* spp. in a CF patient.

4. Microbiological diagnosis

Samples that reach the laboratory are mainly of respiratory origin (sputum, pleural fluid or its biopsy specimen, BAL and lung biopsy specimen). They can also be from skin or other locations if infection is disseminated.

With the staining methods - Ziehl-Neelsen or auramine fluorescence -, there are features on the AFB in terms of their number, shape, and grouping, that characterize the different NTM.

Bacterial overgrowth, especially with *P. aeruginosa*, is problematic and leads to difficulties in isolating mycobacteria from respiratory secretions and sputum. Therefore, together with the classical decontamination process using 0.25% N-acetylcysteine and 1% NaOH, addition of 5% oxalic acid is recommended (Whittier et al., S. 1997)

Samples are cultured in solid (Löwenstein-Jenssen or other) and liquid media (radiometric BACTEC 460 and nonradiometric BACTEC 9050 and 960, Becton Dickinson, or other). Some NTM have specific requirements for culture, such as temperature (MAC 42ºC) and time (RGM grow in less than 7 days, whereas others in 10-14 days).

Colonies may be identified phenotypically in most cases (Kent & Kubica, 1983, Metchock et al., 1999) and be confirmed by molecular typing methods, using commercial RNA/DNA probes (AccuProbe, GenProbe, San Diego, Ca) (Cousins et al.,1996, Wallace et al., 1998) and other techniques (Zhang et al., 1997). The different species included in the MABSC are distinguished by *rpoB* sequencing (AdéKambi et al., 2003). Molecular identification of the mycobacteria also helps in differentiating between relapse and reinfection, and in determining whether an outbreak is secondary to a common origin or not.

Chromatography techniques (Butler & Guthertz, 2001) are less used, since they are more complex and less precise (Leite et al., 2005). Serologic diagnosis, such as determining the presence of IgG immunoglobulin against antigen A 60 (Oliver et al., 2001), has been discarded due to its low sensitivity and specificity (Pottumarthy et al., 2000). Tuberculin skin testing may be positive in patients infected with NTM, since *M. tuberculosis* shares antigens with various species, but generally the induration induced is less than 10 mm in diameter (Field & Cowie, 2006). Techniques based on lymphocyte interferon gamma (IFN-γ) production have been developed and can be useful in distinguishing between infection by *M. tuberculosis*, NTM, or BCG vaccination (Scholvink et al., 2004).

There is controversy over the systematic use of susceptibility testing of NTM, since there is no clear correlation to the clinical therapeutic response. At least for clarithromycin in the case of MAC disease there are some recommendations (Wayne, 2000). RGM are intrinsically resistant to classic antituberculous drugs and have variable antimicrobial susceptibility profile. Clinically significant isolates should be tested against amikacin, cefoxitine, ciprofloxacin, clarithromycin, doxycycline, imipenem, trimethoprim/sulfamethoxazole and recently, linezolid (Woods, 2000). Synergy studies with two or more antibiotics can also be done. Methods used include dilution, diffussion (E-test) and automated techniques.

5. Treatment and evolution

5.1 General aspects

No guidelines exist for the treatment of NTM pulmonary diseases in the CF population. Given the natural tendency of these bacteria to seek refuge in macrophages and to the fact that *in vitro* susceptibility tests do not show true antibiotic concentration, combined therapy may favour synergy and minimize the appearance of resistance. It is difficult to determine a treatment of choice since experience is limited and results are variable, and *in vitro* tests do not always correlate to *in vivo* response. Duration of treatment is also variable, depending on the NTM to be treated, the severity and extent of disease, and the clinical and immune status of the patient. In any case, treatment compliance is difficult since it is long lasting, antibiotics have adverse effects and interactions with other drugs, in particular with immunesuppressors in the case of transplant recipients. A close clinical and microbiological surveillance of the patients is necessary, to watch out for possible relapses, dissemination or risk of graft rejection in the case of transplantation (Morales et al, 2007; Morales et al., 2011).

We will focus on the treatment of MAC and *M. abscessus*, the most frequent NTM in CF patients. Treatment of the less common mycobacteria requires individualized considerations, keeping as a basic principle the combination of two or three active drugs.

5.2 Treatment of MAC

Transmission of the mycobacteria included in the MAC is varied, but mainly through birds and water (Marras et al., 2005). Infection has been related to recreational hot-tubs and can cause a hypersensitivity pneumonitis like syndrome in exposed patients (Embril et al., 1997; Rickman et al., 2002; Hanak et al., 2006).

Mycobacteria included in the MAC are resistant to first-line antituberculous drugs - rifampicin, isoniazid and streptomycin - except for ethambutol, and are usually susceptible to amikacin and macrolides, in particular clarithromycin.

Initial treatment includes ethambutol, clarithromycin or azithromycin and a third drug according to susceptibility test results. Duration of treatment is from 6 to 9 months for small lesions and up to 12-24 months in case of dissemination. Combination of ethambutol, a macrolide and rifampicin has been used successfully due to their synergism and good tolerance (Field & Cowie, 2003). Some authors recommend maintenance of the macrolide 12 more months once patients convert to negative, thus reducing the number of relapses (ATS, 1997). The importance of macrolides relies on the intracellular penetrance of both, the antibiotic and the bacteria. First recommendations included clarithromycin (Field & Cowie, 2003) and then azithromycin (Griffith et al., 2001), but always in combination and not in monotherapy as initial drugs.

M. avium is the most common cause of immune reconstitution inflammatory syndrome caused by NTM (Field & Cowie, 2006). IFN-γ is a macrophage activator in response to mycobacteria. Patients with disseminated MAC infection, with relapses or poor prognosis, respond favorably to inhaled IFN-γ (Holland et al., 1994; Hallstrand et al., 2004).

In exceptional cases, when infection is localized and with persistent lung affection, surgery has been applied. Post-operative morbidity and complications that include hemorrhages, bronchopleural fistula and empyema are possible.

5.3 Treatment of *M. abscessus* and other RGM

This group of mycobacteria is ubiquitous and can survive in adverse conditions. They can grow in any culture media used in bacteriology in less than 7 days, with the risk of not being evaluated or being considered as contaminants. Although it includes various species, the most relevant and virulent in CF patients is *M. abscessus*. This mycobacterium can cause skin infection, lung disease or even disseminate. Its treatment is difficult due to its multiresistance, not only to the classic, already mentioned antituberculous drugs, including ethambutol, but also to ampicillin, amoxicillin-clavulanate, cefoxitin, ciprofloxacin, erythromycin, sulfamethoxazole and tobramycin. It is universally susceptible to amikacin, and a recommended treatment is the combination of amikacin, clarithromycin and imipenem for 6 to 9 months (Yang et al., 2003). There can be initial improvement, but relapses are very frequent, in which case, therapy should be extended and/or a drug should be changed according to susceptibility testing. Other alternative therapeutic agents include the new oxazolidinone, linezolid, that is active against RGM (Wallace et al., 2001) with good therapeutic results (Morales et al, 2007). An open line includes the new quinolones gatifloxacin and moxifloxacin.

In the presence of big lung abscesses, a very rare presentation, surgical drainage might be necessary and can potentially lead to extrapulmonary seeding of the infecting mycobacteria and be an added risk if lung transplantation is needed.

Recommended suppressive therapy includes oral clarithromycin and aerosolized amikacin (Cullen et al., 2000; Colin AA, 2000). Monotherapy must always be avoided, since the most common cause of macrolide resistance is the use of clarithromycin as single drug in patients with CF and disseminated cutaneous infection (Wallace et al., 1996).

6. Prophylaxis

Given the extensive and varied presence of NTM in the environment and their variable susceptibility to antibiotics, the inevitable environmental exposure of CF patients and the lack of person-to-person transmission, primary chemoprophylaxis is not indicated. The only situation in which clarithromycin or azithromycin would be recommended is in HIV positive patients over 6 years of age and with a CD4 count of less than 50/μL, with risk of MAC infection (American Academy of Pediatrics, 2006).

Clinical and radiological monitoring is important, including intensive and selective search for NTM, in pulmonary samples from suspected foci, especially in young adults with impaired lung disease, *Aspergillus* spp. and steroid treatment.

On the other hand, it is important to take into consideration the life style of the patient, with a watchful attitude towards surrounding environment, being aware that it constitutes an unavoidable but reducible risk. Recently, a practical and excellent guideline in this regard has been published (Avery et al., 2009)

7. Peri-transplant considerations

7.1 Pre-transplant

As has been discussed, NTM infections must be kept in mind in the differential diagnosis of any lung disease in CF patients, especially when approaching an indication of LTx. Identification and *in vitro* susceptibility of the mycobacteria are required to ensure proper treatment and to achieve complete recovery before transplantation.

In particular, so difficult is the treatment of *M. abscessus* infection, that it has been considered a strong relative contraindication to LTx (Orens et al., 2006). Recently, Gilljama et al., reported their experience in three double LTx CF patients with ongoing therapy, and a fourth with recent treatment for *M. abscessus* lung infection. The first three developed skin infection and abscesses. Recovery was finally accomplished and pulmonary function was re-established after a prolonged 7 years long follow-up. With this, they conclude that LTx is feasible but may involve severe complications.

7.2 Post-Transplant

Infection and graft rejection in organ recipients are the two main causes of morbidity and mortality. Transplant may lead to the reactivation of a previously undetected infection, to its dissemination or to its initial onset. NTM have emerged as important pathogens in these patients, especially in LTx, causing pulmonary and extrapulmonary infections (Malouf & Glanville, 1999). These bacteria have also been identified as a potential cause of graft dysfunction and mortality by themselves or together with other opportunistic pathogens, which is a very common situation. In particular, infection by *M. abscessus* may be fatal

(Sanguinetti et al., 2001; Fairhurst et al., 2002) or resolve even when disseminated (Morales et al, 2007)

7.3 Donor

Even though we have not found any documented case of NTM infection in the organ donor, mycobacteriosis would be hypothetically a relative contraindication for transplantation. Systematic search of NTM in the bronchoaspirate of donors must be done to introduce treatment as soon as possible.

8. Final considerations

- Life expectancy and quality of life have improved in CF patients and their treatments have turned/become more aggressive.
- NTM cause frequent pulmonary infection especially related to advancing age and lung function deterioration. *M. abscessus* and MAC are the most frequently isolated NTM.
- Early clinical suspicion is important. The routine or selective mycobacterial search according to known risk factors is an important decision. No comparative studies indicate which option is the most effective.
- NTM must be decontaminated, cultured and typified thoroughly, since species identification is crucial for treatment and other clinical considerations.
- When a NTM is isolated from a sputum sample, both clinician and microbiologist will determine whether it should be considered a contaminant, colonization or infective agent, with the consequent attitude.
- It is important to perform correctly the *in vitro* susceptibility tests and to try new antibiotics against NTM.
- Ensure treatment compliance, since it will prevent the emergence of antibiotic resistance, infection relapse and poor outcome.
- Since there are no primary chemoprophylaxis recommendations, patients should be oriented to a healthy life style.
- If the moment for the lung transplant arrives, all the previously mentioned considerations should be taken very seriously, since the probability for infection and dissemination are greater due to the immunosuppressive therapy.
- These processes pose significant social and health burdens (school absenteeism, work and family limitations, doctor visits, hospitalization, diagnostic testing and treatment) with the resulting economic impact.

Future should rely on early suspicion and adequate search for NTM, the use of modern microbiological techniques applied directly on the sample, safer and more active antibiotics, research of mycobacterial virulence factors and the determinants for persistence of infection.

9. References

AdéKambi, T., Colson, P., & Drancourt M. 2003. *rpoB*-based identification of nonpigmented and late-pigmenting rapidly growing mycobacteria. *J Clin Microbiol*, Vol 41, No 12,(December,2003),pp. 5699-5708.

Adékambi, T., Reynaud -Gaubert, M., Greub, G., Gevaudan, MJ., La Scola, B., Raoult, D., & and Drancourt, M. 2004. Amoebal coculture of *Mycobacterium massiliense* sp. nov. from the sputum of a patient of hemoptoic pneumonia. *J Clin Microbiol,* Vol 42, No 12, (December, 2004), pp. 5493-5501.

Adékambi, T., Berger, P., Raoult, D., & Drancourt, M. 2006. *rpo*B gene sequence based characterization of emerging non-tuberculous mycobacteria with description of *Mycobacterium bolletii* sp. nov., *Mycobacterium phocaicum* sp. nov. and *Mycobacterium aubagnense* sp. nov. *Int J Syst Evol Microbiol* Vol 56, Pt 1, (January, 2006), pp. 133-143.

American Academy of Pediatrics. 2006. Micobacterias no tuberculosas, enfermedades. In: Pickening LK., Baker, CJ., Long SS. And McMillan JA. Eds. *Red book:Enfermedades infecciosas en Pediatría.* 27ª ed.Editorial Médica Panamericana, Madrid, Spain, 2007, pp.757-763. ISBN 978-950-06-0548-9

American Thoracic Society. Diagnosis and treatment of disease caused by nontuberculous mycobacteria. *Am J Respir Crit Care Med,* Vol 156, No 2, Pt2, (August, 1997), pp. S1-S25.

Avery, RK., Michaels, MG., & AST Infectious Diseases Community of Practice. 2009. Strategies for safe-living following solid organ transplantation. *Am J Transplant,* Vol 9, No 4 Suppl, (December 2009), pp. S252-S257.

Boxerbaum, B. 1980. Isolation of rapidly growing mycobacteria in patients with cystic fibrosis. *J Pediatr,* Vol 96, No 4, (April,1980), pp. 689-691.

Brown-Elliot, BA, Griffith, DE., & Wallace RJ Jr. 2002. Newly described or emerging human species of non tuberculous mycobacteria. *Infect Dis Clin North Am,* Vol 16, No 1 (Mars, 2002), pp. 187-220.

Burns, JL., Emerson, J., Stapp, JR., Yim, DL., Krzewinski, J., Louden, L., Ramsey, BW., & Clausen, CR. 1998. Microbiology of sputum from patients at cystic fibrosis centers in the United States. *Clin Infect Dis,* Vol 27, No 1 (July,1998), pp. 158-163.

Burns, JL.,& Saiman L. 1999. *Burkholderia cepacia* infections in cystic fibrosis. *Pediatr Infect Dis,* Vol 18, No 2, (February, 1999), pp. 155-156.

Butler WR & Guthertz, LS. 2001. Mycolic acid analysis by high-performance liquid chromatography for identification of Mycobacterium species. *Clin Microbiol Rev,* Vol 14, No 4,(October, 2001), pp. 704-726.

Colin, AA. 2000. Erradication of *Mycobacterium abscessus* in a chronically infected patient with cystic fibrosis. *Pediatr Pulmonol,* Vol 30, No 3, (September,2000),pp.267-268.

Cousins, D., Francis, B., & Dawson, D. 1996. Multiplex PCR provides a low-cost alternative to DNA probe methods for rapid identification of *Mycobacterium avium* and *Mycobacterium intracellulare,* Vol 34, No 9, (September, 1996), pp. 2331-2333.

Cullen, AR., Cannon CL., Mark EJ., & Colin, AA. 2000. *Mycobacterium abscessus* infection in CF. *Am J Respir Crit Care,* Vol 161, No 2, Pt 1, (February,2000),pp. 641-645.

Daley, CL. & Griffith, DE. 2002. Pulmonary disease caused by rapidy growing mycobacteria. *Clin Chest Med,* Vol 23, No 3, (September, 2002), pp. 623-632.

Davis, PB., Drumm, M., & Konstan, MW. 1996. Cystic Fibrosis. *Am J Respir Crit Care Med,* Vol 154, No 5 (November,1996), pp. 1229-1256.

Embril, J., Warren, P., Yakrus, M., Stark, R., Corne, S., Forrest, D., & Hershfield, E. 1997. Pulmonary illness associated with exposure to *Mycobacterium-avium* complex in hot tub water: hypersensitivity pneumonitis or infection?. *Chest*, Vol 111, No 3, (Mars, 1997), pp. 813-816.

Erasmus, JJ., McAdams, HP.,Farrell MA., & Patz, EFJr. 1999. Pulmonary nontuberculous mycobacterial infection: radiologic manifestations. Radiographics, Vol 19, No 6, (November-December,1999), pp. 1487-1505.

Esther, CR Jr., Esserman DA, Gilligan P, Kerr A, & Noone PG. 2010. Chronic *Mycobacterium abscessus* infection and lung function decline in cystic fibrosis. *J Cyst Fibros*, Vol 9, No 2, (March, 2010),pp.117-123.

Fairhurst, RM., Kubak, BM., Shpiner, RB., Levine, MS., Pegues, DA., & Ardehali, A. 2002. *Mycobacterium abscessus* empyema in a lung transplant recipient. *J Heart Lung Transplant*, Vol 21, No 3, (Mars, 2002),pp. 391-394.

Fauroux, B., Delaisi, B., Clement A., Saizou, C., Moissenett, D., Truffot-Pernot, C., Tournier, G., & Vu, T. 1997. Mycobacterial lung disease in cystic fibrosis : a prospective study. *Pediatr Infect Dis*, Vol 16, No 4, (April,1997),pp. 354-358.

Field, SK., & Cowie, RL. 2003. Treatment of *Mycobacterium avium*-intracellulare complex lung disease with a macrolide, ethambutol, and clofazimine. *Chest*, Vol 124, No 4,(October, 2003),pp. 1482-1486.

Field, SK., & Cowie RL. 2006. Lung disease due to the more common nontuberculous mycobacteria. *Chest*, Vol 129, No 6, (June, 2006),pp.1653-1672.

FitzSimmons, SC. 1993. The changing epidemiology of cystic fibrosis. *J Pediatr*, Vol 122, No 1, (January,1993), pp. 1-9.

Gilljama, M., Schersténb, H., Silverbornb, M., Jönssonc, B., & Hollsingd, AE. 2010. Lung transplantation in patients with cystic fibrosis and *Mycobacterium abscessus* infection. *J Cyst Fibros*, Vol 9, No 4, (July, 2010),pp.272-276.

Goo, JM., & Im, J-G. 2002. CT of tuberculosis and nontuberculous mycobacterial infections. *Radiol Clin North Am*, Vol 40, No 1,(January, 2002),pp. 73-87.

Griffith, DE., Girard, WM., & Wallace RJ Jr. 1993. Clinical features of pulmonary disease caused by rapidly growing mycobacteria. An analysis of 154 patients. *Am Rev Respir Dis*, Vol 147, No 5, (May,1993),pp. 1271-1278.

Griffith, DE. 2003. Emergence of nontuberculous mycobacteria as pathogens in cystic fibrosis. *Am J Respir Crit Care Med*, Vol 167, No 6, (Mars, 2003), pp. 810-812.

Griffith, DE., Brown, BA., Girard, WM., Griffith, BE., Couch, LA., & Wallace RJ Jr. Azythromycin-containing regimens for treatment of *Mycobacterium avium* complex lung disease. *Clin Infect Dis*, Vol 32, No 11, (June, 2001), pp. 1547-1553.

Griffith, DE., Aksamit, T.,Brown-Elliot, BA., Catanzaro, A., Daley, C., Gordin, F., Holland, SM., Horsburgh, R., Huitt, G., Iademarco, MF., Iseman, M., Olivier, K., Ruoss, S., von Reyn, CF., Wallace, RJ Jr., & Winthrop, K; ATS mycobacterial diseases subcommitte; American Thoracic Society; Infectious Disease Society of America. 2007. An official ATS/IDSA statement:diagnosis, treatment and prevention on non tuberculous mycobacterial diseases. *Am J Respir Crit Care Med*, Vol 175, No 4, (February, 2007),pp. 367-416.

Hallstrand, TS., Ochs HD., Zhu Q, & Liles, WC. 2004. Inhaled IFN- gamma for persistent nontuberculous mycobacterial pulmonary disease due to functional IFN-gamma deficiency. *Eur Respir J*, Vol 24, No 3,(September, 2004),pp.367-370.

Hanak, V., Kalra, S., Aksamit TR., Hartman, TE., Tazelaar HD., & Ryu, JH. 2006. Hot tub lung: presenting features and clinical course of 21 patients. *Respir Med*, Vol 100, No 4,(April, 2006), pp.610-615.

Hayes, D Jr. 2005. *Mycobacterium abscessus* and other nontuberculous mycobacteria: evolving respiratory pathogens in cystic fibrosis: a case report and review. *South Med J*, Vol 98, No 6, (June, 2005),pp. 657-661.

Hjelte, L., Petrini, B., Kaellenenius, G., & Strandvik, B. 1990. Perspective study of mycobacterial infections in patients with cystic fibrosis. *Thorax*, Vol 45, No 5, (May, 1990), pp. 397-400.

Holland, SM., Eisenstein, EM., Kuhns, DB., Turner, ML., Fleisher, TA., Strober, W., & Gallin, JL.1994. Treatment of refractary disseminated infection with interferon gamma: A preliminary report. *N Eng Jmed*, Vol 330, No 19, (May, 1994), pp. 1348-1355.

Huang, JH., Kao, PN., Adi, V., & Ruoss, SJ. 1999. *Mycobacterium avium-intracellulare* pulmonary infection in HIV-negative patients without preexisting lung disease: diagnostic and management limitations. *Chest*, Vol 115, No 4, (April,1999), pp. 1033-1040.

Jönsson, BE., Gilljam, M., Lindblad, A., Ridell, M., Wold, AE., & Welinder-Olsson, C. 2007. Molecular biology of *Mycobacterium abscessus* with focus on cystic fibrosis. *J Clin Microbiol*, Vol 45, No 5, (May, 2007), pp. 1497-1504.

Kent, PT., & Kubica, GP. 1983. Public health mycobacteriology: a guide for the level III laboratory. Atlanta. Centers for Disease Control.

Kim, HY, Yun, YJ., Park, CG., Lee, DH., Cho, YK., Park, BJ., Joo, SI., Kim, EC., Hur, YJ, Kim, BJ., & KooK, YH. 2007. Outbreak of *Mycobacterium massiliense* infection associated with intramuscular injections.*J Clin microbiol*, Vol 45, No 9, (September, 2007), pp.3127-3130.

Leite, CQ., da Silva Rocha, A., de Andrade Leite, SR., Ferreira, RM., Suffys, PN, de Souza Fonseca, L., & Saad, MH. 2005. A comparison of mycolic acid analysis for nontuberculous mycobacteria identification by thin-layer chromatography and molecular methods. *Microbiol Immunol*, Vol 49, No 7,(2005), pp.571-578.

Levy, I., Grisaru-Soen, G., Lerner-Geva, L., Kerem, E., Blau, H., Bentur, L., Aviram, M., Rivlin, J., Picard, E., Lavy, A., Yahav, Y., & Rahav, G. 2008. Multicenter cross-sectional study of nontuberculous mycobacterial infections among cystic fibrosis patientes, Israel. *Emerg Infect Dis*, Vol 14, No 3, (Mars, 2008), pp. 378-374.

Lynch,DA., Simone, PM., Fox, MA, Bucher, BL., & Heinig, MJ.1995. CT features of pulmonary *Mycobacterium avium* complex infection. *J Comput Assist Tomogr*, Vol 19, No 3, (May-June, 1995), pp.353-360.

Malouf, MA., & Glanville, AR. 1999. The spectrum of mycobacterial infection after lung transplantation. Am J Respir Crit Care Med, Vol 160, No 5 Pt 1, (November, 1999), pp. 1611-1616.

Marras, TK., Wallace, RJ Jr., Koth, LL, Stulbarg, MS., Cowl, CT., & Daley, CL.2005. Hypersensitivity pneumonitis reaction to *Mycobacterium avium* in household water. *Chest,* Vol 127, No 2, (February, 2005), pp. 664-671.

Maycher, B., O´Connor, R., & Long, R. 2000. Computed tomographic abnormalities in Mycobacterium avium complex lung disease include the mosaic pattern of reduced lung attenuation. *Can Assoc Radiol J,* Vol 51, No 2, (April,2000), pp. 93-102.

Metchock, BG., Nolte FS., & Wallace, RJ Jr. 1999. Mycobacterium. In: Murray PR, Baron EJ, Pfaller MA, Tenover FC, Yolken RH, editors. Manual of clinical microbiology. Washington, DC: ASM Press, 1999, pp., 399-437.

Morales, P., Ros JA, Blanes, M., Pérez-Enguix, D., Saiz, V., & Santos. M. 2007. Successful recovery after disseminated infection due to *Mycobacterium abscessus* in a lung transplant patient: subcutaneous nodule as first manifestation- a case report. *Transplant Proc,* Vol 39, No 7, (September, 2007), pp. 2413-2415.

Morales,P., Santos, M., Hadjilidis, D., & Aris, RM. Mycobacterial infections in cardiothoracic transplantation. pp. 161-173. In ISHLT. Monograph Series: Diagnosis and Management of Infectious diseases in Cardiothoracic Transplantation and mechanical ciculatory support. Mooney, ML., Hannan, MM., Husain, S, Kirklin, JK. (Eds). 2011. Elsevier Ed. Philadelphia,P.A. ISSN-1930-2134.

Mussaffi, H., Rivlin, J., Shalit, I., Ephros, M., & Blau, H. 2005. Nontuberculous mycobacteria in cystic fibrosis associated with allergic bronchopulmonary aspergillosis and steroid therapy. *Eur Respir* J, Vol 25, No 2, (February, 2005),pp. 324-328.

Oliver, A., Maiz, L., Cantón, R., Escobar, H., Baquero, E., & Gómez-Mampaso, E. 2001. Nontuberculous mycobacteria in patients with cystic fibrosis. *CID,* Vol 32, No 9, (May, 2001), pp. 1298-1303.

Olivier, KN., Yankaskas, JR., & Knowles, MR. 1996. Nontuberculous mycobacterial pulmonary disease in cystic fibrosis. *Semin Respir Infect,* Vol 11, No 4, (December ,1996), pp. 272-284.

Olivier, KN., Weber, DJ., Wallace, RJ Jr., Faiz, AR., Lee JH., Zhang, Y., Brown-Elliot, BA., Handler, A., Wilson, RW., Schechter, MS., Edwards, LJ., Chakraborti, S., & Knowles, R., for the Nontuberculous Mycobacteria in Cistic Fibrosis Study Group. 2003. Nontuberculous Mycobacteria. I: Multicenter prevalence study in Cystic Fibrosis. *Am J Respir Crit Care Med,* Vol 167, No 6, (Mars , 2003), pp. 828-834.

Orens, JB., Estenne, M., Arcasoy,S., Conte, JV., Corris, P., Egan, JJ., Egan, T., Keshavjee, S., Knoop, C., Kotloff, R., Martinez, FJ., Nathan, S., Palmer, S., Patterson, A., Singer, L., Snell, G., Studer, S., Vachiery, JL., Glanville, AR.; Pulmonary Scientific Council of the International Society for Heart and Lung Transplantation. 2006. International guidelines for the selection of lung transplant candidates: 2006 Update—A consensus report from the pulmonary scientific council of the international society for heart and lung transplantation. J Heart Lung Transplant Vol 25, No 7, (July, 2006), pp. 745–755.

Parker, BC., Ford, MA., Gruft H., & Falkinham JO III. 1983. Epidemiology of infection by nontuberculous mycobacteria.IV.Preferential aerosolization of *Mycobacterium intracellulare* from natural water. *Am Rev Respir Dis,* Vol 128, No 4 (October, 1983),pp.652-656.

Pottumarthy, S., Wells, VC., & Morris, AJ. 2000. A comparison of seven tests for serological diagnosis of tuberculosis. *J Clin Microbiol,* Vol 38, No 6,(June,2000), pp. 2227-2231.

Pierre-Audigier, C., Ferroni, A., Sermet-Gaudelus, I., Le Bourgeois, M., Offredo, C., Vu-Thien, H., Fauroux, B., Mariani, P., Munck, A., Bingen, E., Guillemot, D., Quesne, G., Vincent, V., Berche, P., & Gaillard, JL. 2005. Age-related prevalence and distribution of nontuberculous mycobacterial species among patients with cystic fibrosis. *J Clin Microbiol,* Vol 43, No 7, (July, 2005), pp. 3467-3470.

Primm, TP., Lucero, CA., & Falkinham, JO III. 2004. Health impacts of environmental mycobacteria. *Clin Microbiol Rev,* Vol 17, No 1 (January, 2004), pp. 98-106.

Prince, DS., Peterson, DD., Steiner, RM., Gottlieb, JE, Scott, R., Israel HL, Figueroa WG., & Fish, JE. 1989. Infection with *Mycobacterium avium* complex in patients without predisposing conditions. *N Eng J Med,* Vol 321,No 13, (September,1989), pp. 863-868.

Ramsey BW. 1996. Management of pulmonary disease in patients with cystic fibrosis. *N Eng J Med,* Vol 335, No 3 (July,1996), pp. 179-188.

Rickman, OB., Ryu, JH., Fidler, ME., & Kalra, S. 2002. Hypersensitivity pneumonitis associated with *Mycobacterium avium* complex and hot tube use. *Mayo Clin Proc,* Vol 77, No 11, (November, 2002), pp.1233-1237.

Rodman, DM., Polis, JM., Heltshe, SL, Sontag MK, Chacon C, Rodman RV, Brayshaw SJ, Huitt GA, Iseman MD, Saavedra MT, Taussig LM, Wagener JS, Accurso FJ, Nick JA. 2005. Late diagnosis defines a unique population of long-term survivors of cystic fibrosis. *Am J Respir Crit Care Med,* Vol 171, No 6, (Mars, 2005), pp. 621-626.

Roux, AL., Catherinot, E., Ripoll, F., Soismier, N., Macheras, E., Ravilly, S, Bellis, G., Vibet, MA., Le Roux E, Lemonnier, L., Gutierrez, C., Vincent, V., Fauroux, B., Rottman, M., Guillemot, D, Gaillard, JL, & Herrman JL., for the OMA Group. 2009. Multicenter study of prevalence of nontuberculous *Mycobacteria* in patients with cystic fibrosis in France. *J Clin Microbiol,* Vol 47,No 12, (December, 2009),pp. 4124-4128.

Runyon, EH. 1959. Anonymous mycobacteria in pulmonary disease. *Med Clin North Am,* Vol 43, No 1, (January, 1959), pp. 273-290.

Sanguinetti, M., Ardito F., Fiscarelli E., La Sorda, M., D'Argenio, P., Ricciotti, G., & Fadda, G. 2001. Fatal pulmonary infection due to multidrug-resistant *Mycobacterium abscessus* in a patient with cystic fibrosis. *J Clin Microbiol,* Vol 39, No 2,(February,2001),pp. 816-819.

Sermet-Gaudelus, I., Le Bourgeois, M., Pierre-Audigier, C., Offredo, C., Guillemot, D., Halley, S., Akoua-Koffi, C., Vincent, V, Sivadon-Tardy, V., Ferroni, A., Berche, P-, Scheinmann, P., Lenoir, G., & Gaillard, JL. 2003. *Mycobacterium abscessus* and children with cystic fibrosis. *Emerg Infect Dis,* Vol 9, No 12, (December, 2003),pp.1587-1591.

Schölvink, E., Wilkinson, KA., Whelan, AO., Martineau, AR., Levin, M., & Wlkinson, RJ. 2004. Gamma interferon-based immunodiagnosis of tuberculosis: comparison between whole-blood and enzyme-linked immunospot methods. *J Clin Microbiol,* Vol 42, No 2, (February, 2004),pp.829-831.

Taylor, JL., & Palmer, SM. 2006. *Mycobacterium abscessus* chest wall and pulmonary infection in a cystic fibrosis lung transplant recipient. *J Heart Lung* Transplant, Vol 25, No 8, (August, 2006), pp. 985-988.

Viana-Niero, C., Lima, KV., Lopes, ML, Rabello, MC., Marsola, IR., Brilhanthe, VC., Durham, AM., & Leao, SC. 2008. Molecular characterization of *Mycobacterium massiliense* and *Mycobacterium bolletii* in isolated collected from outbreaks of infections after laparoscopic surgeries cosmetic procedures. *J Clin Microbiol,* Vol 46, No 3, (Mars,2008),pp.850-855.

Wallace, RJ Jr., Brown, BA., Griffith, DE., Girard, WM., & Murphy, DT. 1996. Clarithromycin regimens for pulmonary *Mycobacterium avium* complex. The first 50 patients. *Am J Respir Crit Care Med,* Vol 153, No 6 Pt 1, (June,1996),pp.1762-1772.

Wallace, RJ Jr., Brown, BA., & Griffith DE. 1998. Nosocomial outbreaks/pseudo-outbreaks caused by nontuberculous mycobacteria. *Annu Rev Microbiol,* Vol, 52, pp. 453-490.

Wallace, RJ Jr., Brown-Elliott, BA., Ward, SC., Crist, CJ., Mann, LB., & Wilson, RW. 2001. Activities of linezolid against rapidly growing mycobacteria. *Antimicrob Agents Chemother,* Vol 45, No 3, (Mars, 2001), pp. 764-767.

Wayne, PA.: National Committee for Clinical Laboratory Standards. 2000. Susceptibility testing of mycobacteria, Nocardia, and other aerobic actinomycetes. 2nd ed. Tentative standard M24-T2.

Welsh, MJ. 1990. Abnormal regulation of ion channels in cystic fibrosis epithelia. *FASEB J,* Vol 4, No 10,(July, 1990), pp. 2718-2725.

Whittier, S., Olivier, K., Gilligan, P., Knowles, M., & Della-Latta, P. 1997. Proficiency testing of clinical microbiology laboratories using modified decontamination procedures for detection of nontuberculous mycobacteria in sputum samples from CF patients. *J Clin Microbiol,* Vol 35, No 10,(October,1997), pp. 2706-2708.

Williams, MM., Yakrus, MA., Arduino, MJ,, Cooksey RC., Crane CB., Banerjee, SN., Hilborn, ED., & Donlan, RM. 2009. Structural analysis of biofilm formation by rapidly and slowly growing nontuberculous mycobacteria. *Appl Environ Microbiol,* Vol 75, No 7, (April, 2009), pp. 2091-2098.

Woods, GL. 2000. Susceptibility testing for mycobacteria. 2000. *Clin Infect Dis,* Vol 31, No 5, (November, 2000), pp.1209-1215.

Yang, SC., Hisueh, PR., Lai, HC., Teng, LJ., Huang, LM., Chen, JM., Wang, SK., Shie, DC., Ho, SW., & Luh, KT. 2003. High prevalence of antimicrobial resistance in rapidly growing mycobacteria in Taiwan. *Antimicrobial Agent Chemother,* Vol 47, No 6, (June,2003),pp 1958-1962.

Zelazny AM, Root JM, Shea YR, Colombo RE, Shamputa IC, Stock F, Conlan S, McNulty S, Brown-Elliott BA, Wallace RJ Jr, Olivier KN, Holland SM, Sampaio EP. 2009. Cohort study of molecular identification and typing of *Mycobacterium abscessus, Mycobacterium massiliense,* and *Mycobacterium bolletii. J Clin Microbiol,* Vol 47, No 7, (July, 2009), pp. 1985-1995.

Zhang, Y., Rajagopalan, M., Brown, BA., & Wallace, RJ Jr. 1997. Randomly amplified polymorphic DNA PCR for comparison of *Mcobacterium abscessus* strains from nosocomial outbreaks. *J Clin Microbiol*, Vol 35, No 12, (December,1997),pp. 3132-3139.

10

Atypical Bacteria in the CF Airways: Diversity, Clinical Consequences, Emergence and Adaptation

Marchandin Hélène[1,2], Michon Anne-Laure[1,2] and Jumas-Bilak Estelle[1,3]
[1]*University Montpellier 1, Equipe Pathogènes et Environnements, UMR 5119 ECOSYM,*
[2]*University Hospital of Montpellier, Bacteriology Laboratory*
[3]*University Hospital of Montpellier, Hygiene Laboratory*
France

1. Introduction

The inventory of atypical[1] bacteria that may be found in the airways of cystic fibrosis (CF) patients besides well-known typical CF pathogens like *Staphylococcus aureus, Haemophilus influenzae, Pseudomonas aeruginosa* and *Burkholderia cepacia* complex has greatly evolved over the past decades. Progressively, species initially considered as atypical in the CF airways, mainly gram-negative bacilli including *Stenotrophomonas maltophilia, Achromobacter xylosoxidans* and non-tuberculous mycobacteria have received more and more attention. They are now considered as usual CF-associated bacteria although their role in the disease progression is not fully elucidated (Beringer *et al.*, 2000; Foweraker, 2009; Hauser *et al.*, 2011). At the same time, other species occasionally identified from the respiratory secretions of CF patients were in turn regarded as atypical species in CF (for a recent review, see Hauser *et al.*, 2011). This resulted from both the increasing number of metagenomic studies conducted on CF airways microbiota and a more systematic use of 16S ribosomal RNA (rRNA) gene sequencing to identify bacteria cultured from CF respiratory tract (CFRT) samples (CFRTS).

Recent findings of "new" atypical bacterial species in CF airways by both cultivation-based and cultivation-independent studies gave novel insights in microbiology of the CFRT. However, pathogenesis and clinical significance of these bacteria remain unclear, i.e. adaptation to the CF airways niche, positive or negative interaction between organisms, impact on the respiratory status of the patients. Similarly, antimicrobial susceptibility pattern is more often not investigated for atypical bacteria.

In this chapter, we propose a review of both published studies and personal findings about atypical bacterial species found in CF airways by both cultivation-based and cultivation-independent studies. Personal data came from our expertise of 16S rRNA gene-based identification of atypical bacteria cultured from CFRTS in patients attending the CF center of

[1]The term "atypical" will be used herein to design bacterial species rarely reported in the literature dealing with the microbiology of respiratory tract in CF patients.

the Montpellier University Hospital[2]. Most of these atypical bacteria are either environmental bacteria or belong to the human respiratory tract microbiota. In this context, examples will be mainly taken from a selected panel of bacteria in our area of expertise, including human anaerobic bacteria and environmental alphaproteobacteria: *Agrobacterium*, acetic acid bacteria, *Ochrobactrum* and *Inquilinus*.

2. CF airways, a niche for environmental opportunistic pathogens

CF airways represent a particular niche in which recent cultivation-based and cultivation-independent studies revealed several atypical microbes, which were recently reviewed by Hauser *et al.* (Hauser *et al.*, 2011). Most of these bacteria are from environmental origin and act as opportunistic pathogens. Some isolates corresponded to unknown taxa when cultivated from CFRTS and supported the description of novel species such as *Inquilinus limosus* (Coenye et al., 2002). Other isolates corresponded to species isolated for the first time in man such as the acetic acid bacteria of the genus *Gluconobacter* previously recovered from environmental and food sources only (Alauzet *et al.*, 2010). We previously reported eight other species detected in CF airways samples but so far described in food or environmental samples only: *Acetobacter fabarum*, *Advenella kashmirensis*, *Aquamicrobium lusatiense*, *Chryseobacterium bovis*, *Phyllobacterium myrsinacearum*, *Pseudomonas brenneri*, *Shinella yambaruensis* and *Sphingomonas pseudosanguinis* (Jumas-Bilak *et al.*, 2011). This diversity suggested that the microbiota of the CF airways niche was far to be fully described. Finally, other isolates were identified as environmental bacteria also known to cause opportunistic infections in immunocompromised patients, for example members of the genera *Agrobacterium* or *Ochrobactrum* (Menuet *et al.*, 2008).

2.1 Atypical bacteria identified by molecular means in our center

The following paragraphs and Table 1 present a summary about the atypical bacterial species cultivated from the respiratory tract of CF patients and identified by 16S rRNA gene sequencing in our center.

Methods performed for bacterial DNA extraction, 16S rRNA gene amplification and sequencing and sequence analysis were described elsewhere; particularly a threshold of 98.7% was considered for species identification (Stackebrandt & Ebers, 2006; Teyssier *et al.*, 2003). A total of 23 atypical taxa were identified in 30 CFRTS from 25 patients. Three patients were colonized by 2 to 3 of these atypical species recovered either in a sample or in two distantly sampled specimens. Fourteen species had never been reported in man before being identified in CF patients, 6 were previously isolated in human clinical samples but were not previously reported in CF patients and 3 species were only isolated in CF patients. Among the taxa not previously isolated in man, four have been found in cultivation-independent studies of human biological samples, *Cupriavidus metallidurans* in skin microbiota (Grice *et al.*, 2009), *Cupriavidus respiraculi* in small intestine microbiota (Franck *et al.*, 2007), *P. myrsinacearum* in vaginal microbiota (Hyman *et al.*, 2005) and *S. pseudosanguinis* in diabetic wound microbiota (Grice *et al.*, 2010). Species subjected to detailed paragraphs were not included in Table 1. They were chosen to complete available recent reviews and/or to give information from personal data.

[2]Caring for more than 200 children and adults each year - 95 adults and 110 children in 2009, the CF center of the Montpellier University Hospital is a large regional French CF center.

Bacterial species (Patient designation)	**Non-human isolation**	**Isolation in non-CF patients**	**Isolation from CF RTS**	**Selected reference**
Advenella kashmirensis (1)	Temperate orchard soil	NPR	NPR	Ghosh *et al.*, 2005
Aquamicrobium lusatiense (2)	Activated sludge	NPR	NPR	Fritsche *et al.*, 1999
Chromobacterium aquaticum (9)	Spring-water	NPR	NPR	Young *et al.*, 2008
Chryseobacterium bovis (**3**)	Cow's milk	NPR	NPR	Hantsis-Zacharov *et al.*, 2008
Comamonas koreensis (**4**)	Forest sediment, wetland	NPR	NPR	Chang *et al.*, 2002
Phyllobacterium myrsinacearum (5)	Leaf nodules of tropical plants	NPR	NPR	Mergaert *et al.*, 2002
Pseudomonas brenneri (**6**)	Natural mineral waters	NPR	NPR	Baïda *et al.*, 2001
Pseudomonas nitroreducens (10)	Rhizospheric soil	NPR	NPR	Korade *et al.*, 2009
Shinella yambaruensis (7)	Soil	NPR	NPR	Matsui *et al.*, 2009
Sphingomonas pseudosanguinis (8)	Water reservoir of air humidifier	NPR	NPR	Kämpfer *et al.*, 2007a
Chryseobacterium indologenes (**3**)	Water, soil, hospital environment	Various	NPR	Lin *et al.*, 2010
Delftia tsuruhatensis (16-18)	Agricultural soil, bioreactor, activated sludge, rhizoplane	Catheter	NPR	Preiswerk *et al.*, 2011
Microbacterium sp.[a] (**3**)	Rhizosphere, mosquito, medical wastes	Various	NPR	Gneiding *et al.*, 2008
Nocardia cyriacigeorgica[b] (12-15)	Soil, animals (bovin, cat, dog)	Various	NPR	Schlaberg *et al.*, 2008
Tsukamurella sp.[c] (**4**)	Activated sludge	Blood, RTS, brain, cornea	NPR	Sheng *et al.*, 2009
Wautersiella falsenii (11)	Poultry	Various	NPR	Kämpfer *et al.*, 2006
Cupriavidus metallidurans (**19**)	Industrial biotopes	NPR	2 isolates	Coenye *et al.*, 2005
Cupriavidus respiraculi (20, 21)	NPR	NPR	23 isolates	Coenye *et al.*, 2005
Pandoraea apista (**22**)	NPR	NPR	22 isolates	Atkinson *et al.*, 2006
Pandoraea pulmonicola (23)	NPR	NPR	2 isolates	Coenye *et al.*, 2000
Bordetella petrii (24)	Polluted soil, river sediment, marine sponges, grass root	Bone, RTS	5 isolates	Spilker *et al.*, 2008
Brevundimonas diminuta (25)	Water, marine soil, petroleum oil, food	Various	1 isolate	Menuet *et al.*, 2008
Nocardia farcinica[b] (**22**)	Activated sludge, animals	Various	3 isolates	Bittar *et al.*, 2010

[a] 16S rRNA gene sequencing did not allow discrimination between *Microbacterium oxydans* and *Microbacterium paraoxydans*.
[b] Species identification was achieved by the Observatoire National des Nocardioses laboratory, Lyon, France, due to lack of discrimination between several nocardial species using 16S rRNA gene sequencing.
[c] No discrimination between *Tsukamurella tyrosinosolvens* and *Tsukamurella pulmonis*.
NPR, not previously reported; RTS, respiratory tract sample
Patients' designation in bold type indicated patients with other samples positive for atypical species listed either in Table 1 or in Table 3.

Table 1. Atypical bacterial species identified by 16S rDNA sequencing in CFRTS from patients attending the center of the University Hospital of Montpellier and general data on isolation in non-human specimens, in non-CF and CF patients.

2.2 *Inquilinus*

I. limosus is a gram-negative bacilli that grew slowly with non-pigmented and extremely mucoid colonies (Figures 1C and 1E) (Coenye *et al.*, 2002). This alphaproteobacteria belongs to the order *Rhodospirillales* and to the family *Rhodospirillaceae* that groups environmental non-sulfur purple bacteria (Table 2). Members of this family were never isolated in man except for *I. limosus* that appeared human-associated. Since its characterization from CFRTS in 2002, *I. limosus* was regularly reported, mainly from CFRT (Bittar *et al.*, 2008a; Chiron *et al.*, 2005; Coenye *et al.*, 2002). Most patients with *Inquilinus* were chronically colonized by *P. aeruginosa* and *Inquilinus* chronic colonization appeared usual in CF patients (Chiron *et al.*, 2005; Hayes *et al.*, 2009; Schmoldt *et al.*, 2006). Typing *Inquilinus* strains by random amplified polymorphic DNA (RAPD) and pulsed-field gel electrophoresis (PFGE) revealed no cross-transmission within centers and a diversity of contamination sources (Chiron *et al.*, 2005; Schmoldt *et al.*, 2006).

In our center, a 21-year-old patient is chronically colonized by *Inquilinus* sp. since the age of 12 years (Chiron *et al.*, 2005). The patient has chronic colonization by a methicillin-susceptible *S. aureus* and was transiently colonized by *P. aeruginosa* (3 *P. aeruginosa* strains isolated since *Inquilinus* recovery and no *P. aeruginosa* isolated since 4 years). *Inquilinus* sp. bacterial load ranged from 10^4 to up to 10^8 CFU/ml depending on the sample, representing the dominant or one of the major species in the sputum samples. Despite environmental investigation, the source for infection remained unknown for this patient. Environmental sources for *Inquilinus* contamination are highly suspected but they were never traced. More generally, no environmental niche for *I. limosus* is detected when screening sequences deposited for environmental clones in the GenBank database (http://www.ncbi.nlm.nih.gov/genbank/).

2.3 Acetic acid bacteria

Members of the genus *Acetobacter*, *Gluconobacter* and *Asaia* were recently isolated from the respiratory tract of CF patients. These gram-negative bacilli belong to the family *Acetobacteraceae,* the second family forming the order *Rhodospirillales* in the alphaproteobacteria together with *Rhodospirillaceae,* the family of *Inquilinus* (Table 2). *Acetobacter*, *Gluconobacter* and *Asaia* are Acetic Acid Bacteria (AAB) characterized by their ability to oxidize alcohols or sugars, leading to the production of acetic acid. AAB are commonly found in soil or are associated with plants. They have been used in industrial food processing throughout human history, especially to convert wine to vinegar and to produce tropical fermented products (Yamada & Yukphan, 2008). The first report of human infection involving AAB dates from 2004, i.e. a case of peritonitis associated with *Asaia bogorensis* (Snyder *et al.*, 2004). Since then, AAB have increasingly been reported as organisms potentially infecting humans and were firstly recognized in a CF patient in 2008 (Alauzet *et al.*, 2010; Bittar *et al.*, 2008a).

We reported four additional AAB isolates in 3 CF patients as follows: (i) successive isolation of an *Asaia* sp. and of two unrelated *Gluconobacter* sp. in a 2-year-old CF patient, (ii) a *Gluconobacter* sp. isolate unrelated to the strains from previous patient and recovered in a 3-year-old CF patient followed at the same CF center, (iii) an *A. fabarum* isolate in a 19.5-year-old CF patient (Alauzet *et al.*, 2010; Jumas-Bilak *et al.*, 2011). In these cases, AAB were recovered at low bacterial load in the sputum samples (≤8 x 10^3 CFU/ml). AAB strains usually grew in 24 to 72 h at 30°C on various agar media selective for gram-negative bacteria except MacConkey agar whereas culture on the same media at 37°C yielded very tiny colonies (Figure 1D) (Alauzet *et al.*, 2010; Bittar *et al.*, 2008a). More generally, reports of *A. fabarum*, an AAB species recently characterized from fermented Ghanaian cocoa beans, and of *Gluconobacter* sp. increased the list of AAB, recently recognized as emerging opportunistic human pathogens, recovered from human samples (Alauzet *et al.*, 2010; Cleenwerck *et al.*, 2008).

2.4 *Agrobacterium*

Members of the order *Rhizobiales* and of the family *Rhizobiaceae*, *Agrobacterium* spp. are gram-negative, non-fastidious, non-fermentative short rods that form mucoid or non-mucoid colonies on agar media (Dunne *et al.*, 1993). *Agrobacterium* are recovered from soil rhizosphere and are well-known plant-associated bacteria that may be phytopathogens. Modified strains of *Agrobacterium tumefaciens* are widely used in plant engineering. In the past two decades, *Agrobacterium radiobacter* has been recognized as an opportunistic human pathogen responsible for nosocomial infections, mainly bacteremia, peritonitis, and urinary tract infections despite virulence considered to be low (Chen *et al.*, 2008; Edmond *et al.*, 1993). In 2002, four *A. radiobacter* strains have been isolated from the respiratory tract of CF patients and it has been suggested that *A. radiobacter* may have the potential to spread from patient to patient (Coenye *et al.*, 2002).

In 2010, we reported 19 additional isolates of *Agrobacterium* sp. from 17 CF patients; strains were analyzed by multilocus sequence typing (MLST) showing 11 different Sequence Types (STs), 17 of the 19 strains belonging to the genovar A7, a genovar that contained only clinical strains and probably adapted to human beings. Diversity in a single ST was demonstrated by PFGE showing that cross-contamination between patients did not occur in our center (Aujoulat *et al.*, 2010). *A. radiobacter* was mainly recognized during transient colonization, no other isolate being recovered in the follow-up of most patients (19 patients out of the 22 currently colonized in our center, 86.4%). Patients' age at *A. radiobacter* isolation ranged from 6 months to 29 years (mean age, 9 years). Successive episodes of colonization occurred in 3 patients, from 2 months to 1.5 year apart. One of these cases was investigated by typing methods showing 2 unrelated isolates recovered 1.5 year apart. In three patients, two *A. radiobacter* isolates with different cultural characteristics were observed in a sample. One of these cases was further investigated showing the patient to be colonized by two genetically different and genomically unrelated strains. Bacterial load in samples was relatively low for most cases comprised between 10^2 and 10^3 CFU/ml except for three samples where the load was higher (from 10^4 to 2 x 10^6 CFU/ml) but *A. radiobacter* was not the dominant species. These samples were taken during scheduled consultation for two patients and during exacerbation attributed to *H. influenzae* for the third patient. Bacterial species mainly co-isolated are the usual pathogens *S. aureus* (9 patients) and *H. influenzae* (5 patients) while co-isolation of *P. aeruginosa* was noted in one patient only. Of note, *A. radiobacter* is usually recovered in highly diversified polymicrobial cultures associated with other rarely isolated organisms like *Acinetobacter* spp., *B. diminuta*, *Comamonas acidovorans*, *C. indologenes*, *C. respiraculi*, *D. tsuruhatensis*, *Enterobacteriaceae* (9 different species), *Ochrobactrum anthropi*, *Tsukamurella* sp. or *Roseomonas* sp. (16 out of 22 patients).

2.5 *Ochrobactrum*

Another member of the order *Rhizobiales* in alphaproteobacteria, the genus *Ochrobactrum* groups bacteria increasingly reported in CF (Menuet *et al.*, 2008; Yagüe-Muñoz *et al.*, 2010). First considered as an emerging pathogen by Menuet *et al.*, *O. anthropi* was responsible for a bacteremia in CF. *Ochrobactrum* spp. are gram-negative non-fermentative oxidase-positive short rods recovered from a wide variety of environmental sources (water, soil, rhizosphere) as well as from plants, animals and human. Five species, *O. anthropi, O. intermedium, O. pseudintermedium, O. haematophilum* and *O. pseudogrignonense* were recovered from human samples; the first two species being increasingly reported as opportunistic pathogens mainly during nosocomial infections, particularly bacteremia and endocarditis (Kämpfer *et al.*, 2007b; Teyssier *et al.* 2005, 2007). *Ochrobactrum* spp. do not present exigent cultural requirements and colony morphology depends on the species (Teyssier & Jumas-Bilak, 2011).

In our center, 14 patients are colonized by *Ochrobactrum* spp. strains (mean age, 3 years [10 months-18 years]) and 35 isolates were recovered (one to 10 isolates per patient). Serial isolates were isolated in seven patients. *O. anthropi* was the major species recovered in CF patients, all the isolates except three being identified as *O. anthropi*. Moreover, *O. intermedium* (n=1) and *O. pseudogrignonense* (n=2) were isolated from patients also colonized by *O. anthropi*. The relative importance of species observed in CF did not reflect the distribution of species in the general population where *O. intermedium* was more frequently represented (Teyssier *et al.*, 2003). In a collection of 66 *Ochrobactrum* spp. from the non-CF population attending the University Hospital of Montpellier, species identified by molecular means were distributed as follows: *O. anthropi* (n=37, 56.1%), *O. intermedium* (n=25, 37.9%), *O. pseudogrignonense* (n=1, 1.5%), and *O. pseudintermedium* (n=3, 4.5%) (unpublished data). Two strains of *O. pseudogrignonense* recovered from human clinical samples (blood and ear) supported the description of the species in 2007, then this recently described species was recovered from CFRTS, two patients attending our center being colonized by unrelated *O. pseudogrignonense* strains. Main associated bacteria were *S. maltophilia* (8 patients), *Enterobacteriaceae* (7 patients), and *S. aureus* and *H. influenzae* (6 patients each). Concomitant isolation of *P. aeruginosa* was observed for 6 samples from 4 patients while co-isolation of atypical species like *A. radiobacter, Acinetobacter* spp., *Alcaligenes* spp., *A. kashmirensis, C. acidovorans, C. indologenes, D. tsuruhatensis* and *S. paucimobilis* was frequently observed. Bacterial load was comprised between 10^2 and 4 x 10^4 CFU of *Ochrobactrum* spp./ml and in most samples *Ochrobactrum* spp. were not the dominant species. Molecular typing based on PFGE and MLST revealed a high level of diversity among isolates showing that no epidemic strains spread occurred in our center (Romano *et al.*, 2009). The same typing methods showed that serial isolates recovered from a patient could correspond to successive colonization by unrelated strains. Such successive episodes of colonization were observed in 5 patients. By contrast, chronic colonization was noted over a 10-month period (4 serial isolates) for one patient with intercurrent isolation of unrelated *O. anthropi* strains and for a 3-year period in a second patient (2 isolates). Complex route of colonization by *Ochrobactrum* spp. in CF is revealed here and warrants further investigation to search for the diversity of sources.

2.6 How unusual are atypical CF-associated bacteria?

2.6.1 Incidence of atypical species in CF

When looking at the isolation frequency of the atypical bacteria described by Hauser *et al.* in our CF center, we found that most of the taxa cited were recovered from sputum samples of the patients thereby underlining that these species were not exceptionally isolated from CFRTS (Hauser *et al.*, 2011).

Strains whose identification was confirmed by 16S rRNA gene sequencing were listed in Table 1. Regarding other taxa detailed herein, AAB have been recovered from the respiratory tract of about 1% of the patients attending our CF center and are still to be considered as an unusual isolation in CF. *Agrobacterium* and *O. anthropi* isolates were found in about 10% and 7% of the patients, respectively and should not be considered anymore as unusual species in CFRT. Other species of *Ochrobactrum* are still to be considered as very unusually isolated in CF. A unique patient was chronically colonized by *Inquilinus* sp. in our CF center (0.5% of the patients) while higher incidence was reported in other CF centers. Notably, a higher incidence is reported in a neighbor region in South of France because *Inquilinus* was reported in 2.8% out of 145 CF patients, incidence varying according to age from 1.2% in children to 4.9% in adult patients (Bittar *et al.*, 2008a). *Inquilinus* sp. was not found in the respiratory tract of non-CF patients (Bittar *et al.*, 2008a). Interestingly, we observed that patients colonized by one of the previous taxa are often simultaneously or successively colonized by other of these species. For example, among the 22 patients with at least one isolate of *Agrobacterium* sp., 9 had at least one episode of colonization by another environmental alphaproteobacteria. The two patients with AAB were also colonized by *A. radiobacter* alone or associated with *O. anthropi* colonization. Other species or genera cited by Hauser *et al.* that were isolated in our center but not detailed here are *Acinetobacter* spp., *Chryseobacterium* spp. and members of the family *Enterobacteriaceae*.

2.6.2 Atypical or underestimated species?

Modification in cultivation and identification methods applied for CFRTS processing may explain an increasing rate of recovery of some species during CF. For example, AAB are increasingly recognized as emerging human opportunistic pathogens and their frequency may probably be underestimated because of their growth characteristics, particularly their faint growth at 37°C, a default temperature setting in routine medical microbiology, and because of the difficulty with identifying these microorganisms. For instance, the recovery of AAB in CF was related to the use of *Burkholderia cepacia* complex selective agar that is incubated for a prolonged incubation time (5 days) at 30°C. Therefore, the recovery of *Asaia* and *Gluconobacter* is enhanced because they resisted to antibiotics included in the medium and they grew in such cultivation conditions while no growth is observed on MacConkey agar plates incubated for 3 days at 30°C or 37°C (Alauzet *et al.*, 2010) (Figure 1D).

Growth of atypical bacteria on different media and at different incubation temperatures is shown in Figure 1.

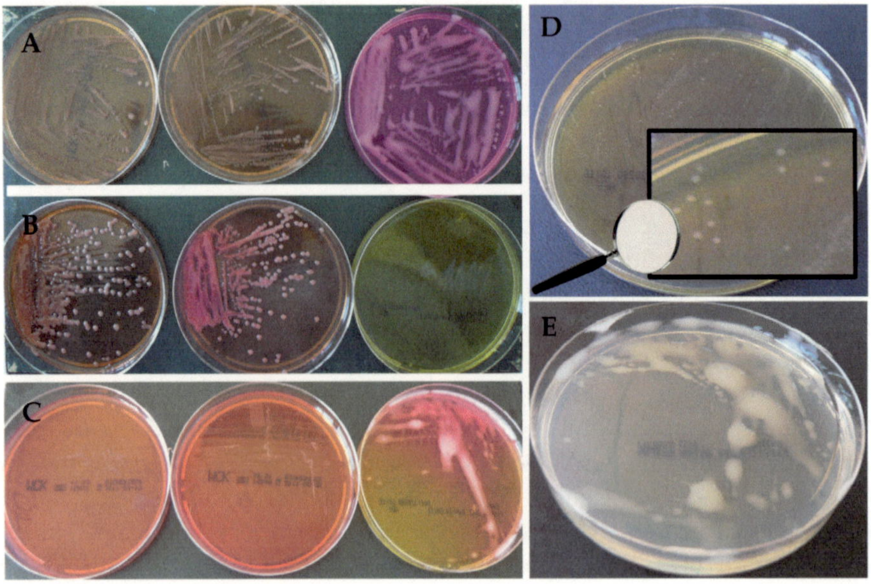

Fig. 1. Growth of *O. anthropi* (A), *A. radiobacter* (B) and *Inquilinus* sp. (C) on MacConkey agar plates (bioMérieux) incubated at 37°C (left) or 30°C (middle) and on the *Burkholderia cepacia*-selective medium Cepacia agar (AES) incubated at 30°C (right); growth of *Gluconobacter* sp. on *B. cepacia*-selective medium Cepacia agar (D), and growth of *Inquilinus* sp. on Mueller-Hinton agar (bioMérieux) (E) (incubation time was 3 days in all cases).

In addition to limitation related to cultivation conditions, recovery of atypical species could also be impaired by the routine practice of CFRT sampling. Indeed, the unique sample usually submitted to bacteriological analysis was shown to be insufficient for recognition of all bacteria that may colonize the patient, including CF pathogens (Rogers *et al.*, 2010).

Regarding identification, molecular-based methods revealed up to 25% of isolates without correct phenotypic identification (Bittar *et al.*, 2008b). *A. radiobacter* strains are accurately identified with API 20NE strip or VITEK2 GN card (bioMérieux) but *A. radiobacter* is named *Rhizobium radiobacter* in API and VITEK2 databases due to confusing taxonomy in these genera (Aujoulat *et al.*, 2010; Otto-Karg *et al.*, 2009; Teyssier *et al.*, 2009). Identification could be more difficult for other taxa. *O. anthropi* is the sole species of the genus included in API and VITEK2 databases. Both systems permit genus-level identification and sequencing of either 16S rRNA gene or another housekeeping gene should be performed for species identification. Although *Inquilinus* sp. showed several notable characteristics that will be discussed below, i.e. mucoid phenotype, characteristic multiresistant pattern to antibiotics and ability to persist in the CF airways, its identification remains difficult. This emerging pathogen was either not detected or misclassified by laboratories (Bittar *et al.*, 2008b; Hogard *et al.*, 2009). Since 2011, a second species has been described in the genus, *Inquilinus ginsengisoli*, isolated from soil (Jung *et al.*, 2011). This species could be differentiated from *I. limosus* by a careful 16S rRNA gene analysis. Similarly, both genera of AAB recovered in CF patients, i.e. *Asaia* and *Gluconobacter* required molecular methods for their identification. However, some closely related species belonging to these genera might remain unidentified despite sequencing housekeeping genes in addition to 16S rRNA gene (Alauzet *et al.*, 2010).

Recently, matrix-assisted laser desorption ionization–time of flight mass spectrometry (MALDI-TOF-MS) was used for identification of non-fermentative gram-negative bacilli isolated from CF patients (Degand *et al.*, 2008). A few atypical species covered by this chapter were included, i.e. 1 *B. hinzii*, 1 *I. limosus*, 1 *C. respiraculi*. The three isolates were correctly identified by the system. Another study evaluating the system for identification of environmental members of the family *Rhizobiaceae* including *Agrobacterium* (= *Rhizobium*) *radiobacter* showed comparable performances to housekeeping gene sequence analysis suggesting that this species might be correctly identified by the system if included in the "CF" database (Ferreira *et al.*, 2011). Additional studies on a larger panel of isolates are needed to precisely evaluate the performance of the system for identifying all the diversity of atypical bacteria that may be encountered in CF samples.

2.7 Taxonomic diversity of atypical bacteria in CF

Atypical taxa isolated from CFRTS in our center and identified by 16S rRNA gene sequencing are distributed among 3 phyla, the phylum *Proteobacteria* being the most represented. The Table 2 gives the taxonomic repartition of the atypical taxa in the 3 major phyla. In the *Proteobacteria*, gram-negative bacilli of the class *Alphaproteobacteria* account for the majority of atypical taxa identified (Table 2). This may suggest that patients are more frequently in contact with the environmental niches of these species and/or that these taxa have an increased potential to colonize the CFRT.

Phylum	Class	Order	Family	Taxon
Actinobacteria	*Actinobacteria*	*Actinomycetales*	*Actinomycetaceae*	*Actinomyces graevenitzii*
			Microbacteriaceae	*Microbacterium* sp.
			Nocardiaceae	*Nocardia* spp.
			Tsukamurellaceae	*Tsukamurella* sp.
Bacteroidetes	*Flavobacteria*	*Flavobacteriales*	*Flavobacteriaceae*	*Chryseobacterium* spp.
				Wautersiella falsenii
Proteobacteria	*Alphaproteobacteria*	*Caulobacterales*	*Caulobacteraceae*	*Brevundimonas diminuta*
		Rhizobiales	*Brucellaceae*	*Ochrobactrum* spp.
			Phyllobacteriaceae	*Aquamicrobium lusatiense*
				Phyllobacterium myrsinacearum
			Rhizobiaceae	*Agrobacterium* sp.
				Shinella yambaruensis
		Rhodospirillales	*Acetobacteraceae*	*Acetobacter fabarum*
				Asaia sp.
				Gluconobacter sp.
			Rhodospirillaceae	*Inquilinus limosus*
		Sphingomonadales	*Sphingomonadaceae*	*Sphingomonas pseudosanguinis*
	Betaproteobacteria	*Burkholderiales*	*Alcaligenaceae*	*Advenella kashmirensis*
				Bordetella spp.
			Burkholderiaceae	*Cupriavidus* spp.
				Pandoraea spp.
			Comamonadaceae	*Comamonas koreensis*
				Delftia tsuruhatensis
		Neisseriales	*Neisseriaceae*	*Chromobacterium aquaticum*
	Gammaproteobacteria	*Pseudomonadales*	*Pseudomonadaceae*	*Pseudomonas brenneri*
				Pseudomonas nitroreducens

Table 2. Taxonomic lineages for atypical bacteria identified from CFRTS in our center using 16S rRNA gene sequencing.

2.8 Unknown cultivated bacterial taxa in CF

Diversity of the cultivable part of the CFRT microbiota remains underestimated. In the past decade, 12 novel species were characterized based on isolates recovered in CFRTS, i.e. 7 *Burkholderia* species, 3 *Ralstonia* species (of which 2 are yet reclassified in the genus *Cupriavidus*), *Advenella incenata* and *I. limosus* (PubMed search on August the 1st, 2011 with key words "sp. nov." and "cystic fibrosis"). In our center, identification based on 16S rDNA revealed 5 potential novel taxa cultivated from CFRTS (Table 3). Of note, 2 patients had other samples positive for atypical species listed in Table 1. Altogether these data illustrate the diversity not fully explored of bacteria that could be cultivated from CFRTS.

Isolate reference	**Patient no.**	**16S rDNA sequence similarity with the closest known species** (%, name of the species)	**Taxonomic interpretation***
29 dec. 2009, 2320	26	96%, *Corynebacterium durum*	Novel species in the genus *Corynebacterium*
15 jun. 2007, 5197	**19**	96.5%, *Cupriavidus metallidurans*	Novel species in the genus *Cupriavidus*
21 jul. 2009, 2477	27	97.6%, *Roseomonas cervicalis*	Probable novel species in the genus *Roseomonas*
20 nov. 2009, 5248	28	98.2%, *Cupriavidus respiraculi*	Probable novel species in the genus *Cupriavidus*
15 apr. 2005, 5138	**6**	98.5%, *Cupriavidus respiraculi*	Probable novel species in the genus *Cupriavidus*

* Isolates showing less than 97% of sequence similarity with the closest known species were considered as novel taxa (Stackebrandt & Goebel, 1994); isolates showing between 97% and 98.7% of sequence similarity with the closest known species were considered as probable novel taxa (Stackebrandt & Ebers, 2006). Bold type indicated patients with other samples positive for atypical species as listed in Table 1.

Table 3. Unknown taxa in the CFRTS from patients attending the CF center of the University Hospital of Montpellier.

3. Atypical pathologic communities in CF

3.1 Microbial diversity in CFRT assessed by cultivation-independent studies

Over the last decade, our knowledge of the bacterial diversity in CFRT microbiota has evolved due to cultivation-independent methods. Terminal Restriction Fragment Length Polymorphism Profiling, Temporal Temperature Gradient gel Electrophoresis or sequencing were employed to characterize 16S ribosomal DNA in CFRT community and revealed both a higher biodiversity than previously presumed and several atypical organisms (Bittar *et al.*, 2008b; Guss *et al.*, 2011; Kolak *et al.*, 2003; Rogers *et al.*, 2004).

Comparison between cultivation-based methods and cultivation independent methods revealed the overlooked part of bacteria present in CFRTS including species recovered from the oral microbiota during health and diseases, atypical species of unknown pathogenicity and well-known bacterial species pathogenic for CF patients (Bittar *et al.*, 2008b; Rogers *et al.*, 2009; van Belkum *et al.*, 2000). For example, Bittar *et al.*, studying 25 CF sputum samples showed that 53 species were found using the PCR-cloning-sequencing approach while only 13 were cultivated (Bittar *et al.*, 2008b). Sixteen species only found by the molecular method corresponded to anaerobes not covered by the cultivation conditions used in the study. Nevertheless, several aerobic and anaerobic species detected by the genomic method corresponded to species unusually or firstly detected in CF (Bittar *et al.*, 2008b).

Additional unexpected bacteria were described in other cultivation-independent studies. For example, Harris *et al.* reported in a 14-year-old CF patient the first occurrence in man of sequences corresponding to the alphaproteobacteria *Chelatococcus asaccharovorans* (Harris *et al.*, 2007). These sequences represented 5% of the total sequences found in the corresponding specimen. Some of the other unexpected bacteria overlooked by cultivation-based methods and revealed by cultivation-independent methods may be clinically relevant in CF. Indeed, CF candidate pathogens were identified by Harris *et al.* comparing microbiota from CF and non-CF patients as follows: *Prevotella denticola*, *Lysobacter* sp., and *Rickettsiales* sp. (Harris *et al.*, 2007). Interestingly, members of the genus *Lysobacter* are gram-negative bacilli showing similar environmental lifestyle as *Agrobacterium* and *Ochrobactrum*, i.e. isolated from soil, rhizosphere and plant-associated samples. *Lysobacter* spp. were also found as dominant species on the human tongue dorsum and recovered from the surface of prosthetic hip joints (Dempsey *et al.*, 2007; Riggio *et al.*, 2008). Unless additional arguments are given, *Lysobacter* sp. should be considered with caution as a CF potential pathogen. Finally, cultivation-independent studies revealed the occurrence of several unknown taxa in the CFRTS like novel members of the order *Rickettsiales* and of the family *Coxiellaceae* (the latter representing 11% of the sequences found in association with those of *Chelatococcus asaccharovorans*) (Harris *et al.*, 2007). Regarding bacterial taxa developed in this chapter, i.e. *Inquilinus*, acetic acid bacteria, *Agrobacterium* and *Ochrobactrum*, sequences of *Inquilinus* sp. were recovered in some cultivation-independent studies while the other taxa were not found (Bittar *et al.*, 2008b). In addition to patients' sampling methods, these taxa may be overlooked in molecular-based approaches due to their minority in the CFRT microbiota, a hypothesis congruent with the low bacterial load observed in culture for these bacteria.

3.2 Dysbiosis in the CF polymicrobial disease and example of anaerobes

Comparison of microbiota diversity in CF patients and in control groups, as well as cultivation-independent studies suggested that CF should be considered as a polymicrobial disease (Klepac-Ceraj *et al.*, 2010; Sibley *et al.*, 2006). A major recent finding revealed that lung function is significantly and positively correlated with the bacterial species richness of the global microbiota (van der Gast *et al.*, 2011). Considering the inter-individual variations in the microbiota composition, van der Gast *et al.* studying microbiota composition of sputum samples from 14 adult CF patients further showed that both core and satellite taxa are significantly correlated with lung function (van der Gast *et al.*, 2011). Moreover, any disequilibrium in the consortium of microorganisms found in the CFRT may have clinical consequences on the clinical status as previously observed in other dysbiosis-associated diseases like bacterial vaginosis (Oakley *et al.*, 2008). Although the total number of bacterial species observed in a population of CF patients was shown significantly more diverse than that observed in a control group including bronchiectasis patients (Bittar *et al.*, 2008b), at the individual level, libraries of lower complexity were observed in CF compared to a control group (Harris *et al.*, 2007). Such a low diversity observed in CF patients may reflect the enrichment of a pathogenic species and/or the consequence of dysbiosis and so possibly signify bacterial involvement in disease (Harris *et al.*, 2007). For example, among the 28 CF patients included in the study, more than the half (53.6%) had less than 5 organisms detected and one of these microorganisms dominated the poorly diversified microbiota (from 63 to 98% of the sequences). For 8 patients, all sequences corresponded to a unique bacterial taxon (*S. aureus*, *Lysobacter* sp., *S. maltophilia*, *P. aeruginosa* and *Mycobacterium abscessus*). Atypical bacteria proposed as CF candidate pathogens and cited above, i.e. *P. denticola*, *Lysobacter* sp., and *Rickettsiales* sp. were all encountered in dysbiotic environment. Indeed, these sequences were each recovered in a CF patient as a major or as the unique sequence among sequences of the patient's microbiota, representing 56%, 100% and 36% of the total sequences, respectively (Harris *et al.*, 2007). Based on the example of *P. denticola*, we will discuss further on the role of anaerobes, particularly those belonging to the genus *Prevotella*, in the dysbiosis that may occur in CF (for a review on anaerobic bacteria infection in cystic fibrosis airway disease, see Lambiase *et al.*, 2010).

In both cultivation-based and cultivation-independent studies, particular attention was recently paid to anaerobic microflora, which had received little attention before (Bittar *et al.*, 2008b; Harris *et al.*, 2007; Tunney *et al.*, 2008). Indeed, anaerobic cultures are not performed in the routine practice of sputum samples and thus anaerobic bacteria are totally ignored except when specifically studied (Jewes & Spencer, 1990). Tunney *et al.* assessing anaerobic bacteria in CF children by means of culture of bronchoalveolar lavage fluid samples demonstrated that anaerobic bacteria are: (i) frequently present in the airway specimens, (ii) in higher numbers than in healthy volunteers, and (iii) generally different species compared with those detected in the non-CF control group (Tunney *et al.*, 2008). Identification of the anaerobes isolated revealed 14 different genera with the genus *Prevotella*, being the most frequently isolated before *Veillonella*, *Propionibacterium*, and *Actinomyces*. *Prevotella* spp. were present in 22% to > 80% of the CF patients depending on the study while found in 10% of healthy patients (Field *et al.*, 2010; Tunney *et al.*, 2008). Based on cultivation-independent methods, Bittar *et al.* showed the anaerobes to represent 30.2% of the detected species in CF sputum specimens (16/53 species) with *Prevotella* sequences being dominant (48.7%) among sequences corresponding to anaerobes (Bittar *et al.*, 2008b). *Prevotella melaninogenica* is usually the most common species identified in these studies. Strict anaerobes are well-known oral species. However, they were not regarded to be simply contaminants because of their diversity and abundance within the CF airways compared to non-CF population (Jones, 2011). Among them, *Prevotella* spp., already known as contributing to the consortia of microorganisms involved in several human pathologies attributed to dysbiosis, may contribute to CF airway disease (Alauzet *et al.*, 2010; Field *et al.*, 2010).

What remains also unknown is how the quantitative and/or qualitative modification in the composition of the microbiota would affect interactions between organisms. These interactions were previously demonstrated in complex microbiota like modulation of *P. aeruginosa* gene expression by host microflora through interspecies communication (Duan *et al.*, 2003; Sibley *et al.*, 2008b). It was hypothesized that *Prevotella* spp. may also modulate *P. aeruginosa* virulence gene expression as well as growth and virulence of the potential CF pathogen of the *Streptococcus milleri* group (Field et al., 2010; Shinzato *et al.*, 1994; Sibley *et al.*, 2008a). Unfortunately, *Prevotella* spp. were not included by Sibley *et al.* in the 40 oropharyngeal species tested for both microbe-microbe and polymicrobe-host interactions in *Drosophila melanogaster* infection model (Sibley *et al.*, 2008b).

4. Pathogenesis and clinical consequences of colonization by atypical bacteria

Harris *et al.* previously hypothesized that atypical bacteria may explain inflammation in the absence of documented pathogens as well as failure to standard treatment in CF (Harris *et al.*, 2007). The clinical significance in CF of bacteria detailed in this chapter remains unclear, as it is still the case for more frequently isolated species like *A. xylosoxidans* (Hauser *et al.*, 2011).

Regarding anaerobes, Worlitzsch *et al.* showed that patients with and without obligate anaerobes in sputum specimens did not differ in lung function (Worlitzsch *et al.*, 2009). AAB, *Agrobacterium*, *Inquilinus* and *Ochrobactrum* members are considered as opportunistic human pathogens, being involved in systemic or severe infections in immunocompromised patients or patients with underlying diseases/conditions (Alauzet *et al.*, 2010; Chen *et al.*, 2008; Cieslak *et al.*, 1996; Kiratisin *et al.*, 2006).

Case reports documented potential virulence in CF for some of these atypical bacteria. For AAB, the first case report in CF documented *Acetobacter indonesiensis* isolation during pneumonia occurring after lung transplant. The bacterium was considered to be the primary cause of the infection because of clinical improvement after adapted antimicrobial therapy (Bittar *et al.*, 2008a). By contrast, *Gluconobacter* and *Asaia* sp. could not be incriminated in the evolution of the disease because of a favorable clinical evolution without any specific treatment (Alauzet *et al.*, 2010). Case reports also witnessed for a potential pathogenic power of *Ochrobactrum* sp. in CF patients because *O. anthropi* was previously involved: (i) in association with *B. diminuta* in a case of acute pneumonia in a 17-year-old CF patient showing clinical improvement after adapted antimicrobial therapy including imipenem and tobramycin (Menuet *et al.*, 2008), (ii) in a case of bacteremia in children (Yagüe-Muñoz *et al.*, 2010). *Inquilinus* isolation was associated either with acute pulmonary exacerbation, respiratory decline without signs of acute exacerbation or stable respiratory status (Chiron *et al.*, 2005; Schmoldt *et al.*, 2006). To date, the patient chronically colonized by *Inquilinus* sp. in our center has stable respiratory status. *Inquilinus* sp. was also responsible for prosthetic valve endocarditis in a tetralogy of Fallot patient (Kiratisin *et al.*, 2006). Additional arguments in favor of pathogenic potential of *Inquilinus* sp. are: (i) specific serum antibody response found in patients with *Inquilinus* sp. (Schmoldt *et al.*, 2006), (ii) mucoid characteristic of *Inquilinus* sp. that could be related to exopolysaccharides, recognised as important virulence factors in lung infections, showing novel structures with usual components and similarity with *P. aeruginosa* exopolysaccharides (Herasimenka *et al.*, 2007). Finally, no clinical data associated with *A. radiobacter* isolation in CF are currently available. From our personal data, *A. radiobacter* was mainly a transient colonizer of the CFRT while *Ochrobactrum* spp. displayed more complex relationships with CF host. These species were usually recovered at low bacterial load and in mixed cultures from the respiratory secretions sampled in patients during scheduled consultations. Their recovery was mainly associated with stable respiratory status but in some cases, respiratory decline with or without signs of acute exacerbation were noted. In these cases, multiple species were simultaneously isolated from the CFRTS, making it difficult to attribute signs and symptoms to a specific bacterium.

Treatment against these species was usually not started except in one case of *A. radiobacter* isolation that was recovered at low bacterial load but in pure culture in a context of respiratory decline in a 4-year-old patient. Trimethoprim/sulfamethoxazole treatment for 15 days led to eradication of the species from the airways and clinical improvement in this patient. In another patient with deteriorated respiratory status, antimicrobial treatment associating ciprofloxacin and trimethoprim/sulfamethoxazole was established. According to the antibiograms, this treatment was effective against all bacteria cultured from the sputum specimen, i.e. *A. radiobacter* but also *D. tsuruhatensis*, two enterobacteria and *S. aureus*, the major species in the sample and showed efficacy on the clinical status of the patient.

Of note, *Agrobacterium* and/or *Ochrobactrum* spp. were relatively frequently isolated after antimicrobial treatment against *P. aeruginosa* or *S. aureus* due to their resistance to amoxicillin/clavulanic acid, ceftazidime, tobramycin and/or colistin. Indeed, as previously described for other mild opportunistic pathogens of environmental origin like *S. maltophilia*; acetic acid bacteria, *Inquilinus* and *Ochrobactrum* spp. displayed a high level of resistance to antibacterial compounds (Alauzet *et al.*, 2010; Berg *et al.*, 2005; Bittar *et* al, 2008a; Thoma *et al.*, 2009) (Figure 2).

Multiresistance-encoding genetic determinant has only been characterized for *O. anthropi* as a chromosomal class C beta-lactamase named OCH-1 while remaining unknown for *Agrobacterium*, AAB, *Inquilinus* sp. and other *Ochrobactrum* species (Nadjar *et al.*, 2001). Moreover, majority of these species displayed intrinsic resistance to colistin. *Agrobacterium* sp. resisted to several drugs used in CF patients like ceftazidime and tobramycin but displayed resistance to less drugs than AAB, *Inquilinus* and *Ochrobactrum*.

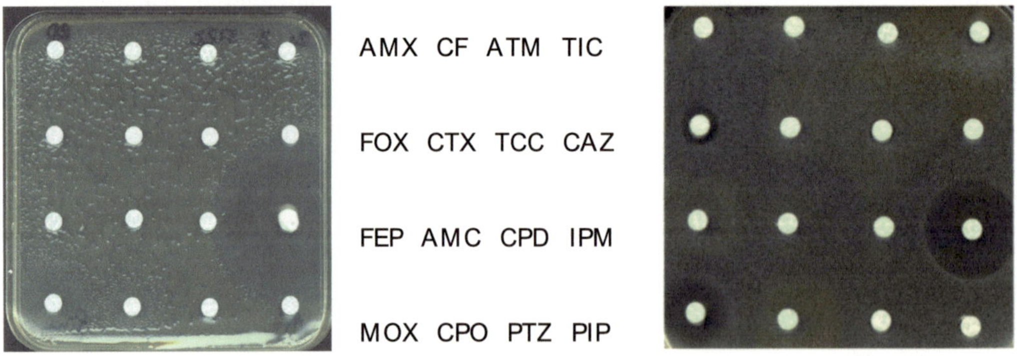

Fig. 2. Multiresistance pattern to β-lactam agents observed for *Inquilinus* sp. (left) and *O. intermedium* (right) by disk diffusion assay (antibiotic disk position is indicated by corresponding drug abbreviation in the middle).

Abbreviations and concentrations for antibiotics indicated according to disk position are: AMX, amoxicillin (25 µg); CF, cephalotin (30 µg); ATM, aztreonam (30 µg); TIC, ticarcillin (75 µg); FOX, cefoxitin (30 µg); CTX, cefotaxime (30 µg); CAZ, ceftazidime (30µg); TCC, ticarcillin/clavulanic acid (75 µg /10 µg); FEP, cefepime (30 µg); AMC, amoxicillin/clavulanic acid (20 µg /10 µg); CPD, cefpodoxime (30 µg); IPM, imipenem (10 µg); MOX, latamoxef (30 µg); CPO, cefpirome (30 µg); PTZ, piperacillin/tazobactam (75 µg /10 µg); PIP, piperacillin (75 µg).

There are too few isolates reported in the literature and even fewer CF case reports involving these atypical bacteria to drawn conclusion on their clinical relevance in CF. Moreover, interactions between these atypical species and other organisms within the CFRT microbiota is unknown. Knowledge on the virulence of these atypical bacteria required rigorous description and follow-up of cases involving such bacteria. Moreover, case control studies will also be needed to determine their clinical implication in CF patients as well as risk factors for acquisition. From our experience, it could be hypothesized that these species may be selected by antimicrobial therapy against pathogens due to their resistance or multidrug resistance. This has been previously suggested for *S. maltophilia,* which has a predilection to infect CF patients with more advanced disease and consequently more frequently exposed to broad-spectrum antibiotics (Hauser *et al.*, 2011). Similarly, the increased use of nebulized colistin in CF patients may select specific colistin-resistant bacteria as previously suggested for *B. diminuta* (Menuet *et al.*, 2008).

Besides intrinsic resistance, several bacteria present in the CFRT microbiota may acquire additional resistance mechanisms. Development of multidrug resistance is a frequent finding in CF and is usually mediated by combination of several resistance mechanisms (Poole, 2011). Acquired multidrug resistance may also be encoded by extended spectrum β-lactamases (ESBLs) and carbapenemases, which are increasingly reported in pathogens commonly found in CF (*P. aeruginosa, S. maltophilia*). *Enterobacteriaceae* can harbor ESBL-encoding genes localized on mobile genetic elements that may be transferable between members of the community. Although such observations remain rare (Cantón *et al.*, 1997; 2 unpublished isolates in our centre), microbiologists have to be aware of multidrug resistant enterobacteria in CF due to pandemic dissemination of some enzymes like CTX-M ESBLs in the global population (Cantón *et al.*, 2006). In this context, atypical bacteria from environmental origin, even transiently colonizing CFRT may constitute a reservoir of resistance determinants that can be mobilized into the microbial community, thereby contributing to the global increase of the microbiota resistance (Wright, 2010). Moreover, antibiotic degrading diffusible enzymes that may be secreted by atypical bacteria are a matter of concern. Indeed, antimicrobial treatment against pathogens associated with these atypical bacteria may become ineffective due to antibiotic hydrolysis by these enzymes. Altogether, bacteria showing multidrug resistance whether this resistance is innate or acquired contribute to the increase of the global resistome of the CFRT microbiota.

5. Adaptation of atypical bacteria to the CF airways niche

5.1 Adaptation to CFRT conditions

Airways of CF patients represent an ecological niche recognized as a model system for studies on bacterial adaptation. Indeed, in this specific niche, the bacteria incoming from the outer environment are submitted to complex selective forces from microbiological, immunological, physiological and biochemical environment of the CF airways that may drive the evolution of the corresponding microorganism (Yang *et al.*, 2011a, 2011b). Several microbial species appear to be well adapted to survival within the CF airways (Hauser *et al.*, 2011). Some species may adapt by forming colony variants, i.e. small-colony variants for *S. aureus* and *P. aeruginosa* or mucoid colony variants for *P. aeruginosa,* favoring resistance to antibiotics, evasion to immune system and then long-term persistence in the CF airways. *P. aeruginosa*, the most studied pathogen, may adapt by a wide range of mechanisms that were recently reviewed (Hauser *et al.*, 2011).

For atypical bacteria considered herein, little is known about the mechanisms of adaptation to host environment i.e. to CFRT. Extrapolating from *P. aeruginosa*, mucoid phenotype (*Inquilinus, Ochrobactrum*), antibiotic resistance (*Inquilinus, Ochrobactrum, Agrobacterium*), modifications in lipopolysaccharide (gram-negative genera) or existence of subsets of host-adapted strains (*Ochrobactrum, Agrobacterium*) are traits that may favor adaptation to CFRT. Although not yet further investigated, we observed diversification in both colonial morphology and antibiotype (susceptibility/resistance to fluoroquinolones) after a 6-year period of *Inquilinus* sp. colonization. Moreover, population genetics revealed lineages of *Agrobacterium* and *O. anthropi* adapted to man but not specifically CF-adapted in contrast to *P. aeruginosa* for which two genotypes were shown as specifically-associated with CF (Aujoulat *et al.*, 2010; Romano *et al.*, 2009; van Mansfeld *et al.*, 2010). In addition, some other mechanisms of adaptation may be suspected for bacteria covered by this chapter. As far as AAB are concerned, it was previously hypothesized that they might specifically colonize the CFRT in relation to their ability to grow in acidic conditions. Indeed, this particular metabolic trait may confer a selective advantage to these bacteria in the acidified CF airways (Alauzet *et al.*, 2010; Poschet *et al.*, 2002).

5.2 Adaptative evolution in the CFRT

CFRT is a compartimentalized niche, which is spatially and temporally heterogeneous according to the anatomic site and to the period of disease evolution. A variable but relatively closed niche could drive diversification and adaptative evolution of the microbiota. In addition, mortality agents such as host immunity, antibiotics and lysogenic phages could lead to the diversification of a bacterial population that contribute to the persistence of the infection, as previously described for *P. aeruginosa* in the CF lung (Brockhurst *et al.*, 2005).

The ability to switch to hypermutable phenotypes by rapid acquisition of mutations at an unusually high rate lead to phenotypic diversification as observed for *H. influenzae, S. aureus* and *P. aeruginosa* (Hauser *et al.*, 2011). Besides hypermutation, genome plasticity is a mechanism for a bacterium to diversify its population and to adapt in various environments. Genomic rearrangements have been described in *P. aeruginosa* to switch from a saprophytic to a pathogenic lifestyle. Large chromosomal inversions are associated with insertion sequences duplication in *P. aeruginosa* strains isolated in CF. These events, by disrupting genes, have been shown to be involved in phenotypic adaptation of the strains to their particular environment (Coyne *et al.*, 2010).

Genomic macrorestriction followed by PFGE is an efficient tool to follow genomic rearrangements, particularly in bacterial species poorly investigated at the genetic level, as atypical species isolated from CFRT. Genomic evolution was previously demonstrated in serial isolates recovered from the respiratory tract of a non-CF patient chronically colonized over a 1.5-year period by *O. intermedium* (Teyssier *et al.*, 2003). The clone evolved *in vivo* by a deletion of a 150 kb-genomic fragment, which included one copy of ribosomal operon. It was suggested that: (i) the new genomic organization gave a selective advantage to the strain *in vivo*, (ii) the genomic reduction may be an adaptative phenomenon of this free-living bacterium to the narrow ecological niche represented by the human respiratory tract. Indeed, the relation between host-restricted lifestyle and a small genome size is patent in bacteria, particularly in alphaproteobacteria (Moreno, 1998). We recently hypothesize that a phenomenon of genomic rearrangement might also be observed in *Inquilinus* sp. strains. Investigation was conducted on 21 serial isolates recovered during the 9-year follow-up of a CF patient chronically colonized by *Inquilinus* sp. PFGE analysis revealed the genomic stability of the strains while showing the existence of two closely related variants. Genomic reduction is suspected in one of the two co-existing variants suggesting that an adaptation process to human host is ongoing in these isolates but this should be further investigated (Teyssier *et al.*, 2011). This hypothesis was supported by comparison of sequential *Inquilinus* isolates recovered in one German patient revealing identical RAPD profiles but slightly different protein patterns. Expression of two antigens disappeared between successively isolated strains and was considered as suggestive of an adaptation of the *Inquilinus* clone during the course of infection (Schmoldt *et al.*, 2006). As observed by PFGE, the two variants co-existed in the respiratory tract.

6. Hypothesis: CFRT is a hotspot for emergence of human pathogens

The emergence of human pathogens from environment involves a dramatic jump in the lifestyle of bacteria. CFRT and atypical bacteria provide examples for different types of lifestyle switches. Bacteria like *Ochrobactrum* spp. have a very versatile behavior with no obvious pathogenicity except in man but with close association with diverse organisms, association that can be as close as symbiosis (Teyssier *et al.*, 2004). In the respiratory tract, *O. intermedium* can evolve by genomic reduction until displaying a genome structure similar to *Brucella*, an intracellular strict pathogen phylogenetically related to *Ochrobactrum* spp. (Teyssier *et al.*, 2003). In some cases, pathogenic microorganisms are capable to cause disease in a variety of organisms that may belong to different biological kingdoms of life. Such cross-kingdom pathogenesis could be illustrated by *A. radiobacter/tumefaciens* that causes both plant and human diseases. The virulence factors involved in phytopathogenicity are not found in clinical strains (unpublished data). However, multi-locus phylogeny showed that the clinical strains belonged to an epidemic clone among the *Agrobacterium* spp. population. This epidemic clone so-called genovar A7 could correspond to a new species in the genus and presented some phenotypic characters such as growth at 40 °C, which is a basic trait for human pathogenicity (Aujoulat *et al.*, 2011). The bacterial lifestyle needs basic requirements such as temperature, water, nutrients and pH optima. In human-associated *Agrobacterium*, growth at high temperature is an emergent character. In other cases, basic requirements may be similar in both pathogenic and harmless members of neighbor clades, hence considered to be pre-existing adaptations. Different members of the *Acetobacteraceae* could infect human suggesting that they shared common traits, such as ability to grow at acidic pH, that permits their opportunistic growth, particularly in CFRT.

One primary condition for colonization and pathogenicity is the probability to meet the bacteria that implies living in close proximity. AAB could be considered as "domestic" for human since they were used for a long time in food processing. This situation differed from that observed for *Inquilinus*, which is the sole genus to include human-adapted bacteria in

Rhodospirillaceae. I. limosus emerged from the family *Rhodospirillaceae*, a group found in soil and plant but totally unrelated to human beings. Association with coral, sponge and cuttlefish is also described, particularly in the neighborhood of the genus *Inquilinus*. It is noteworthy that, when associated with animals, *Rhodospirillaceae* are found in mucous or gelatinous environment, such as the egg capsule in sepia. 16S rDNA sequences of *I. ginsengisoli* described from the soil of ginseng fields differed slightly from that of *I. limosus* type strain (Jung *et al.*, 2011). 16S rDNA-based phylogeny showed a short robust branch (bootstrap value at 85) that groups all the clinical isolates and only one environmental isolate from roots of a perennial grass of Thar Desert in India (Figure 3). In a rooted tree, this branch appeared as supporting the most recently emerging species in the *Inquilinus* genus (data not shown). Finally, no relationship with human or other mammals was found for bacteria in the phylogenetic neighborhood of *Inquilinus*. Therefore, we could hypothetize that the association of *I. limosus* with CFRT resulted from a recent emergence by a speciation process of a human-adapted species from a group that experimented life in mucous environment.

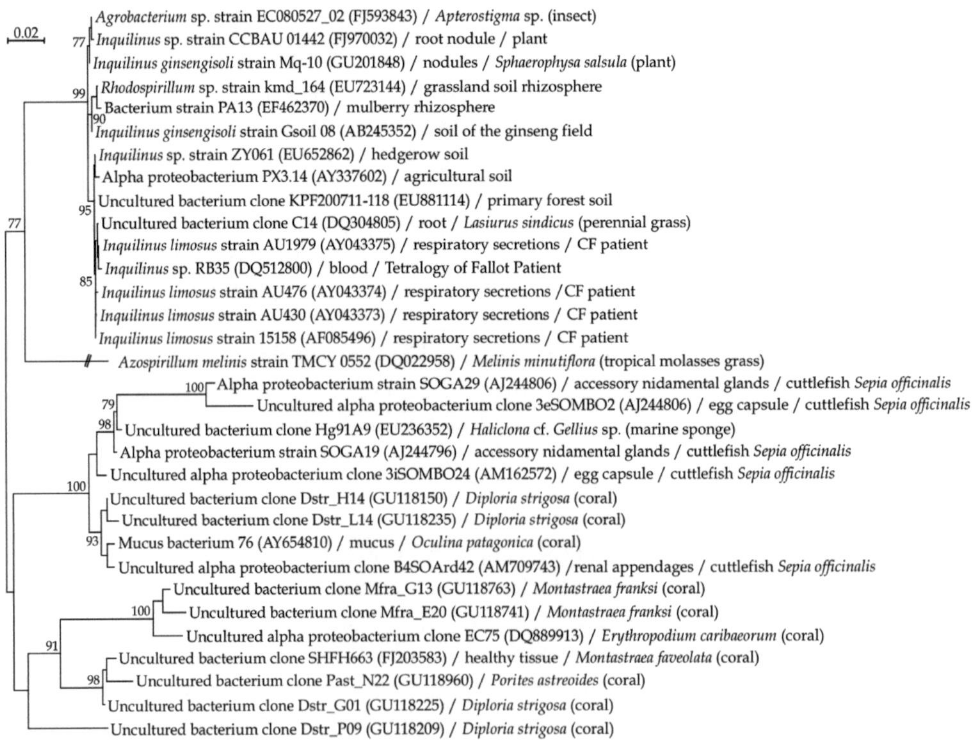

Fig. 3. Maximum-likelihood phylogenetic tree based on partial 16S rRNA gene sequences showing relationship among members of the genus *Inquilinus* and between *Inquilinus* spp. and selected close relatives from the family *Rhodospirillaceae*. Genbank accession numbers, isolation source and host follow sequence names. Numbers at nodes indicate percentage bootstrap support, based on analysis of 100 replicates. They are indicated for major nodes when >70. Bar, 0.02 substitutions per site.

We showed that the manner that CFRT niche drive the speciation and the adaptative evolution of bacteria is not univocal. However, the CFRT formed an abnormal human niche with basic conditions that allow the installation of environmental bacteria generally unrelated to human beings. Bacteria associated with CFRT, occupy two types of anatomical regions: i) the lower regions of the respiratory tract that are normally free of bacteria ii) the upper regions of the respiratory tract that are normally colonized by a resident microbiota. In CFRT, both dysbiosis and colonization by atypical environmental bacteria lead to a modified ecosystem where bacterial interactions may be unbalanced. The CFRT could be considered as an ecosystem with an emerging community where many bacteria belonging to different phyla interact and exchange genes at an increased rate. Lateral gene exchange is recognized as main innovation source for bacteria. They can acquire new genomic repertoires from which clonal specialists could emerge. Hotspots of interaction and exchange such as amoeba and rhizosphere have been previously described (Berg *et al.*, 2005; Saisongkorh *et al.*, 2010). The hypothesis that CFRT could play this role is reinforced by the number of atypical bacteria observed in this niche and by the probable emergence of specific sub-populations or species. Thus, emergence of opportunistic human pathogens from environmental origin may be first recognized from the CF airways model, a niche for bacterial adaptation and emergence (Yang *et al.*, 2011b).

7. Conclusion

Atypical bacteria are increasingly recognized in CF. These bacteria may be considered as emerging from both biological and methodological points of view in CF. Recognition of these atypical bacteria should be encouraged in the perspective of a more complete description of their prevalence, relative importance of encountered species, antimicrobial susceptibility patterns and clinical relevance.

Despite some candidate pathogens were proposed, the role of these atypical bacteria in the disease evolution is unknown. More than considering individual pathogenic species, the diversity of the microbiota is more and more considered as an important marker in the evolution of the disease. Klepac-Ceraj *et al.* recently suggested that community composition might be a better predictor of disease progression than the presence of *P. aeruginosa* alone (Klepac-Ceraj *et al.*, 2010) and van der Gast *et al.* showed that taxa richness decreased with a reduction in lung function (van der Gast *et al.*, 2011). From this point of view, each taxon contributing to increase the global diversity of the microbiota appeared important whatever its identification.

Finally, whether these species may interact with other members of the CFRT microbiota and with more common pathogens to influence the onset and/or the evolution of colonization/infection by typical pathogens like *P. aeruginosa* are great questions for future advances in CF-associated infectious diseases.

8. Acknowledgments

The authors sincerely thank Dr Corinne Teyssier and Fabien Aujoulat for their help with data summary. We are also very grateful to Linda Aleyrangues, Marie-Pierre Servent and Isabelle Zorgniotti for their excellent technical assistance in isolating and identifying atypical bacteria. Finally, we thank Dr Raphaël Chiron, pulmonary physician specialist for CF, for fruitful collaboration.

9. References

Alauzet, C.; Teyssier, C.; Jumas-Bilak, E.; Gouby, A.; Chiron, R.; Rabaud, C.; Counil, F.; Lozniewski, A. & Marchandin, H. (2010). *Gluconobacter* as well as *Asaia* species, newly emerging opportunistic human pathogens among acetic acid bacteria. *Journal of Clinical Microbiology*, Vol.48, No.11, (November 2010), pp. 3935-3942, ISSN 1098-660X

Atkinson, RM.; Lipuma, JJ.; Rosenbluth, DB. & Dunne, WM Jr. (2006). Chronic colonization with *Pandoraea apista* in cystic fibrosis patients determined by repetitive-element-sequence PCR. *Journal of Clinical Microbiology*, Vol.44, No.3, (March 2006), pp. 833-836, ISSN 1098-660X

Aujoulat, F.; Jumas-Bilak, E.; Masnou, A.; Sallé, F.; Faure, D.; Segonds, C.; Marchandin, H. & Teyssier, C. (2011). Multilocus sequence-based analysis delineates a clonal population of *Agrobacterium (Rhizobium) radiobacter (Agrobacterium tumefaciens)* of human origin. *Journal of Bacteriology*, Vol.193, No.10, (May 2011), pp. 2608-2618, ISSN 1098-5530

Baïda, N.; Yazourh, A.; Singer, E. & Izard, D. (2001). *Pseudomonas brenneri* sp. nov., a new species isolated from natural mineral waters. *Research in Microbiology*, Vol.152, No.5, (June 2001), pp. 493-502, ISSN 0923- 2508

Beringer, PM. & Appleman, MD. (2000). Unusual respiratory bacterial flora in cystic fibrosis: microbiologic and clinical features. *Current Opinion in Pulmonary Medicine*, Vol.6, No.6, (November 2000), pp. 545-550, ISSN 1531-6971

Berg, G.; Eberl, L. & Hartmann, A. (2005). The rhizosphere as a reservoir for opportunistic human pathogenic bacteria. *Environmental Microbiology*, Vol.7, No.11, (November 2005), pp. 1673-1685, ISSN 1462-2920

Bittar, F.; Reynaud-Gaubert, M.; Thomas, P.; Boniface, S.; Raoult, D. & Rolain JM. (2008). *Acetobacter indonesiensis* pneumonia after lung transplant. *Emerging Infectious Diseases*, Vol.14, No.6, (June 2008), pp. 997-998, ISSN 1080-6059

Bittar, F.; Richet, H.; Dubus, JC.; Reynaud-Gaubert, M.; Stremler, N.; Sarles, J.; Raoult, D. & Rolain, JM. (2008). Molecular detection of multiple emerging pathogens in sputa from cystic fibrosis patients. *Public Library of Science One*, Vol.3, No.8, (August 2008), e2908, ISSN 1932-6203

Bittar, F.; Stremler, N.; Audié, JP.; Dubus, JC.; Sarles, J.; Raoult, D. & Rolain, JM. (2010). *Nocardia farcinica* lung infection in a patient with cystic fibrosis: a case report. *Journal of Medical Case Reports*, Vol.4, (March 2010), p. 84, ISSN 1752-1947

Brockhurst, MA.; Buckling, A. & Rainey, PB. (2005) The effect of a bacteriophage on diversification of the opportunistic bacterial pathogen, *Pseudomonas aeruginosa*. *Proceedings in Biological Sciences*, Vol.272, No.1570 (July 2005), pp. 1385-1391, ISSN 1471-2954.

Cantón, R.; Morosini, MI.; Ballestero, S.; Alvarez, ME.; Escobar, H.; Máiz, L & Baquero, F. (1997). Lung colonization with *Enterobacteriaceae* producing extended-spectrum beta-lactamases in cystic fibrosis patients. *Pediatric Pulmonology*, Vol.24, No.3, (September 1997), pp. 213-217, ISSN 1099-0496

Cantón, R. & Coque, TM. (2006). The CTX-M beta-lactamase pandemic. *Current Opinion in Microbiology*, Vol.9, No.5, (October 2006), pp. 466-75, ISSN 1879-0364

Chang, YH.; Han, JI.; Chun, J.; Lee, KC.; Rhee, MS.; Kim, YB. & Bae, KS. (2002). *Comamonas koreensis* sp. nov., a non-motile species from wetland in Woopo, Korea. *International*

Journal of Systematic and Evolutionary Microbiology, Vol.52, No.2, (March 2002), pp. 377-381, ISSN 1466-5034

Chen, CY.; Hansen, KS. & Hansen, LK. (2008). *Rhizobium radiobacter* as an opportunistic pathogen in central venous catheter associated bloodstream infection: case report and review. *Journal of Hospital Infection*, Vol.68, No.3, (March 2008), pp. 203-207, ISSN 1532-2939

Chiron, R.; Marchandin, H.; Counil, F.; Jumas-Bilak, E.; Freydière, A-M.; Bellon, G.; Husson, M-O.; Turck, D.; Brémont, F.; Chabanon, G. & Segonds, C. (2005). Clinical and microbiological features of *Inquilinus* sp. isolates from five patients with cystic fibrosis. *Journal of Clinical Microbiology*, Vol.43, No.8, (August 2005), pp. 3938-3943, ISSN 1098-660X

Cieslak, TJ.; Drabick, CJ. & Robb, ML. (1996). Pyogenic infections due to *Ochrobactrum anthropi*. Clinical Infectious Diseases, Vol.22, No.5, (May 1996), pp. 845-847, ISSN 1537-6591.

Cleenwerck, I.; Gonzalez, A.; Camu, N.; Engelbeen, K.; De Vos, P.& De Vuyst, L. (2008). *Acetobacter fabarum* sp. nov., an acetic acid bacterium from a Ghanaian cocoa bean heap fermentation. *International Journal of Systematic and Evolutionary Microbiology*, Vol.58, No.9, (September 2008), pp. 2180-2185, ISSN 1466-5034

Coenye, T.; Falsen, E.; Hoste, B.; Ohlén, M.; Goris, J.; Govan, JR.; Gillis, M. & Vandamme, P. (2000). Description of *Pandoraea* gen. nov. with *Pandoraea apista* sp. nov., *Pandoraea pulmonicola* sp. nov., *Pandoraea pnomenusa* sp. nov., *Pandoraea sputorum* sp. nov. and *Pandoraea norimbergensis* comb. nov. *International Journal of Systematic and Evolutionary Microbiology*, Vol.50, No.2, (March 2000), pp. 887-899, ISSN 1466-5034

Coenye, T.; Goris, J.; Spilker, T.; Vandamme, P. & LiPuma, JJ. (2002). Characterization of unusual bacteria isolated from respiratory secretions of cystic fibrosis patients and description of *Inquilinus limosus* gen. nov., sp. nov *Journal of Clinical Microbiology*, Vol.40, No.6, (June 2002), pp. 2062-2069, ISSN 1098-660X

Coenye, T.; Spilker, T.; Reik, R.; Vandamme, P. & Lipuma, JJ. (2005). Use of PCR analyses to define the distribution of *Ralstonia* species recovered from patients with cystic fibrosis. *Journal of Clinical Microbiology*, Vol.43, No.7, (July 2005), pp. 3463-3466, ISSN 1098-660X

Coyne, S.; Courvalin, P. & Galimand, M. (2010). Acquisition of multidrug resistance transposon Tn*6061* and IS*6100*-mediated large chromosomal inversions in *Pseudomonas aeruginosa* clinical isolates. *Microbiology*,Vol.156, No.5, (May 2010), pp. 1448-1458, ISSN 1465-2080

Degand, N.; Carbonnelle, E.; Dauphin, B.; Beretti, JL.; Le Bourgeois, M.; Sermet-Gaudelus, I.; Segonds, C.; Berche, P.; Nassif, X. & Ferroni, A. (2008). Matrix-assisted laser desorption ionization-time of flight mass spectrometry for identification of nonfermenting gram-negative bacilli isolated from cystic fibrosis patients. *Journal of Clinical Microbiology*, Vol.46, No.10, (October 2008), pp. 3361-3367, ISSN 1098-660X

Dempsey, KE.; Riggio, MP.; Lennon, A.; Hannah, VE.; Ramage, G.; Allan, D. & Bagg, J. (2007). Identification of bacteria on the surface of clinically infected and non-infected prosthetic hip joints removed during revision arthroplasties by 16S rRNA gene sequencing and by microbiological culture. *Arthritis Research and Therapy*, Vol.9, No.3, (May 2007), R46, ISSN 1478-6354

Duan, K.; Dammel, C.; Stein, J.; Rabin, H. & Surette, MG. (2003). Modulation of *Pseudomonas aeruginosa* gene expression by host microflora through interspecies communication. *Molecular Microbiology*, Vol.50, No.5, (December 2003), pp. 1477-1491, ISSN 1365-2958

Dunne, WM. Jr; Tillman, J. & Murray, JC. (1993). Recovery of a strain of *Agrobacterium radiobacter* with a mucoid phenotype from an immunocompromised child with bacteremia. *Journal of Clinical Microbiology*, Vol.31, No.9, (September 1993), pp. 2541-2543, ISSN 1098-660X

Edmond, MB.; Riddler, SA.; Baxter, CM.; Wicklund, BM. & Pascuile, AW. (1993). *Agrobacterium radiobacter* a recently recognized opportunistic pathogen. *Clinical Infectious Diseases*, Vol.16, No.3, (March 1993), pp. 388-391, ISSN 1537-6591

Ferreira, L.; Sánchez-Juanes, F.; García-Fraile, P.; Rivas, R.; Mateos, PF.; Martínez-Molina, E.; González-Buitrago, JM. & Velázquez, E. (2011). Maldi-tof mass spectrometry is a fast and reliable platform for identification and ecological studies of species from family *rhizobiaceae*. *Public Library of Science One*, Vol.6, No.5, (May 2011), e20223, ISSN 1932-6203

Field, TR.; Sibley, CD.; Parkins, MD.; Rabin, HR. & Surette, MG. (2010). The genus *Prevotella* in cystic fibrosis airways. *Anaerobe*, Vol.16, No.4, (August 2010), pp. 337-344, ISSN 1075-9964

Foweraker, J. (2009). Recent advances in the microbiology of respiratory tract infection in cystic fibrosis. *British Medical Bulletin*, Vol.89, (January 2009), pp. 93-110, ISSN 1468-5833

Frank, DN.; St Amand, AL.; Feldman, RA.; Boedeker, EC.; Harpaz, N. & Pace, NR. (2007). Molecular-phylogenetic characterization of microbial community imbalances in human inflammatory bowel diseases. *Proceedings of the National Academy of Sciences of the United States of America*, Vol.104, No.34, (August 2007), pp. 13780-13785, ISSN 1091-6490

Fritsche, K.; Auling, G.; Andreesen, JR. & Lechner, U. (1999). *Defluvibacter lusatiae* gen. nov., sp. nov., a new chlorohenol-degrading member of the alpha-2 subgroup of proteobacteria. *Systematic and Applied Microbiology*, Vol.22, No.2, (May 1999), pp. 197-204, ISSN 0723-2020

Ghosh, W.; Bagchi, A.; Mandal, S.; Dam, B. & Roy, P. (2005). *Tetrathiobacter kashmirensis* gen. nov., sp. nov., a novel mesophilic, neutrophilic, tetrathionate-oxidizing, facultatively chemolithotrophic betaproteobacterium isolated from soil from a temperate orchard in Jammu and Kashmir, India. *International Journal of Systematic and Evolutionary Microbiology*, Vol.55, No.5, (September 2005), pp. 1779-1787, ISSN 1466-5034

Gneiding, K.; Frodl, R. & Funke, G. Identities of *Microbacterium* spp. encountered in human clinical specimens. (2008). *Journal of Clinical Microbiology*, Vol.46, No.11, (November 2008), pp. 3646-3652, ISSN 1098-660X

Grice, EA.; Kong, HH.; Conlan, S.; Deming, CB.; Davis, J.; Young, AC.; NISC Comparative Sequencing Program; Bouffard, GG.; Blakesley, RW.; Murray, PR.; Green, ED.; Turner, ML. & Segre, JA. (2009). Topographical and temporal diversity of the human skin microbiome. *Science*, Vol.324, No.5931, (May 2009), pp. 1190-1192, ISSN 1095-9203

Grice, EA.; Snitkin, ES.; Yockey, LJ.; Bermudez, DM.; NISC Comparative Sequencing Program; Liechty, KW. & Segre, JA. (2010). Longitudinal shift in diabetic wound microbiota correlates with prolonged skin defense response. *Proceedings of the National Academy of Sciences of the United States of America*, Vol.107, No.33, (August 2010), pp. 14799-14804, ISSN 1091-6490

Guss, AM.; Roeselers, G.; Newton, IL.; Young, CR.; Klepac-Ceraj, V.; Lory, S. & Cavanaugh, CM. (2011). Phylogenetic and metabolic diversity of bacteria associated with cystic fibrosis. *ISME Journal*, Vol.5, No.1 (January 2011), pp. 20-29, ISSN 1751-7370

Hall V. (2008). *Actinomyces*--gathering evidence of human colonization and infection. *Anaerobe*, Vol.14, No.1, (February 2008), pp. 1-7, ISSN 1075-9964

Hantsis-Zacharov, E.; Senderovich, Y. & Halpern, M. (2008). *Chryseobacterium bovis* sp. nov., isolated from raw cow's milk. *International Journal of Systematic and Evolutionary Microbiology*, Vol.58, No.4, (April 2008), pp. 1024-1028, ISSN 1466-5034

Harris, JK.; De Groote, MA.; Sagel, SD.; Zemanick, ET.; Kapsner, R.; Penvari, C.; Kaess, H.; Deterding, RR.; Accurso, FJ. & Pace, NR. (2007). Molecular identification of bacteria in bronchoalveolar lavage fluid from children with cystic fibrosis. *Proceedings of the National Academy of Sciences of the United States of America*, Vol.104, No.51, (December 2007), pp. 20529-20533, ISSN 1091-6490

Hauser, AR.; Jain, M.; Bar-Meir, M. & McColley, SA. (2011). Clinical significance of microbial infection and adaptation in cystic fibrosis. *Clinical Microbiology Reviews*, Vol.24, No.1, (January 2011), pp. 29-70, ISSN 1098-6618

Hayes, D Jr.; Murphy, BS.; Kuhn, RJ.; Anstead, MI. & Feola, DJ. (2009). Mucoid *Inquilinus limosus* in a young adult with cystic fibrosis. *Pediatric Pulmonology*, Vol.44, No.6, (June 2009), pp. 619-621, ISSN 1099-0496

Herasimenka, Y.; Cescutti, P.; Impallomeni, G. & Rizzo R. (2007). Exopolysaccharides produced by *Inquilinus limosus*, a new pathogen of cystic fibrosis patients: novel structures with usual components. Carbohydrate Research, Vol.342, No.16, (November 2007), pp. 2404-2415, ISSN 0008-6215

Hogardt, M.; Ulrich, J.; Riehn-Kopp, H. & Tümmler, B. (2009). EuroCareCF quality assessment of diagnostic microbiology of cystic fibrosis isolates. *Journal of Clinical Microbiology*, Vol.47, No.11, (November 2009), pp. 3435-3438, ISSN 1098-660X

Hyman, RW.; Fukushima, M.; Diamond, L.; Kumm.; Giudice, LC. & Davis, RW. (2005). Microbes on the human vaginal epithelium. *Proceedings of the National Academy of Sciences of the United States of America*, Vol.102, No.22, (May 2005), pp. 7952-7957, ISSN 1091-6490

Jewes, LA. & Spencer RC. (1990). The incidence of anaerobes in the sputum of patients with cystic fibrosis. *Journal of Medical Microbiology*, Vol.31, No.4, (April 1990), pp. 271-274, ISSN 1473-5644

Jones, AM. (2011). Anaerobic bacteria in cystic fibrosis: pathogens or harmless commensals? *Thorax*, Vol.66, No.7, (July 2011), pp. 558-599, ISSN 1468-3296

Jumas-Bilak, E.; Chiron, R.; Michon, AL.; Filleron, A.; Aleyrangues, L.; Teyssier, C. & Marchandin, H. (2011). CF airways, a particular ecological niche for bacterial species as-yet non-reported in man. 34th European Cystic Fibrosis Conference, Hamburg, Germany, June 2011

Jung, HM.; Lee, JS.; Bae, HM.; Yi, TH.; Kim, SY.; Lee, ST. & Im, WT. (2011). *Inquilinus ginsengisoli* sp. nov., isolated from soil of a ginseng field. *International Journal of*

Systematic and Evolutionary Microbiology, Vol.61, No.1, (January 2011), pp. 201-204, ISSN 1466-5034

Kämpfer P.; Avesani, V.; Janssens, M.; Charlier, J.; De Baere, T. & Vaneechoutte, M. (2006). Description of *Wautersiella falsenii* gen. nov., sp. nov., to accommodate clinical isolates phenotypically resembling members of the genera *Chryseobacterium* and *Empedobacter*. *International Journal of Systematic and Evolutionary Microbiology*, Vol.56, No.10, (October 2006), pp. 2323-2329, ISSN 1466-5034

Kämpfer, P.; Meurer, U.; Esser, M.; Hirsch, T. & Busse, HJ. (2007). *Sphingomonas pseudosanguinis* sp. nov., isolated from the water reservoir of an air humidifier. *International Journal of Systematic and Evolutionary Microbiology*, Vol.57, No.6, (June 2007), pp. 1342-1345, ISSN 1466-5034

Kämpfer, P.; Scholz, HC.; Huber, B.; Falsen, E. & Busse, H. (2007). *Ochrobactrum haematophilum* sp. nov. and *Ochrobactrum pseudogrignonense* sp. nov., isolated from human clinical specimens. *International Journal of Systematic and Evolutionary Microbiology*, Vol.57, No.11, (November 2007), pp. 2513-2518, ISSN 1466-5034

Kiratisin, P.; Koomanachai, P.; Kowwigkai, P.; Pattanachaiwit, S.; Aswapokee, N. & Leelaporn, A. (2006). Early-onset prosthetic valve endocarditis caused by *Inquilinus* sp. *Diagnostic Microbiology and Infectious Disease*, Vol.56, No.3, (November 2006), pp. 317-320, ISSN 0732-8893

Klepac-Ceraj, V.; Lemon, KP.; Martin, TR.; Allgaier, M.; Kembel, SW.; Knapp, AA.; Lory, S.; Brodie, EL.; Lynch, SV.; Bohannan, BJ.; Green, JL.; Maurer, BA. & Kolter, R. (2010). Relationship between cystic fibrosis respiratory tract bacterial communities and age, genotype, antibiotics and *Pseudomonas aeruginosa*. *Environmental Microbiology*, Vol.12, No.5, (May 2010), pp. 1293-1303, ISSN 1462-2920

Kolak, M.; Karpati, F.; Monstein, HJ. & Jonasson, J. (2003). Molecular typing of the bacterial flora in sputum of cystic fibrosis patients. *International Journal of Medical Microbiology*, Vol.293, No.4, (August 2003), pp. 309-317, ISSN 1438-4221

Korade, DL. & Fulekar, MH. (2009). Rhizosphere remediation of chlorpyrifos in mycorrhizospheric soil using ryegrass. *Journal of Hazardous Materials*, Vol.172, No.2-3, (December 2009), pp.1344-50, ISSN 1873-3336

Lambiase, A.; Catania, MR. & Rossano, F. (2010). Anaerobic bacteria infection in cystic fibrosis airway disease. *New Microbiologica*, Vol.33, No.3, (July 2010), pp. 185-194, ISSN 1121-7138

Lin, YT.; Jeng, YY.; Lin, ML.; Yu, KW.; Wang, FD. & Liu, CY. (2010). Clinical and microbiological characteristics of *Chryseobacterium indologenes* bacteremia. *Journal of Microbiology, Immunology and Infection*, Vol.43, No.6, (December 2010), pp. 498-505, ISSN 1995-9133

Matsui, T.; Shinzato, N.; Tamaki, H.; Muramatsu, M. & Hanada, S. (2009). *Shinella yambaruensis* sp. nov., a 3-methyl-sulfolane-assimilating bacterium isolated from soil. *International Journal of Systematic and Evolutionary Microbiology*, Vol.59, No.3, (March 2009), pp. 536-539, ISSN 1466-5034

Menuet, M.; Bittar, F.; Stremler, N.; Dubus, JC.; Sarles, J.; Raoult, D. & Rolain, J-M. (2008). First isolation of two colistin-resistant emerging pathogens, *Brevundimonas diminuta* and *Ochrobactrum anthropi*, in a woman with cystic fibrosis: a case report. *Journal of Medical Case Reports*, Vol.2, (December 2008), p. 373, ISSN 1752-1947

Mergaert, J.; Cnockaert, MC. & Swings, J. (2002). *Phyllobacterium myrsinacearum* (subjective synonym *Phyllobacterium rubiacearum*) emend. *International Journal of Systematic and Evolutionary Microbiology*, Vol.52, No.5, (September 2002), pp. 1821-1823, ISSN 1466-5034

Moreno, E. (1998). Genome evolution within the alpha Proteobacteria: why do some bacteria not possess plasmids and others exhibit more than one different chromosome? *FEMS Microbiology Reviews*, Vol.22, No.4, (October 1998), pp. 255–275, ISSN 1574-6976

Nadjar, D.; Labia, R.; Cerceau, C.; Bizet, C.; Philippon, A. & Arlet, G. (2001). Molecular characterization of chromosomal class C beta-lactamase and its regulatory gene in *Ochrobactrum anthropi*. *Antimicrobial Agents and Chemotherapy*, Vol.45, No.8, (August 2001), pp. 2324-2330, ISSN 1098-6596

Oakley, BB.; Fiedler, TL.; Marrazzo, JM. & Fredricks, DN. (2008). Diversity of human vaginal bacterial communities and associations with clinically defined bacterial vaginosis. *Applied and Environmental Microbiology*, Vol.74, No.15, (August 2008), pp. 4898-4909, ISSN 1098-5336

Otto-Karg, I.; Jandl, S.; Müller, T.; Stirzel, B.; Frosch, M.; Hebestreit, H. & Abele-Horn, M. (2009). Validation of Vitek 2 nonfermenting gram-negative cards and Vitek 2 version 4.02 software for identification and antimicrobial susceptibility testing of nonfermenting gram-negative rods from patients with cystic fibrosis. *Journal of Clinical Microbiology*, Vol.47, No.10, (October 2009), pp. 3283-3288, ISSN 1098-660X

Poole, K. (2011). *Pseudomonas aeruginosa*: resistance to the max. *Frontiers in Microbiology*, Vol.2, (April 2011), 65, ISSN 1664-302X

Poschet, J.; Perkett, E. & Deretic, V. (2002). Hyperacidification in cystic fibrosis: links with lung disease and new prospects for treatment. *Trends in Molecular Medicine*, Vol.8, No.11, (November 2002), pp. 512-519, ISSN 1471-4914

Preiswerk, B.; Ullrich, S.; Speich, R.; Bloemberg, GV. & Hombach, M. (2011). Human infection with *Delftia tsuruhatensis* isolated from a central venous catheter. *Journal of Medical Microbiology*, Vol.60, No.2, (February 2011), pp. 246-248, ISSN 1473-5644

Riggio, MP.; Lennon, A.; Rolph, HJ.; Hodge, PJ.; Donaldson, A.; Maxwell, AJ. & Bagg, J. (2008). Molecular identification of bacteria on the tongue dorsum of subjects with and without halitosis. *Oral Diseases*, Vol.14, No.3, (April 2008), pp. 251-258, ISSN 1354-523X

Rogers, GB.; Carroll, MP.; Serisier, DJ.; Hockey, PM.; Jones, G. & Bruce, KD. (2004). Characterization of bacterial community diversity in cystic fibrosis lung infections by use of 16s ribosomal DNA terminal restriction fragment length polymorphism profiling. *Journal of Clinical Microbiology*, Vol.42, No.11, (November 2004), pp. 5176-5183, ISSN 1098-660X

Rogers, GB.; Daniels, TW.; Tuck, A.; Carroll, MP.; Connett, GJ.; David, GJ. & Bruce, KD. (2009). Studying bacteria in respiratory specimens by using conventional and molecular microbiological approaches. *BMC pulmonary medicine*, Vol.9, (April 2009), 14, ISSN 1471-2466

Rogers, GB.; Skelton, S.; Serisier, DJ.; van der Gast, CJ. & Bruce KD. (2010). Determining cystic fibrosis-affected lung microbiology: comparison of spontaneous and serially induced sputum samples by use of terminal restriction fragment length polymorphism profiling. *Journal of Clinical Microbiology*, Vol.48, No.1, (January 2010), pp. 78-86, ISSN 1098-660X

Romano, S.; Aujoulat, F.; Jumas-Bilak, E.; Masnou, A.; Jeannot, JL.; Falsen, E.; Marchandin, H. & Teyssier C. (2009). Multilocus sequence typing supports the hypothesis that *Ochrobactrum anthropi* displays a human-associated subpopulation. BMC Microbiology, Vol.9, No.267 (December 2009), ISSN 1471-2180

Saisongkorh, W.; Robert, C.; La Scola, B.; Raoult, D. & Rolain, JM. (2010). Evidence of transfer by conjugation of type IV secretion system genes between *Bartonella* species and *Rhizobium radiobacter* in amoeba. *Public Library of Science One*, Vol.5, No.9, (September 2010), e12666, ISSN 1932-6203

Schlaberg, R.; Huard, RC. & Della-Latta, P. (2008). *Nocardia cyriacigeorgica*, an emerging pathogen in the United States. *Journal of Clinical Microbiology*, Vol.46, No.1, (January 2008), pp. 265-273, ISSN 1098-660X

Schmoldt, S.; Latzin, P.; Heesemann, J.; Griese, M.; Imhof, A. & Hogardt M. (2006). Clonal analysis of *Inquilinus limosus* isolates from six cystic fibrosis patients and specific serum antibody response. *Journal of Medical Microbiology*, Vol.55, No.19, (October 2006), pp. 1425-1433, ISSN 1473-5644

Sheng, WH.; Huang, YT.; Chang, SC.& Hsueh, PR. (2009). Brain abscess caused by *Tsukamurella tyrosinosolvens* in an immunocompetent patient. *Journal of Clinical Microbiology*, Vol.47, No.5, (May 2009), pp. 1602-1604, ISSN 1098-660X

Shinzato, T. & Saito, A. (1994). A mechanism of pathogenicity of "*Streptococcus milleri* group" in pulmonary infection: synergy with an anaerobe. *Journal of Medical Microbiology*, Vol.40, No.2, (February 1994), pp. 118-123, ISSN 1473-5644

Sibley, CD.; Rabin, H. & Surette, MG. (2006). Cystic fibrosis: a polymicrobial infectious disease. *Future Microbiology*, Vol.1, No.1, (June 2006), pp. 53-61, ISSN 1746-0913

Sibley, CD.; Parkins, MD.; Rabin, HR.; Duan, K.; Norgaard, JC. & Surette, MG. (2008). A polymicrobial perspective of pulmonary infections exposes an enigmatic pathogen in cystic fibrosis patients. *Proceedings of the National Academy of Sciences of the United States of America*, Vol.105, No.39, (September 2008), pp. 15070-15075, ISSN 1091-6490

Sibley, CD.; Duan, K.; Fischer, C.; Parkins, MD.; Storey, DG.; Rabin, HR. & Suretten MG. (2008). Discerning the complexity of community interactions using a *Drosophila* model of polymicrobial infections. *Public Library of Science One* Pathogens, Vol.4, No.10, (October 2008), e1000184, ISSN 1553-7374

Snyder, RW.; Ruhe, J.; Kobrin, S.; Wasserstein, A.; Doline, C.; Nachamkin, I. & Lipschutz JH. (2004). *Asaia bogorensis* peritonitis identified by 16S ribosomal RNA sequence analysis in a patient receiving peritoneal dialysis. *American Journal of Kidney Diseases*, Vol.44, No.2, (August 2004), e15-17, ISSN 1523-6838

Spilker, T.; Liwienski, AA. & LiPuma, JJ. (2008). Identification of *Bordetella* spp. in respiratory specimens from individuals with cystic fibrosis. *Clinical Microbiology and Infection*, Vol.14, No.5, (May 2008), pp. 504-506, ISSN 1469-0691

Stackebrandt, E. & Goebel, BM. (1994). Taxonomic note: a place for DNA–DNA reassociation and 16S rRNA sequence analysis in the present species definition in bacteriology. *International Journal of Systematic Bacteriology*, Vol.44, No.4, (October 1994), pp. 846-849, ISSN 0020-7713

Stackebrandt, E. & Ebers, J. (2006). Taxonomic parameters revisited: tarnished gold standards. *Microbiology Today*, Vol.33, (November 2006), pp. 152-155, ISSN 1464-0570

Teyssier, C.; Marchandin, H.; Siméon de Buochberg, M.; Ramuz, M. & Jumas-Bilak E. (2003). Atypical 16S rRNA gene copies in *Ochrobactrum intermedium* strains reveal a large genomic rearrangement by recombination between *rrn* copies. *Journal of Bacteriology*, Vol.185, No.9, (May 2003), pp. 2901-2909, ISSN 1098-5530

Teyssier, C.; Marchandin, H. & Jumas-Bilak, E. (2004). The genome of alpha-proteobacteria : complexity, reduction, diversity and fluidity. *Canadian Journal of Microbiology*, Vol.50, No.6, (June 2004), pp. 383-396, ISSN 1480-3275

Teyssier, C.; Marchandin, H.; Jean-Pierre, H.; Diego, I.; Darbas, H.; Jeannot, JL.; Gouby, A. & Jumas-Bilak, E. (2005). Molecular and phenotypic features for identification of the opportunistic pathogens *Ochrobactrum* spp. *Journal of Medical Microbiology*, Vol.54, No.10, (October 2005), pp. 945-953, ISSN 1473-5644

Teyssier, C.; Marchandin, H.; Jean-Pierre, H.; Masnou, A.; Dusart, G. & Jumas-Bilak E. (2007). *Ochrobactrum pseudintermedium* sp. nov., a novel member of the family *Brucellaceae*, isolated from human clinical samples. *International Journal of Systematic and Evolutionary Microbiology*, Vol.57, No.5, (May 2007), pp. 1007-1013, ISSN 1466-5034

Teyssier, C.; Jumas-Bilak, E.; Counil, F.; Masnou, A.; Aleyranges, L.; Chiron, R. & Marchandin H. (2009). *Ochrobactrum* and *Agrobacterium* spp.: emerging opportunistic pathogens in cystic fibrosis patients? 32nd European Cystic Fibrosis Conference, Brest, France, June 2009

Teyssier, C. & Jumas-Bilak, E. (2011). *Ochrobactrum*, In: *Molecular detection of human bacterial pathogens*, Liu D., pp. 659-670, CRC press, ISBN 978-1-4398-1238-9, USA

Teyssier, C.; Kypraios, S.; Aujoulat, F.; Chiron, R.; Jumas-Bilak, E. & Marchandin H. (2011). Remarkable persistence of genomically stable isolates of *Inquilinus* sp. in the respiratory tract of a cystic fibrosis patient. 4th congress of the Federation of European Microbiological Societies, Genève, Switzerland, June 2011

Thoma, B.; Straube, E.; Scholz, HC.; Al Dahouk, S.; Zöller, L.; Pfeffer, M.; Neubauer, H. & Tomaso, H. (2009). Identification and antimicrobial susceptibilities of *Ochrobactrum* spp. *International Journal of Medical Microbiology*, Vol.299, No.3, (March 2009), pp. 209-220, ISSN 1438-4221

Tunney, MM.; Field, TR. & Moriarty, TF. (2008). Detection of anaerobic bacteria in high numbers in sputum from patients with cystic fibrosis. *American Journal of Respiratory and Critical Care Medicine*, Vol.177, No.9, (May 2008), pp. 995-1001, ISSN 1535-4970

van Belkum, A.; Renders, NH.; Smith, S.; Overbeek, SE. & Verbrugh, HA. (2000). Comparison of conventional and molecular methods for the detection of bacterial pathogens in sputum samples from cystic fibrosis patients. *FEMS immunology and medical microbiology*, Vol.27, No.1, (January 2000), pp. 51-57, ISSN 1574-695X

van der Gast, CJ.; Walker, AW.; Stressmann, FA.; Rogers, GB.; Scott, P.; Daniels, TW.; Carroll, MP.; Parkhill, J. & Bruce, KD. (2011). Partitioning core and satellite taxa from within cystic fibrosis lung bacterial communities. *The ISME journal*, Vol.5, No.5, (May 2011), pp. 780-789, ISSN 1751-7370 van Mansfeld, R.; Jongerden, I.; Bootsma, M.; Buiting, A.; Bonten, M. & Willems, R. (2010). The population genetics of *Pseudomonas aeruginosa* isolates from different patient populations exhibits high-level host specificity. *Public Library of Science One*, Vol.5, No.10, (October 2010), e13482, ISSN 1932-6203

Worlitzsch, D.; Rintelen, C.; Böhm, K.; Wollschläger, B.; Merkel, N.; Borneff-Lipp, M. & Döring, G. (2009). Antibiotic-resistant obligate anaerobes during exacerbations of cystic fibrosis patients. *Clinical Microbiology and Infection*, Vol.15, No.5, (May 2009), pp. 454-460, ISSN 1469-0691

Wright, GD. (2010). Antibiotic resistance in the environment: a link to the clinic? *Current Opinion in Microbiology*, Vol.13, No.5, (October 2010), pp. 589-594. ISSN 1879-0364

Yagüe-Muñoz, A.; Gregori-Roig, P.; Valls-López, S. & Pantoja-Martínez, J. (2010). *Ochrobactrum anthropi* bacteremia in a child with cystic fibrosis. *Enfermedades Infecciosas y Microbiología Clínica*, Vol.28, No.2, (February 2010), pp. 137-138, ISSN 0213-005X

Yamada, Y. & Yukphan P. (2008). Genera and species in acetic acid bacteria. *International Journal of Food Microbiology*, Vol.125, No.1, (June 2008), pp. 15–24, ISSN 0168-1605

Yang, L.; Jelsbak, L.; Marvig, RL.; Damkiær, S.; Workman, CT.; Rau, MH.; Hansen, SK.; Folkęsson, A.; Johansen, HK.; Ciofu; O.; Høiby, N.; Sommer, MO. & Molin, S. (2011). Evolutionary dynamics of bacteria in a human host environment. *Proceedings of the National Academy of Sciences of the United States of America*, Vol.108, No.18, (May 2011), pp. 7481-7486, ISSN 1091-6490

Yang, L.; Jelsbak, L. & Molin, S. (2011). Microbial ecology and adaptation in cystic fibrosis airways. *Environmental Microbiology*, Vol.13, No.7, (July 2011), pp. 1682-1689, ISSN 1462-2920

Young, CC.; Arun, AB.; Lai, WA.; Chen, WM.; Chou, JH.; Shen, FT.; Rekha, PD. & Kämpfer P. (2008). *Chromobacterium aquaticum* sp. nov., isolated from spring water samples. *International Journal of Systematic and Evolutionary Microbiology*, Vol.58, No.4, (April 2008), pp.877-880, ISSN 1466-5034

11

Viral Respiratory Tract Infections in Cystic Fibrosis

Dennis Wat
Adult Cystic Fibrosis Unit, Papworth Hospital, Cambridge, United Kingdom

1. Introduction

Cystic Fibrosis (CF) is the most commonly inherited potentially lethal disease amongst Caucasian children and young adults. In Europe, approximately 35,000 children and adults are affected by CF. The prevalence in the US and in Canada is approximately 30,000 and 3,000, respectively. CF is an autosomal recessive disorder and is caused by mutations in the Cystic Fibrosis Transmembrane Conductance Regulator gene (CFTR) (Riordan, Rommens et al. 1989). The main function of CFTR in many tissues is to regulate and participate in the transport of chloride ions across epithelial cell membranes. To date, more than 1,800 mutations have been described in this gene, but the most common mutation worldwide is caused by deletion of phenylalanine at position 508 (Delta F508) of the CFTR on chromosome 7. The dramatic improvement in survival from CF has taken great strides over the past 40 years with the introduction of specialist centre care, optimising nutritional status and preventing pulmonary inflammation. The median survival of children born in the 1990s is estimated to exceed 40 years of age with more than 85% of them achieving adulthood. CF is a multisystem disorder and is characterised by chronic suppurative lung disease and by exocrine pancreatic insufficiency which affects gastrointestinal function and causes restricted growth and maturation. CF also causes obstructive azoospermia and thus male infertility. However, in most individuals with CF the major burden is on the lungs. The absence of CFTR in airway epithelium leads to malfunction of chloride conductance and subsequent airway surface liquid (ASL) volume reduction, mucins are concentrated, the periciliary liquid depleted, and mucous clearance by ciliary and cough dependent mechanisms diminished, which leads to airflow obstruction and eventually bacterial colonisation. Bacteria implicated in the morbidity and mortality of CF include *Pseudomonas aeruginosa, Burkholderia cepacia complex, Achromobacter xylosoxidans, Staphylococcus aureus, Haemophilus influenzae, Stenotrophomonas maltophilia* and *non-tuberculous mycobacteria.* However despite the appropriate use of antibiotic therapy, chronic obstructive airway disease continues to develop in patients with CF and is the major cause of morbidity and mortality.

However, the use of appropriate antibiotic therapy has had a limited effect in slowing the progression of pulmonary disease. As a result, recent studies have hypothesised that respiratory viral infection may be a contributing factor to pulmonary exacerbations. Respiratory viruses implicated in the respiratory exacerbations of CF include *influenza A and*

B, respiratory syncytial virus (RSV), parainfluenza virus (PIV) types 1 to 4, rhinovirus, metapneumovirus, coronavirus and *adenovirus*.

The role of respiratory viruses in the aetiology of respiratory exacerbations in CF is not fully understood and may have been underestimated as many previous studies have used insensitive techniques to isolate respiratory viruses, therefore undermining their prevalence. New viral detection techniques have further enhanced the awareness of respiratory viral aetiology in CF exacerbations. A recent in vitro study illustrating the interaction of respiratory virus and *P. aeruginosa* may contribute to the pathogenesis of CF exacerbations. No doubt more work will be required in this area to further understand their relationship so as to allow the development of potential novel treatment. If respiratory viruses do lead to secondary bacterial infection in CF, this may rationalize the treatment of CF in future. Although there are commercially available vaccines and anti-virals for the prevention and treatment of respiratory viral infections, they are mainly limited to influenza viral infection. A number of studies are currently underway looking at the development of new vaccines and anti-virals, hopefully it will not be long before treatment becomes available for different types of respiratory viruses.

This chapter will provide an overview on the epidemiology of respiratory viruses in CF, the available detection techniques for viruses and their differences in sensitivities, the clinical implications of viral infection in CF, the interaction between viruses and bacteria, and the management of viral infections.

CF is the most commonly inherited, potentially lethal disease amongst Caucasian children and young adults (Mearns 1993). Pathological changes occur in all exocrine glands (Vawter and Shwachman 1979), however, in most individuals with CF the major impact is on the lungs (Oppenheimer and Esterly 1975). Chronic lung infections may start very early in the lives of patients with CF. It has been hypothesised that impaired mucociliary clearance and low airway surface liquid (ASL) volume is pivotal for the pathogenesis of lung infections. These in turn lead to impaired bacterial clearance from respiratory epithelial cells (Saiman and Siegel 2004). Pulmonary infections remain to be the greatest cause of morbidity and mortality leading to premature death in CF (Rajan and Saiman 2002).

The incidence of CF in the United Kingdom is around 1 in 2500 live births and 1 in 25 of the population carry a mutation in their CF genes (Dodge, Morison et al. 1993). CF is a multisystem disorder and is characterised by chronic suppurative lung disease and by exocrine pancreatic insufficiency which affects gastrointestinal function and causes restricted growth and maturation. CF also causes obstructive azoospermia and thus male infertility.

CF is an autosomal recessive disorder and is caused by mutations in the CFTR (Riordan, Rommens et al. 1989). The main function of CFTR in many tissues is to regulate and participate in the transport of chloride ions across epithelial cell membranes (Barasch and al-Awqati 1993). So far more than 1,800 mutations have been described in this gene (http://genet.sickkids.on.ca/cgi-bin/WebObjects/MUTATION), but the most common mutation worldwide is caused by deletion of phenylalanine at position 508 (Delta F508) of the CFTR on chromosome 7.

Survival from CF is increasing rapidly as exemplified by the median life expectancy of CF children born in 1990 to be around 40 years which is double that of 20 years ago (Elborn, Shale et al.). The prolonged life expectancy might be attributed to multi-disciplinary care, improved nutritional status, use of antibiotics and better understanding of disease pathology.

CF pulmonary exacerbations represent decreased host defences within the lungs leading to alterations in airway microbiology, airway obstruction related to increased sputum production and ventilatory failure (Goss and Burns 2007). Pulmonary exacerbations are associated with acquisition of new organisms and increased concentration of airway flora (Aaron, Ramotar et al. 2004). The presences of some organisms including S. aureus, P. aeruginosa and B. cepacia in the airways have been shown to lead to clinical deterioration (Thomassen, Demko et al. 1985; Nixon, Armstrong et al. 2001; Sawicki, Rasouliyan et al. 2008). The new acquisitions of *P. aeruginosa* in CF have been demonstrated to occur in the winter months coinciding with the peak of respiratory viral infections (Johansen and Hoiby 1992). *Influenza* is a substantial health threat, it is associated with approximately >36,000 deaths and 220,000 hospitalisations in the United States yearly (Thompson, Shay et al. 2004). The emergence of novel *influenza virus (H1N1)* further heightened the awareness of influenza-like illness. CF Pulmonary exacerbation rates have been shown to be significantly increased during the winter and are highly associated with the influenza season (Ortiz, Neuzil et al. 2010).

2. Viral respiratory infections in CF

Early studies looking at respiratory viruses in CF relied on repeated serological testing, either alone (Petersen, Hoiby et al. 1981) or in combination with viral cultures for viral detection (Wang, Prober et al. 1984; Ramsey, Gore et al. 1989; Pribble, Black et al. 1990; Armstrong, Grimwood et al. 1998; Hiatt, Grace et al. 1999). These methods are relatively insensitive and more recent studies have utilised PCR based methodologies (Smyth, Smyth et al. 1995; Collinson, Nicholson et al. 1996; Punch, Syrmis et al. 2004; Olesen, Nielsen et al. 2006; Wat, Gelder et al. 2008). All these studies produced different results in terms of prevalence of respiratory viruses in CF. The differences can be due to different methodologies. There are also likely to be differences in the populations studied as the prognosis for CF has improved with each successive birth cohort.

The viruses implicated in causing respiratory symptoms in CF include *RSV, adenovirus, PIV (Types 1 to 4) , influenza A&B, rhinovirus* (Ramsey, Gore et al. 1989; Smyth, Smyth et al. 1995; Collinson, Nicholson et al. 1996; Wat, Gelder et al. 2008) and more recently *metapneumovirus* (Garcia, Hiatt et al. 2007). RSV represents 9-58% of all reported viral infection in CF, with the highest incidence in young children (Armstrong, Grimwood et al. 1998). It is possible that RSV precipitates in the initial infection by *P. aeruginosa* of the CF airway(Petersen, Hoiby et al. 1981), the proposed mechanism of which will be discussed later. A new subtype of human *rhinovirus* was recently identified, *rhinovirus* C, and was shown by de Almeida et al (de Almeida, Zerbinati et al. 2010) that it is significantly associated with respiratory exacerbations in children with CF (Odd ratio- 1.213). *Influenza A and B* take 12-27%, but in one small study, it comprised of 77% of positive samples (Hordvik, Konig et al. 1989). *PIV* are found in lower frequencies with only one study showing a detection rate of 43% from positive samples (Petersen, Hoiby et al. 1981). *Metapneumovirus* has recently been detected in nasopharyngeal aspirates taken from hospitalised children and infants with respiratory tract infections who had signs and symptoms similar to those of RSV infection (van den Hoogen, de Jong et al. 2001). This virus is also associated with lower respiratory tract infections in patients with CF (Garcia, Hiatt et al. 2007).

It is now nearly 30 years since Wang et al (Wang, Prober et al. 1984) described the relationship between respiratory viral infections and deterioration in clinical status in CF. In this 2 year prospective study (Wang, Prober et al. 1984), viruses were identified through repeated serology and nasal lavage for viral isolation in 49 patients with CF (mean age 13.7 years). Although the CF patients had more respiratory illnesses than sibling controls (3.7 versus 1.7/year), there were no differences in virus identification rates (1.7/year). The rate of proven virus infection was significantly correlated with the decline in lung functions, radiology score, and frequency and duration of hospitalisation.

More recent studies suggest no difference in the frequency of either upper respiratory tract illness (URTI) episodes (Hiatt, Grace et al. 1999) or proven respiratory viral infections (Ramsey, Gore et al. 1989) between children with CF and healthy controls, but children with CF have significantly more episodes of lower airway symptoms than controls (Ramsey, Gore et al. 1989; Hiatt, Grace et al. 1999). Ramsey et al (Ramsey, Gore et al. 1989) prospectively compared the incidence and effect of viral infections on pulmonary function and clinical scores in 15 school-age patients with CF aged between 5 to 21 years and their healthy siblings. Over a two-year period, samples were taken at regular two monthly intervals and during acute respiratory illnesses (ARI) for pharyngeal culture and serology for respiratory viruses. There was a total of 68 ARI episodes occurred in the patients with CF and in 19 episodes there was an associated virus identified. A total of 49 infective agents were identified either during ARIs or at routine testing in the patients with CF; 14 were identified on viral isolation (*rhinovirus* on 11 occasions), whilst 35 were isolated on seroconversion (*PIV* on 12, *RSV* on 9 and *M. pneumoniae* on 6 occasions). There was no significant difference in the rate of viral infections between the patients with CF and their sibling controls, as measured either by culture or serology. The rate of viral infections was higher in younger children (both CF and controls), and the rate of decline in pulmonary function was greater in the younger children with CF with more viral infections. At the time of an ARI, the virus isolation and seroconversion (fourfold increase in titres) rates were 8.8% and 19.1%, respectively in children with CF compared to 15.0% and 15.0% respectively for the non-affected siblings. In contrast the rates of virus isolation and seroconversion at routine 2 monthly visits were 5.6% and 16.2 % respectively for children with CF and 7.7% and 20.2% respectively for the healthy siblings.

Similarly Hiatt (Hiatt, Grace et al. 1999) assessed respiratory viral infections over three winters in 22 infants less than two years of age with CF (30 patient seasons), and 27 age matched controls (28 patient seasons). The average number of acute respiratory illness per winter was the same in the control and CF groups (5.0 versus 5.0). However, only 4 of the 28 control infants had lower respiratory tract symptoms in association with the respiratory tract illness, compared with 13 out of the 30 infants with CF (Odd ratio- 4.6; 95% confidence interval 1.3 and 16.5; p-value <0.05). 7 of the infants with CF cultured *RSV*, of whom 3 required hospitalisation. In contrast, none of the controls required hospitalisation. Pulmonary function measured by rapid chest compression technique was significantly reduced in the infants with CF after the winter months and was associated with two interactions; *RSV* infection with lower respiratory tract infection and male sex with lower respiratory tract infection.

From previous reports, two viral agents appear to have the greatest effect on respiratory status in CF, namely *RSV and influenza,* possibly because the uses of viral culture and serology have underestimated the effects of rhinovirus. In younger children, *RSV* is a major pathogen resulting in an increased rate of hospitalisation. Abman et al (Abman, Ogle et al. 1991) prospectively followed up 48 children with CF diagnosed through newborn screening and documented the effect of *RSV* infection. Eighteen of the infants were admitted into hospital a total of 30 times over a mean follow-up of 28 months (range 5-59). In seven of these infants *RSV* was isolated, and their clinical course was severe with 3 requiring mechanical ventilation and 5 necessitating chronic oxygen therapy. Over the next 2 years these infants had significantly more frequent respiratory symptoms and lower Brasfield chest radiograph (Brasfield, Hicks et al. 1979) scores than *non-RSV* infected counterparts. Brasfield scores air trapping on the lateral chest film, and linear markings, nodular cystic lesions, large lesions, and general severity on the posteroanterior chest film. Twenty five points represent a normal chest radiograph with lower scores indicating increasing disease severity.

In older children and adults with CF, *influenza* seems to have the greatest effect. Pribble et al (Pribble, Black et al. 1990) assessed acute pulmonary exacerbation isolates from 54 patients with CF. Over the year of the study, 80 exacerbations were identified, of which 21 episodes were associated with an identified viral agent (*influenza A*- 5 episodes; *influenza B*- 4 episodes; *RSV*- 3 episodes) with most agents identified on serology. Compared to other respiratory viruses, infection with *influenza* was associated with a more significant drop in pulmonary function (FEV_1 declined by 26% compared with 6%). There were also a higher proportion of patients with a greater than 20% drop in FEV_1 within the *influenza* infected cohort. A retrospective study in older patients with chronic *P. aeruginosa* infection reported an acute deterioration in clinical status in association with *influenza A* virus infection (Conway, Simmonds et al. 1992).

Over a 1-year period, Smyth et al (Smyth, Smyth et al. 1995) prospectively investigated 108 patients with CF (mean age of 7.9 years) using a combination of viral immunofluorescence, culture and seroconversion (fourfold increase in titres) to identify respiratory viruses. With the exception of *rhinovirus,* a seminested reverse transcriptase PCR technique was used. During the study, 76 subjects had 157 respiratory exacerbations (1.5 episodes/patient/year) and a viral agent was identified in 44 episodes, 25 of which were *rhinovirus* and an equal distribution of other viruses identified almost always on seroconversion. Identification of a respiratory virus during the course of the year was associated with a significantly greater decline in Shwachman score (Shwachman and Kulczycki 1958) and days of intravenous antibiotics use. The Shwachman scoring system is an objective measurement of the clinical status of cystic fibrosis patients. This score is based on clinical and radiological evaluation and represented a milestone in the history of CF. Patients with scores of 90 to 100 are classified as 'excellent', 80 to 89 as 'good', 70 to 79 as 'fair', and 50 to 69 reflects a 'poor' clinical status. In addition, those children in whom a non-rhinovirus was identified had a significantly greater decrease in FEV_1 over the year of the study.

Collinson et al (Collinson, Nicholson et al. 1996) followed 48 children with CF over a 15 month period using viral cultures for viral detection, with the exception of *picornaviruses* where PCR was used. 38 children completed the study and there were 147 symptomatic upper respiratory tract infections (2.7 episodes/child/year), with samples available for 119 episodes. *Picornaviruses* were identified in 51 (43%) of these episodes, of which 21 (18%) were *rhinoviruses.* In those children old enough to perform spirometry, there were significant reduction in both FVC and FEV_1 in association with URTIs, with little difference in severity of reduction whether a picornavirus was identified or not. Maximal mean drop in FEV_1 was 16.5%, at 1-4 days after onset of symptoms, but a deficit of 10.3% persisted at 21-24 days. Those with more URTIs appeared to have greater change in total Shwachman score (Shwachman and Kulczycki 1958) and Chrispin-Norman score (Chrispin and Norman 1974) over the study. Chrispin-Norman score (Chrispin and Norman 1974)is a standardized scoring system to assess the severity of CF lung disease on chest radiograph and to allow longitudinal follow-up. Six children isolated a *P.aeruginosa* for the first time during the study, 5 at the time of a URTI and only 1 was asymptomatic at the time of first isolation. However, the data from this study has to be handled with care as the term 'upper respiratory tract illness-URTI' did not necessarily imply a positive viral isolation.

Punch et al (Punch, Syrmis et al. 2004) used a multiplex reverse transcriptase PCR (RT-PCR) assay combined with an enzyme-linked amplicon hybridization assay (ELAHA) for the identification of seven common respiratory viruses in the sputum of 38 CF patients. 53 sputum samples were collected over 2 seasons and 12 (23%) samples from 12 patients were positive for a respiratory virus (4 for *influenza B,* 3 for *parainfluenza type 1,* 3 for *influenza A* and 2 for *RSV*). There were no statistical associations between virus status and demographics, clinical variables or isolation rates for *P. aeruginosa, S. aureus or A. fumigatus.*

Olesen and colleagues (Olesen, Nielsen et al. 2006) obtained sputum/laryngeal aspirates from children with CF over a 12 month period in outpatient clinics. They achieved a viral detection rate of 16%, with *rhinovirus* being the most prevalent virus. FEV_1 was significantly reduced during viral infection (-12.5%, p=0.048), with the exception of *rhinovirus* infection. The authors were not able to demonstrate a positive correlation between respiratory viruses and bacterial infections in their studied population as the type or frequency of bacterial infection during or after viral infections were not altered. They also concluded that clinical viral symptoms had a very poor predictive value (0.39) for a positive viral test.

Wat et al (Wat, Gelder et al. 2008) utilised 'real-time' Nucleic Acid Sequenced Based Amplification to examine the role of respiratory viruses in CF. They achieved the highest detection rate of 46% amongst all existing literature concerning respiratory viruses in the CF population during reported episodes of respiratory illness. The results compare favourably with previous studies and this may be that earlier studies relied heavily on repeated serological testing, either alone(Petersen, Hoiby et al. 1981) or in combination with viral isolation (Wang, Prober et al. 1984; Ramsey, Gore et al. 1989; Pribble, Black et al. 1990; Armstrong, Grimwood et al. 1998; Hiatt, Grace et al. 1999). They also achieved a viral detection rate of 18.3% from routine nasal samples and this is comparable to the seroconversion rate of 12.3% as reported by Wang et al(Wang, Prober et al. 1984). This value is similar to the seroconversion rate of 16.2% from asymptomatic samples achieved by Ramsey and colleagues(Ramsey, Gore et al. 1989). Amongst stable asthmatic children, Johnston et al (Johnston, Pattemore et al. 1995) found a viral detection rate of 12% by PCR. Therefore, a laboratory method with a higher sensitivity for viral detection used in this study has not increased the detection rate in asymptomatic samples, implying that the high detection rate of respiratory viruses during exacerbations reinforces their pathogenicity. The authors also demonstrated that *influenza A and B* viruses are major viruses in causing respiratory exacerbations in CF and both viruses are more commonly detected during pulmonary exacerbations. 22 of 88 (23%) viruses found in this study are *influenza viruses (A & B)*. The result is consistent with majority of the previous studies which showed that *influenza* virus represented between 12 to 27% of all viruses detected. In relation to *influenza* vaccination, the uptake rate was up to 70% during the 2003/4 season (Wat, Gelder et al. 2008) and the significance is that the *influenza* detection rate in this study could easily have been higher had the vaccination uptake rate in the study not been this high.

In 2009, a novel swine pandemic *influenza A virus (H1N1)* was identified. To date very little data exists regarding its impact on patients with CF. Nash et al (Nash, Whitmill et al. 2011) showed the symptoms of CF patients infected with H1N1 tend to be mild. There was no significant reduction in FEV_1 % predicted, FVC % predicted and body mass index regardless of whether the patients were positive or negative for *H1N1*. Colombo et al (Colombo, Battezzati et al. 2011) performed a multi-centre survey showed that diagnostic testing did not identify clinical characteristics specifically associated with *H1N1* infections. Similarly, they did not show a significant decline in lung function associated with this infection.

Experimental data on the effects of viral infections in CF are limited. Toll-like receptors (TLRs) have recently been identified as key mediators of the innate response and they recognise pathogens through detection of conserved microbial structures that are absent from the host. Kurt-Jones et al (Kurt-Jones, Popova et al. 2000) found that *RSV* persisted longer in the lungs of infected TLR4-deficient mice compared to normal mice. Haynes et al (Haynes, Moore et al. 2001) also demonstrated that TLR4-deficient mice when challenged with *RSV* exhibited impaired natural killer cell trafficking and impaired virus clearance compared to normal ones. Limited human studies have demonstrated the important role of TLRs in host response against many major groups of mammalian pathogens(Qureshi and Medzhitov 2003). The relationship between TLR and respiratory virus including *RSV* in humans will require further studies before it can be established.

Some studies have suggested a higher viral replication when there is an impairment of the innate host defence in CF. *Influenza* titres were significantly increased in a mouse model which were chronically infected with *P. aeruginosa* compared to control model (Seki, Higashiyama et al. 2004). Increased virus replication was also found after *PIV* infection of CF human airway epithelial cells, compared to controls (Zheng, De et al. 2003). One of the possible causes of increased virus replication and of virus persistence might be a reduced production of respiratory nitric oxide (NO), which is a vital part of innate antiviral defence mechanism (Zheng, Xu et al. 2004). Increased production of NO protects against viral infections. In CF patients, expression of the NO producing enzyme NO synthase type 2 (NOS2) is considerably reduced.

3. Detection of respiratory viruses

The principal laboratory methods of respiratory virus diagnosis rely on their detection in respiratory secretions and another important factor in respiratory viral diagnosis is to submit an appropriate sample for testing. Inappropriate specimen collection and transport account for the largest source of error in the accuracy of viral detection results (Nutting, Main et al. 1996). Nasal swabs, nasopharyngeal aspirates, nasal wash and sputum specimens are generally considered as the specimens of choice for the detection of respiratory viruses (Hall and Douglas 1975; Schmid, Kudesia et al. 1998; Covalciuc, Webb et al. 1999; Punch, Syrmis et al. 2004). Performing a nasopharyngeal aspirate or suction can be unpleasant and requires the use of a suction device by a trained individual, which makes it unattractive in widespread clinical applications. In contrast, the collection of a nasal swab is simple, painless and quick and it does not require special equipment and skilled personnel. A prospective study by Heikkinen et al showed that the sensitivity of nasal swabs was comparable to nasopharyngeal aspirates for the detection of all major respiratory viruses by tissue culture with the exception of RSV (Heikkinen, Marttila et al. 2002). In non-sputum producing patients with CF, it has been shown that throat swab is not inferior to nasopharyngeal suction in detecting pathogens (Taylor, Corey et al. 2006).

Molecular techniques have superseded many 'conventional' methods utilised for respiratory viral detection such as viral culture and serology analysis due to their rapid turn-around of results. Traditional virus culture and serology analysis may require 1 to 2 weeks before results are available and direct antigen detection can have variable sensitivity and specificity (Swierkosz, Erdman et al. 1995). Molecular assays also have particular advantages where the starting material available is acellular (swab) or where surveillance samples have a low copy number of the viral target. The rapid turn-over of results allowing diagnostic virology to have an impact on patient management, avoiding the inappropriate prescription of antibiotics and allowing the proper use of anti-virals. It may also play an important role in infection control in the hospital setting.

More recently, Virochip has been shown to be a pan-virus microarray platform that is capable of detection of known as well as novel viruses in a single assay simultaneously (Chiu, Rouskin et al. 2006). The Virochip is very much a research tool at present, and several issues must be addressed before it can be used on a routine basis for virus detection in the clinical setting. These issues include cost, accuracy, reproducibility, and sensitivity/specificity for virus detection in comparison with traditional laboratory techniques. In addition, the implication of novel viruses in the human respiratory tract is not yet defined.

4. Interaction between respiratory viruses and bacteria

In a 25 year retrospective review from the Danish CF clinic, the first isolation of *P. aeruginosa* was most likely between October and March (Johansen and Hoiby 1992) coinciding with the peak of the *RSV* season. These findings must be interpreted with caution by the design of the study, as there are a number of other possible agents that would broadly fit the *RSV* season, most notably *influenza, rhinovirus* and *metapneumovirus*.

An increase in immunoglobulin A (IgA) antibodies to the O-antigen of *P. aeruginosa* is noted in 62% of viral infections (Przyklenk, Bauernfeind et al. 1988). This suggests a possible 'microbial synergism' between bacterial infections and infections with respiratory viruses in CF.

The first bacterial isolation of a given organism in CF has also been shown to often follow a viral infection. In the 17 month prospective study reported by Collinson et al (Collinson, Nicholson et al. 1996), five of the six first isolations of *P. aeruginosa* were made during the symptomatic phase of an upper respiratory tract infection or three weeks thereafter. In contrast only one of the six initial infections with *P. aeruginosa* was identified during the asymptomatic period. Similarly, *H. influenzae* was recovered for the first time from 3 children within 3 weeks of an upper respiratory tract infection and the one new *S. aureus* infection was identified immediately following a viral infection.

Armstrong and colleagues have reported that 50% of CF respiratory exacerbations requiring hospitalisation are associated with isolation of a respiratory virus (Armstrong, Grimwood et al. 1998). In their prospective study of repeated bronchoalveolar lavage (BAL) in infants over a 5 year period, a respiratory virus was identified in 52% of infants hospitalised for a respiratory exacerbation, most commonly *RSV*. 11 of the 31 hospitalised infants (35%) acquired *P. aeruginosa* in the subsequent 12-60 month follow up, compared to 3 of 49 (6%) non-hospitalised infants (Relative risk 5.8).

Respiratory viruses can disrupt the airway epithelium and precipitate bacterial adherence. *Influenza A* infection has been shown to cause epithelial shedding to basement membrane with submucosal oedema and neutrophil infiltrate (Walsh, Dietlein et al. 1961), while both influenza and adenovirus have a cytopathic effect on cultured nasal epithelium leading to destruction of the cell monolayer (Winther, Gwaltney et al. 1990). This epithelial damage results in an increase in the permeability of the mucosal layer (Igarashi, Skoner et al. 1993; Ohrui, Yamaya et al. 1998) and possibly facilitating bacterial adherence. Bacteria can also utilise viral glycoproteins and other virus induced receptors on host cell membrane as bacterial receptors in order to adhere to virus infected cells (Sanford, Shelokov et al. 1978; Raza, Essery et al. 1999).

Kim et al (Kim, Battaile et al. 2008) found that invariant natural killer T cells induce a type of macrophage activation driving the secretion of interleukin-13 leading to the production of globlet cell metaplasia and airway hyperactivity following infection with Sendai virus. The term 'invariant' stems from the fact that all invariant natural killer T cells in humans and mice use a unique T cell receptor that is essential for interaction with CD1d. CD1d molecules present lipid antigens to T lymphocytes rather than peptide antigens as in the case of major histocompatibility-complex (MHC) class I and II molecules. Historically, MHC class II dependent CD4 and T lymphocytes, through their response to stimulation by environmental allergens, are keys to the pathogenesis of human asthma. The findings by the authors lead to the notion of the use of anti-interleukin-13 therapy as a potential therapy in patients.

Viral infections might predispose to secondary bacterial infections by impairing mucociliary function and triggering host inflammatory receptors (Wilson and Cole 1988; Murphy and Sethi 1992). This phenomenon has been demonstrated both in vivo and in vitro (Jiang, Nagata et al. 1999; White, Gompertz et al. 2003). Avadhanula et al (Avadhanula, Rodriguez et al. 2006) showed that different respiratory viruses use different mechanisms to enhance the adherence of bacteria to respiratory epithelial cells. In particular *RSV* and *PIV type 3* upregulate intercellular adhesion molecule-1 (ICAM-1), carcinoembryonic adhesion molecule 1 (CEACAM1) and platelet activating factor receptor (PAFr) but not mucin on the surfaces of A549, BEAS-2B and NHBE but not SAE cell lines. Much of the increased bacterial adhesion following *RSV* infection could be blocked by antibodies directed against these receptors. A549 and BEAS-2B are transformed cell lines derived from type II alveolar and normal bronchial cells, respectively. NHBE and SAE cells and primary epithelial cells obtained from bronchi and distal bronchial tree and are likely to include a heterogeneous population of cells.

Mechanisms independent of the expression of conventional receptors for bacteria, such as binding to viral proteins, could be responsible for enhanced adhesion (Hament, Kimpen et al. 1999). Immunofluorescence microscopy demonstrates that bacteria binding to *RSV* infected A549 cells adhere not only to these cells expressing viral antigens but also to uninfected epithelial cells. These data suggest that the ability to augment bacterial adhesion may result from a factor served by infected cells that exert a paracrine effect on adjacent epithelium. Cytokines or other inflammatory molecules are potential good candidates for such a mediator.

Rhinovirus has been shown to potentiate bacterial infections by inhibiting the secretion of TNF alpha and interleukin-8 by macrophages in vitro following co-infection with gram negative bacterial products, lipopolysaccharide (LPS), and gram positive bacterial products, lipoteichoic acid (LTA) (Oliver, Lim et al. 2008). This rhinovirus dependent impairment of the macrophage immune response was not mediated by autocrine production of the anti-inflammatory cytokines interleukin-10 and PGE2, or by downregulation of the cell surface receptor for LTA and LPS. In addition, the authors also show that rhinovirus inhibit the phagocytosis of bacterial products by macrophages. These findings support the notion that *rhinovirus* exposure resulted in a reduced ability to innate and adaptive immune responses against bacterial products, hence promoting the occurrence of bacterial and viral co-infections.

The lower respiratory tract is protected by local mucociliary mechanisms that involve the integration of the ciliated epithelium, periciliary fluid and mucus. Mucus acts as a physical and chemical barrier onto which particles and organisms adhere. Cilia lining the respiratory tract propel the overlying mucus to the oropharynx where it is either swallowed or expectorated. *Influenza* viral infection has been shown to precipitate the loss of cilial beat, and shedding of the columnar epithelial cells generally within 48 hours of infection (Thompson, Barclay et al. 2006). Pittet et al (Pittet, Hall-Stoodley et al.) showed that a prior *influenza* infection of tracheal cells in vivo does not increase the initial number of *pneumococci* found during the first hour of infection, but it does significantly reduce mucociliary velocity, and thereby reduces *pneumococcal* clearance during the first 2 hours after *pneumococcal* infection at both 3 and 6 days after an *influenza* infection. The defects in *pneumococcal* clearance were greatest at 6 days after *influenza* infection. Changes to the tracheal epithelium induced by *influenza* virus may increase susceptibility to a secondary *S. pneumoniae* infection by increasing *pneumococcal* adherence to the tracheal epithelium and/or decreasing the clearance of *S. pneumoniae* via the mucociliary escalator of the trachea, and thus increasing the risk of secondary bacterial infection.

De Vrankrijker et al (de Vrankrijker, Wolfs et al. 2009) showed that mice that were co-infected with *RSV* and *P. aeruginosa* had a 2,000 times higher colony-forming units (CFU) counts of Pseudomonas aeruginosa in the lung homogenates compared to mice that were infected with *P. aeruginosa* alone. Co-infected mice also had more severe lung function changes. These results suggest that *RSV* can facilitate the initiation of acute *P. aeruginosa* infection.

Another study also showed that *H. influenzae* and *S. pneumoniae* bind to both free *RSV* virions and epithelial cells transfected with cell membrane-bound G protein, but not to secreted G protein. Pre-incubation with specific anti-G antibody significantly reduce bacterial adhesion to G protein-transfected cells (Avadhanula, Wang et al. 2007).

Stark et al (Stark, Stark et al. 2006) showed that mice that were exposed to *RSV* had significantly decreased *S. pneumonia, S. aureus* or *P. aeruginosa* clearance 1 to 7 days after *RSV* exposure. Mice that were exposed to both *RSV* and bacteria had a higher production of neutrophil-induced peroxide but less production of myeloperoxidase compared to mice that were exposed to *S. pneumoniae* alone. This suggests that functional changes in the recruited neutrophils may contribute to the decreased bacterial clearance.

More recently, Chattoraj et al (Chattoraj, Ganesan et al., 2011) demonstrated that acute infection of primary CF airway epithelial cells with rhinovirus liberates planktonic bacteria from biofilm. Superinfection with *rhinovirus* stimulates robust chemokine responses from CF airway epithelial cells that were pretreated with mucoid *P. aeruginosa*. The authors also showed that these chemokine responses lead to a liberation of bacteria from mucoid *P. aeruginosa* biofilm and transmigration of planktonic bacteria from the apical to the basolateral surface of mucociliary-differentiated CF airway epithelial cells. Planktonic bacteria, which are more proinflammatory than their biofilm counterparts, stimulate increased chemokine responses in CF airway epithelial cells which, in turn, may contribute to the pathogenesis of CF exacerbations and subsequent prolonged intravenous antibiotic use and hospitalisation.

Taken together, these findings suggest that respiratory viruses may lead to epithelial disruption, increased or decreased cytokine production, neutrophil influx, inhibition of macrophage phagocytosis, destruction of mucociliary escalator, increased cytokine production, and increased neutrophil induced peroxide release, indirectly facilitating bacterial infection of the airway.

5. Prevention and treatment for respiratory viruses

The existence of diverse viral serotypes in causing infection has made vaccine preparation very difficult. Frequent mutations of viral proteins of RNA viruses (for example genetic drift and shift of *influenza*) have further hampered the prevention of the illness.

Influenza associated death is between 13,000 to 20,000 per year in the winter months in the UK (Fleming 1996), though some of the deaths may be attributed to *RSV*. *Influenza* vaccines are the only commercially available vaccines against common respiratory viruses. They have been used since mid 1940s and they now have an established role in prevention of *influenza A and B* infections. Inactivated *influenza* vaccine is effective even in young children including those younger than 2 years (Heinonen, Silvennoinen et al. 2010). The waning of vaccine-induced immunity over time requires annual re-immunisation even if the vaccine antigens are unchanged.

Recent vaccines contain antigens of two *influenza A* subtypes, strains of the currently circulating *H3N2 and H1N1 (Swine flu)* subtypes, and one *influenza B* virus. The current recommendation for *influenza* vaccination in the UK is to offer it to those over the age of 65, those with chronic heart, respiratory (including CF) or renal diseases and those who are diabetic or immunosuppressed.

Wat et al (Wat, Gelder et al. 2008) recently showed that *influenza* vaccination provides protection against *influenza* acquisition in patients with CF, with 1 of 41 patients vaccinated had a positive nasal swab for influenza compared to 4 of the 22 non-vaccinated patients (p=0.046). Although *influenza* vaccination does not appear to have any impact on respiratory exacerbation rates, it does have a role in preventing live infections. In this study, respiratory exacerbation rates in the preceding 10 months before the study between the vaccinated and non-vaccinated groups were similar, indicating that these were unlikely to be the reasons influencing the decision on immunisation. The decision may be down to a combination of patient/ parent education, social background, awareness of vaccination and accessibility of vaccination.

Due to the lack of randomised controlled studies looking at the efficacy of *influenza* vaccine in CF, the Cochrane review recommends clinicians to make their own judgements on the benefits and risks of this therapy in this cohort of patients (Dharmaraj and Smyth 2009). In addition to vaccine, neuraminidase inhibitors have been shown to have a role in preventing *influenza A and B* infections (Harper, Bradley et al. 2009).

Rhinovirus has more than 100 serotypes; it is unlikely that a unifying vaccine will be developed. VP4, one of the nonenveloped capsids, is highly conserved among all of the rhinoviruses; anti-VP4 antibodies have recently been generated and been shown to have the potential for future vaccine development(Katpally, Fu et al. 2009).

The development of an *RSV vaccine* has been hampered by the experience with formalin-inactivated whole *RSV* vaccine in the 1960s, as it caused 80% of *RSV* vaccinees to become hospitalised compared with 5% of controls, as well as two fatalities (Kim, Canchola et al. 1969). Current major research work has focused on a prophylaxis using a humanised mouse monoclonal antibody, Palizivumab. In patients with CF, monthly Palizivumab injection significantly reduce the hospitalisation rate for acute respiratory illness during the *RSV* season compared to those who were not immunised ($p<0.05$). The former group also had fewer hospital days for acute respiratory illness (Giebels, Marcotte et al. 2008).

There is currently no licensed *PIV* vaccine to date. The formalin-inactivated vaccine generated in the 1960s was not able to prevent *PIV* infection and was soon abandoned. Recently, recombinant bovine *PIV type 3* and human *PIV type 3* attenuated vaccines are being evaluated in animal models as vectors for the delivery of other viral antigens such as *RSV*-G and *RSV*-F proteins. This bivalent vaccine combination provides high level of resistance to challenges with *PIV type 3* and *RSV* in animal models (Schmidt, McAuliffe et al. 2001).

The conventional methods of vaccination are via the intramuscular and subcutaneous routes. Mucosal immunisation has recently been explored as it represents an attractive manner of delivering vaccines. It is fast, simple, non-invasive and can be carried out by unskilled individuals. The use of mucosal vaccination seems logical in that most of respiratory viral infections initially start at the mucosal sites and therefore inducing local immunity.

So far, there has been inconclusive evidence to support the use of vitamin C and extracts of the plant Echinacea in common cold prevention. Daily supplementation with large doses of vitamin C does not seem to prevent common colds, however there seems to be a modest (8 to 9%) reduction in the number of symptom days in individuals with established cold symptoms, with larger doses having greater effect (Douglas, Chalker et al. 2000). In vitro studies have shown that Echinacea can activate macrophages, increase phagocytosis, enhance cytokine production (Sharma, Arnason et al. 2006), and natural killer cell activity, and improve lymphocyte and monocyte cell counts (Goel, Lovlin et al. 2005). Current data is available in the adult population and has reported positive findings both in the treatment and prevention of upper respiratory tract infection. However, variations in the design of the clinical trial and in Echinacea preparations have to be taken into account (Giles, Palat et al. 2000).

Zinc has been shown to possess anti-viral properties in vitro and different preparations of zinc have been proposed for the treatment of common cold. Postulated mechanisms in the common cold include interfering with rhinovirus protein cleavage or capsid binding to ICAM-1 in nasal epithelium (Novick, Godfrey et al. 1996). Zinc lozenges appeared to have positive effects on adults but negative effects on children in terms of duration and severity of common cold symptoms (Macknin, Piedmonte et al. 1998; Marshall 2000). Higher doses were found to have a greater impact in reduction of symptom duration and reduced symptom severity (Godfrey, Conant Sloane et al. 1992; Mossad, Macknin et al. 1996). Zinc nasal spray appears to reduce the total symptom score but has no effect on the duration of common cold (Belongia, Berg et al. 2001). Irritation by nasal sprays limits their use; they also seem to have lower concentrations in the nasopharynx (Godfrey 1988).

Amantadine has been the conventional anti-viral against *influenza*. However it is strain specific as it is only effective against *influenza A* and has common side-effects such as insomnia, poor concentration and irritability. It is now largely being replaced by neuraminidase inhibitors such as Zanamivir and Oseltamivir which are licensed for the treatment of *influenza A and B*, including *avian flu H5N1* and *swine flu H1N1*. However, Amantadine still has a role in dealing with Oseltamivir resistant H1N1 virus. In children and adults, early initiation of neuraminidase inhibitors within 48 hours of the onset of symptoms can reduce the duration of flu-like symptoms by 0.5 to 2.5 days (Shun-Shin, Thompson et al. 2009). Early use of these medications can also reduce development of complications such as pneumonia (Yu, Liao et al. 2010). The 2009 pandemic *H1N1* virus remains susceptible to neuraminidase inhibitors, and Oseltamivir has been used extensively for treatment related to this viral infection. Resistance to Oseltamivir has been reported with *H1N1* viral infection but this is mainly restricted to immunocompromised individuals (Bautista, Chotpitayasunondh et al. 2010). Zanamivir has a poor oral bioavailability, and intranasal application has been shown to be effective in treating experimental *influenz*a infection with the reduction in symptoms caused, virus shedding and development of otitis media (Hayden, Treanor et al. 1996). Intravenous use of Peramivir or Zanamivir could be lifesaving in critically ill patients with *influenza* infection (Birnkrant and Cox 2009; Harter, Zimmermann et al. 2010).

Ribavarin, a synthetic guanosine nucleoside that has a broad spectrum of antiviral activity, has been used for treatment of infections related to *RSV, metapneumovirus, and parainfluenza and influenza viruses* (Yin, Brust et al. 2009). Potential benefits of ribavarin therapy include the inhibition of RSV-specific IgE production in nasal secretions, which has been associated with the development of hypoxaemia and wheezing (Rosner, Welliver et al. 1987) and it has improved pulmonary functions (Hiatt 1990). Controlled studies also show that the use of ribavarin is effective in reducing the clinical severity score, duration of mechanical ventilation, supplemental oxygen use and days of hospitalisation (Smith, Frankel et al. 1991). Aerosolised ribavarin has been used for the treatment of *RSV* related bronchiolitis and pneumonia. Intravenous formulation could be used for treatment of severe pneumonia, caused by infection *RSV, metapneumovirus, or parainfluenza virus*, on the basis of experience in immunocompromised patients (Hopkins, McNeil et al. 2008). Bonney et al has shown that *metapneumovirus* can be successfully treated with a combination of intravenous ribavarin and immunoglobulin (Bonney, Razali et al. 2009).

Although *rhinovirus* is the major cause of colds, its vast amount of serotypes has made development of anti-virals against it problematic. 90% of *rhinovirus* serotypes gain entry into epithelial cells using ICAM-1 cellular receptors and blockade of these receptors in experimental studies have shown reduced infection severity (Turner, Wecker et al. 1999), but further study is required before this treatment option becomes widely available. Macrolide antibiotics, Bafilomycin A1 and Erythromycin have been shown to inhibit ICAM-1 epithelial expression and hypothesis about their potential as anti-inflammatory agents have yet to be definitive, as clinical proof is either negative or inconclusive (Suzuki, Yamaya et al. 2002).

Recently, an anti-rhinoviral agent known as Plecoranil, which acts by inhibiting the uncoating of Picornaviruses (Ledford, Patel et al. 2004), the RV 3C protease inhibitor, Ruprintrivir(Hayden, Turner et al. 2003) and soluble ICAM-1, Tremacamra(Turner, Wecker et al. 1999) have shown promising results in early-stage clinical trials, but each of these medications was derailed by a combination of cost, pharmacokinetics, toxicity, drug interactions, and limited efficacy (Turner 2005).

6. Conclusion

With the available knowledge regarding the impact of respiratory viruses in the exacerbation of CF, screening for respiratory viruses during pulmonary exacerbations should be implemented as part of routine clinical assessment. This assessment should include obtaining specimens from the respiratory tract and using molecular viral detection methods to reach a rapid diagnosis. The identification of respiratory viruses may allow appropriate anti-virals to be used.

With gene therapy still undergoing further research with regards to its validity and specificity, gaining further understanding in the pathogenesis of virus induced respiratory exacerbations in CF may allow the development of new therapeutic techniques. If viral infection does predispose to bacterial infection, then influencing the interaction between viruses and bacteria could be a next pathway to diminish respiratory morbidity in patients with CF. The development of novel therapies will be exciting and this may further prolong the lifespan of patients with CF and more importantly improve their quality of life.

In light of the above, future research in respiratory viruses in CF is urgently required to address a number of important questions: 1) What is the optimal way for viral sampling? 2) What is the most efficient and rapid method to detect a range of respiratory viruses? 3) How do respiratory viruses influence bacterial behaviour in chronically infected airways? 4) What is the efficacy of *influenza* vaccination in CF? 5) What are the roles of anti-virals in CF?

Further understanding in the pathogenesis of viral infection in CF would be beneficial as this may provide insight to the above unresolved mysteries. At the moment it appears that *influenza* vaccination remains the mainstay of management of viral infections in CF.

7. References

Aaron, S. D., K. Ramotar, et al. (2004). "Adult cystic fibrosis exacerbations and new strains of Pseudomonas aeruginosa." *Am J Respir Crit Care Med* 169(7): 811-5.

Abman, S. H., J. W. Ogle, et al. (1991). "Early bacteriologic, immunologic, and clinical courses of young infants with cystic fibrosis identified by neonatal screening." *J Pediatr* 119(2): 211-7.

Armstrong, D., K. Grimwood, et al. (1998). "Severe viral respiratory infections in infants with cystic fibrosis." *Pediatr Pulmonol* 26(6): 371-9.

Avadhanula, V., C. A. Rodriguez, et al. (2006). "Respiratory viruses augment the adhesion of bacterial pathogens to respiratory epithelium in a viral species- and cell type-dependent manner." *J Virol* 80(4): 1629-36.

Avadhanula, V., Y. Wang, et al. (2007). "Nontypeable Haemophilus influenzae and Streptococcus pneumoniae bind respiratory syncytial virus glycoprotein." *J Med Microbiol* 56(Pt 9): 1133-7.

Barasch, J. and Q. al-Awqati (1993). "Defective acidification of the biosynthetic pathway in cystic fibrosis." *J Cell Sci Suppl* 17: 229-33.

Bautista, E., T. Chotpitayasunondh, et al. (2010). "Clinical aspects of pandemic 2009 influenza A (H1N1) virus infection." *N Engl J Med* 362(18): 1708-19.

Belongia, E. A., R. Berg, et al. (2001). "A randomized trial of zinc nasal spray for the treatment of upper respiratory illness in adults." *Am J Med* 111(2): 103-8.

Birnkrant, D. and E. Cox (2009). "The Emergency Use Authorization of peramivir for treatment of 2009 H1N1 influenza." *N Engl J Med* 361(23): 2204-7.

Bonney, D., H. Razali, et al. (2009). "Successful treatment of human metapneumovirus pneumonia using combination therapy with intravenous ribavirin and immune globulin." *Br J Haematol* 145(5): 667-9.

Brasfield, D., G. Hicks, et al. (1979). "The chest roentgenogram in cystic fibrosis: a new scoring system." *Pediatrics* 63(1): 24-9.

Chattoraj, S. S., S. Ganesan, et al. (2011) "Rhinovirus infection liberates planktonic bacteria from biofilm and increases chemokine responses in cystic fibrosis airway epithelial cells." *Thorax* 66(4): 333-9.

Chiu, C. Y., S. Rouskin, et al. (2006). "Microarray detection of human parainfluenzavirus 4 infection associated with respiratory failure in an immunocompetent adult." *Clin Infect Dis* 43(8): e71-6.

Chrispin, A. R. and A. P. Norman (1974). "The systematic evaluation of the chest radiograph in cystic fibrosis." *Pediatr Radiol* 2(2): 101-5.

Collinson, J., K. G. Nicholson, et al. (1996). "Effects of upper respiratory tract infections in patients with cystic fibrosis." *Thorax* 51(11): 1115-22.

Colombo, C., P. M. Battezzati, et al. (2011). "Influenza A/H1N1 in patients with cystic fibrosis in Italy: a multicentre cohort study." *Thorax* 66(3): 260-1.

Conway, S. P., E. J. Simmonds, et al. (1992). "Acute severe deterioration in cystic fibrosis associated with influenza A virus infection." *Thorax* 47(2): 112-4.

Covalciuc, K. A., K. H. Webb, et al. (1999). "Comparison of four clinical specimen types for detection of influenza A and B viruses by optical immunoassay (FLU OIA test) and cell culture methods." *J Clin Microbiol* 37(12): 3971-4.

de Almeida, M. B., R. M. Zerbinati, et al. (2010). "Rhinovirus C and respiratory exacerbations in children with cystic fibrosis." *Emerg Infect Dis* 16(6): 996-9.

de Vrankrijker, A. M., T. F. Wolfs, et al. (2009). "Respiratory syncytial virus infection facilitates acute colonization of Pseudomonas aeruginosa in mice." *J Med Virol* 81(12): 2096-103.

Dharmaraj, P. and R. L. Smyth (2009). "Vaccines for preventing influenza in people with cystic fibrosis." *Cochrane Database Syst Rev*(4): CD001753.

Dodge, J. A., S. Morison, et al. (1993). "Cystic fibrosis in the United Kingdom, 1968-1988: incidence, population and survival." *Paediatr Perinat Epidemiol* 7(2): 157-66.

Douglas, R. M., E. B. Chalker, et al. (2000). "Vitamin C for preventing and treating the common cold." *Cochrane Database Syst Rev*(2): CD000980.

Elborn, J. S., D. J. Shale, et al. (1991). "Cystic fibrosis: current survival and population estimates to the year 2000." *Thorax* 46(12): 881-5.

Fleming, D. M. (1996). "The impact of three influenza epidemics on primary care in England and Wales." *Pharmacoeconomics* 9 Suppl 3: 38-45; discussion 50-3.

Garcia, D. F., P. W. Hiatt, et al. (2007). "Human metapneumovirus and respiratory syncytial virus infections in older children with cystic fibrosis." *Pediatr Pulmonol* 42(1): 66-74.

Giebels, K., J. E. Marcotte, et al. (2008). "Prophylaxis against respiratory syncytial virus in young children with cystic fibrosis." *Pediatr Pulmonol* 43(2): 169-74.

Giles, J. T., C. T. Palat, 3rd, et al. (2000). "Evaluation of echinacea for treatment of the common cold." *Pharmacotherapy* 20(6): 690-7.

Godfrey, J. C. (1988). "Zinc for the common cold." *Antimicrob Agents Chemother* 32(4): 605-6.

Godfrey, J. C., B. Conant Sloane, et al. (1992). "Zinc gluconate and the common cold: a controlled clinical study." *J Int Med Res* 20(3): 234-46.

Goel, V., R. Lovlin, et al. (2005). "A proprietary extract from the echinacea plant (Echinacea purpurea) enhances systemic immune response during a common cold." *Phytother Res* 19(8): 689-94.

Goss, C. H. and J. L. Burns (2007). "Exacerbations in cystic fibrosis. 1: Epidemiology and pathogenesis." *Thorax* 62(4): 360-7.

Hall, C. B. and R. G. Douglas, Jr. (1975). "Clinically useful method for the isolation of respiratory syncytial virus." *J Infect Dis* 131(1): 1-5.

Hament, J. M., J. L. Kimpen, et al. (1999). "Respiratory viral infection predisposing for bacterial disease: a concise review." *FEMS Immunol Med Microbiol* 26(3-4): 189-95.

Harper, S. A., J. S. Bradley, et al. (2009). "Seasonal influenza in adults and children--diagnosis, treatment, chemoprophylaxis, and institutional outbreak management: clinical practice guidelines of the Infectious Diseases Society of America." *Clin Infect Dis* 48(8): 1003-32.

Harter, G., O. Zimmermann, et al. (2010). "Intravenous zanamivir for patients with pneumonitis due to pandemic (H1N1) 2009 influenza virus." *Clin Infect Dis* 50(9): 1249-51.

Hayden, F. G., J. J. Treanor, et al. (1996). "Safety and efficacy of the neuraminidase inhibitor GG167 in experimental human influenza." *Jama* 275(4): 295-9.

Hayden, F. G., R. B. Turner, et al. (2003). "Phase II, randomized, double-blind, placebo-controlled studies of ruprintrivir nasal spray 2-percent suspension for prevention and treatment of experimentally induced rhinovirus colds in healthy volunteers." *Antimicrob Agents Chemother* 47(12): 3907-16.

Haynes, L. M., D. D. Moore, et al. (2001). "Involvement of toll-like receptor 4 in innate immunity to respiratory syncytial virus." *J Virol* 75(22): 10730-7.

Heikkinen, T., J. Marttila, et al. (2002). "Nasal swab versus nasopharyngeal aspirate for isolation of respiratory viruses." *J Clin Microbiol* 40(11): 4337-9.

Heinonen, S., H. Silvennoinen, et al. (2010). "Effectiveness of inactivated influenza vaccine in children aged 9 months to 3 years: an observational cohort study." *Lancet Infect Dis* 11(1): 23-9.

Hiatt, P. T., D Laber, L (1990). "Pulmonary function (PF) following treatment with ribavarin in infants hospitalised with RSV bronchiolitis." *Am Rev Respir Dis* 141: A624.

Hiatt, P. W., S. C. Grace, et al. (1999). "Effects of viral lower respiratory tract infection on lung function in infants with cystic fibrosis." *Pediatrics* 103(3): 619-26.

Hopkins, P., K. McNeil, et al. (2008). "Human metapneumovirus in lung transplant recipients and comparison to respiratory syncytial virus." *Am J Respir Crit Care Med* 178(8): 876-81.

Hordvik, N. L., P. Konig, et al. (1989). "Effects of acute viral respiratory tract infections in patients with cystic fibrosis." *Pediatr Pulmonol* 7(4): 217-22.

http://genet.sickkids.on.ca/cgi-bin/WebObjects/MUTATION.

Igarashi, Y., D. P. Skoner, et al. (1993). "Analysis of nasal secretions during experimental rhinovirus upper respiratory infections." *J Allergy Clin Immunol* 92(5): 722-31.

Jiang, Z., N. Nagata, et al. (1999). "Fimbria-mediated enhanced attachment of nontypeable Haemophilus influenzae to respiratory syncytial virus-infected respiratory epithelial cells." *Infect Immun* 67(1): 187-92.

Johansen, H. K. and N. Hoiby (1992). "Seasonal onset of initial colonisation and chronic infection with Pseudomonas aeruginosa in patients with cystic fibrosis in Denmark." *Thorax* 47(2): 109-11.

Johnston, S. L., P. K. Pattemore, et al. (1995). "Community study of role of viral infections in exacerbations of asthma in 9-11 year old children." *Bmj* 310(6989): 1225-9.

Katpally, U., T. M. Fu, et al. (2009). "Antibodies to the buried N terminus of rhinovirus VP4 exhibit cross-serotypic neutralization." *J Virol* 83(14): 7040-8.

Kim, E. Y., J. T. Battaile, et al. (2008). "Persistent activation of an innate immune response translates respiratory viral infection into chronic lung disease." *Nat Med* 14(6): 633-40.

Kim, H. W., J. G. Canchola, et al. (1969). "Respiratory syncytial virus disease in infants despite prior administration of antigenic inactivated vaccine." *Am J Epidemiol* 89(4): 422-34.

Kurt-Jones, E. A., L. Popova, et al. (2000). "Pattern recognition receptors TLR4 and CD14 mediate response to respiratory syncytial virus." *Nat Immunol* 1(5): 398-401.

Ledford, R. M., N. R. Patel, et al. (2004). "VP1 sequencing of all human rhinovirus serotypes: insights into genus phylogeny and susceptibility to antiviral capsid-binding compounds." *J Virol* 78(7): 3663-74.

Macknin, M. L., M. Piedmonte, et al. (1998). "Zinc gluconate lozenges for treating the common cold in children: a randomized controlled trial." *Jama* 279(24): 1962-7.

Marshall, I. (2000). "Zinc for the common cold." *Cochrane Database Syst Rev*(2): CD001364.

Mearns, M. (1993). Cystic fibrosis: the first 50 years: a review of the clinical problems anf theit management. *Cystic Fibrosis Current Topics.* J. A. Dodge, D. J. H. Brock and J. H. Widdicombe, John Wiley and Sons Ltd. 1.

Mossad, S. B., M. L. Macknin, et al. (1996). "Zinc gluconate lozenges for treating the common cold. A randomized, double-blind, placebo-controlled study." *Ann Intern Med* 125(2): 81-8.

Murphy, T. F. and S. Sethi (1992). "Bacterial infection in chronic obstructive pulmonary disease." *Am Rev Respir Dis* 146(4): 1067-83.

Nash, E. F., R. Whitmill, et al. (2011). "Clinical outcomes of pandemic (H1N1) 2009 influenza (swine flu) in adults with cystic fibrosis." *Thorax* 66(3): 259.

Nixon, G. M., D. S. Armstrong, et al. (2001). "Clinical outcome after early Pseudomonas aeruginosa infection in cystic fibrosis." *J Pediatr* 138(5): 699-704.

Novick, S. G., J. C. Godfrey, et al. (1996). "How does zinc modify the common cold? Clinical observations and implications regarding mechanisms of action." *Med Hypotheses* 46(3): 295-302.

Nutting, P. A., D. S. Main, et al. (1996). "Toward optimal laboratory use. Problems in laboratory testing in primary care." *Jama* 275(8): 635-9.

Ohrui, T., M. Yamaya, et al. (1998). "Effects of rhinovirus infection on hydrogen peroxide-induced alterations of barrier function in the cultured human tracheal epithelium." *Am J Respir Crit Care Med* 158(1): 241-8.

Olesen, H. V., L. P. Nielsen, et al. (2006). "Viral and atypical bacterial infections in the outpatient pediatric cystic fibrosis clinic." *Pediatr Pulmonol* 41(12): 1197-204.

Oliver, B. G., S. Lim, et al. (2008). "Rhinovirus exposure impairs immune responses to bacterial products in human alveolar macrophages." *Thorax* 63(6): 519-25.

Oppenheimer, E. H. and J. R. Esterly (1975). "Pathology of cystic fibrosis review of the literature and comparison with 146 autopsied cases." *Perspect Pediatr Pathol* 2: 241-78.

Ortiz, J. R., K. M. Neuzil, et al. (2010). "Influenza-associated cystic fibrosis pulmonary exacerbations." *Chest* 137(4): 852-60.

Petersen, N. T., N. Hoiby, et al. (1981). "Respiratory infections in cystic fibrosis patients caused by virus, chlamydia and mycoplasma--possible synergism with Pseudomonas aeruginosa." *Acta Paediatr Scand* 70(5): 623-8.

Pittet, L. A., L. Hall-Stoodley, et al. "Influenza virus infection decreases tracheal mucociliary velocity and clearance of Streptococcus pneumoniae." *Am J Respir Cell Mol Biol* 42(4): 450-60.

Pribble, C. G., P. G. Black, et al. (1990). "Clinical manifestations of exacerbations of cystic fibrosis associated with nonbacterial infections." *J Pediatr* 117(2 Pt 1): 200-4.

Przyklenk, B., A. Bauernfeind, et al. (1988). "Viral infections in the respiratory tract in patients with cystic fibrosis." *Serodign Immunother Infect Dis*(2): 217-25.

Punch, G., M. W. Syrmis, et al. (2004). "Method for detection of respiratory viruses in the sputa of patients with cystic fibrosis." *Eur J Clin Microbiol Infect Dis.*

Qureshi, S. T. and R. Medzhitov (2003). "Toll-like receptors and their role in experimental models of microbial infection." *Genes Immun* 4(2): 87-94.

Rajan, S. and L. Saiman (2002). "Pulmonary infections in patients with cystic fibrosis." *Semin Respir Infect* 17(1): 47-56.

Ramsey, B. W., E. J. Gore, et al. (1989). "The effect of respiratory viral infections on patients with cystic fibrosis." *Am J Dis Child* 143(6): 662-8.

Raza, M. W., S. D. Essery, et al. (1999). "Infection with respiratory syncytial virus and water-soluble components of cigarette smoke alter production of tumour necrosis factor alpha and nitric oxide by human blood monocytes." *FEMS Immunol Med Microbiol* 24(4): 387-94.

Riordan, J. R., J. M. Rommens, et al. (1989). "Identification of the cystic fibrosis gene: cloning and characterization of complementary DNA." *Science* 245(4922): 1066-73.

Rosner, I. K., R. C. Welliver, et al. (1987). "Effect of ribavirin therapy on respiratory syncytial virus-specific IgE and IgA responses after infection." *J Infect Dis* 155(5): 1043-7.

Saiman, L. and J. Siegel (2004). "Infection control in cystic fibrosis." *Clin Microbiol Rev* 17(1): 57-71.

Sanford, B. A., A. Shelokov, et al. (1978). "Bacterial adherence to virus-infected cells: a cell culture model of bacterial superinfection." *J Infect Dis* 137(2): 176-81.

Sawicki, G. S., L. Rasouliyan, et al. (2008). "The impact of incident methicillin resistant Staphylococcus aureus detection on pulmonary function in cystic fibrosis." *Pediatr Pulmonol* 43(11): 1117-23.

Schmid, M. L., G. Kudesia, et al. (1998). "Prospective comparative study of culture specimens and methods in diagnosing influenza in adults." *Bmj* 316(7127): 275.

Schmidt, A. C., J. M. McAuliffe, et al. (2001). "Recombinant bovine/human parainfluenza virus type 3 (B/HPIV3) expressing the respiratory syncytial virus (RSV) G and F proteins can be used to achieve simultaneous mucosal immunization against RSV and HPIV3." *J Virol* 75(10): 4594-603.

Seki, M., Y. Higashiyama, et al. (2004). "Acute infection with influenza virus enhances suspectibility to fatal pneumonia following Streptococcus pneumoniae infection in mice with chronic pulmonary colonisation with Psudomonas aeruginosa." *Clin Exp Immunol* 137(1): 35-40.

Sharma, M., J. T. Arnason, et al. (2006). "Echinacea extracts modulate the pattern of chemokine and cytokine secretion in rhinovirus-infected and uninfected epithelial cells." *Phytother Res* 20(2): 147-52.

Shun-Shin, M., M. Thompson, et al. (2009). "Neuraminidase inhibitors for treatment and prophylaxis of influenza in children: systematic review and meta-analysis of randomised controlled trials." *BMJ* 339: b3172.

Shwachman, H. and L. L. Kulczycki (1958). "Long-term study of one hundred five patients with cystic fibrosis; studies made over a five- to fourteen-year period." *AMA J Dis Child* 96(1): 6-15.

Smith, D. W., L. R. Frankel, et al. (1991). "A controlled trial of aerosolized ribavirin in infants receiving mechanical ventilation for severe respiratory syncytial virus infection." *N Engl J Med* 325(1): 24-9.

Smyth, A. R., R. L. Smyth, et al. (1995). "Effect of respiratory virus infections including rhinovirus on clinical status in cystic fibrosis." *Arch Dis Child* 73(2): 117-20.

Stark, J. M., M. A. Stark, et al. (2006). "Decreased bacterial clearance from the lungs of mice following primary respiratory syncytial virus infection." *J Med Virol* 78(6): 829-38.

Suzuki, T., M. Yamaya, et al. (2002). "Erythromycin inhibits rhinovirus infection in cultured human tracheal epithelial cells." *Am J Respir Crit Care Med* 165(8): 1113-8.

Swierkosz, E. M., D. D. Erdman, et al. (1995). "Isolation and characterization of a naturally occurring parainfluenza 3 virus variant." *J Clin Microbiol* 33(7): 1839-41.

Taylor, L., M. Corey, et al. (2006). "Comparison of throat swabs and nasopharyngeal suction specimens in non-sputum-producing patients with cystic fibrosis." *Pediatr Pulmonol* 41(9): 839-43.

Thomassen, M. J., C. A. Demko, et al. (1985). "Pseudomonas cepacia colonization among patients with cystic fibrosis. A new opportunist." *Am Rev Respir Dis* 131(5): 791-6.

Thompson, C. I., W. S. Barclay, et al. (2006). "Infection of human airway epithelium by human and avian strains of influenza a virus." *J Virol* 80(16): 8060-8.

Thompson, W. W., D. K. Shay, et al. (2004). "Influenza-associated hospitalizations in the United States." *JAMA* 292(11): 1333-40.

Turner, R. B. (2005). "New considerations in the treatment and prevention of rhinovirus infections." *Pediatr Ann* 34(1): 53-7.

Turner, R. B., M. T. Wecker, et al. (1999). "Efficacy of tremacamra, a soluble intercellular adhesion molecule 1, for experimental rhinovirus infection: a randomized clinical trial." *Jama* 281(19): 1797-804.

van den Hoogen, B. G., J. C. de Jong, et al. (2001). "A newly discovered human pneumovirus isolated from young children with respiratory tract disease." *Nat Med* 7(6): 719-24.

Vawter, G. F. and H. Shwachman (1979). "Cystic fibrosis in adults: an autopsy study." *Pathol Annu* 14 Pt 2: 357-82.

Walsh, J. J., L. F. Dietlein, et al. (1961). "Bronchotracheal response in human influenza. Type A, Asian strain, as studied by light and electron microscopic examination of bronchoscopic biopsies." *Arch Intern Med* 108: 376-88.

Wang, E. E., C. G. Prober, et al. (1984). "Association of respiratory viral infections with pulmonary deterioration in patients with cystic fibrosis." *N Engl J Med* 311(26): 1653-8.

Wat, D., C. Gelder, et al. (2008). "Is there a role for influenza vaccination in cystic fibrosis?" *J Cyst Fibros* 7(1): 85-8.

Wat, D., C. Gelder, et al. (2008). "The role of respiratory viruses in cystic fibrosis." *J Cyst Fibros* 7(4): 320-8.

White, A. J., S. Gompertz, et al. (2003). "Chronic obstructive pulmonary disease . 6: The aetiology of exacerbations of chronic obstructive pulmonary disease." *Thorax* 58(1): 73-80.

Wilson, R. and P. J. Cole (1988). "The effect of bacterial products on ciliary function." *Am Rev Respir Dis* 138(6 Pt 2): S49-53.

Winther, B., J. Gwaltney, et al. (1990). "Respiratory virus infection of monolayer cultures of human nasal epithelial cells." *Am Rev Respir Dis.* 141(4 Pt 1): 839-45.

Yin, M., J. Brust, et al. (2009). Antiherpes, anti-hepatitis virus, and anti-respiratory virus agents. *Clinical virology, 3rd edition.* D. Richman, R. Whiyley and F. Hayden. Washington, ASM Press: 217-64.

Yu, H., Q. Liao, et al. (2010). "Effectiveness of oseltamivir on disease progression and viral RNA shedding in patients with mild pandemic 2009 influenza A H1N1: opportunistic retrospective study of medical charts in China." *BMJ* 341: c4779.

Zheng, S., B. De, et al. (2003). "Impaired innate host defense causes suspectibility to respiratory virus infections in cystic fibrosis." *Immunity* 18(5): 619-30.

Zheng, S., W. Xu, et al. (2004). "Impaired nitirc oxide synthase-2 signaling pathway in cystic fibrosis airway epithelium." *Am J Physiol Lung Cell Mol Physiol* 287(2): L374-81.

12

Immune Dysfunction in Cystic Fibrosis

Yaqin Xu and Stefan Worgall
Weill Cornell Medical College, Department of Pediatrics, New York, NY, USA

1. Introduction

Absence of the cystic fibrosis transmembrane regulator (CFTR) function leads to chronic lung disease characterized by inflammation and persistent infections. The mechanisms for the increased susceptibility of the respiratory tract for infections in CF are most likely complex and only partially understood. Most attention has been focused on the effect of the defective expression of CFTR in epithelial cells and submucosal gland cells and the increased susceptibility of the respiratory tract to infections was was mostly thought to be related to the abnormal chloride channel function (Welsh MJ, 2011, Ratjen F 2003). However, numerous studies over the past years have shown that the absence of CFTR affects the immune system and that dysfunctional immune responses contribute to pathological processes in the CF lung. In addition, it has become increasingly evident that the chloride channel dysfunction alone cannot completely explain the pathology of CF lung disease and that other pathways known to be regulated by CFTR play a role in the immune dysregulation in the CF lung (Mehta A 2008). This chapter reviews both soluble factors in the CF milieu that modify immune cell function and specific alterations in the cellular components of the innate and adaptive immune system that contribute to the impaired immune defense in CF lung disease.

2. The role of immune responses in CF

Innate host defenses are defective in CF. It is still not entirely clear how defective CFTR results in an impaired host response in the CF lung. Three general components comprise the innate and adaptive immune defenses in the respiratory tract: (1) the mucociliary escalator; (2) a humoral component of surfactant proteins, defensins, and other antimicrobial compounds; and (3) a cellular component that includes epithelial cells, neutrophils, macrophages, monocytes, dendritic cells, and lymphocytes.

2.1 Abnormal humoral responses in CF

The respiratory tract epithelium and the cells of the submucosal glands in the airways constitute a major part of the innate immune defense system of the lung that responds primarily to incoming pathogens with the release of various mediators. They are influenced and/or amplified in their responses by factors such as cytokines derived from neighboring inflammatory and immune cells (Bartlett J 2008). The defective chloride channel function in CF leads to alterations in the physical properties of the airway mucus and the composition of the airway surface liquid that are linked to impairment of innate defense mechanisms. These affect the shield of antimicrobial factors such as lysozyme, lactoferrin, defensins, and other antimicrobial peptides, as well as disturb the mechanical clearance of inhaled particles and pathogens by the mucociliary escalator. **Table 1** summarizes the known alterations in soluble innate immune factors in the CF lung. One school of thought has pursued the concept that alterations in the chloride secretion and sodium hyperabsorption in the airways lead to the subsequent entrapment of pathogens that then lead to recruitment and activation of neutrophils and macrophages. This has also been supported by the lung phenotype of a mouse model with genetic over-expression of the sodium channel ENac that mimics CF with thick mucus and inflammation in the absence of infection (Mall MA 2010). Salt-sensitive antimicrobials such as defensins were initially thought to be defective in the human CF lung. However, as the exact concentrations of chloride and sodium in the airway liquid are still not entirely clear, and so the degree of impairment of these innate defense mechanisms in CF is not exactly known.

Mediator	Abnormality	Reference
Defensins	Impaired activity	Goldman MJ *et al.* 1997, Bals R *et al.* 2001
Surfactant proteins	Decreased or inactive	Hartl D, Griese M 2006, Meyer KC *et al.* 2000, Noah TL *et al.* 2003
Antioxidants	Reduced glutathione availability in airways	Gao L *et al.* 1999, Roum JH *et al.* 1993, Day BJ 2005, Childers M *et al.* 2007, Hudson VM 2001
Opsonins	Proteolytic degradation	Eichler I *et al.* 1989
Cytokines		
IFN-γ [1]	Decreased secretion	Moss RB *et al.*1996 and 2000
IL-1[2]	Increased secretion	Bonfield TL *et al.* 1995
IL-4[3]	Increased secretion	Moss RB *et al.*1996 and 2000, Mueller C *et al.*2010
IL-6[4]	Increased secretion	Black HR *et al.* 1998, Becker MN *et al.* 2004, Andersson C *et al.* 2007, Vandivier RW *et al.* 2009,
IL-8[5]	Increased secretion	Bonfield TL *et al.* 1995, Black HR *et al.* 1998, Becker MN *et al.* 2004, Vandivier RW *et al.* 2009,
IL-10[6]	Altered secretion	Bonfield TL *et al.* 1995, Moss RB *et al.* 1996 and 2000, Armstrong DS *et al.* 2005
IL-13[7]	Increased secretion	Mueller C *et al.*2010
IL-17[8]	Increased secretion	McAllister F *et al.*2005, Tan HL *et al.*2011
TNF- α[9]	Increased secretion	Bonfield TL *et al.* 1995, Andersson C *et al.* 2007,
Chemokines		
MIP-1β[10]	Increased secretion	Brennan S *et al.* 2009
MCP-1[11]	Increased secretion	Brennan S *et al.* 2009

Notes: [1] IFN-γ (interferon-gamma); [2] IL-1β (interleukin-1 beta), [3] IL-4 (interleukin-4), [4] IL-6 (interleukin-6), [5] IL-8 (interleukin-8), [6] IL-10 (interleukin-10), [7] IL-13 (interleukin-13), [8] IL-17(interleukin-17), [9] TNF-α (tumor necrosis factor-alpha), [10] MIP-1β (macrophage inflammatory protein-1 beta), [11] MCP-1 (macrophage chemotactic protein-1)

Table 1. Altered humoral mediators in the respiratory tract in CF

2.1.1 Soluble mediators

Numerous humoral factors that affect pulmonary innate immune response have been studied in the CF lung. These include the collectins and surfactant proteins (Hartl D 2006, Noah TL 2003, Meyer KC 2000), defensins (Goldman MJ 1997, Bals 2001), glutathione (Gao TJ 1999, Kogan I 2003, Roum JH 1993, Hudson VM 2001) and antiproteases such as secretory leukoprotease inhibitor (SLPI) and tissue inhibitor of metalloproteinase 1 (TIMP-1) (Gaggar 2007, Cantin AM 1991, Vandivier 2002). Initially, it was thought that defensins in the CF lung were impaired due to the altered salt concentration in the CF airway (Goldmann 1997). Subsequent studies showed the impairment of defensins is not only related to an altered salt concentration, but also to increased inflammation (Bals 2001, Chen CI 2004). The Levels of β-defensin were even found to be similar in bronchial brushings in CF and non CF patients (Dauletbaev N 2002). Surfactant proteins, besides their surface-tension regulating properties, also have immuno-modulatory and anti-inflammatory functions were shown to be degraded (Hartl D 2006, Noah TL 2003) and structurally altered in CF (Meyer KC 2000). Glutathione, a critical component of the antioxidant defense system in the lung, was found to be reduced in the CF lung (Roum JH 1993). Importantly, this seemed to be directly related to the function of CFTR as a channel for the transmembrane transport of glutathione (Gao 1999, Kogan 2003). As glutathione deficiency also leads to activation of nucleic factor kappa B (NFκB)-mediated inflammation, aerosolized glutathione has been studied as a potential anti-inflammatory therapeutic in CF (Roum 1999).

Antiprotease, which plays an important role in the lung to counter the proteolytic products released by activated neutrophils, did not seem to be altered in the CF lung at baseline (Cartin AM 1991). However, these normal baseline levels were probably insufficient to neutralize the massive invasion of neutrophils and have thus been considered to be relatively deficient in the CF lung.

2.1.2 Defective CFTR leads to release of inflammatory cytokines

One of the dominant features of CF lung disease is the exaggerated inflammatory response. Numerous studies have linked the CFTR defect to activation of inflammatory cytokines, in particular interleukin-8 (IL-8). IL-8 is closely related to the CF inflammation as it is one of the major chemoattractants for neutrophils. Neutrophils dominate the inflammatory milieu in the CF lung. The importance of the vast number of neutrophils has been underscored by the successful use of recombinant DNAse to break down DNA released from neutrophils as one of the few effective therapeutics to ameliorate CF lung disease (Suri R 2002). Although it is still debated if inflammation precedes infection in the lungs of infants and young children with CF, it is undisputed that CFTR is linked to the NFκB pathway, a crucial transcription activator for inflammatory and immune responses. These intrinsic activations of NFκB and cytokines, such as IL-8 and tumor necrosis factor alpha (TNF-α), have been observed both in naïve lung macrophages from CFTR knockout mice (CF mice) and in un-stimulated human macrophages with decreased CFTR expression (Bruscia EM 2008, Xu Y 2010). It seems that the intrinsic activation of NFκB-mediated inflammatory cytokine release is independent of the chloride channel function of the CFTR protein. Neutrophil elastase and other products of neutrophils, that are abundant in the CF lung, also induce IL-8 expression in epithelial cells (McElvaney NG 1992). Besides an increase in inflammatory cytokines, the CFTR defect has also been associated with a decrease in the anti-inflammatory cytokine interleukin-10 (IL-10). Increased susceptibility to CF pathogens such as *Pseudomonas aeruginosa* (*P. aeruginosa*) has been demonstrated in IL-10 deficient mice (Soltys J 2002).

2.2 Abnormal cellular immune response in CF

Cells of the innate and adaptive immune system have been studied in CF. The main findings are outlined in **Table 2**. As the role of epithelial cells in CF will be discussed in other chapters, the following details the functions and abnormalities seen in the neutrophils, macrophages, monocytes, dendritic cells, and lymphocytes that are likely playing a part in the pathogenesis of CF lung disease.

2.2.1 Neutrophils

Neutrophils are the dominating cell type in the inflammatory milieu of the CF airways. The content of their granules and products, in particular DNA and neutrophil elastase, contribute significantly to the CF lung damage. The increase in the serum and lung cytokine levels, especially of IL-8, preactivates neutrophils and lowers their threshold for granule release (Swain SD 2002). A number of abnormalities have been observed in CF neutrophils, including defective phagocytosis and oxidative burst (Alexis NE 2006), increased degranuation (myeloperoxidase) (Koller DY 1995), augmented proteolytic activity with elevated elastase and matrix metalloprotein release (Brockbank S 2005, Ratjen F 2002, Sagel SD 2005), increased apoptosis and chemotaxis (Brennan S 2001, Watt AP 2005), decreased acidification of phagolysosomes and reduced antimicrobial activity (Painter RG 2006), defective protein kinase C (Graff I 1991), and dysregulated cytokine secretion (Corvol H 2003).Blood neutrophils from CF patients were impaired in chlorination of ingested bacteria due to defective hypochlorous acid (HOCl) production within phagolysosomes, whereas extracellular HOCl production was normal (Painter RG 2006). Profound functional and signaling changes have been shown in viable inflammatory neutrophils collected from airways of CF patients compared to their blood counterparts (Tirouvanziam R 2007). On CF airway neutrophils, the surface expression of phagocytosis receptors CD16 and CD14 was lost, whereas other lineage markers such as CD80 and MHCII appeared, indicating potential functional reprogramming (Tirouvanziam R 2007).

The study by Hartl D *et al.* has provided another pathophysiologic mechanism showing unopposed proteolytic cleavage of chemokine receptor CXCR1 on CF neutrophils and subsequent failure of their bacterial-killing capacity (Hartl D 2007). One of the most important features of the neutrophils in CF is their delayed apoptosis, which could be even measured in CF heterozygous individuals (Moriceau S 2010).

Toll-like receptors (TLRs) play crucial roles in the innate host defense against *P. aeruginosa* Neutrophils express all human TLRs except for TLR3. TLR2 and TLR5 present the main TLRs for the recognition of *P. aeruginosa*. TLR2 and TLR4 are involved in the cytokine response to *P. aeruginosa* infection. Intact flagellin/TLR5 signaling is a prerequisite for an efficient clearance of acute *P. aeruginosa* infection. The expression levels of TLRs in CF neutrophils have been investigated (Koll B 2008, Petit-Bertron AF 2008). Circulating and airway neutrophils from CF patients displayed a distinct pattern of surface markers as compared to the cells from healthy controls (Petit-Bertron AF 2008). CF blood neutrophils

Cell type	Function	Reference
Epithelial cells	Bacterial killing	Moskwa P *et al.* 2007
	Transport of GSH[1]	Velsor LW *et al.* 2001
	Redox balance	Xu Y *et al.* 2006
	Cytokine production	Tabary O *et al.* 2000
Neutrophils	Phagocytosis	Morris MR *et al.* 2005, Alexis NE *et al.* 2006
	Degranulation	Gaggar A *et al.* 2007, Koller DY *et al.* 1995, Brockbank S *et al.* 2005, Ratjen F *et al.* 2002, Sagel SD *et al.* 2005
	Apoptosis	Vandivier RW *et al.* 2002, Watt AP *et al.* 2005
	Chemotaxis	Brennan S *et al.* 2001
	Chlorination of phagolysosomes	Painter RG *et al.* 2006
	Anti-microbial activity	Painter RG *et al.* 2006, Moraes TJ *et al.* 2006
	Cytokine production	Corvol H *et al.* 2003, Tirouvanziam R *et al.* 2007
	CXCR1[2] cleavage	Hartl D *et al.* 2007
	TLR[3]-2, 4, 5 expression	Petit Bertron AF *et al.* 2008
Macrophages	Clearance of apoptotic cells	Vandiview RW *et al.* 2002a, 2002b
	Cytokine production	Bonfield TL *et al.* 1995, Bruscia EM *et al.* 2009, Brennan S *et al.* 2009, Xu Y *et al.* 2010
	Phagocytosis	Knight RA *et al.* 1997, Di A *et al.* 2006
	Acidification of lysosomes	Di A *et al.* 2006, Haggie PM, Verkman AS 2007 and 2009
	Antigen presentation	Knight RA *et al.* 1997
	PPAR[4]/LXR[5] regulation	Andersson C *et al.* 2007
Dendritic cells	CD1d-restricted natural killer T cells activation	Rzemienaik SE *et al.* 2010
	Differentiation and maturation	Xu Y *et al.* 2009
	Activation, antigen presentation, and cytokine secretion	Roghanian A *et al.* 2006, Xu Y *et al.* 2009
Monocytes	Phagocytosis	del Fresno C *et al.* 2009
	Antigen presentation	Sorio C *et al.* 2011
	MHCII expression	del Fresno C *et al.* 2008
	TREM-1[6] expression	del Fresno C *et al.* 2008
	Cytokine production	del Fresno C *et al.* 2008
	Toll-2, 4 expression	Sturge N C *et al.* 2010
Lymphocytes	Chloride channel function	McDonald TV *et al.*1992, Dong YJ *et al.*1995, Moss RB *et al.*1996
	Cytokine production	Knutsen AP *et al.*1989 and 1990, Lahat N *et al.*1989, Moss RB *et al.*1996 and 2000, Hubeau C *et al.*2004, Hartl D *et al.*2005 Muller C *et al.*2010, Tan HL *et al.*2011

Notes: [1] GSH (glutathione); [2] CXCR (C-X-C chemokine receptor), [3] TLR (toll like receptor), [4] PPAR (peroxisomal proliferator activated receptors), [5] LXR (liver X receptors), [6] TREM-1 (triggering receptor expressed on myeloid cells-1)

Table 2. Cellular immune dysfunction in CF

expressed elevated levels of CD64, an activation marker, and lower levels of TLR2 compared to blood neutrophils from healthy controls (Petit-Bertron AF 2008). In contrast, CF airway neutrophils expressed an elevated level of TLR4 and spontaneously released IL-8 that was neither enhanced by microbial activators nor inhibited by recombinant human IL-10, indicating intrinsic resistance to anti-inflammatory signals delivered by IL-10 (Petit-Bertron AF 2008). A similar study by Koller B *et al.* investigated the expression levels of TLR2, TLR4, TLR5, and TLR9 on airway neutrophils compared to circulating neutrophils in CF patients infected with *P. aeruginosa*. TLR5 was the only TLR that was significantly higher expressed in CF airway neutrophils compared to the controls (Koller B 2008).

2.2.2 Macrophages

Alveolar macrophages (AM) are important as a first line host defense in the lung. Besides the phagocytosis of inhaled pathogens and apoptotic cells and the release of inflammatory mediators they play an important role in orchestrating innate immune defenses (Takabayshi 2006). One of the important regulatory functions of AM may be to dampen immune responses (Lambrecht 2006), so that dysfunction of AM in CF could be related to increased inflammation. The antigen-presenting capacity of AM is low, compared to other macrophages and a majority of their function is related to phagocytosis. Dysfunctional CFTR in macrophages has been linked to impaired clearance of apoptotic cells, pro-inflammatory cytokines production, deficient antigen presentation, abnormal TLR4 trafficking, decreased bactericidal activity, and defective phagocytosis (Bonfield TL 1995, Bruscia EM 2009 and 2011, del Porto P 2011, Di A 2006, Knight RA 1997, Vandivier RW 2002a and 2002b, Xu Y 2010). Lipopolysaccharide (LPS) stimulated peritoneal macrophages from CF mice showed increased TNF-α and IL-6 secretion as well as NFκB p65 activity. It also demonstrated attenuated induction of peroxisomal proliferator activated receptors (PPAR) and liver X receptors (LXR), those are two mediators known as the inhibitory regulators of pro-inflammatory cytokines (Andersson C 2007). Bruscia *et al.* showed that macrophages directly contributed to the exaggerated inflammatory response following LPS administration in CF mice with increased secretion of cytokines including IL-6 and keratinocyte chemoattractant (Bruscia EM 2009). The same group also demonstrated that abnormal trafficking and degradation of TLR4 might underlie the elevated inflammatory response in CF (Bruscia EM 2011). Macrophages isolated from lavage samples from CF patients were not able to stimulate allogeneic lymphocytes and to present antigen, while peripheral blood monocytes from the same patients were functional in both assays (Knight RA 1997). Macrophages derived from peripheral blood from CF patients did not differ in phagocytic activity when infected with *P. aeruginosa*, whereas the percentage of surviving bacteria was significantly higher inside CF cells compared to the controls (del Porto P 2011). As AM in human CF lungs are highly activated by the inflammatory milieu, our group assessed the direct influence of CFTR on the function of AM by knockdown CFTR expression in normal human AM with siRNA silencing. A pro-inflammatory phenotype and increased apoptosis were seen in human AM with defective CFTR, possibly due to increased expression of the lipid raft protein Caveolin-1 (Xu Y 2010). The CFTR defect has been linked to augmented apoptosis with an abnormal cellular ceramide composition which is thought to be dependant on alteration in the lipid rafts in CF cells (Becker KA 2010). Altered pH of lysosome in CF macrophages has been suggested to induce defective acidification and bactericidal activity (Di A 2006). These findings have been disputed by others as the pH in the CF lysosomes was not altered using pH sensitive fluorescent probes (Haggie PM 2007 and 2009).

Macrophages may be part of an abnormal priming process in CF during fetal development. This has been suggested by the analysis of fetal lungs for early features of immune dysregulation, which showed that the number of macrophages in the lung was higher in CF fetal lungs compared to non-CF lungs during the later stages of lung development (Hubeau 2001). Findings in the lungs of young infants with CF also point to the presence of increased macrophages as the macrophage recruiting CC chemokines elevated (Brennan S 2008; Starner 2003).

2.2.3 Monocytes

Peripheral blood monocytes, the precursors of AM, represent a pool of cells available to migrate to the lungs in response to bacterial infection. Abnormal functions of monocytes in peripheral blood from CF patients have been shown despite of absence of systemic infection in CF (del Fresno C 2008 and 2009, Sturges NC 2010, Zaman MM 2004). Augmented IL-8 secretions at baseline and in response to LPS were seen in monocytes of adult subjects heterozygous for ΔF508 mutation, with no increased expression of LPS receptors including CD14 and TLR4 but possible association with alterations in mitogen activated phosphate kinase (MAPK) signaling (Zaman MM 2004). Blood peripheral monocytes isolated from CF patients were found to be locked in an endotoxin tolerance state in comparison to those exacted from healthy volunteers, not due to a deficient TLR activation but likely resulted from down-regulation of Triggering Receptor Expressed on Myeloid cells-1 (TREM-1) (del Fresno C 2008). Further investigation demonstrated potent phagocytic activity with impaired antigen presentation in LPS-tolerant monocytes from CF patients, possible by reason of decreased expression of MHCII and co-stimulatory molecules CD80, CD83, and CD86 (del Fresno C 2008). Contradictory to Zaman's finding, Sturge *et al.* have shown enhanced expression of TLR4 but similar TLR2 levels in monocytes from young CF patients with median age of 3.3 compared to healthy controls (Sturges NC 2010). The conflicting results may be due to difference in the age of subjects, and longitudinal studies are required to determine TLR4 expression as CF lung disease progresses.

2.2.4 Dendritic cells

Dendritic cells (DC), the most potent antigen presenting cells, are critical at the interface of innate and adaptive immune response. It is not known if DC function is affected in CF in humans. Only one study assessed blood-derived DC from CF patients in their capacity to activate CD1d-restricted natural killer T cells (NKT cells). The finding was that CF and non CF DC could comparably stimulate NKT cells with no apparent impact from defective CFTR chloride channel function (Rzemieniak SE 2010). Normal murine bone marrow derived DC (BMDC) were cultured in sputum from CF patients. These DC showed down-regulated expression of co-stimulatory molecules CD40, CD80, and CD86 (but not MHCII), inhibited LPS-induced activation, and defective antigen-presenting ability, partially owing to the inflammatory mediator neutrophil elastase (Roghanian A 2006). In our study, BMDC from CF mice expressed CFTR but were delayed in the early phase of differentiation. The expression levels of a number of genes related to lipid metabolism including caveolin-1, 3β-hydroxysterol-Δ7 reductase (Dhcr7), and stearoyl-CoA desaturase 2 (Scd2) were altered (Xu Y 2009). The roles of pulmonary DC, crucial in orchestrating innate and adaptive immune responses, have been investigated in lungs from CF mice in our laboratory (Xu Y 2009).

Phenotypic and functional abnormalities in CF lung DC were found including decreased numbers, altered maturation and activation profiles, and an impaired T cell-stimulation capacity. In response to respiratory syncytial virus infection, recruitment to the lung and T cell stimulatory potential of lung DC of CF mice were impaired in comparison to controls (Xu Y 2009). The dysfunctional CFTR might play a direct role in impaired lung DC. Indirect influence from the environment, where DC reside, on the phenotype and function of lung DC could not be excluded, although inflammation in lungs of CF mice at baseline is considerably mild compared to lungs of CF patients. Further investigation is undertaken to elucidate the mechanism of mal-functional DC in CF lungs.

2.2.5 Lymphocytes

Like the other immune cells, lymphocytes express CFTR and CF lymphocytes have a defective cAMP-regulated chloride channel function (Dong YJ 1995, McDonald TV 1992). B-lymphocytes from CF patients produced similar amounts of IgG compared to non-CF cells, but showed resistance to dexamethasone. This was proposed as a potential factor for the susceptibility to bacterial bronchopulmonary infections (Emilie D 1990). Selective cytokine dysregulation has been shown in CF $CD4^+$ T cells after maximal activation with anti-CD3 or phorbol myristate acetate. It included decreased IFN-γ secretion and reduced IL-10 production, whereas the levels of IL-2, IL-4, and IL-5 remained similar to controls (Moss RB 1996 and 2000). IL-2 has been known to stimulate the growth, differentiation and survival of antigen-selected cytotoxic T cells. IL-4 is a cytokine that induces differentiation of naïve helper T cells (Th0 cells) to Th2 cells. The functions of IL-5 are to stimulate B cell growth and increase immunoglobulin secretion.

Lymphocytes from CF patients or CF mice showed a profile skewed towards T_H2 (Hartl D 2005, Mueller C 2010). In CF patients with *P. aeruginosa* infection, the prevalence of a pulmonary T_H2 immune response has been shown with higher levels of $CCR4^+CD4^+$ (T_H2) cells, increased levels of IL-4, IL-13, and lower levels of IFN-γ compared with non-infected patients with CF and healthy controls (Hartl D 2005). Comparably, CF mice mounted an exaggerated IgE response upon *Aspergillus fumigatus* infection in the lung with increased levels of IL-4 and IL-13, mimicking both the T_H2 biased immune responses seen in CF patients (Mueller C 2010). Similar findings are also reported in studies with peripheral blood derived monocytes or whole blood cultures from CF patients infected with *P. aeruginosa* (Brazova J 2005, Moser C 2000). A dysregulated $T_H1/2$ response might contribute to the impaired clearance of pathogens in CF.

Recently, more attention has been focused on the role of T_H17 cells and interleukin-17 (IL-17) in the CF lung disease (McAllister F 2005, Tan HL 2011). IL-17 receptor signaling is critical for pulmonary neutrophil recruitment and host defense against Gram-negative bacteria through the coordinated release of granulocyte-colony stimulating factor (G-CSF) and CXC chemokine elaboration (Steinman L 2007, Bettelli 2007). Significantly elevated levels of IL-17A, IL-17F and IL-17R were found in the sputum of patients with CF who were colonized with *P. aeruginosa* at the time of pulmonary exacerbation. These levels were declined with therapy directed against *P. aeruginosa* (McAllister F 2005). T_H17 lymphocytes and other T_H17^+ cells, including neutrophils, γδ T cells, and natural killer T cells, have been shown to be present in the airway sub-mucosa in CF patients even in a young, newly diagnosed group. Highest levels of IL-17 were found in bronchoalveolar lavage from established CF compared to the controls, with a significant correlation between IL-17 and neutrophil counts as well as IL-4 (Tan HL 2011). IL-17 pathway could serve as a new therapeutic candidate for CF, while the exact pathogenic mechanisms of IL-17 in CF still remain to be elucidated.

3. Conclusion

Augmented inflammation, increased susceptibility of the respiratory tract for infections and lack of efficient clearance of the pathogens are features of a defective immune function. Abnormal CFTR chloride channel function (and potentially associated sodium hyperabsorption) in epithelial and mucous gland cells in the lung can only partially explain the pathophysiology of CF lung disease. Members of the innate and adaptive immune system are clearly affected by the milieu created by the altered salt and water composition. There is also evidence that CFTR dysfunction directly affects immune responses, probably beyond the stimulation of inflammatory cytokines. CFTR is expressed and is functional in a variety of immune cells. CFTR-related abnormalities have been shown in neutrophils, macrophages, monocytes, dendritic cells, and lymphocytes independent of exposure to the CF milieu of the respiratory tract as demonstrated in **Fig 1.** Thus, direct CFTR-mediated dysfunction of these cells may play a role in the enigmatic CF lung disease.

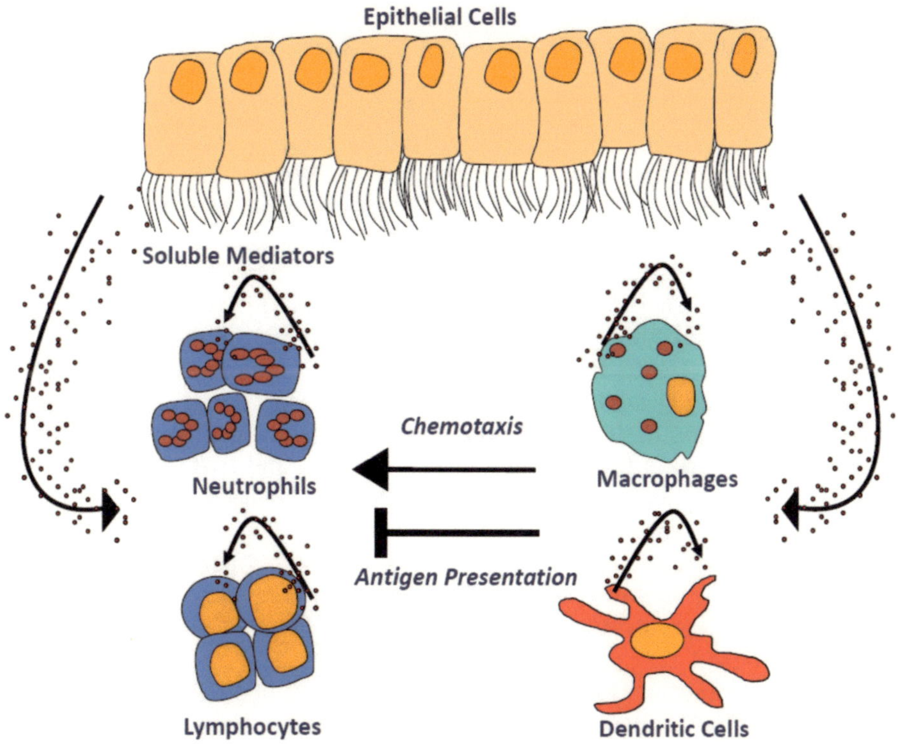

Fig. 1. Model of abnormal humoral and cellular immune responses in the CF lung. Altered humoral responses are comprised of soluble mediators including cytokines, chemokines, antioxidants, and antiproteases. Neutrophils, macrophages, dendritic cells, and lymphocytes are either affected by the altered soluble mediators from the CFTR-deficient epithelial and immune cells or by their own defective CFTR function.

4. Acknowledgment

We thank Ms. Christine Filner for excellent assistance in the preparation of this manuscript. Our studies were supported by R21 HL077557 and the Cystic Fibrosis Foundation XU09F0, Bethesda, MD.

5. References

Alexis, N.E., M.S.Muhlebach, D.B.Peden, and T.L.Noah. (2006). Attenuation of Host Defense Function of Lung Phagocytes in Young Cystic Fibrosis Patients. *Journal of Cystic Fibrosis* 5:17-25. ISSN 1569-1993

Andersson, C., M.M.Zaman, A.B.Jones, and S.D.Freedman. (2008). Alterations in Immune Response and PPAR/LXR Regulation in Cystic Fibrosis Macrophages. *Journal of Cystic Fibrosis* 7:68-78. ISSN 1569-1993

Armstrong, D.S., S.M.Hook, K.M.Jamsen, G.M.Nixon, R.Carzino, J.B.Carlin, C.F.Robertson, and K.Grimwood. (2005). Lower Airway Inflammation in Infants with Cystic Fibrosis Detected by Newborn Screening. *Pediatr. Pulmonol.* 40:500-510. ISSN 8755-6863

Armstrong, D., K.Grimwood, J.Carlin, R.Carzino, J.Gutièrrez, J.Hull, A.Olinsky, E.Phelan, C.Robertson, and P.Phelan. (1997). Lower Airway Inflammation in Infants and Young Children with Cystic Fibrosis. *Am. J. Respir. Crit. Care Med.* 156:1197-1204. ISSN 1073-449X

Assef, Y.A., A.E.Damiano, E.Zotta, C.Ibarra, and B.A.Kotsias. (2003). CFTR in K562 Human Leukemic Cells. *Am J Physiol Cell Physiol* 285:C480-C488. ISSN 0363-6143

Bals, R., D.J.Weiner, R.L.Meegalla, F.Accurso, and J.M.Wilson. (2001). Salt-independent Abnormality of Antimicrobial Activity in Cystic Fibrosis Airway Surface Fluid. *Am. J. Respir. Cell Mol. Biol.* 25:21-25. ISSN:1044-1549

Bals, R., D.J.Weiner, and J.M.Wilson. (1999). The Innate Immune System in Cystic Fibrosis Lung Disease. *J Clin Invest* 103:303-307. ISSN 0021-9738

Bartlett J, Fischer A, and J.McCray PB. (2008). Innate Immune Functions of the Airway Epithelium. *In* Trends in Innate Immunity.Contrib Microbiol. Egesten A, Schmidt A, and Herwald H, editors. S Karger, ISBN 3805585489, Basel. 147-163.

Bhattacharyya, S., U.Gutti, J.Mercado, C.Moore, H.B.Pollard, and R.Biswas. (2010). MAPK Signaling Pathways Regulate IL-8 mRNA Stability and IL-8 Protein Expression in Cystic Fibrosis Lung Epithelial Cells Lines. *Am J Physiol Lung Cell Mol Physiol* doi:10.1152/ajplung.00051.2010. ISSN 1040-0605

Black, H.R., J.R.Yankaskas, L.G.Johnson, and T.L.Noah. (1998). Interleukin-8 Production by Cystic Fibrosis Nasal Epithelial Cells after Tumor Necrosis Factor-alpha and Respiratory Syncytial Virus Stimulation. *Am. J. Respir. Cell Mol. Biol.* 19:210-215. ISSN:1044-1549

Bonfield, T.L., J.R.Panuska, M.W.Konstan, K.A.Hilliard, J.B.Hilliard, H.Ghnaim, and M.Berger. (1995). Inflammatory Cytokines in Cystic Fibrosis Lungs. *Am. J. Respir. Crit. Care Med.* 152:2111-2118. ISSN: 1073-449X

Brazova, J., A.Sediva, D.Pospisilova, V.Vavrova, P.Pohunek, J.Macek, J.Bartunkova, and H.Lauschmann. (2005). Differential Cytokine Profile in Children with Cystic Fibrosis. *Clin Immunol* 115:210-215. ISSN:1521-6616

Brennan, S., D.Cooper, and P.D.Sly. (2001). Directed Neutrophil Migration to IL-8 is Increased in Cystic Fibrosis: a Study of the Effect of Erythromycin. *Thorax* 56:62-64. ISSN 0040-6376

Brennan, S., P.D.Sly, C.L.Gangell, N.Sturges, K.Winfield, M.Wikstrom, S.Gard, J.W.Upham, and on behalf of AREST CF. (2009). Alveolar Macrophages and CC Chemokines are Increased in Children with Cystic Fibrosis. *European Respiratory Journal* 34:655-661. ISSN 0903-1936

Brennan, S. (2008). Innate Immune Activation and Cystic Fibrosis. *Paediatric Respiratory Reviews* 9:271-280. ISSN 1526-0542

Brockbank, S., D.Downey, J.S.Elborn, and M.Ennis. (2005). Effect of Cystic Fibrosis Exacerbations on Neutrophil Function. *International Immunopharmacology* 5:601-608. ISSN 1567-5769

Bruscia, E.M., P.X.Zhang, A.Satoh, C.Caputo, R.Medzhitov, A.Shenoy, M.E.Egan, and D.S.Krause. (2011). Abnormal Trafficking and Degradation of TLR4 Underlie the Elevated Inflammatory Response in Cystic Fibrosis. *J Immunol* 186:6990-6998. ISSN 0022-1767

Bruscia, E.M., P.X.Zhang, E.Ferreira, C.Caputo, J.W.Emerson, D.Tuck, D.S.Krause, and M.E.Egan. (2008). Macrophages Directly Contribute to the Exaggerated Inflammatory Response in CFTR-/- Mice. *Am. J. Respir. Cell Mol. Biol.* 40:295-304. ISSN 1044-1549

Bubien, J. (2001). CFTR may Play a Role in Regulated Secretion by Lymphocytes: a New Hypothesis for the Pathophysiology of Cystic Fibrosis. *Pflugers Arch* 443:S36-S39. ISSN 0031-6768

Buchanan, P.J., R.K.Ernst, J.S.Elborn, and B.Schock. (2009). Role of CFTR, Pseudomonas aeruginosa and Toll-like Receptors in Cystic Fibrosis Lung Inflammation. *Biochem Soc Trans* 37:863-867. ISSN 0300-5127

Cantin, A.M., S.Lafrenaye, and R.O.Begin. (1991). Antineutrophil Elastase Activity in Cystic Fibrosis Serum. *Pediatr. Pulmonol.* 11:249-253. ISSN 8755-6863

Chen CI, Schaller-Bals S, Paul KP, Wahn U, and Bals R. (2004). Beta-defensins and LL-37 in Bronchoalveolar Lavage Fluid of Patients with Cystic Fibrosis. *Journal of Cystic Fibrosis* 3:45-50. ISSN 1569-1993

Childers, M., G.Eckel, A.Himmel, and J.Caldwell. (2007). A New Model of Cystic Fibrosis Pathology: Lack of Transport of Glutathione and its Thiocyanate Conjugates. *Medical Hypotheses* 68:101-112. ISSN 0306-9877

Conese, M. (2011). Cystic Fibrosis and the Innate Immune System: Therapeutic Implications. *Endocr. Metab Immune. Disord. Drug Targets.* 11:8-22. ISSN 1871-5303

Corvol, H., C.Fitting, K.Chadelat, J.Jacquot, O.Tabary, M.Boule, J.M.Cavaillon, and A.Clement. (2003). Distinct Cytokine Production by Lung and Blood Neutrophils from Children with Cystic Fibrosis. *American Journal of Physiology - Lung Cellular and Molecular Physiology* 284:L997-L1003. ISSN 1522-1504

Day, B.J. (2005). Glutathione: a Radical Treatment for Cystic Fibrosis Lung Disease? *Chest* 127:12-14. ISSN 0012-3692

Deriy, L.V., E.A.Gomez, G.Zhang, D.W.Beacham, J.A.Hopson, A.J.Gallan, P.D.Shevchenko, V.P.Bindokas, and D.J.Nelson. (2009). Disease Causing Mutations in the Cystic Fibrosis Transmembrane Conductance Regulator Determine the Functional Responses of Alveolar Macrophages. *Journal of Biological Chemistry*. ISSN 0021-9258 del Fresno, C., F.Garcia-Rio, V.Gomez-Pina, A.Soares-Schanoski, I.Fernandez-Ruiz, T.Jurado, T.Kajiji, C.Shu, E.Marin, A.Gutierrez del Arroyo, C.Prados, F.Arnalich, P.Fuentes-Prior, S.K.Biswas, and E.Lopez-Collazo. (2009). Potent Phagocytic Activity with Impaired Antigen Presentation Identifying Lipopolysaccharide-tolerant Human Monocytes: Demonstration in Isolated Monocytes from Cystic Fibrosis Patients. *J Immunol* 182:6494-6507. ISSN 0022-1767

del Fresno, C., V.Gomez-Pina, V.Lores, A.Soares-Schanoski, I.Fernandez-Ruiz, B.Rojo, R.varez-Sala, E.Caballero-Garrido, F.Garcia, T.Veliz, F.Arnalich, P.Fuentes-Prior, F.Garcia-Rio, and E.Lopez-Collazo. 2008. Monocytes from Cystic Fibrosis Patients are Locked in an LPS Tolerance State: Down-Regulation of TREM-1 as Putative Underlying Mechanism. *PLoS ONE* 3:e2667. ISSN 1932-6203

Di, A., M.E.Brown, L.V.Deriy, C.Li, F.L.Szeto, Y.Chen, P.Huang, J.Tong, A.P.Naren, V.Bindokas, H.C.Palfrey, and D.J.Nelson. (2006). CFTR Regulates Phagosome Acidification in Macrophages and Alters Bactericidal Activity. *Nat Cell Biol* 8:933-944. ISSN 1465-7392

dib-Conquy, M., T.Pedron, A.F.Petit-Bertron, O.Tabary, H.Corvol, J.Jacquot, A.Clement, and J.M.Cavaillon. (2008). Neutrophils in Cystic Fibrosis Display a Distinct Gene Expression Pattern. *Mol Med* 14:36-44. ISSN 1432-1440

Dong, Y.J., A.C.Chao, K.Kouyama, Y.P.Hsu, R.C.Bocian, R.B.Moss, and P.Gardner. (1995.) Activation of CFTR Chloride Current by Nitric Oxide in Human T Lymphocytes. *EMBO J* 14:2700-2707. ISSN 0261-4189

Gaggar, A., A.Hector, P.E.Bratcher, M.A.Mall, M.Griese, and D.Hartl. (2011). The Role of Matrix Metalloproteinases in Cystic Fibrosis Lung Disease. *European Respiratory Journal* 38:721-727. 0903-1936

Gaggar, A., Y.Li, N.Weathington, M.Winkler, M.Kong, P.Jackson, J.E.Blalock, and J.P.Clancy. (2007). Matrix Metalloprotease-9 Dysregulation in Lower Airway Secretions of Cystic Fibrosis Patients. *American Journal of Physiology Lung Cellular and Molecular Physiology* 293:L96-L104. ISSN 1040-0605

Gao, L., K.J.Kim, J.R.Yankaskas, and H.J.Forman. (1999). Abnormal Glutathione Transport in Cystic Fibrosis Airway Epithelia. *American Journal of Physiology - Lung Cellular and Molecular Physiology* 277:L113-L118. ISSN 1040-0605

Goldman, M.J., G.M.Anderson, E.D.Stolzenberg, U.P.Kari, M.Zasloff, and J.M.Wilson. (1997). Human [beta]-Defensin-1 Is a Salt-Sensitive Antibiotic in Lung That Is Inactivated in Cystic Fibrosis. *Cell* 88:553-560. ISSN 0092-8674

Haggie, P.M. and A.S.Verkman. (2009). Unimpaired Lysosomal Acidification in Respiratory Epithelial Cells in Cystic Fibrosis. *J Biol Chem* 284:7681-7686. ISSN 0021-9258

Hampton, T.H. and B.A.Stanton. (2010). A Novel Approach to Analyze Gene Expression Data Demonstrates that the {Delta}F508 Mutation in CFTR Downregulates the Antigen Presentation Pathway. *Am J Physiol Lung Cell Mol Physiol* 298:L473-L482. ISSN 1040-0605

Hartl, D. and M.Griese. (2006). Surfactant Protein D in Human Lung Diseases. *European Journal of Clinical Investigation* 36:423-435. ISSN 1526-0542

Hartl, D., M.Griese, M.Kappler, G.Zissel, D.Reinhardt, C.Rebhan, D.J.Schendel, and S.Krauss-Etschmann. (2006). Pulmonary TH2 Response in Pseudomonas aeruginosa-infected Patients with Cystic Fibrosis. *J Allergy Clin Immunol* 117:204-211. ISSN 0091-6749

Hauber, H.P., M.K.Tulic, A.Tsicopoulos, B.Wallaert, R.Olivenstein, P.Daigneault, and Q.Hamid. (2005). Toll-like Receptors 4 and 2 Expression in the Bronchial Mucosa of Patients with Cystic Fibrosis. *Can. Respir J* 12:13-18. ISSN 1198-2241

Hausler, M., K.Schweizer, S.Biesterfeld, T.Opladen, and G.Heimann. (2002). Peripheral Decrease and Pulmonary Homing of CD4+CD45RO+ Helper Memory T cells in Cystic Fibrosis. *Respiratory Medicine* 96:87-94. ISSN 0954-6111

Hubeau, C., E.Puchelle, and D.Gaillard. (2001). Distinct Pattern of Immune Cell Population in the Lung of Human Fetuses with Cystic Fibrosis. *Journal of Allergy and Clinical Immunology* 108:524-529. ISSN 0091-6749

Hudson, V.M. (2001). Rethinking Cystic Fibrosis Pathology: the Critical Role of Abnormal Reduced Glutathione (GSH) Transport Caused by CFTR Mutation. *Free Radical Biology and Medicine* 30:1440-1461. ISSN 0891-5849

Jacquot, J., O.Tabary, P.Le Rouzic, and A.Clement. (2008). Airway Epithelial Cell Inflammatory Signalling in Cystic Fibrosis. *The International Journal of Biochemistry & Cell Biology* 40:1703-1715. ISSN 1357-2725

Kerby, G.S., V.Cottin, F.J.Accurso, F.Hoffmann, E.D.Chan, V.A.Fadok, and D.W.H.Riches. (2002). Impairment of Macrophage Survival by NaCl: Implications for Early Pulmonary Inflammation in Cystic Fibrosis. *American Journal of Physiology - Lung Cellular and Molecular Physiology* 283:L188-L197. ISSN 1040-0605

Khan, T.Z., J.S.Wagener, T.Bost, J.Martinez, F.J.Accurso, and D.W.Riches. (1995). Early Pulmonary Inflammation in Infants with Cystic Fibrosis. *Am. J. Respir. Crit. Care Med.* 151:1075-1082. ISSN 1073-449X

Knight, R.A., S.Kollnberger, B.Madden, M.Yacoub, and M.E.Hodson. (1997). Defective Antigen Presentation by Lavage Cells from Terminal Patients with Cystic Fibrosis. *Clin Exp Immunol* 107:542-547. ISSN 0009-9104

Knutsen, A.P. and R.G.Slavin. (1989). In vitro T cell Responses in Patients with Cystic Fibrosis and Allergic Bronchopulmonary Aspergillosis. *J Lab Clin Med.* 113:428-435. ISSN 0022-2143

Knutsen, A.P., K.R.Mueller, P.S.Hutcheson, and R.G.Slavin. (1990). T- and B-cell Dysregulation of IgE Synthesis in Cystic Fibrosis Patients with Allergic Bronchopulmonary Aspergillosis. *Clinical Immunology and Immunopathology* 55:129-138. ISSN 0090-1229

Kogan, I., M.Ramjeesingh, C.Li, J.F.Kidd, Y.Wang, E.M.Leslie, S.P.C.Cole, and C.E.Bear. (2003). CFTR Directly Mediates Nucleotide-regulated Glutathione Flux. *EMBO J* 22:1981-1989. I SSN 0261-4189

Koller, B., M.Kappler, P.Latzin, A.Gaggar, M.Schreiner, S.Takyar, M.Kormann, M.Kabesch, D.Roos, M.Griese, and D.Hartl. (2008). TLR Expression on Neutrophils at the Pulmonary Site of Infection: TLR1/TLR2-Mediated Up-Regulation of TLR5 Expression in Cystic Fibrosis Lung Disease. *J Immunol* 181:2753-2763. ISSN 0022-1767

Koller, D.Y., R.Urbanek, and M.Gotz. (1995). Increased Degranulation of Eosinophil and Neutrophil Granulocytes in Cystic Fibrosis. *Am J Respir Crit Care Med* 152:629-633. ISSN 1073-449X

Lahat, N., J.Rivlin, and T.C.Iancu. (1989). Functional Immunoregulatory T-cell Abnormalities in Cystic Fibrosis Patients. *J Clin Immunol* 9:287-295. ISSN 0271-9142

Mall, M.A., B.Button, B.Johannesson, Z.Zhou, A.Livraghi, R.A.Caldwell, S.C.Schubert, C.Schultz, W.K.O'Neal, S.Pradervand, E.Hummler, B.C.Rossier, B.R.Grubb, and R.C.Boucher. (2010). Airway Surface Liquid Volume Regulation Determines Different Airway Phenotypes in Liddle Compared with betaENaC-overexpressing Mice. *Journal of Biological Chemistry* 285:26945-26955. ISSN 0021-9258

McAllister, F., A.Henry, J.L.Kreindler, P.J.Dubin, L.Ulrich, C.Steele, J.D.Finder, J.M.Pilewski, B.M.Carreno, S.J.Goldman, J.Pirhonen, and J.K.Kolls. (2005). Role of IL-17A, IL-17F, and the IL-17 Receptor in Regulating Growth-Related Oncogene-+¦ and Granulocyte Colony-Stimulating Factor in Bronchial Epithelium: Implications for Airway Inflammation in Cystic Fibrosis. *J Immunol* 175:404-412. ISSN 022-1767

McDonald, T.V., P.T.Nghiem, P.Gardner, and C.L.Martens. (1992). Human Lymphocytes Transcribe the Cystic Fibrosis Transmembrane Conductance Regulator Gene and Exhibit CF-defective cAMP-regulated Chloride Current. *Journal of Biological Chemistry* 267:3242-3248. ISSN 0021-9258

McElvaney, N.G., H.Nakamura, P.Birrer, C.A.H+¬bert, W.L.Wong, M.Alphonso, J.B.Baker, M.A.Catalano, and R.G.Crystal. (1992). Modulation of Airway Inflammation in Cystic Fibrosis. In vivo Suppression of Interleukin-8 Levels on the Respiratory Epithelial Surface by Aerosolization of Recombinant Secretory Leukoprotease Inhibitor. *J Clin Invest* 90:1296-1301.ISSN 0021-9738

Meyer, K.C., A.Sharma, R.Brown, M.Weatherly, F.R.Moya, J.Lewandoski, and J.J.Zimmerman. (2000). Function and Composition of Pulmonary Surfactant and Surfactant-derived Fatty Profiles are Altered in Young Adults with Cystic Fibrosis. *Chest* 118:164-174. ISSN 0012-3692

Meyer, M., F.Huaux, X.Gavilanes, S.van den Brule, P.Lebecque, S.Lo Re, D.Lison, B.Scholte, P.Wallemacq, and T.Leal. (2009). Azithromycin Reduces Exaggerated Cytokine Production by M1 Alveolar Macrophages in Cystic Fibrosis. *Am. J. Respir. Cell Mol. Biol.* 41:590-602. ISSN 1044-1549

Moraes, T.J., J.Plumb, R.Martin, E.Vachon, V.Cherepanov, A.Koh, C.Loeve, J.Jongstra-Bilen, J.H.Zurawska, J.V.Kus, L.L.Burrows, S.Grinstein, and G.P.Downey. (2006). Abnormalities in the Pulmonary Innate Immune System in Cystic Fibrosis. *Am. J. Respir. Cell Mol. Biol.* 34:364-374. ISSN 1044-1549

Morris, M.R., I.J.M.Doull, S.Dewitt, and M.B.Hallett. (2005). Reduced iC3b-mediated Phagocytotic Capacity of Pulmonary Neutrophils in Cystic Fibrosis. *Clinical & Experimental Immunology* 142:68-75. ISSN 1365-2249

Moskwa, P., D.Lorentzen, K.J.D.A.Excoffon, J.Zabner, P.B.McCray, Jr., W.M.Nauseef, C.Dupuy, and B.Banfi. (2007). A Novel Host Defense System of Airways is Defective in Cystic Fibrosis. *Am. J. Respir. Crit. Care Med.* 175:174-183. ISSN 1073-449X

Moss, R.B., R.C.Bocian, Y.P.Hsu, Y.J.Dong, M.KEMNA, T.WEI, and P.Gardner. (1996). Reduced IL-10 Secretion by CD4+ T Lymphocytes Expressing Mutant Cystic Fibrosis Transmembrane Conductance Regulator (CFTR). *Clinical & Experimental Immunology* 106:374-388. ISSN 1365-2249

Moss, R.B., Y.P.Hsu, and L.Olds. (2000). Cytokine Dysregulation in Activated Cystic Fibrosis (CF) Peripheral Lymphocytes. *Clinical & Experimental Immunology* 120:518-525. ISSN 1365-2249

Mueller, C., S.A.Braag, A.Keeler, C.Hodges, M.Drumm, and T.R.Flotte. (2010). Lack of Cftr in CD3+ Lymphocytes Leads to Aberrant Cytokine Secretion and Hyper-inflammatory Adaptive Immune Responses. *Am. J. Respir. Cell Mol. Biol.*doi:10.1165/rcmb.2010-0224OC. ISSN 1044-1549

Noah, T.L., P.C.Murphy, J.J.Alink, M.W.Leigh, W.M.Hull, M.T.Stahlman, and J.A.Whitsett. (2003). Bronchoalveolar Lavage Fluid Surfactant Protein-A and Surfactant Protein-D Are Inversely Related to Inflammation in Early Cystic Fibrosis. *Am. J. Respir. Crit. Care Med.* 168:685-691. ISSN 1073-449X

Nurlan Dauletbaev, Roswitha Gropp, Michaela Frye, Stefan Loitsch, Thomas-Otto-Friedrich Wagner, and Joachim Bargon. (2002). Expression of Human Beta Defensin (HBD-1 and HBD-2) mRNA in Nasal Epithelia of Adult Cystic Fibrosis Patients, Healthy Individuals, and Individuals with Acute Cold. *Respiration* 69:46-51. ISSN 1423-0356

Painter, R.G., R.W.Bonvillain, V.G.Valentine, G.A.Lombard, S.G.LaPlace, W.M.Nauseef, and G.Wang. (2008). The Role of Chloride Anion and CFTR in Killing of Pseudomonas aeruginosa by Normal and CF Neutrophils. *J Leukoc Biol* 83:1345-1353. ISSN 0741-5400

Petit-Bertron, A.F., O.Tabary, H.Corvol, J.Jacquot, A.Clqment, J.M.Cavaillon, and M.dib-Conquy. (2008). Circulating and Airway Neutrophils in Cystic Fibrosis Display Different TLR Expression and Responsiveness to Interleukin-10. *Cytokine* 41:54-60. ISSN 1043-4666

Ratjen, F. and G.Doring. (2003). Cystic Fibrosis. *The Lancet* 361:681-689. ISSN 0140-6736

Roghanian, A., E.M.Drost, W.MacNee, S.E.M.Howie, and J.M.Sallenave. (2006). Inflammatory Lung Secretions Inhibit Dendritic Cell Maturation and Function via Neutrophil Elastase. *Am. J. Respir. Crit. Care Med.* 174:1189-1198. ISSN 1073-449X

Roum, J.H., R.Buhl, N.G.McElvaney, Z.Borok, and R.G.Crystal. (1993). Systemic Deficiency of Glutathione in Cystic Fibrosis. *Journal of Applied Physiology* 75:2419-2424. ISSN 8750-7587

Rzemieniak, S.E., A.F.Hirschfeld, R.E.Victor, M.A.Chilvers, D.Zheng, P.Van Den Elzen, and S.E.Turvey. (2010). Acidification-dependent Activation of CD1d-restricted Natural Killer T cells is Intact in Cystic Fibrosis. *Immunology* 130:288-295. ISSN 1365-2567

Sagel, S.D., R.K.Kapsner, and I.Osberg. (2005). Induced Sputum Matrix Metalloproteinase-9 Correlates with Lung Function and Airway Inflammation in Children with Cystic Fibrosis. *Pediatr. Pulmonol.* 39:224-232. ISSN 1099-0496

Soltys, J., T.Bonfield, J.Chmiel, and M.Berger. (2002). Functional IL-10 Deficiency in the Lung of cystic fibrosis (cftr-/-) and IL-10 Knockout Mice causes Increased Expression and Function of B7 Costimulatory Molecules on Alveolar Macrophages. *J Immunol* 168:1903-1910. ISSN 0022-1767

Sturges, N.C., M.E.Wikstrim, K.R.Winfield, S.E.Gard, S.Brennan, P.D.Sly, and J.W.Upham. (2010). Monocytes from Children with Clinically Stable Cystic Fibrosis Show Enhanced Expression of Toll-like Receptor 4. *Pediatr. Pulmonol.* 45:883-889. ISSN 8755-6863

Suri, R., L.J.Marshall, C.Wallis, C.Metcalfe, A.Bush, and J.K.Shute. (2002). Effects of Recombinant Human DNase and Hypertonic Saline on Airway Inflammation in Children with Cystic Fibrosis. *Am. J. Respir. Crit. Care Med.* 166:352-355. ISSN 1073-449X

Tabary, O., S.Escotte, J.Couetil, D.Hubert, D.Dusser, E.Puchelle, and J.Jacquot. (2001). Relationship Between IkappaBa Deficiency, NFkappaB Activity and Interleukin-8 Production in CF Human Airway Epithelial Cells. *Pflugers Archiv European Journal of Physiology* 443:S40-S44. ISSN 0031-6768

Tan, H.L., N.Regamey, S.Brown, A.Bush, C.M.Lloyd, and J.C.Davies. (2011). The Th17 Pathway in Cystic Fibrosis Lung Disease. *Am. J. Respir. Crit. Care Med.* 184:252-258. ISSN 1073-449X

Tirouvanziam, R. (2006). Neutrophilic Inflammation as a Major Determinant in the Progression of Cystic Fibrosis. *Drug News Perspect.* 19:609-614. ISSN 0214-0934

Vandivier, R.W., V.A.Fadok, P.R.Hoffmann, D.L.Bratton, C.Penvari, K.K.Brown, J.D.Brain, F.J.Accurso, and P.M.Henson. (2002a). Elastase-mediated Phosphatidylserine Receptor Cleavage Impairs Apoptotic Cell Clearance in Cystic Fibrosis and Bronchiectasis. *Journal of Clinical Investigation* 109:661. ISSN 0021-9738

Vandivier, R.W., V.A.Fadok, C.A.Ogden, P.R.Hoffmann, J.D.Brain, F.J.Accurso, J.H.Fisher, K.E.Greene, and P.M.Henson. (2002b). Impaired Clearance of Apoptotic Cells From Cystic Fibrosis Airways. *Chest* 121:89S. ISSN 0012-3692

Velsor, L.W., A.van Heeckeren, and B.J.Day. (2001). Antioxidant Imbalance in the Lungs of Cystic Fibrosis Transmembrane Conductance Regulator Protein Mutant Mice. *American Journal of Physiology - Lung Cellular and Molecular Physiology* 281:L31-L38. ISSN 1522-1504

Watt, A.P., J.Courtney, J.Moore, M.Ennis, and J.S.Elborn. (2005). Neutrophil Cell Death, Activation and Bacterial Infection in Cystic Fibrosis. *Thorax* 60:659-664. ISSN 0040-6376

Welsh MJ, Ramsey BW, Accurso F, and Cutting GR. (2011). Cystic Fibrosis. *In* the Online Metabolic & Molecular Bases of Inherited Disease. Charles R.Scriver, editor. McGraw-Hill, ISBN 0079130356, New York.

Xu, Y., C.Liu, J.C.Clark, and J.A.Whitsett. (2006). Functional Genomic Responses to Cystic Fibrosis Transmembrane Conductance Regulator (CFTR) and CFTRdeltaF508 in the Lung. *Journal of Biological Chemistry* 281:11279-11291. ISSN 0021-9258

Xu Y, Krause A, Wu W, Joh J, Limberis MP, and Worgall S. Characterization of Pulmonary Dendritic Cell in the Lung Disease of Cystic Fibrosis Mice following Respiratory Syncytial Virus Infection. American Thoracic Society 2009 International Conference. The American Journal of Respiratory and Critical Care Medicine ISSN 1535-4970, San Diego, California, USA, May 15-20, 2009.

Xu, Y., A.Krause, H.Hamai, B.G.Harvey, T.S.Worgall, and S.Worgall. (2010). Proinflammatory Phenotype and Increased Caveolin-1 in Alveolar Macrophages with Silenced CFTR mRNA. *PLoS. One.* 5:e11004. ISSN 1932-6203

Xu, Y., C.Tertilt, A.Krause, L.Quadri, R.Crystal, and S.Worgall. (2009). Influence of the CysticFibrosis Transmembrane Conductance Regulator on Expression of Lipid Metabolism-related Genes in Dendritic Cells. *Respir Res* 10:26.ISSN 1465-9921

Zaman, M.M., A.Gelrud, O.Junaidi, M.M.Regan, M.Warny, J.C.Shea, C.Kelly, B.P.O'Sullivan, and S.D.Freedman. (2004). Interleukin 8 Secretion from Monocytes of Subjects Heterozygous for the deltaF508 Cystic Fibrosis Transmembrane Conductance Regulator Gene Mutation is Altered. *Clin Diagn Lab Immunol* 11:819-824. ISSN 1071-412X

Part 4

Therapeutic Options

13

Channel Replacement Therapy for Cystic Fibrosis

John M. Tomich, Urška Bukovnik, Jammie Layman and Bruce D. Schultz
Departments of Biochemistry and Anatomy and Physiology
Kansas State University, Manhattan, Kansas
USA

1. Introduction

Epithelial monolayers act as barriers to the movement of small solute molecules - including both inorganic ions and drugs - between body compartments. Ions traverse epithelial apical and basolateral membranes *via* a combination of tightly regulated ion-specific transporters and channels. Compromised function of any component leads to electrolyte and fluid imbalances resulting in morbidity and potentially, mortality. In the case of cystic fibrosis (CF) the defect lies in various genotypes that result in suboptimal synthesis, folding, transport, or gating of the CF transmembrane conductance regulator (CFTR; an anion channel that has other reported cellular functions). Many of the current therapies involve palliative interventions that address infections, inflammation, nutrition and mucus viscosity issues in patients. While these approaches have increased the life span of CF patients by reducing the rate of decline in lung functions or other health issues, none of them addresses the underlying cause of the disease at the cellular or tissue level, namely reduced anion conductance that sets the chemiosmotic driving force for both paracellular and transcellular fluid movement.

Many recent studies focus on small molecule approaches to rescue some forms of CFTR that are defective with respect to folding, intracellular trafficking, or activity. Of particular note has been the identification of VX-770, a small molecule that restores CFTR activity in patients harboring the G551D mutation. Results of a phase 3 clinical trial showed that VX-770 improved lung function by 10.5 percent over the placebo and achieved all secondary goals of the study (Accuroso et al., 2010). This is the first drug to show improvement in lung function in patients with the G551D mutation. Unfortunately, such profound effects of this drug have not been realized when tests were conducted with patients harboring other CFTR mutations. Other small molecules that may affect other forms of CFTR (e.g., ataluren for premature stop codons) are in the pipeline, although none appears to be as advanced as VX-770.

The idea of using small pore-forming peptides to treat various channelopathies has been an ongoing objective since identifying the pore-defining M2 transmembrane (TM) segment in the α-subunit of the spinal cord glycine receptor (GlyR) Cl^- channel in the early 1990's (Reddy et al., 1993). The parent sequence, M2GlyR, is the pore-forming segment of the Cl^-

selective human spinal cord glycine receptor. In Wallace et al., (1992), we first suggested that inserting exogenous Cl^- channel-forming peptides into the apical membranes of airway epithelial cells of CF patients may aid in restoring the ability of these cells to secrete fluid. This was the rationale for developing synthetic Cl^--conducting channel-forming peptides as potential therapeutic agents. We have since developed synthetic peptides that form pores with varying degrees of anion conduction and selectivity. A guiding goal has been the *de novo* generation of a pore that could be used as a general therapeutic for CF since it would not require genotyping of individual patients. This novel therapeutic intervention, which would provide a new conductance pathway for selected anions, lies midway between conventional drug therapy and gene therapy. The primary target tissue, airway epithelium is accessible to aerosolized formulations such that the therapeutic peptides could be delivered easily.

The ideal therapeutic channel-forming peptide should: 1) have high aqueous solubility as a monomer; 2) have no detectable antigenicity; 3) bind to and then partition into biological membranes rapidly at low solution concentrations; 4) undergo supramolecular assembly in the membrane to form pores with measurable ion throughput; and 5) show physiologically relevant anion selectivity. All of these targeted outcomes have been achieved with the exception of the final goal, anion selectivity. In this regard, we are exploring distinct approaches to raise the permselectivity for Cl^- (P_{Cl}) relative to both Na^+ and K^+.

Cells exposed to our *de novo* peptides that form membrane pores appear to tolerate them well, with net anion flux controlled by the natural regulation of counter-ion transport and/or anion loading. Using a combination of peptide synthesis, electrophysiology, structural biology and computer simulations we are endeavoring to prepare highly anion-selective channels. Numerous studies have been performed that switch anion to cation selectivity and vice-versa (see review-Keramidasa et al., 2004). Our studies targeting enhanced anion selectivity are novel and will yield a lead compound for treating CF as well as aid in our understanding of anion selectivity in channel proteins. The work is being accomplished by preparing sequences with rational alterations to the residues that dictate the chemical composition and structure of the pore.

This chapter will review our extensive exploration of the permissible amino acid replacements in the M2GlyR sequence based on knowledge of Cl^- binding motifs and channel architecture. Modifications to the channel forming peptides were based on a wealth of data obtained from the fields of inorganic chemistry, channel physiology, structural determinations and computer modeling. The channel-forming peptides discovered during this project are remarkable in several ways: 1) they are small and easily synthesized; 2) they are water soluble and can be delivered to membrane surfaces without added organic solvents; 3) most are predominantly monomeric in solution; 4) when inserted into membranes, all peptides are expected to be oriented in the same direction due to the highly positively charged N-terminus; 5) all assembled pores are composed with a parallel orientation of the helices; 6) functional ion conducting pores are formed that can provide information on various channel properties; and 7) the small size of the peptides and the assembled pores facilitate concerted efforts for structural analyses and computer modeling that can produce informative structures.

To our knowledge no other membrane/peptide system offers such flexibility for design and analysis. Many TM sequences have been and are being studied by others (Marsh, 1996). However, for the most part, incorporation into bilayers leads to a mixed orientation with helical dipoles present in both directions. Such mixing of dipole orientations is prevented in our oligo-lysine adducted M2GlyR peptide system. This review will describe our understanding of how these peptides form channels with a range of anion selectivity and conductance properties, through a combination of electrophysiology, biophysical structural studies and computer simulations.

2. Current CF therapies

While a number of therapies for CF are currently in development, many of the treatment options presently available to patients are palliative in nature, addressing one or more symptoms of the condition and acting to reduce the severity of these effects and their associated risks.

Diet/nutritional supplements Proper diet and nutrition may reduce the impact and risk of CF-related conditions such as diabetes and osteoporosis. The lungs of CF patients appear to have fewer natural antioxidants than those without the condition, which may contribute to repeated infection and persistent inflammation. Patients may benefit from an increase in their intake of antioxidants through diet or supplements to fight this inflammation. Further promise may lie in drugs that work to build antioxidants in the lungs. AquADEKs® by Yasoo Health, Inc. is a vitamin supplement specifically formulated to meet the antioxidant needs of those with CF, and is commercially available. It has been shown to improve lung function, normalize vitamin levels in plasma and reduce neutrophilic inflammation (Sagel et al., 2011).

Enzyme replacement therapies Pancreatic enzyme products work to increase the digestion and absorption of fats, proteins, and starches while promoting the absorption of certain vitamins in those with CF, who often suffer from malnutrition due to enzyme deficiencies. The U.S. Food and Drug Agency (FDA) has approved a number of these products, including Zennen® (Eurand Pharmaceuticals), Creon® (Abbott Laboratories) and Pancreaze™ (Ortho-McNeil Pharmaceutical), while others, such as Pancrecarb® (DCI) and Ultrase® (Axcan Scandipharm) are still awaiting clinical trials. Liprotamase® (Alnara Pharmaceuticals) is a non-porcine pancreolipase enzyme therapy, which has completed a phase 3 clinical trial. However, the new drug application submitted by Alnara was rejected by the FDA on the grounds of insufficient data demonstrating the efficacy of the drug (Lowry, 2011).

Antibiotics/anti-infectives Due to the increased risk of disease caused by the excess and/or viscous mucus that is characteristic of CF, patients are often treated with antibiotics to circumvent chronic infections, such as that of *Pseudomonas aeruginosa*. Antibiotics can be administered orally, intravenously, via inhalation through devices such as metered dose inhalers (MDIs), or through implanted devices such as a port or Peripherally Inserted Central Catheter (PICC) (Gibson et al. 2003). TOBI® (tobramycin solution for inhalation) and recently developed Cayston® (aztreonam solution for inhalation) are two approved and commonly prescribed antibiotics for patients with CF, and both are effective against *P. aeruginosa*. TOBI® is approved to treat P. aeruginosa infections by concentrating the delivery of the antibiotic to the airways. Developed by Novartis Pharmaceuticals and widely used worldwide since its FDA approval in 1997, TOBI® has been successful in improving overall lung function while reducing hospital stays for CF patients (Cheer et al., 2003). TIP (TOBI® Inhalation Powder) is a new form of tobramycin that takes less time to administer via a Podhaler® and exhibits the same efficacy as the original formulation. It has been approved for use in Canada (http://www.pharmiweb.com/pressreleases/pressrel.asp?ROW_ID=23942 and http://www.novartis.com/newsroom /media-releases/en/2010/1446760.shtml). Cayston® (formerly GS9310/11) by Gilead Sciences is a newly developed version of the antibiotic aztreonam lysine in aerosol form. It was approved by the FDA and has been available to CF patients since February of 2010 (http://www.accessdata.fda.gov/scripts/cder/drugsatfda/ index.cfm?fuseaction=Search.DrugDetails).

The macrolide antibiotic azithromycin (Pfizer, Inc.) has been shown, when administered orally, to fight *P. aeruginosa* infection and improve pulmonary function in CF patients aged 6 years and older. Further studies are required to determine efficacy of prolonged treatment and in treating those under 6 years of age (Saiman et al., 2003). Further, azithromycin (Delete "the common antibiotic") was shown in phase 3 trials to preserve healthy lung function in CF patients (Saiman et al., 2010). Several other anti-infective agents, which are presently being evaluated, are discussed in brief below. Mpex Pharmaceuticals has recently developed MP-376, an aerosol form of levofloxacin, used to treat *P. aeruginosa* infections in the lungs. Phase 3 trials are currently underway (http://www.mpexpharma.com/mp-376.html). Insmed Incorporated recently completed phase 2 trials of Arikace™, a version of the FDA-approved antibiotic amikacin in a liposomal formulation that is inhaled using a nebulizer. It was shown in animal studies to decrease the pathogenicity of *P. aeruginosa* and has demonstrated success in permeating human sputum in the lungs. Phase 3 trials are set to begin in late 2011 (http://www.insmed.com/arikace.php). Bayer Schering Pharmaceuticals' BAY Q3939, was developed as a new inhaled version of the drug ciprofloxacin to more effectively treat infections in air passages. Phase 2 trials for the drug are currently underway (http://clinicaltrials.gov/ct2/show/NCT00645788).

Mucolytics/Airway-Rehydrating Agents Since viscous mucus build-up in the lungs can promote bacterial infections, many therapies are directed toward reducing the symptom by restoring the liquid necessary to hydrate the mucus or the underlying layer to facilitate expectoration (Pettit and Johnson, 2011) or, in the case of Pulmozyme® and other agents, to reduce mucus viscosity. Pulmozyme® by Genentech is a Dornase alfa (recombinant human deoxyribonuclease) treatment used to break down the DNA responsible for thickening pulmonary mucus and thus to reduce viscosity, promote mucus clearing, and ultimately restrict (delete "to", replace "reduce" with "restrict") the environment that supports bacterial growth. Approved in 1993 and introduced in 1994, Pulmozyme® is currently in use as a mucolytic for patients with CF and has been shown to increase lung function by about 6% and reduce the risk of infection by 27% (Fuchs et al., 1994; http://www.pulmozyme.com/hcp/prescribing-info.jsp#table1). Moli1901 by Lantibio stimulates alternative Cl^- channels in order to compensate for the deficiencies of CFTR in the pulmonary epithelium of patients. In phase 2 European trials, Moli1901 was well tolerated in most patients (one participant experienced a transient decrease in pulmonary function). Those receiving treatment of 2.5 mg daily of inhaled Moli1901 showed significant improvement in lung function measured as forced expiratory volume in one second (FEV_1; Grasemann et al., 2007).Initially promising, Denufosol, a P2Y2 agonist developed by Inspire, was believed to rehydrate the airway surface liquid, bypassing the basic CFTR protein defect, producing improvement in pulmonary function (Kellerman et al., 2008). However, the most recent clinical trial found it to be without effect. GS9411 by Gilead is an epithelial Na^+ channel (ENaC) inhibitor, which blocks Na^+ absorption in airways to reduce mucus dehydration. A phase 1 trial of GS9411 has been completed and the drug was shown to be safe and well tolerated (Sears et al., 2011; http://clinicaltrials.gov/ct2/show/NCT00999531).

An Australian clinical trial showed that a mist of hypertonic saline delivered via nebulizer twice daily for one year helped to improve lung function and reduce lung infections. The study included participants 6 years of age and older with mild or moderate lung disease (however, those with *Burkholderia cepacia* were not included in the study). The study tested two groups, one receiving "normal saline" solution at 0.9%, and the other receiving the "hypertonic saline" solution at 7% salt. While both groups showed improvement in pulmonary function during the study, those receiving hypertonic saline exhibited significantly greater improvement than those on normal saline. Elkins et al. (2006) reported that hypertonic saline also caused a reduction in exacerbations from the lungs, and Donaldson et al. (2008) hypothesized that this was due to the "protection" by hypertonic saline of non-obstructed airways from further mucus build-up and bacterial infection.

Similarly, an inhaled version of mannitol was shown to help clear CF airways and improve pulmonary function by an average of 7.3% (FEV_1) and forced airway flow by 15.5%. Mannitol works by drawing water into the lungs osmotically and thus helping to clear mucus. No serious adverse side effects were observed and it appeared to be well tolerated by patients (Jaques et al., 2008; Bilton et al., 2011). Phase 3 trials have been completed and the therapy is currently being marketed in Europe, and Pharmaxis hopes to submit a new drug application for Bronchitol to the FDA (http://www.pharmaxis.com.au/assets/pdf/2010/15122010).

Anti-Inflammatories Due to the recruitment of macrophages and neutrophils during rounds of bacterial infection, collateral damage to host airway cells by nuclear factor (NF)-*kappa* B activation and elevated pro-inflammatory cytokines leads to scarring and fibrosis. A number of anti-inflammatory agents are currently being used or studied to determine their efficacy in reducing inflammation in the pulmonary passages of CF patients. The over-the-counter drug, ibuprofen, taken orally twice daily at dosages adjusted to give peak plasma concentrations of 50 to 100 micrograms per milliliter, reportedly reduced the decline of lung function (Konstan et al., 1995). Oral N-acetylcysteine (PharrmaNAC, BioAdvantex Pharma, Inc.) was shown in clinical trials to reduce inflammation and increase pulmonary function by restoring glutathione in neutrophils. A phase 2 trial has completed enrolling subjects recently (Tirouvanziam et al., 2006; Atkuri et al., 2007). In a similar approach, inhaled doses of glutathione have completed phase 2 trials in Germany and data will be available in late 2011 (Retsch-Bogart, 2007). A University of Massachusetts study was conducted to test the efficacy of adding the fatty acid docosahexaenoic acid (DHA) to fortify infant formula in reducing CF pathogenicity. This work is based on the observation that an imbalance in fatty acids can lead to inflammation. It is hypothesized that an increase in DHA can help reduce inflammation that occurs with CF-related imbalances. Results of the study will be available in 2011. Genzyme Corp., which has licensed the patent as a treatment for CF, is considering new and more effective means of delivering DHA (Freedman et al., 1999; 2004). KB001 produced by Kalobios Pharmaceuticals reduces local inflammation from the virulence factor of *P. aeruginosa*. *P. aeruginosa* uses the structure of its Type Three Secretion System (TTSS) to break through cellular membranes and release toxins. KB001 binds to the PcrV protein essential to TTSS and inhibits its activity, reducing pathogenicity and preserving the immune defense of the host against *P. aeruginosa*. Though KB001 may reduce pathogenicity of *P. aeruginosa*, thereby preventing inflammation, it does not appear to affect in vivo growth of the bacteria, and thus is not classified as an anti-infective (Baer et al., 2008; http://www.kalobios.com/kb_pipeline_001.php). A recent report showed that an inhaled phosphodiesterase type 5 inhibitor, sildenafil, increased Cl^- transport in mice (Lubamba et al., 2011). Further research at the University of Wales suggested that sildenafil may assist in intracellular trafficking of the ΔF508-CFTR gene protein (Dormer et al., 2005). The corticosteroid, GSK SB 656933 manufactured by GlaxoSmithKline is an inhaled dose of fluticasone propionate used to treat lung inflammation was shown to be safe and tolerated in CF patients in phase 1 clinical trials (Lazar et al., 2011; http://www.clinicaltrials.gov/ct2/show/NCT00903201?term=656933&rank=5NLM Identifier: NCT00903201). The drug is currently used to reduce pulmonary inflammation in chronic obstructive pulmonary disease (COPD).

Experimental CF Therapies Aside from gene therapy, some new experimental approaches are aimed at modifying the folding or translocation of the endogenous mutant CFTR proteins in order to generate a functional channel protein at the cell surface. Correcting these defects would re-establish transcellular flow of Cl^-, Na^+, and water to clinically relevant levels to provide appropriate airway surface liquid volume and composition (http://www.cff.org/treatments/Pipeline/).

CF Gene Therapy is directed toward correcting the channelopathy by incorporating DNA that encodes for the full-length wild-type CFTR protein. Research suggests that CFTR gene expression is required at a mere 5% of the normal level in order to improve pulmonary function (Ramalho et al., 2002). There are a number of gene therapy protocols currently under investigation with the frontrunners discussed below.

Compacted DNA (PLASmin®): (unbold. Inconsistent) One problem in developing a treatment for CF through gene therapy is that non-viral DNA must be condensed, which is commonly achieved through the use of polycations. However, this often results in a complex that is too large to cross the cellular membrane effectively and deliver DNA to the affected cells. Cleveland-based Copernicus Therapeutics, Inc. developed a compacted DNA/DNA nanoparticle therapy (PLASmin®) that decreases the volume of the complex by up to 1000-fold, to a single molecule small enough to permeate the membrane and nuclei of target cells. The complex contains only one copy of the DNA to be delivered, increasing the stability and efficacy of the treatment (Chen et al., 2007). In phase 1a trials, plasmid DNA nanoparticles with the gene responsible for encoding CFTR were applied intra-nasally with lysine peptides substituted with polyethylene glycol. About two-thirds of the participants in the study showed a significant improvement and results persisted for up to 6 days. No adverse side effects of considerable severity were observed as a result of the compacted DNA. However, this trial presented no demonstration of gene expression (Konstan et al., 2004). More recently, Copernicus has experienced greater success with the level and duration of CFTR expression in animal models (http://www.thefreelibrary.com/Copernicus+ Receives+Milestone+Payment+from+Cystic+ Fibrosis+Foundation...-a0172302400).

VX-770 (Ivacaftor; Vertex Pharmaceuticals) is a novel therapy that seeks to augment CFTR activity in patients harboring the G551D mutation. This small molecule is a CFTR "potentiator" that increases function of faulty CFTR proteins by holding the defective channels in the open conformation. This treatment has completed phase 1 and phase 2 trials, which have shown efficacy in reducing sweat Cl^- concentrations and increasing nasal potential difference measures as well as improvements in general lung health. VX-770 replicated these results in two phase 3 trials - one for ages 12 and above (adult) and one for ages 6-11 (child). Both trials showed relevant increases in FEV_1 of 10.6% and 12.5% for each age group respectively over the placebo groups. VX-770 also helped patients in the trials gain weight - nearly 7 pounds on average for the adult trial and about 8 pounds for the children's trial. Finally, the phase 3 trials also showed increases in general lung health, indicated the treatment was well tolerated, and demonstrated lower sweat Cl^- levels. This closer to normal Cl^- range is very important to note as it provides empirical evidence that VX-770 is effectively treating the cause of CF and not just its symptoms. Vertex plans to submit a new drug application (NDA) to the FDA in late 2011 for VX-770 (Sheridan, 2011).

VX-809 in conjunction with VX-770: VX-809 is a novel small molecule CFTR "corrector" being developed by Vertex Pharmaceuticals that seeks to augment channel activity in CF patients with the ΔF508 CFTR mutation when used in conjunction with VX-770. The ΔF508 mutation affects 87% of CF patients in the United States (48% of patients have both mutant alleles while 39% have one). Misfolding of the mutated protein interferes with cytosolic trafficking such that the protein never reaches the apical membrane, precluding any anion secretion. VX-809 partially corrects the defect by promoting the trafficking of CFTR proteins to its proper location in the apical membrane. ΔF508 CFTR has a reduced open probability. Thus, VX-809 is paired with VX-770, the CFTR "potentiator", in the hopes of increasing total protein function for maximum effect on the disease. A phase 2 trial testing various dose combinations of the two compounds met its primary endpoints of safety and efficacy in the first part of the trial. Patients harboring the ΔF508 mutation were given VX-809 or a placebo for 14 days and then a combination VX-809 and VX-770 or a placebo for 7 more days. The drugs were well tolerated, though about half of patients did report some adverse respiratory events, none of which were deemed serious. Furthermore, the most effective combination regiment showed significant total reductions in the sweat Cl^- levels of 13 mmol/L from a baseline of ~100 mmol/L. The 14 days of solely VX-809 reduced sweat Cl^- by 4 mmol/L. This is strong evidence that, first, VX-809 is able to direct CFTR to its operational location and, second, that VX-770 is able to increase the function of this most common mutated form of CFTR once it has been moved to that location. The final part of this study will begin at the end of 2011 (Pollack, 2011; and http://investors.vrtx.com/releasedetail.cfm?releaseid= 583683).

Ataluren (formerly known as PTC124®) is a protein restoration therapy that helps produce working copies from mutated forms of CFTR that harbor nonsense mutations (nmCF). Pioneered by PTC Therapeutics, Ataluren® is a small molecule compound that has shown clinical promise through phase 2 trials in the alleviation of several genetic disorders caused by nonsense mutations, including nmCF. Exclusively targeting nonsense mutations, ataluren® overrides the premature stop codons symptomatic of these mutations to allow for the completion of the desired protein. In the case of nmCF, a small (19 participant) phase 2 trial showed an ability to produce viable, working copies of CFTR via this "ribosomal read through" mechanism. The study showed significant improvements in total Cl^- channel activity, measured by nasal transepithelial potential difference, which increased over time and led to improved pulmonary function and coughing. Ataluren was able to do this without interfering with other properly functioning stop codons, allowing the CFTR protein to be translated as initially designed and making the compound safe to administer. All trials of the compound have shown it to be well tolerated in humans with side effects mild and sparse to date. Ataluren®is currently in a 48 week CF phase 3 trial seeking statistically significant increased lung function, measured by FEV_1 as its primary endpoint with safety and drug activity as secondary endpoints. Ataluren has orphan status from the FDA and European Commission as well as Subpart E for expedited development from the FDA. The phase 3 trial data will become available in the first half of 2012 (Wilschanski et al., 2011; and http://www.ptcbio.com/3.1.1_genetic_disorders.aspx).

3. Channel replacement therapy

As indicated above, there are numerous approaches to treating this channelopathy. Combinations of these treatment modalities have increased the lifespan of those afflicted from 4, to now greater than 35 years of age. Perhaps the most significant of these therapies has been the use of pancreatic enzyme replacements, anti-inflammatories and powerful antibiotics. While restoration of CFTR activity has been an ultimate goal through CFTR rescue and in particular gene therapy, these therapeutic approaches have helped only limited numbers of patients. We have advocated another approach: *peptide-based channel replacement therapy.* Under this scenario a channel-forming peptide is applied to the apical surface of CF airway tissues to promote anion secretion and surface hydration. Gene therapy, to date, has involved the delivery of a CFTR-encoding DNA segment encased in a viral capsid to the affected epithelial tissues. There are serious problems with the gene therapy delivery vectors, transformation efficiency and CFTR production and delivery. Also airway epithelial cells have limited half-lives and the airway would need to undergo gene therapy on a regular basis to maintain expression. The new approach described here is much simpler (administered at home) and places the therapeutic directly on the target membrane (**Fig. 1**). Our efforts have been focused on developing a membrane-active peptide that can be delivered efficiently, assemble into a Cl^- selective pore, trigger fluid secretion and elicit no detectable immune or inflammatory responses. The remainder of this chapter traces the development of this treatment modality. While many of the desired properties have been incorporated into this therapy some hurdles remain. These will be discussed later in the chapter.

Chloride Channels Ion channels are usually multi-subunit protein molecules that have gated water-lined pores and an ion selectivity filter. Channels are individually gated by a variety of signals including ligands, non-covalent and covalent modifications, voltage, and/or mechanical stimuli. In most biological fluids, the most relevant physiological cations and anions are Na^+, K^+, and Ca^{2+}; and Cl^-, and HCO_3^-, respectively. An extensive literature is available to clearly document the high selectivity of naturally occurring cation channels in both excitable and non-excitable tissues (e.g., K_v, Na_v, ENaC, Ca_v, etc.). Three major classes of Cl^- channels have been cloned and studied. These include 1) the ligand gated channels typified by inhibitory post-synaptic glycine, glutamate and GABA receptors; 2) CFTR, which is an ABC transporter family member exhibiting complex nucleotide-dependent gating; and 3) ClC channels, which appear to be ubiquitous and are both voltage and metabolically gated. Ion channel classes display significant structural differences in the conductive pathway.

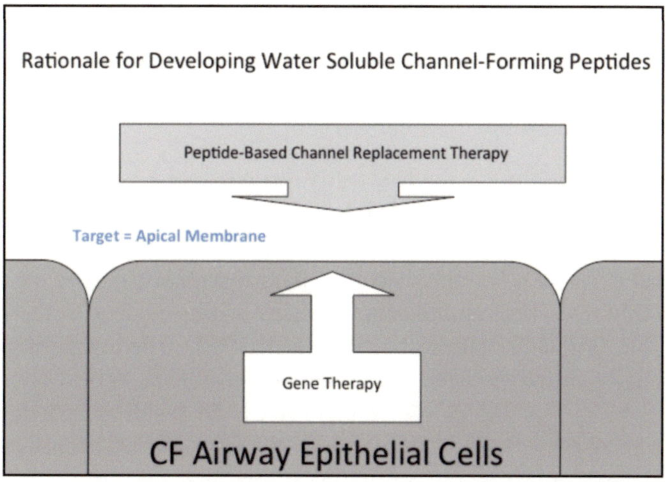

Fig. 1. The channel-forming peptide is delivered as an aerosol to the apical surface of CF airway cells. Upon binding to the surface it assembles to form an anion selective pathway to raise fluid secretion into the airway lumen thus rehydrating the airway surface fluid layer to allow proper cilia mediated airway clearance.

Class 1, the cys-loop ligand-gated ion channel superfamily of neurotransmitter receptors, includes the anion-selective inhibitory post-synaptic glycine (GlyR) and γ–aminobutyric acid type A (GABAAR) receptors, as well as cation selective nicotinic acetylcholine (nAChR), and 5-hydroxytryptamine type 3 (5-HT3R) receptors (Jensen et al., 2005; Sine and Engel, 2006) and the invertebrate post-synaptic glutamate receptor (Sunesen et al., 2006). These related structures all have a simple central pore defined by the parallel association of the second TM or 'M2' segments contributed by each of the five assembled subunits. Structural features common across members of this superfamily include the presence of heteropentameric bundles of subunits that are each composed of four hydrophobic TM segments, M1-M4, along with various sizes of intracellular and extracellular domains. Each M2 contributes a pore lining helix to form the channel. Unwin and co-workers (Unwin, 2003; Miyazawa et al., 2003; Unwin, 2005) published a 4 Å density map of the nAChR from *Torpedo marmorata.* The pentameric pore forms an hourglass-shaped pathway with the narrowest part at the middle of the lipid bilayer. The cation-conducting pathway, which is 40 Å long and extends beyond the lipid bilayer, is formed by parallel helices that are aligned, in registry, such that the same residues in different helices form rings that define discrete microenvironments. S266, E262, T244, E241, S248, and S252 form polar rings and hydrophobic residues V255 and L251 form the narrowest portion of the pore. It is important to note that in this barrel and stave type pore, amino acids possessing R-groups with a full charge are present. These negatively charged R groups are located as sites where the hourglass geometry is more open. McCammon and co-workers (Ivanov et al., 2007) modeled the α1-GlyR pore by threading the GlyR M2 helical segments onto the Unwin structure. Then, using molecular dynamics, they simulated the water density profile and Cl^- translocation. A number of relevant conclusions were presented: the GlyR M2 pore is fully hydrated indicating that permeating Cl^- is fully hydrated as well, no hydrophobic barrier was observed that would help in dehydrating the anion, and that the pore at its narrowest had a radius of 2.5 Å. These observations are in agreement with data that we have observed with our anion selective pores, which will be presented later. The McCammon group did not take into account any contribution of the M1-M2 loop toward anion selectivity. This extracellular loop, through mutational analyses, has been implicated in selectivity by several groups (Gunthorpe and Lummis, 2001; Jensen et al., 2005).

Hilf and Dutzler (2008) published the first x-ray structure of a bacterial cys-loop channel at 3.3 Å resolution in a presumed "closed-state". This channel protein shares 16% sequence identity with the *Torpedo* nAChRα protein. It is strictly a cation channel although there is little selectivity between Na^+, K^+, and Ca^{2+}. It differs significantly from the mammalian cys-loop channels in that no helical cytoplasmic domain is present. The authors were unable to identify any ion binding sites within the pore itself. This structure is of great significance since it provides key parameters such as the handedness of the helical bundle (left) and the tilt angle of the helices. The TM pore-forming helix is 25 residues in length with the pore lined by residues S226, E229, T233, T236, T240, A243, Y247 and I251. This structure provides key spatial coordinates for our modeling studies.

GlyR α_1-subunits alone have been shown to form homopentameric channels, when expressed in *Xenopus* oocytes, with properties similar to the parent channels (Schmeiden et al., 1989). The ability of this channel to function as a homo-pentameric array made it an attractive candidate for probing ion selectivity and permeation.

Class 2 is represented by CFTR, the only channel member of the ABC transporter superfamily, which has 12 TM segments divided between two different halves each containing a nucleotide binding domain and linked by a regulatory domain (Riordan, 2008; Zhang et al., 2011). In a collaborative study with M. Montal, we identified four segments (M2, M6, M10, and M12) that assembled in synthetic bilayers to form a Cl^- conducting pore (Montal, et al., 1994). Since that time other TM segments (M1, M3, M5 and M11) have been implicated in participating in pore assembly (Zhang et al., 2000; Linsdell, 2006). Others have suggested that the active channel is composed of a homo-dimer (Zerhusen et al., 1999). The selectivity filter is believed to reside in the M6 segment (Zhou et al., 2002). Mutational studies in M6 support this assignment (Beck et al., 2008; Alexander et al., 2009). Clearly, this channel structure is more complex than that observed for the GlyR in that the CFTR pore requires the assembly of multiple non-identical TM segments.

Dawson and co-workers (Mansoura et al., 1998; Dawson et al., 1999; Smith et al., 2001; Liu et al., 2001) examined the selectivity properties of the CFTR channel, and proposed that reducing the dielectric of the pore is enough to cause anion selectivity. They prefaced their remarks by saying that the CFTR channel is probably a more primitive channel than the Class 1 channel types. CFTR exhibits lyotropic anion selectivity such that anions that are more readily dehydrated than Cl- are preferentially selected and show higher permeability rates. Their model predicts that larger anions, like SCN^-, although they experience weaker interactions (relative to Cl^-) with water and the channel, are more permeant than Cl^- (but with a smaller conductance). They appear to have a smaller net energy cost entering the channel relative to that of Cl^-. That is, the reduced energy of hydration allows the net transfer energy (the well depth) to be more negative. The net positive charge of the pore lining residues also contributes to selectivity.

Class 3 is the ClC channel family, which includes ClC-0, through ClC-7 in vertebrate species. This is the only family for which detailed structural assignments have been generated. Several bacterial ClC channels have been crystallized and analyzed with regard to the pore structure and the Cl^- selectivity filter (Dutzler, et al., 2002; Dutzler et al., 2003). The active protein is a homo-dimer assembled from subunits that contain two identical anti-parallel domains. Each subunit contributes one channel to make a double-barreled channel structure. Each pore is made up of numerous anti-parallel helices of various lengths and contains two gating regions and a Cl^- binding site. More recent crystallographic and mutational data suggest that there are three anion-binding sites within the open state of each pore in the highly conserved ClC family of channels and transporters (Lobet and Dutzler, 2006). The proposed central selectivity filter is composed, in part, using amide nitrogens from three different helices (N, F and D) pointing toward the anion-binding site. These amides are more positively charged because of the helix dipoles. The site also contains S107 and T445 (Corry and Chung, 2006). The amides and hydroxyls of these atoms are oriented such that they could form hydrogen bonds with Cl^-. The serine side chain appears to be activated since the serine hydroxyl oxygen is also hydrogen bound to the amide nitrogen of I109. The anion never appears to interact with full positive charge from residues such as lysine or arginine. More recently three other residues have been implicated in selectivity through mutational studies K149, G352, and H401 in ClC-0 (Zhang et al., 2006). This class of channels is structurally distinct from the class 1 ligand-gated channels that contain a single pentameric array of parallel M2 helices of identical length. Despite these significant differences, the central ClC Cl^- selectivity filter offers insight into the types of binding interactions that are utilized by Cl^- selective channels.

4. M2GlyR studies

Early studies regarding first generation M2GlyR sequences When it became apparent that CFTR was a Cl^- selective channel, finding and inserting an alternative Cl^- conductive pathway into airway epithelia as a potential treatment modality became a realizable goal. Having already observed Cl^- selectivity in synthetic phospholipid bilayers (Reddy et al., 1993) with the M2 segment from the glycine receptor as both the free peptide (M2GlyR) and as a four-helix bundle (T_4-M2GlyR) built with a template strategy (Mutter et al., 1989; Iwamoto et al., 1994), this sequence was an obvious choice to begin studying its effects on epithelial monolayers. Due to the complexity of synthesizing and purifying the template sequence, the studies focused on the more tractable monomeric form.

The initial ion permeation studies in epithelial monolayers were conducted with the sequence PARVGLGITTVLTMTTQSSGSRA, corresponding to amino acids 250-272 in the glycine receptor protein, using confluent Madin-Darby canine kidney (MDCK) monolayers. When suspended at 100 μM in water containing 1% DMSO, the peptide caused a 1 μAcm^{-1} increase in short circuit current (I_{sc}), an extremely sensitive indicator of net ion flux. The increase in I_{SC}

occurred slowly with the net change being observed 30 minutes after peptide addition and this increase was observed only in 24 of 37 monolayers tested, suggesting inconsistencies in delivering the sequence to the membrane and then having it insert properly. In addition to the poor efficiency value, other drawbacks included limited solubility of the sequence and the inability to control the orientation of the inserted peptide in the bilayer.

To decrease these deficiencies, the M2GlyR sequence was modified systematically by adding up to six lysyl or diaminopropionic acid (DAP) residues to either the C- or N-terminus (Tomich et al., 1998). This study examined a number of physical, pharmacological and physiological characteristics of the adducted sequences. Increasing the positive charge at either terminus increased solubility dramatically and also directed the orientation of the peptide within the bilayer. The effect was more dramatic for the C-terminus additions (**Fig. 2**) with 5 lysines giving a peptide that showed solubility at saturation, in Ringer solution, of 56.1 mM. Placing four lysines at either the C- or N-terminus appeared to be optimal in that these modified sequences yielded larger I_{SC} values, greater aqueous solubility and exhibited nearly 100 percent efficiency in generating measurable changes in I_{SC}. The resulting I_{SC} was sensitive to bumetanide, a diuretic that blocks the activity of the $Na^+/K^+/2Cl^-$ cotransporter that is responsible for anion loading at the basolateral membrane, and to a non-selective Cl^- channel blocker, DPC. The aqueous solubility increased from 1.4 mM for the unmodified sequence to 27.5 and 13.4 mM for the CK_4- and NK_4-M2GlyR sequences, respectively. I_{SC} for CK_4- and NK_4-M2GlyR were larger by 2.7- and 1.2-fold, respectively.

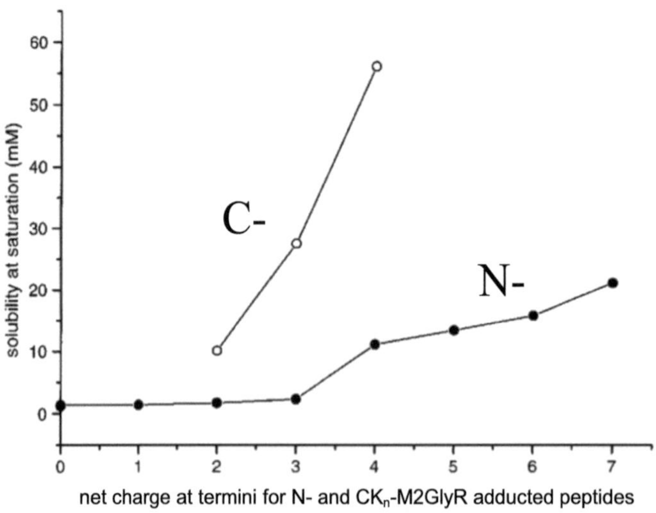

Fig. 2. Solubility as a function of net charge by the addition of lysines to either the C- or N-terminus of M2GlyR

Given the fact that adding lysines to either end improved solubility and showed increased magnitudes of net ion transport, studies were initiated to more fully describe the effects of CK_4-M2GlyR on MDCK cell monolayers primarily because placing lysines at the C-terminus yielded a pore that had an orientation, relative to the cell membrane, that was identical to the native GlyR channel. Additionally, the presence of the C-terminal lysines would be expected to stabilize the helix dipole. The helix dipole is important in the packing of adjacent helices such as those found in the helical bundle formed by the supramolecular assembly of the M2 peptides.

CK_4-M2GlyR significantly increased I_{SC}, hyperpolarized transepithelial potential difference, and induced fluid secretion. In 28 monolayers, CK_4-M2GlyR (100 μM) significantly increased I_{SC} from 0.8 ± 0.1 to 3.3 ± 0.4 μAcm^{-2} and hyperpolarized transepithelial voltage (V_{te}) from 1.5 ± 0.4 to 3.5 ± 0.6 mV (apical bath negative). Transepithelial electrical resistance (R_{te}; a composite indicator of the transcellular and paracellular permeation pathways) decreased from 1,399 ± 341 to 1,013 ± 171 Ω cm^2. In other experiments the increase in I_{SC} was inhibited by bumetanide (100 μM) and by some Cl^- channel inhibitors. The effectiveness of the channel blockers followed the sequence niflumic acid ≥ 5-nitro-2- (3-phenylpropylamino) benzoate (NPPB) > diphenylamine-2-carboxylate (DPC) > glibenclamide. The effect of the peptide was not inhibited by 4,4′- diisothiocyanostilbene-2, 2′-disulfonic acid (DIDS). Removing Cl^- from the bathing solutions also abrogated the effect of the peptide. The Cl^- efflux pathway induced by CK_4-M2GlyR differs from the native adenosine 3′, 5′-cyclic monophosphate (cAMP)-mediated pathway that can be activated by adrenergic agonists and by forskolin. First, intracellular cAMP levels were unaffected and second, the concentration of DPC required to inhibit the effect of the peptide was much lower than that needed to block the forskolin response (100 μM vs. 3 mM). These results support the hypothesis that the synthetic peptide, CK_4-M2GlyR, can form Cl^--selective channels in the apical membrane of secretory epithelial cells and can induce sustained transepithelial Cl^- secretion that can drive fluid secretion. I_{SC} remained relatively constant for the first 2 h after the addition of the peptide. After 3 h, the CK_4-M2GlyR-stimulated current was 90% of the current recorded at 60 min and decreased to 55% after 4 h. In washout experiments (n = 3), I_{SC} was measured after removing CK_4-M2GlyR from the bath. One hour after removal of the peptide, 39% of the CK_4-M2GlyR-induced current remained, and, after 2 h, there was no persisting effect of the peptide.

In a separate series of experiments (Wallace et al., 2000), transport of Cl^- through the CK_4-M2GlyR conductive pathway was modulated by basolateral K^+ efflux through Ca^{2+}-dependent K^+ channels. Application of CK_4-M2GlyR to the apical surface of T84 cell monolayers (derived from human colon) generated a sustained increase in I_{SC} and caused net fluid secretion. The current was reduced by clotrimazole, an inhibitor of SK and IK channels, and by charybdotoxin, a more selective and potent inhibitor of the *KCNN4* gene product, KCa3.1, a Ca^{2+}-dependent K^+ channel. Direct activation of these channels with 1-ethyl-2-benzimidazolinone (1-EBIO) greatly amplified the Cl^- secretory current induced by CK_4-M2GlyR. The effect of the combination of CK_4-M2GlyR and 1-EBIO on I_{SC} was significantly greater than the sum of the individual effects of the two compounds and was independent of cAMP. Treatment with 1-EBIO also increased the magnitude of fluid secretion induced by the peptide. The cooperative action of CK_4-M2GlyR and 1-EBIO on I_{SC} was attenuated by Cl^- transport inhibitors, by removing Cl^- from the bathing solution, and by basolateral treatment with K^+ channel blockers. These results indicate that apical membrane insertion of Cl^- channel-forming peptides such as CK_4-M2GlyR and direct activation of basolateral K^+ channels with benzimidazolones may coordinate the apical Cl^- conductance and the basolateral K^+ conductance, thereby providing a pharmacological approach to modulate Cl^- and fluid secretion by human epithelia deficient in CFTR.

Changes in the electrical properties of epithelial monolayers exposed to both 1-EBIO and CK_4-M2GlyR were observed. Basolateral addition of 1-EBIO (600 μM) induced a small increase in I_{SC} and doubled V_{te} with only a nominal decrease in R_{te}. Apical exposure of the 1-EBIO-treated monolayers to CK_4-M2GlyR (100 μM) caused an eight-fold increase in I_{SC} from 2.1 ± 0.2 to 16.5 ± 0.9 μAcm^{-2}, hyperpolarized V_{te} hyperpolarized by 7.3±0.5 mV and reduced R_{te} by 1.53±0.33 $K\Omega cm^2$. In two experiments, the response to 1-EBIO and CK_4-M2GlyR was monitored for 5 h. I_{SC} remained relatively constant during the first 60 min; however, I_{SC} had decreased to 73% of this current at 2 h, 53% at 3 h, 41% at 4 h and 29% of the current at 5 h. In washout experiments (n=2), the current generated by the additions of 1-EBIO and CK_4-M2GlyR was monitored for a set period of time, then CK_4-M2GlyR was washed out of the chamber. The removal of CK_4-M2GlyR from the medium decreased I_{SC} by 39%, whereas the subsequent removal of 1-EBIO decreased I_{SC} to the control level.

The addition of 1-EBIO increases the secretion of fluid induced by the apical application of CK_4-M2GlyR to T84 cell monolayers. T84 cell monolayers were grown in four groups of 10 monolayers, to test for the effects on the rate of transcellular fluid transport. Group I was incubated for 12 h in control medium, group II was exposed apically to CK_4-M2GlyR (500 μM), group III was exposed to 1-EBIO (300 μM) and group IV was exposed to both CK_4-M2GlyR and 1-EBIO. Monolayers incubated in control medium secreted fluid at a rate of 130 ± 40 $nLh^{-1}cm^{-2}$, a value that was not significantly different from monolayers exposed to 1-EBIO (180 ± 30 $nLh^{-1}cm^{-2}$). Monolayers exposed to just CK_4-M2GlyR exhibited a significantly greater rate of fluid secretion, 250 ± 20 $nLh^{-1}cm^{-2}$ and a combination of CK_4-M2GlyR and 1-EBIO increased the rate of fluid secretion further to 330 ± 20 $nLh^{-1}cm^{-2}$. These results demonstrated that anion secretion induced by the apical membrane insertion of CK_4-M2GlyR drives the secretion of fluid and that the direct activation of basolateral K^+ channels by 1-EBIO potentiates this effect on the rate of secretion.

In other experiments, it was determined that the increase in Cl^- and fluid secretion induced by combining CK_4-M2GlyR and 1-EBIO was independent of intracellular cAMP levels since the addition of the two compounds did not significantly affect cAMP content. This implies that CK_4-M2GlyR and 1-EBIO had minimal effect on CFTR Cl^- conductance or other cAMP-dependent processes. Therefore, we propose that the major action of 1-EBIO is to activate the Ca^{2+}-dependent K^+ channels and that the increase in the Cl^- secretory current is due to increasing the electrochemical driving force for Cl^- efflux through synthetic Cl^- channels generated by the membrane insertion of CK_4-M2GlyR. In summary, we have demonstrated that the synthetic Cl^- channel-forming peptide, CK_4-M2GlyR, induces Cl^- and fluid secretion by T84 cells, which are derived from human intestine. Activators and inhibitors of a basolateral Ca^{2+}-dependent K^+ conductance modulated the magnitude of this response. We propose that the combination of the novel synthetic Cl^- channel-forming peptide, CK_4-M2GlyR, and agents like 1-EBIO may have pharmacological benefits for inducing and modulating transepithelial Cl^- and fluid secretion independent of the cAMP-dependent Cl^- secretion that is impaired in CF.

In a subsequent study we examined whether CK_4-M2GlyR could exert effects on whole cell Cl^- conductance in isolated epithelial cells, and if the observed effects were the result of formation of a novel Cl^- conductance pathway, modulation of endogenous Cl^- channel activity, or a combination of these effects. The outcomes indicated that extracellular application of CK_4-M2GlyR to isolated MDCK, T84, and IB3-1 cells resulted in increased permeability of the cells to Cl^-. The experimental evidence suggested a direct mechanism of action. Studies looking at the effects of the oligo-lysine portion of the sequence suggested that a poly-lysine modified K_4-helical peptide was not sufficient to activate endogenous CFTR through an electrostatic mechanism.

The ability of CK_4-M2GlyR to induce a time- and voltage-independent current in the IB3-1 cell line, which lacks functional CFTR, suggested that CK_4-M2GlyR does not increase Cl^- current by activating CFTR. Furthermore, the pharmacological profile of the induced current supports this conclusion. Specifically, the CK_4-M2GlyR-induced currents do not share biophysical characteristics of the hyperpolarization activated current associated with ClC-2 as determined with and without antisense ClC-2 cDNA, the swelling-activated current associated with Volume-Sensitive Organic Osmolyte/Anion Channels (VSOAC), with and without tamoxifen, and the Ca^{2+}-dependent Cl^- current activated by CaM Kinase II, with and without KN-62. Together, these results support the premise that the M2GlyR peptides increase I_{SC} across epithelial monolayers by forming a novel permeation pathway for Cl^- rather than by activation of endogenous Cl^- conductances.

In some of the most compelling work done to test the validity of the peptide-based channel replacement therapy, nasal potential difference (PD) studies were performed at the Gregory Fleming James Cystic Fibrosis Center at the University of Alabama, Birmingham, under the direction of Dr. Eric Sorscher. More than 40 mice were tested for effects of either CK_4-M2GlyR or NK_4-M2GlyR. A standardized protocol that employs transitions to amiloride, Cl^--free medium, and exposure to adrenergic stimuli was employed. The ΔF508 homozygous transgenic mouse nasal epithelia exhibit ion transport defects identical to those in CF human airways and, thus, are an excellent model to test for potential therapeutic effects. Ion transport was assessed by repeated nasal PD measurements in both transgenic and wild-type mice (Brady et al., 2001). Key data from a double-blind study employing both CK_4-M2GlyR and NK_4-M2GlyR are summarized in **Fig. 3**. As expected, isoproterenol, in a Cl^--free medium containing amiloride, caused a positive shift in nasal PD of CF mice (CF control) while causing a negative shift in the nasal PD of wild-type (WT) littermates. Importantly, following exposure of CF nasal epithelia to either CK_4-M2GlyR or NK_4-M2GlyR (500 μM) the effect of isoproterenol more closely resembled the effect in the WT animals than in the CF animals that received no peptide or were exposed to either of two control peptides that were expected to have no effect. Control #1 was too short to span the bilayer of a cell membrane and Control #2 (NK_4-Sc) has its transmembrane segment randomized, although computer modeling was employed to maximize helical propensities while minimizing the amphipathic character of the helix. Sustained Cl^- conductance was observed for up to 6 h after a single application of peptide in solution. While this outcome is very encouraging, this type of treatment would have to be administered one or more times per day for optimal clinical results.

Concurrent exposure to 1-EBIO changed the direction for the development of M2GlyR channel-forming peptides. Initially, most studies were performed using CK_4-M2GlyR. However, CK_4-M2GlyR and NK_4-M2GlyR behaved differently in the presence of the K^+-channel opener. N-terminal modification of a channel-forming peptide increases capacity for epithelial anion secretion. In Ussing chamber experiments, apical exposure of MDCK and T84 cell monolayers to NK_4-M2GlyR (250 μM) increased I_{SC} by 7.7 ± 1.7 and 10.6 ± 0.9 μAcm-

[2], respectively (Broughman et al., 2001). These values are significantly greater than those previously reported for the same peptide modified by adding the lysines at the C- terminus (Wallace et al., 1997). NK_4-M2GlyR caused a concentration-dependent increase in I_{SC} ($k_{1/2}$ = 190 μM) that was potentiated two- to threefold by 1-EBIO (300 μM). NK_4-M2GlyR-mediated increases in I_{SC} were insensitive to changes in apical cation species. Pharmacological inhibitors of endogenous Cl^- conductances (glibenclamide, DPC, NPPB, DIDS, and niflumic acid) had little effect on NK_4-M2GlyR-mediated I_{SC}. Whole cell membrane patch-voltage clamp studies revealed an NK_4-M2GlyR-induced anion conductance that exhibited modest outward rectification and modest time- and voltage-dependent activation. Planar lipid bilayer studies indicated that NK_4-M2GlyR forms a 50-pS anion conductance with a $k_{1/2}$ for Cl^- of 290 mEq. NK_4-M2GlyR was similar to the previously characterized analog, CK_4-M2GlyR, in that both sequences elicited increases in the anion-selective current in lipid bilayers, whole cell membrane patches, and epithelial monolayers. When employed at similar concentrations, NK_4-M2GlyR provided for greater anion secretion across epithelial cell monolayers than any related channel-forming peptide tested to this point. Effects for NK_4-M2GlyR were observed with as little as 25–30 μM, and maximal effects were observed with about 500 μM (**Table 1** and **Fig. 4**; Broughman et al., 2002a).

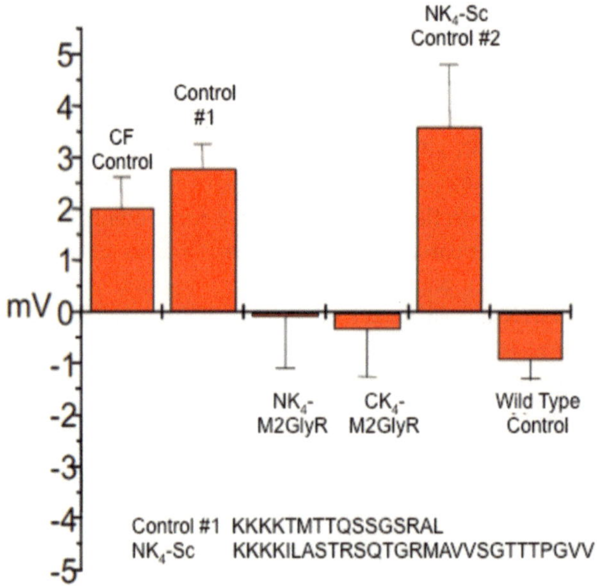

Fig. 3. Isoproterenol-induced change in nasal PD of ΔF508 homozygous mice and wild-type littermates in the absence or presence of indicated peptides.

Sequence	name	Mr (Da)	Sol.(mM)	n	I_{MAX} (μA/cm2)	$k_{1/2}$ (μM)
1. PARVGLGITTVLTMTTQSSGSRA	M2GlyR	2304.7	1.4	N/A	N/A	N/A
2. PARVGLGITTVLTMTTQSSGSRAKKKK	CK_4-M2GlyR	2817.4	27.5	2.7 ± 0.9	102.5	>500
3. KKKKPARVGLGITTVLTMTTQSSGSRA	NK_4-M2GlyR	2817.4	13.4	1.52 ± 0.55	24.3 ± 0.5	319 ± 192

Table 1. Characterization of M2GlyR peptides with C- and N-terminal oligo-lysine adducts.

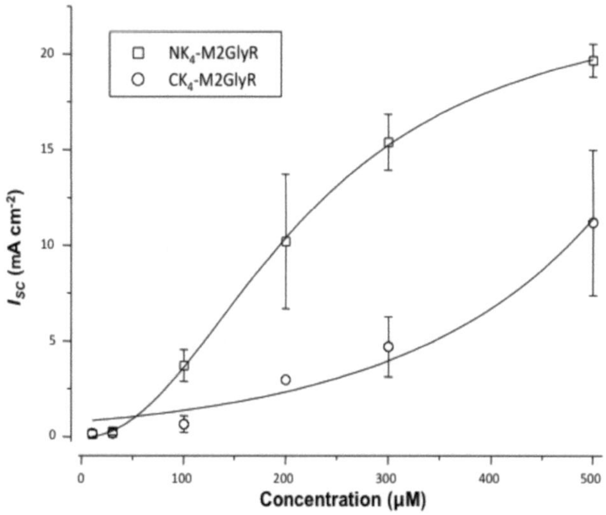

Fig. 4. The dependence of I_{SC} of MDCK monolayers on NK4-M2GlyR and CK4-M2GlyR concentration in the presence of 1-EBIO. Solid lines represent the best fit of a modified Hill equation to the data sets.

The resulting parameters for NK4-M2GlyR (I_{max} = 25.2 ± 10.4 μAcm^{-2}, $k_{1/2}$ = 319 ± 192 μM, n (Hill coefficient) = 1.52 ± 0.55) are similar to those reported above , I_{max} = 24.3 ± 0.5 μAcm^{-2}, $k_{1/2}$ = 208 ± 6 μM, and n = 2.6 ± 0.1). This degree of cooperativity suggests that a multi-step process is required to form functional channel assemblies. Whether the cooperative step involves membrane partitioning, assembly of the helical bundles into structures, or a combination of these necessary steps for channel formation is not known. The concentration dependence of CK4-M2GlyR is right-shifted compared to that of NK4-M2GlyR, with the response at the greatest concentration tested (500 μM) showing no indication of saturation. The experimental data for CK4-M2GlyR, when fitted by the modified Hill equation, resulted in a substantially greater value for I_{max} than that observed for a variety of agonists and pore-forming peptides (25–30 μA cm^{-2}). When employed at similar concentrations, NK4-M2GlyR provides for greater anion secretion across epithelial cell monolayers than any related channel-forming peptide tested thus far. These results indicate that NK4-M2GlyR forms an anion-selective channel in epithelial monolayers and again showed its therapeutic potential for the treatment of hyposecretory disorders such as CF.

One of the early applications of NK4-M2GlyR included a study looking at the effect of exogenously applied peptide to the surface of immortalized human tracheal epithelial cells from a homozygous ΔF508 CFTR CF patient (Yankaskas et al., 1993). CF is characterized by defective epithelial Cl^- transport with damage to the lungs occurring, in part, via chronic inflammation and oxidative stress. Glutathione, a major antioxidant in the airway lining fluid, is decreased in CF airway due to reduced glutathione efflux (Gao et al., 1999). This observation prompted a study to examine the question of whether exposure to channel-forming peptides would also restore glutathione secretion (Gao et al., 2001). Addition of the Cl^- channel-forming NK4-M2GlyR (500 μM) and a K^+ channel activator (chlorzoxazone, 500 μM) increased Cl^- secretion, measured as bumetanide-sensitive I_{SC}, and/or glutathione efflux, measured by high-performance liquid chromatography, in a human CF airway epithelial cell line (CFT1). Addition of the peptide alone increased glutathione secretion (181 ± 8% of the control value), whereas chlorzoxazone alone did not significantly affect glutathione efflux; however, chlorzoxazone potentiated the effect of the NK_4-M2GlyR on glutathione release (359 ± 16% of the control value). CK_4-M2GlyR has decreased efficacy compared with NK_4-M2GlyR in both I_{SC} and GSH efflux assays. The addition of 1-EBIO also amplified the effect of NK_4-M2GlyR (500 μM) on GSH efflux (286 ± 1 % of control values). These studies demonstrated that glutathione efflux can be modulated by channel-forming peptides and is likely associated with Cl^- secretion, not necessarily with CFTR per se, and the defect of glutathione efflux in CF can be overcome pharmacologically.

Both orientations of the M2GlyR helix within the membrane form anion-selective pores. However, differences in solubility, solution associations and channel-forming activity for the oligo-lysyl adducted forms were observed. While deciding on which of the oligo-lysine adducted M2GlyR peptides to develop further, we began a study utilizing chemical cross-linking, NMR and molecular modeling to determine how the positioning of the lysyl residues affected the channel properties and structural characteristics. These sequences are amphipaths with distinct clusters of hydrophobic and hydrophilic residues. In aqueous solution, hydrophobic patches associate and hydrophilic ones are solvent exposed. This property generally leads to aggregation through a concentration dependent process. This model predicts that multiple higher molecular weight assemblies, which do not readily interact with membranes, would be formed (**Fig. 5**). Evidence indicating aggregate formation is discussed below. A preferred outcome, however, would be to have a peptide that remained predominantly monomeric in solution while retaining its membrane binding and insertion activities. The actual sequence of insertion and assembly events leading to a functional channel are still unresolved. We do know that much of the process is slowly reversible based on perfusion washout experiments (indicated by the double ended arrows). Two possible routes are shown. One (right) has the peptide inserting and folding as a single step followed by assembly. The second (left) has peptide folding occurring at the surface followed by assembly as a prerequisite for insertion. A mixture of the two pathways could also be possible. Optimization of the channel-forming structure included modifications to reduce solution oligomerization and thereby increase the concentration of peptide that could insert and form active assemblies. CK_4-M2GlyR and NK_4-M2GlyR formed aggregates in aqueous solutions to differing degrees, as shown in **Fig. 6**. A cross-linking reagent was used to trap solution aggregates that were visualized using sodium dodecyl sulfate - polyacrylamine gel electrophoresis (SDS-PAGE) (Broughman et al., 2002b). Bis [Sulfosuccinimidyl] suberate (BS^3), a water-soluble homo-bifunctional cross-linking reagent that reacts with free amino groups in the lysine adducts was employed. The cross-linking reactions were carried out in 10 mM 4-(2-hydroxyethyl) piperazine-1-ethanesulfonic acid (HEPES) buffer, pH 6.5, at selected peptide concentrations in the presence of a 40-fold molar excess of cross-linking reagent. The results from a typical experiment are shown in **Fig. 6**. Lanes 5 and 9, show the electrophoretic mobility of non-cross-linked CK_4-M2GlyR and NK_4-M2GlyR boiled in 10% SDS, respectively. Under these conditions both sequences are monomeric, indicating that the solution associations that are trapped with the cross-linking reagent (in the adjoining lanes) are dissociated in the presence of the anionic detergent. The cross-linked molecular weight profiles for the two sequences are strikingly different. CK_4-M2GlyR forms lower molecular weight associations with monomer through trimer being the most prevalent. NK_4-M2GlyR forms many more associated forms, starting with monomer and going beyond 20-mers. Comparing the relative concentration of monomer to the higher species for each of the sequences, monomer is the most abundant species for CK_4-M2GlyR while in NK_4-M2GlyR the monomer accounts for less than 50% of the captured species. This result was somewhat surprising since NK_4-M2GlyR has considerably more activity per peptide concentration even though there is apparently a smaller percentage of monomer able to bind and insert into the membrane.

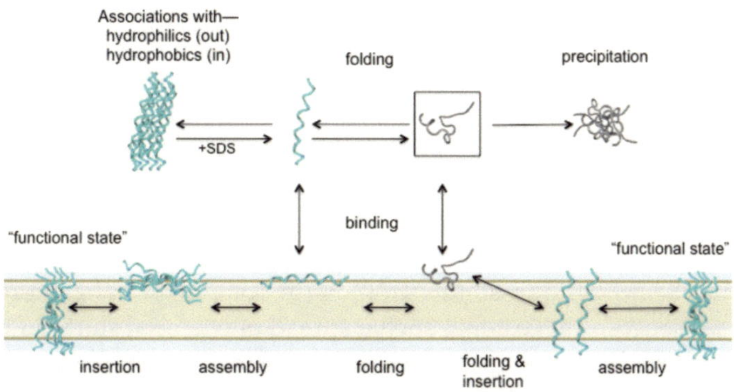

Fig. 5. Solution and membrane inserted states for channel-forming peptides.

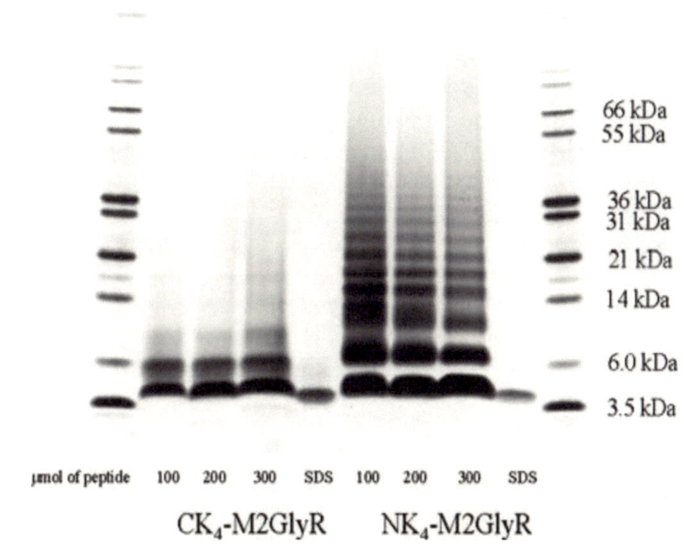

Fig. 6. Silver-stained polyacrylamide gel of cross-linked NK_4-M2GlyR and CK_4-M2GlyR.

Assuming that the energy barrier for the translocation of the four-lysyl residues across the hydrophobic membrane is prohibitive (Vogt et al., 2000), either orientation (NH_2 or COOH terminal towards extracellular surface) can insert into the membrane and assemble into an anion-conducting pore. However, based on the observation that the concentration required to produce 50% of the maximum increase in I_{SC} ($k_{½}$) for NK_4-M2GlyR is one-third less than that required for CK_4-M2GlyR (319 μM vs. 553 μM, respectively), the efficiency of the insertion or the assembly of these two peptides into channel-forming structures is not equivalent. Furthermore, the concentration-dependent effects of the peptides on I_{SC} show a smaller Hill coefficient for NK_4-M2GlyR than CK_4-M2GlyR (n = 1.5 vs. 2.3, respectively). This suggests that one or more of the steps required for channel assembly (e.g., insertion, oligomerization) is/are more cooperative in the case of CK_4-M2GlyR. Alternatively, as NK_4-M2GlyR is less soluble than CK_4-M2GlyR in aqueous solution, the hydrophobic driving force for the insertion of NK_4-M2GlyR into the membrane is greater. In either case, structural differences between the lysine-modified peptides result in altered channel-forming activity.

A series of one- and two-dimensional NMR experiments were performed on NK_4- and CK_4-M2GlyR. TOCSY NMR spectra were recorded for each (Broughman et al., 2002b). Data presented in **Fig. 7** show the fingerprint region (NH to Cα and side chain proton connectivity) for 500 MHz 1H 2D-experiments for both peptides recorded in water containing 30% deuterated trifluoroethanol (TFE) at 30°C (assignments are shown for the lysine residues). The extent of chemical-shift dispersion of the backbone proton resonances, particularly of the lysine residue amide protons (in spite of the oligomeric nature of the lysines in these sequences), suggest that such a spread of chemical shift can be induced only by secondary structure. However, in comparing the chemical shifts for the lysine residues in the two TOCSY spectra, it is clear that the environments for these basic amino acids in the two peptides are distinct. For the NH_2-terminal lysine adducted peptide the dispersion range of the TOCSY chemical shifts for 3 of the 4 lysines was 8.55 to 8.1 ppm. The fourth lysine could not be assigned. In contrast, the COOH-terminal-adducted peptide had a dispersion range of chemical shifts that spanned 8.15–7.72 ppm. All four of the CK_4-M2GlyR lysine resonances were assigned. Greater dispersion in the chemical shift pattern observed with NK_4-M2GlyR indicates that these residues are more mobile and solvent exposed while the lysine residues adducted to the COOH-terminus are hydrogen bonded intramolcularly.

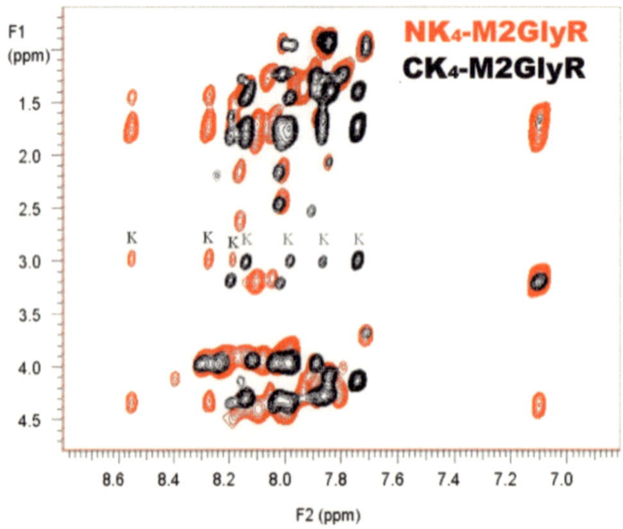

Fig. 7. TOCSY NMR spectra (500 MHz) of NK4-M2GlyR and CK4-M2GlyR.

The NMR coordinates for CK_4-M2GlyR and NK_4-M2GlyR were modeled using a combination of energy based minimizations and molecular-dynamics simulations. The lysine residues of CK_4-M2GlyR form a C-cap by extensive H-bonding interactions with the helix backbone, which remain fairly static throughout the molecular dynamics simulation period. The side chain ε-amino group of K24 of CK_4-M2GlyR forms a capping structure that stabilizes the helix by forming H-bonds with the backbone carbonyl groups of S21, R22 and A23, fulfilling H-bonding interactions that are absent in the COOH terminal residues of an α-helix. The ε-amino group of K25 of CK_4-M2GlyR forms H-bonds with the backbone carbonyl groups of T16 and K-27 and the hydroxyl side chain of T16. The ε-amino groups of K26 and K27 of CK_4-M2GlyR form hydrogen bonds to the backbone carbonyl of K25 and the side chain carbonyl of Q17, respectively. The side chain ε-amino groups of K1 and K4 of NK_4-M2GlyR do not form H-bonds, as the lysyl residues' side chains extend away from the helix backbone. There was very little motion of the helix backbone of CK_4-M2GlyR during the simulation period. In contrast, the lysine residues of NK_4-M2GlyR remained mostly extended away from the helix during the simulation, interacting minimally with the M2GlyR backbone. These differences in dynamics could affect the rates of assembly and pore geometries. Large differences are predicted for the dipoles of NK_4-M2GlyR and CK_4-M2GlyR (**Fig. 8** left and right structures, respectively). Note the similarities, both in magnitude and in orientation, between the dipoles of the unmodified M2GlyR sequence and NK_4-M2GlyR. The dipole of CK_4-M2GlyR is shifted by nearly 90 degrees and is less than 2% of the magnitude of the dipole for the parent compound. This perturbation of the dipole could play a role in the differences observed in peptide-peptide association and channel activity of the CK_4-M2GlyR peptide.

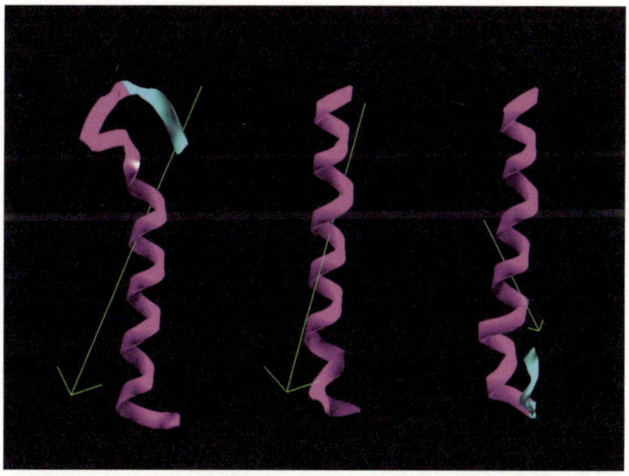

Fig. 8. The dipole moments of NK_4-M2GlyR (left), M2GlyR (center) and CK_4-M2GlyR (right) are shown as ribbon structures (magenta is helix and cyan is random coil) with the dipoles represented by green arrows. For this representation, the dipoles of NK_4-M2GlyR and M2GlyR were scaled down by a factor of 20, while the dipole for CK_4-M2GlyR was scaled up by a factor of 3.

To identify the portion of the M2GlyR molecule that was promoting the solution assemblies of NK_4-M2GlyR, channel activity and cross-linking experiments were performed on various truncated forms of CK_4-M2GlyR and NK_4-M2GlyR. The results (**Figs. 9 and 10**) suggested that a nucleation site for self-association of the peptide is located near the COOH-terminus of the M2GlyR sequence since removal of five residues (SGSRA) from the C-terminus of NK_4-M2GlyR resulted in a reduction of higher molecular weight species. Importantly, there was little loss of ion transport activity. Removal of additional C-terminal residues led to a progressive decrease in I_{SC}, although there was a slight reduction in apparent solubility to 11.1 mM. Measurable activity was observed with even 11 residues removed from the C-terminus. In contrast, the nucleation site is likely masked by the oligo-lysine tail at the COOH-terminus, which prevents formation of higher order assemblies by CK_4-M2GlyR and removal of residues from the N-terminus of CK_4-M2GlyR had little effect on the various low molecular weight associations. However, these truncated forms exhibited substantially less ion transport activity. The truncated NK_4 sequence, referred to as NK_4-M2GlyR-p22, became the lead compound for further development. Removing the five residues greatly reduced the cost of synthesizing a purer peptide with fewer failed sequences.

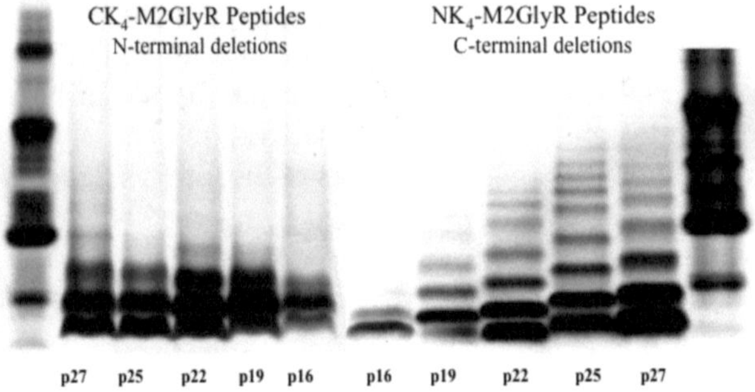

Fig. 9. Silver-stained Tricine polyacrylamide gel of cross-linking patterns for truncated CK_4-M2GlyR and NK_4-M2GlyR treated with a 40-fold excess of crosslinking reagent.

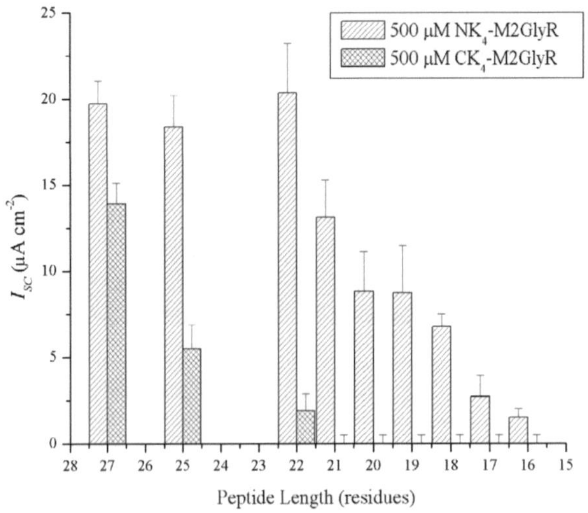

Fig. 10. I_{SC} induced by the full length and truncated NK_4-M2GlyR and CK_4-M2GlyR peptides (500 µM) on MDCK epithelial monolayers. Symbols represent the mean and standard error of three to seven observations.

Results described thus far indicate that the native M2 sequence that forms the GlyR pore can be employed to form de novo anion selective channels in epithelial cell membranes. Further, the structure can be optimized to enhance aqueous solubility and to decrease solution aggregation, which increases effective bioavailable concentration. Lysyl-adduction at the amino terminus appeared to be preferred based upon outcomes with truncated peptides. An additional and exciting outcome of these truncation studies was that shorter peptides might be used to achieve the therapeutic goal, which provides for many potential benefits in design and delivery of this therapeutic modality.

Studies on the second generation of NK_4-M2GlyR-p22 sequences In the process of truncating the NK_4-adducted M2GlyR sequence, a number of hydrophilic residues were eliminated as defined by the Wimley and White hydrophobicity scales developed for TM sequences (Wimley and White, 1996; Wimley and White, 1999; Wimley and White, 2000; Jayasinghe et al., 2001). The increase in hydrophobicity was reflected in reduced solubility for the deletion peptides. Among the residues removed was R22 in the C-terminus of the parent M2 sequence. It has been postulated, based on solution NMR studies in dodecyl phosphatidylcholine micelles, that the registry of the wild-type TM segment is defined by residues R3 and R22, thereby defining an 18-residue TM segment (Tang et al., 2002; Yushmanov et al., 2003). Arginine is often located at the water/lipid interface in TM segments (Vogt et al., 2000; Harzel and Bechinger, 2000; Mitaku et al., 2002). Without the C-terminal R in the NK_4-M2GlyR-p22 sequence, both ion selectivity and positioning, and registry of the TM segment within the acyl lipid core are potentially compromised. Therefore, a study was initiated to evaluate the effects on channel transport properties of reintroducing an R at positions near the new carboxyl-terminus. Arginine residues were introduced individually at positions 18 through 22 and in subsequent experiments double amino acid replacements were generated with aromatic amino acids placed at or near the C-terminus along with R at positions 19-22. MDCK monolayers were used to assess peptide-dependent ion transport.

A series of five individual C-terminal R substitutions were made placing R at the following positions: M18R, T19R, T20R, Q21R and S22R (Shank et al., 2006). With the exception of M18R, the substituted peptides generally exhibited similar concentration dependent I_{SC} profiles in MDCK monolayers (**Table 2**). Substitution of an R enhanced solubility by 50% or more, did not affect the Hill coefficient (**n**), showed similar half maximal activity ($k_{1/2}$) values and had similar helical content as judged by circular dichroism recorded using 50 μM peptide in 10 mM sodium dodecyl sulfate (SDS). Cross-linking experiments using BS^3 revealed that all of these substituted sequences showed solution aggregation patterns similar to that seen for NK_4-M2GlyR-p22 (e.g., see **Fig. 9**).

Rather than rely simply on an R to define the lipid-water boundary at the truncated end of M2GlyR, a W was used to replace the C-terminal serine. A propensity for tryptophans residing at the aqueous/lipid interface also had been observed and tested by others (Braun and von Heijne, 1999; Mall et al., 2000; Demmers et al., 2001; de Planque et al., 2003; Granseth et al., 2005; van der Wel et al., 2007; Hong et al., 2007). Placing a W at the C-terminus sets the registry of the TM segment that spans the bilayer. In the absence of an R or aromatic residue at or near the C-terminus, the peptide could rise up and down within the fluid bilayer thereby affecting the depth of peptide insertion into the membrane and tilt angle of the peptide. By limiting mobility, the degrees of freedom for the TM registry of the peptide are reduced. During the assembly process this allows the annealing peptides to find their preferred interfacial contacts faster and at a lower concentration. **Fig. 11** shows the concentration dependence on I_{SC} for the full length and the truncated M2GlyR peptides when applied to the apical membrane of MDCK cells in the presence of 1-EBIO (Cook et al., 2004). The solid lines represent the best fit of a modified Hill equation to each data set. In paired monolayers both NK_4-M2GlyR-p27 and NK_4-M2GlyR-p22 peptides (previously characterized in Broughman et al., 2002a) displayed similar concentration dependency curves and induced similar I_{SC} at each concentration tested. Introduction of the W in NK_4-M2GlyR-p22 S22W yielded a curve with a reduced I_{MAX} (13.0 ± 1.0 μAcm^{-2}) but more importantly a significantly reduced $k_{1/2}$ (44 ± 6 μM) with a considerably greater Hill coefficient of 5.4 ± 2.9. The sum effect of changes in the three kinetic parameters (I_{MAX}, $k_{1/2}$, and Hill coefficient) is a substantial reduction in the peptide concentration required to yield maximal anion secretion.

Sequence	Substitu-tion	Mr (Da)	Sol.(mM)	n	I_{MAX} (μA/cm^2)	$k_{1/2}$ (μM)
1. KKKKPARVGLGITTVLTMTTQS	none	2358.9	11.1	1.9 ± 0.6	23.7 ± 5.6	210 ± 70
2. KKKKPARVGLGITTVLTMTTQR	S22R	2427.9	15.6	2.7 ± 0.9	24.1 ± 5.3	290 ± 60
3. KKKKPARVGLGITTVLTMTTRS	Q21R	2387.0	19.7	2.2 ± 1.1	31.0 ± 18.0	390 ± 220
4. KKKKPARVGLGITTVLTMTRQS	T20R	2414.0	18.7	1.3 ± 0.5	28.5 ± 14.8	310 ± 227
5. KKKKPARVGLGITTVLTMRTQS	T19R	2414.0	18.3	0.7 ± 0.6	16.3 ± 3.5	120 ± 40
6. KKKKPARVGLGITTVLTRTTQS	M18R	2383.9	23.3	0.6 ± 2.6	3.0 ± 4.0	840 ± 200

Table 2. Characterization of M2GlyR-p22 derived peptides with C-terminal Arginines.

We then assessed the solution associations of the selected NK_4-M2GlyR peptides using a silver-stained gel following cross-linking reactions. In **Fig. 12**, lane 1 (consistent with 34:9-11) contained a mobility standard to indicate relative molecular weights. Lanes 2 through 9 contain the indicated peptides that were suspended in aqueous buffer in the absence and presence of a twenty-fold excess of BS3, as indicated The cross-linker revealed the presence of higher molecular weight homo-oligomers. Without the addition of cross-linker and after boiling the sample in SDS containing loading buffer, only monomer was observed. The W substituted sequence, however, appeared to be predominantly monomeric in solution under either experimental condition. These results indicated that NK_4-M2GlyR-p22 S22W (150 μM) forms essentially no aggregates in aqueous solution and the entire suspended mass is capable of membrane interaction.

It is unclear whether the left shift in $k_{½}$ observed for the W containing peptide in **Fig. 11** is due solely to an increase in concentration of the membrane active monomeric species or includes a contribution from the C-terminal W limiting the possible orientations of the peptide within the bilayer. The change in the Hill coefficient is likely due to the addition of the membrane anchor that facilitates the supramolecular assembly of the peptides into an active oligomeric pore. We speculated that the anchor reduces the degrees of freedom for the TM segment making alignment more favorable during assembly. An alternative explanation could be that in the absence of the tryptophan there is both positive and negative cooperativity. Addition of the tryptophan eliminates the negative cooperativity and we see the level of positive cooperativity that might be expected for the assembly of a pentameric structure. The presence of the fluorescent tryptophan also provides both a convenient method for determining the concentration of the peptide solution and a sensitive tool for probing the environment surrounding the indole.

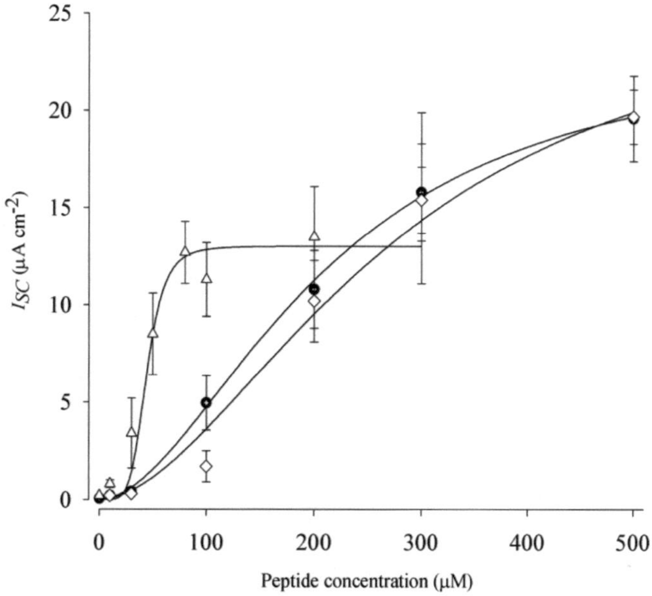

Fig. 11. Concentration-dependence of I_{SC} induced by NK_4-M2GlyR derived peptides on MDCK epithelial monolayers. The NK_4-M2GlyR derived peptides concentration dependent I_{SC} curves are as follows: NK_4-M2GlyR p27(◊), NK_4-M2GlyR p22 WT (●) and NK_4-M2GlyR p22 S22W (Δ).

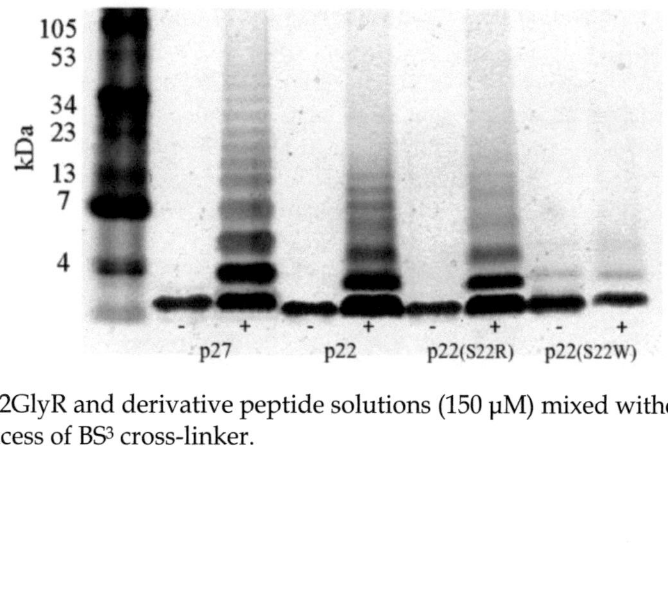

Fig. 12. NK_4-M2GlyR and derivative peptide solutions (150 μM) mixed without (-) and with (+) a 20-fold excess of BS^3 cross-linker.

NMR structural and computer modeling studies were carried out on 40% deuterated TFE solutions of NK_4-M2GlyR-p22 and NK_4-M2GlyR-p22 S22W to determine how the substituted C-terminal W potentially influences solution associations of the peptide (Cook et al., 2004). A measurement of the NK_4-M2GlyR-p22 (WT) peptide structure shows that the length of the entire TM segment is greater than 32 Å, more than enough to span the hydrophobic core of the membrane (**Fig. 13,** left structure). This structure is similar to the results shown in micelle studies done on the wild-type glycine receptor α_1 subunit (Tang et al., 2002; Yushmanov et al., 2003). An identical segment of the peptide was determined to be helical when incorporated in SDS micelles. The rest of the peptide was unstructured and flexible, including the C-terminus. The outcomes indicated that the structured portion of the peptide is restricted to residues 8 to 22 regardless of the length of the peptide. The WT structure resembles other TM segments observed in the x-ray crystal structure of a ClC chloride channel. In that structure, the Cl^- binding TM segments are made up of shorter helices that do not completely span the width of the membrane (Dutzler et al., 2002; Esrévez and Jentsch, 2002).

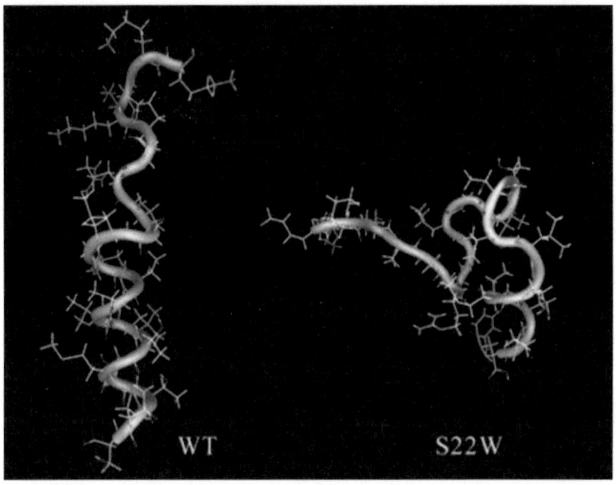

Fig. 13. Calculated models of NK_4-M2GlyR-p22 and NK_4-M2GlyR-p22 S22W in TFE.

The structured C-terminus of NK_4-M2GlyR-p22 S22W is made up of a single-turn helix (residues 11 - 14), a stretched beta-like turn (residues 14 - 17), and then another two-turn helix (residues 15 - 21). The observed structure indicated a helical content of about 40%, which was in good agreement with CD data for the S22W containing 22-residue peptide. This backbone structure allows the peptide to loop or fold over into a closed structure (**Fig. 13**). This fold sequesters the hydrophobic residues such that the acyl side chains have reduced solvent exposure. The structure likely has little relevance to a TM segment where the aliphatic side chains would be fully exposed and interacting with the lipid acyl chains in the membrane bilayer. Nonetheless, the C-terminal fold of NK_4-M2GlyR-p22 S22W explains why the peptide remains in the monomeric form in solution, since the hydrophobic groups are less exposed and unable to associate with hydrophobic groups from other peptides. While TFE is not added to peptide stock solutions used for assessing channel activity, it is clear that this monomer-inducing fold is sampled with enough frequency that the higher molecular weight forms do not occur. Based on the CD spectra obtained using 10 mM SDS micelles, the peptide is able to adopt a more helical structure, much like the WT peptide.

NMR studies in SDS (**Fig. 14**) confirmed the CD results (Herrera et al., 2010). These atomic structures clearly show that both NK_4-M2GlyR-p22 (WT) and NK_4-M2GlyR-p22 S22W are linear and mostly helical from residues 6–20 in SDS micelles. The N-terminal lysines are largely unstructured and apparently exhibit substantial flexibility. These lysine residues are expected to be out of the micelle floating in the aqueous environment and/or interacting with the sulfate groups. The hydrophobic and hydrophilic side chains are segregated to different sides of the helix, as expected for channel forming TM segments.

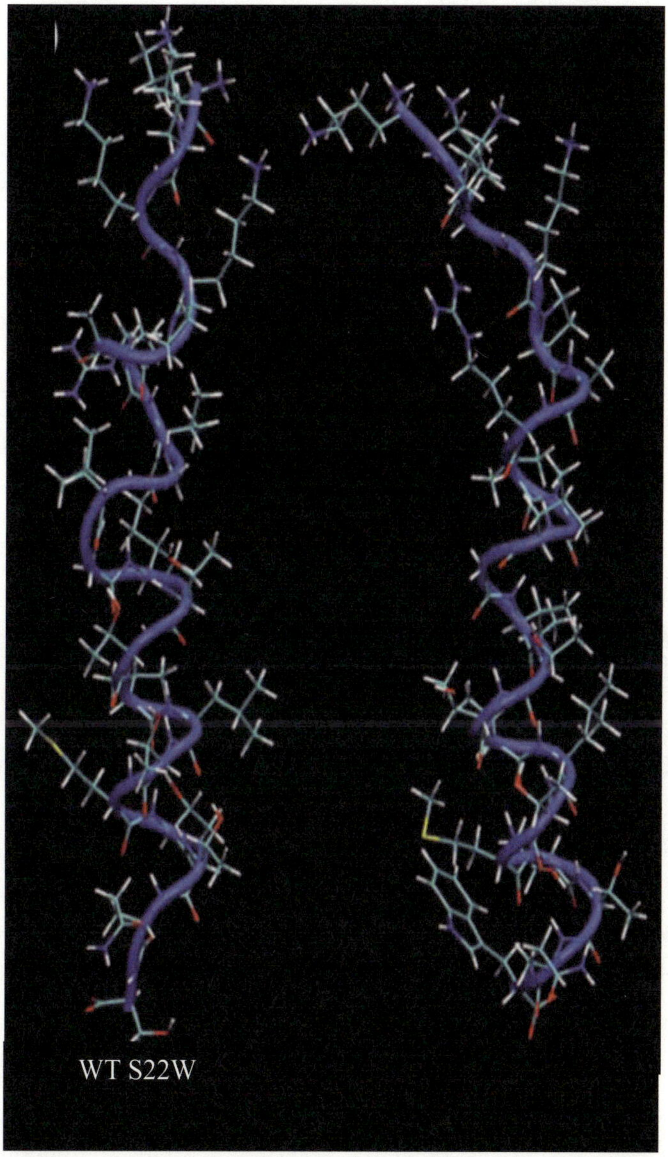

Fig. 14. Average structures of NK_4-M2GlyR-p22 and NK_4-M2GlyR-p22 S22W after MD refinement in an implicit membrane. Backbones are shown as a blue tube with licorice side chains.

NMR structures, along with a range of additional experimental data and theoretical considerations, were utilized to assemble the monomer structure into channels, including oligomerization state, pore-lining interface, helix packing distance, and tilt angle. In particular, experimental identification of the pore-lining residues greatly reduces uncertainty of the channel assembly and allows the construction of reliable initial structural models. All-atom molecular dynamics (MD) simulations in fully solvated 1-palmitoyl-2-oleoyl-*sn*-glycero-3-phosphocholine (POPC) bilayers were subsequently carried out to refine these structural models and to characterize and validate the structural and dynamical properties of the channels (**Fig. 15**). The results demonstrate that the channel structures as constructed are adequately stable within the simulation time frame (up to 20 ns) and remain sufficiently open for ion conductance. All initial structures relax to transiently stable structures within a few nanoseconds. Analysis of the relaxed structures of NK_4-M2GlyR-p22 WT and NK_4-M2GlyR-p22 S22W reveal important differences in their structural and dynamical properties, providing a basis for understanding the differences in channel activities. Specifically, the structural characterization supports the initial postulation that the S22W substitution in NK_4-M2GlyR-p22 helps to anchor the peptide in the membrane and reduces the flexibility of the whole assembly. The implied increased stability of the NK_4-M2GlyR-p22 S22W channel potentially explains the steeper short circuit current-concentration slope measured experimentally. Furthermore, introduction of the C-terminal W appears to lead to global changes of the channel structure. The NK_4-M2GlyR-p22 S22W channel maintains a smaller opening at the narrowest region and throughout the rest of the pore compared with the NK_4-M2GlyR-p22 channel. The smaller size of NK_4-M2GlyR-p22 S22W could effectively reduce its ion throughput or conductance by a magnitude that is consistent with a nearly 50% reduction in measured I_{MAX}. The ability to recapitulate these differences in key physiological properties observed experimentally is an important validation of the proposed structural models.

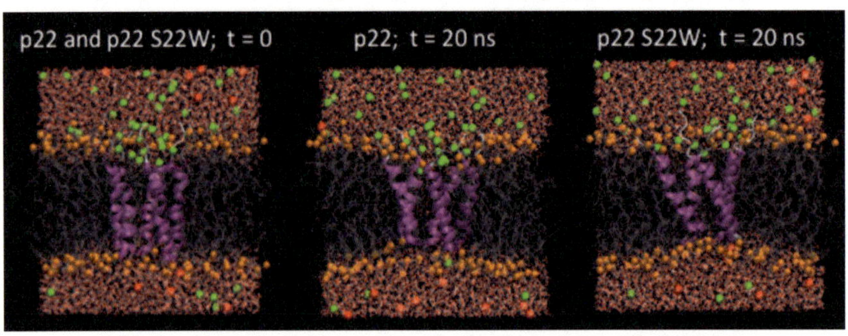

Fig. 15. Snapshots of NK_4-M2GlyR-p22 and NK_4-M2GlyR-p22 S22W left-handed channels in a fully solvated POPC bilayer before and after the 20 ns production simulation. Both peptides have identical structures at t = 0.The protein is shown in purple cartoon and lipid molecules shown in the grey licorice with phosphorus atoms shown as orange spheres.

Development of third generation NK_4-M2GlyR-p22 derived sequences From a drug delivery perspective, adding the W at the C-terminus yields a compound that can be delivered from solution at a stable accurate concentration and at considerably lower dosages. Both having the peptide predominantly as the monomer and treating with lower dosages dramatically reduce the cost of the treatment. For the third generation sequences substitutions were made based on increasing conductance and anion selectivity. In an attempt to enhance anion selectivity by reintroducing a charged residue at or near the C-terminus of the W-substituted sequence, a series of doubly substituted peptides were prepared. Restoration of a positive charge near the C-terminus of the 22-residue peptide was first tested with regard to increasing throughput rates. A helical wheel projection of the M2GlyR-p22 helix revealed an even distribution of the polar residues. Not knowing where to optimally substitute an R, a series of M2GlyR peptides was prepared with R replacing one amino acid in each of the four C-terminal sequence positions.

NK_4-M2GlyR-p22 displayed concentration-response relationships similar to those observed with the 27 residue full-length CK_4-M2GlyR and NK_4-M2GlyR peptides. **Table 3** presents the summarized ion transport kinetic constants associated with the fitted lines presented in **Fig. 16**. NK_4-M2GlyR-p22 displayed a concentration-dependent response similar to that observed with the 27 residue full-length CK_4-M2GlyR and NK_4-M2GlyR peptides. NK_4-M2GlyR-p22 provided benchmark values for I_{MAX} of 23.7 ± 5.6 μAcm^{-2}, $k_{1/2}$ of 210 ± 70 μM, and Hill coefficient of 1.9 ± 0.6.

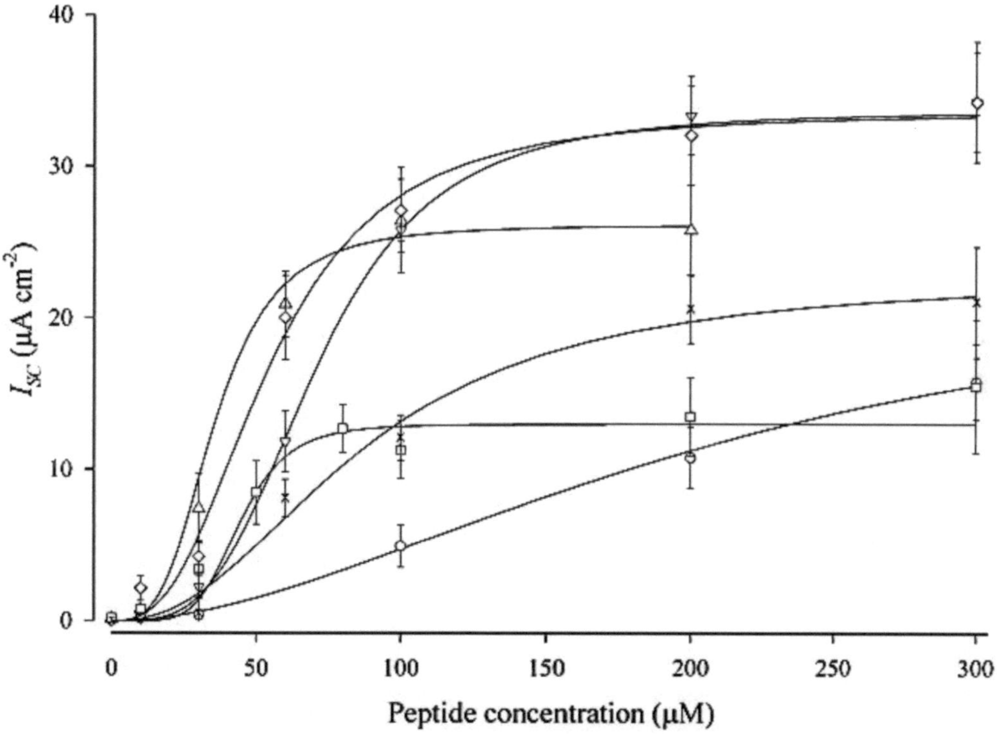

Fig. 16. Concentration-dependence of I_{SC} induced by NK_4-M2GlyR-p22 derived peptides with W and R amino acid substitutions on MDCK epithelial monolayers. Symbols represent the mean and standard error of 6 or greater observations for each concentration tested. Solid lines represent the best fit of a modified Hill equation to each data set. The NK_4-M2GlyR derived peptides concentration dependent I_{SC} curves are as follows: NK_4-M2GlyR-p22 (O), NK_4-M2GlyR-p22 S22W (□), NK_4-M2GlyR-p22 Q21R,S22W(Δ), NK_4-M2GlyR-p22 T20R,S22W(×), NK_4-M2GlyR-p22 T19R, S22W (∇) and NK_4-M2GlyR-p22 Q21W, S22R(◊).

Sequence	Replace-ment	Mr (Da)	Sol.(mM)	n	I_{MAX} (µA/cm²)	$k_{1/2}$ (µM)
KKKKPARVGLGITTVLTMTTQS	none	2358.9	11.1	1.9 ± 0.6	23.7 ± 5.6	210 ± 70
KKKKPARVGLGITTVLTMTTQW	S22W	2458.0	1.9	5.4 ± 2.9	13.0 ± 1.0	45
KKKKPARVGLGITTVLTMTTRW	Q21R, S22W	2486.1	4.9	3.3 ± 1.6	26.5 ± 3.2	36 ± 5
KKKKPARVGLGITTVLTMTRQW	T20R, S22W	2513.1	5.2	2.3 ± 0.8	22.7 ± 2.7	87 ± 15

Table 3. Characterization of M2GlyR derived peptides with W and R substitutions.

Introduction of a W in the presence and absence of the added R had a dramatic effect on the concentration required for half-maximal ion transport activity. The left-shifted $k_{1/2}$ values ranged from 36 to 87 µM as compared with the 210 µM observed for NK_4-M2GlyR-p22. Three of the doubly substituted sequences exhibited similar left shifts in the $k_{1/2}$ for anion transport when compared to NK_4-M2GlyR-p22 S22W. NK_4-M2GlyR-p22 T20R, S22W did not show this dramatic left-shift. The simplest interpretation is that the sequences with left-shifted $k_{1/2}$ values form homo-oligomeric supramolecular assemblies at lower concentrations than the benchmark peptide.

With regard to I_{MAX}, the doubly substituted sequences exhibited greater maximal transport rates relative to either NK_4-M2GlyR-p22 or C-terminal W substituted NK_4-M2GlyR-p22 S22W peptides. In the doubly substituted sequences the position of the R relative to the W also had an effect on I_{MAX}. The sequences which introduced R at positions 20 or 21, exhibited a greater I_{MAX} (22.7 ± 2.7 and 26.2 ± 3.2 µAcm^{-2}, respectively) than was observed with the W alone substituted sequence. These I_{MAX} values are similar to that seen for M2GlyR-p22. Introduction of the R at position 19 and inverting the R - W pair of sequence NK_4-M2GlyR-p22 Q21R, S22W to W - R resulted in even larger I_{MAX} values of 33.7 ± 1.3 and 33.6 ± 2.2 µAcm^{-2}, respectively. Most importantly, R substituted sequences showed greatly enhanced efficacy with I_{SC} values equaling I_{MAX} for M2GlyR-p22 with concentrations at or below 50 µM. The sum effect of changes in the kinetic parameters (I_{MAX} and $k_{1/2}$) is a substantial reduction in the peptide concentration required to attain ion transport rates that will likely be relevant in future basic and applied applications. With the exception of NK_4-M2GlyR-p22 T20R, S22W all of the other W and R containing sequences have greater Hill coefficients (3.3 ± 1.6 to 5.4 ± 2.9) than that calculated for NK_4-M2GlyR-p22 (2.1 ± 0.8). M2GlyR-p22 T20R, S22W had a Hill coefficient (2.8 ± 0.8) similar to that seen with NK_4-M2GlyR-p22. The increase in the Hill coefficients to values approaching five suggests that association/dissociation mechanisms in the bilayer are sensitive to structural changes in the peptide and consistent with the prediction that the channel pore is a homo-oligomeric supramolecular assembly that assembles by a complex or multistep mechanism.

As assessed in the Ussing chamber experiments, reintroduction of an R near the C-terminus in conjunction with the added W contributes another factor that influences the minimum concentrations required for assembly of a functional channel. Introduction of an R at, at any of the tested positions slightly decreases the Hill coefficient, suggesting that there is an energetic cost in forcing the R (transiently) across the acyl core of the phospholipids. Placing R either at position 19 or just outside the membrane appears to be optimal with regard to I_{MAX}, while an R placed at position 21 appears to be optimal with regard to $k_{1/2}$. Placing R at position 20 seems to be the least optimal position since the Hill coefficient, $k_{1/2}$ and I_{MAX}

show the lowest values within this peptide series. Computer modeling studies indicated that the R in any of the internal C-terminal positions could snorkel back toward the membrane to form a second membrane anchor. There is no evidence that the R in any of these substituted peptides is positioned with the side chain pointed into the water-filled lumen of the assembled pore.

In a parallel set of experiments designed to assess the role of the indole group in altering n, I_{MAX} and $k_{1/2}$ values (Derived from **Fig. 17** and summarized in **Table 4**), sequences were prepared that replaced the W with either F or Y. The F or Y substituted sequences, which also contain a second R substitution, exhibited greater solubility compared to their W-containing counterparts, with the exception of NK$_4$-M2GlyR-p22 Q21F, S22R. All of the aromatic amino acid containing sequences had lesser amounts of higher molecular weight associations in aqueous environments compared to the aromatic-free sequence. Predominantly monomer, with some dimer, is present in the cross-linked aromatic sequences.

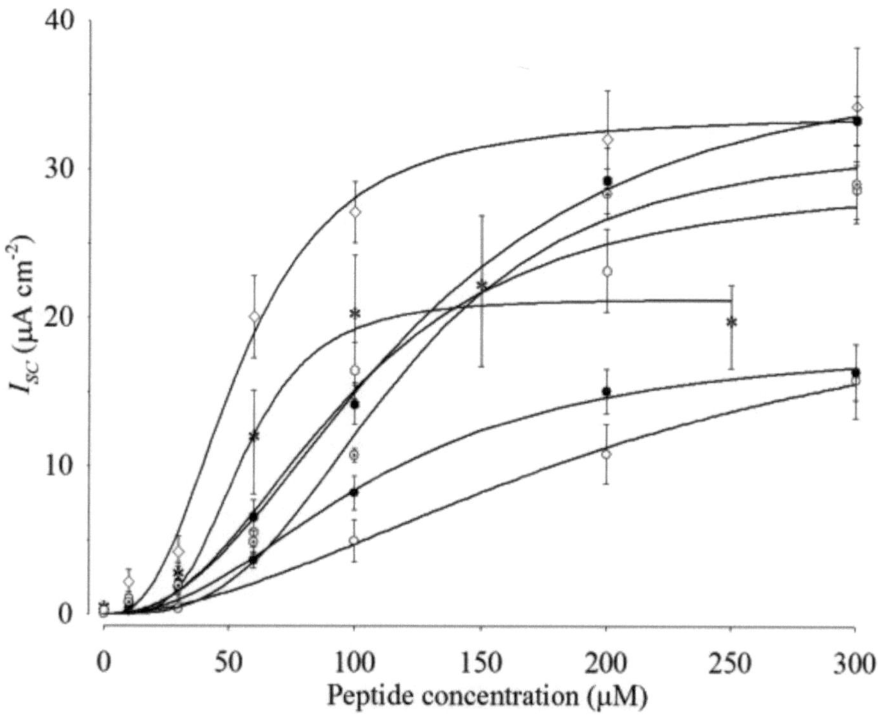

Fig. 17. Concentration-dependence of I_{SC} induced by NK$_4$-M2GlyR-p22 derived peptides with either F or Y and W amino acid substitutions on MDCK epithelial monolayers. Symbols represent the mean and standard error of 4 or greater observations for each concentration tested. Solid lines represent the best fit of a modified Hill equation to each data set. The NK$_4$-M2GlyR derived peptides dose dependent I_{SC} curves are as follows: NK$_4$-M2GlyR-p22 (O), NK$_4$-M2GlyR-p22 Q21W, S22R (◊), NK$_4$-M2GlyR-p22 Q21R, S22F (*), NK$_4$-M2GlyR-p22 T19R, S22F (closed hexagon), NK$_4$-M2GlyR-p22 Q21F, S22R (⊕), NK$_4$-M2GlyR-p22 Q21R, S22Y (open hexagon) and NK$_4$-M2GlyR-p22 T19R, S22Y (●).

Sequence	Replace-ment	Mr (Da)	Sol.(mM)	n	I_{MAX} (μA/cm²)	$k_{1/2}$ (μM)
KKKKPARVGLGITTVLTMTTRF	Q21R, S22F	2447.1	6.1	3.8 ± 2.5	21.3 ± 2.5	56 ± 8
KKKKPARVGLGITTVLTMRTQF	T19R, S22F	2474.1	12.2	2.3 ± 0.3	38.0 ± 2.3	120 ± 14
KKKKPARVGLGITTVLTMTTFR	Q21F, S22R	2447.1	21.0	3.1 ± 0.6	31.8 ± 3.6	120 ± 10

Table 4. Characterization of M2GlyR derived peptides with F/Y and R Substitutions.

The secondary structures of these peptides were measured in SDS micelles. CD spectra contained minima at 208 and 222 nm, similar to those seen for all other sequences, which indicate predominantly helical structures. Considering the lack of solution aggregation and similar CD profiles, we concluded that these sequences formed a similar hydrophobic fold (in solution) that prevents association or aggregation in aqueous solution, similar to that described above for other structures. In addition to stabilizing the concentration of monomer in aqueous solutions, inclusion of any C-terminal aromatic residue provided a lipid/water interfacial anchor. As was seen with W, F residues are commonly present (and Y to a lesser extent) at the hydrophobic/hydrophilic interface for TM segments of membrane proteins (Braun and von Heijne, 1999; Mall et al., 2000; Demmers et al., 2001; de Planque et al., 2003; Granseth et al., 2005; van der Wel et al., 2007; Hong et al., 2007). The data for sequences NK_4-M2GlyR-p22 and NK_4-M2GlyR-p22 Q21W, S22R are included as reference values. Comparing the F substituted sequences to those containing the paired W, the F-containing peptides displayed similar I_{MAX} but have right-shifted $k_{1/2}$ values. The Y variants gave mixed results relative to their W counterparts. NK_4-M2GlyR-p22 Q21R, S22Y showed a higher I_{MAX}, but had a right-shifted $k_{1/2}$ value while sequence NK_4-M2GlyR-p22 T19R, S22Y was inferior in both respects. With the exception of NK_4-M2GlyR-p22 Q21R, S22F, the $k_{1/2}$ values for the Y and F containing peptides are right-shifted relative to the W-containing peptides but left-shifted relative to the unmodified M2GlyR-p22.

Comparing all of the summarized data in **Tables 3 and 4** and the profiles shown in **Figs. 16 and 17**, the sequences displaying the highest ion transport activity and the second and third most left-shifted $k_{1/2}$ values are both W containing peptide sequences, NK_4-M2GlyR-p22 T19R, S22W and NK_4-M2GlyR-p22 Q21W, S22R. Based on the concentrations required for $k_{1/2}$, a rank ordering of the assembly-promoting effects of the C-terminal aromatic substitutions are as follows W > F >>Y. Given that when the R is placed at the C-terminus in NK4-M2GlyR-p22 Q21W, S22R will most likely cause further thinning of the membrane upon insertion (see **Fig. 17**), the sequence NK_4-M2GlyR-p22 T19R, S22W was chosen as a lead sequence for further analysis and modification.

Before committing to *in vivo* animal studies and preclinical trials, a few questions had to be addressed—did the lysine adduction and amino acid substitutions at T19R and S22W of the peptide alter its selectivity as an anion channel and did these modifications generate a potentially immunogenic structure?

NK_4-M2GlyR-p22 T19R, S22W was administered at clinically relevant dosages to the nasal passages of specific-pathogen-free female C57/BL6 mice to test for the induction of an immune response with or without cholera toxin (CT) a strong mucosal adjuvant. Lipopolycaccharide (LPS)-free peptide, when administered alone, induced very little peptide-specific immunity based on analyses of peptide-specific antibodies by enzyme-linked immunosorbent and enzyme-linked immunospot assays, induction of cytokine production, and delayed-type hypersensitivity (DTH) responses. The administration of NK_4-M2GlyR-p22 T19R, S22W with CT induced peptide-specific immunoglobulin G (IgG) antibodies, DTH responses and a Th2-dominant cytokine response. Co-administration of CT induced a systemic NK_4-M2GlyR-p22 T19R, S22W-specific IgG response but not a mucosal peptide-specific antibody response. The lack of peptide-specific immunity and specifically mucosal immunity should allow repeated NK_4-M2GlyR-p22 T19R, S22W peptide applications to epithelial surfaces to correct ion channelopathies (van Ginkel et al., 2008).

Results indicate that additional modifications are necessary to achieve the desired anion selectivity. NK_4-M2GlyR-p22 T19R, S22W was tested in artificial bilayers composed of **1-palmitoyl-2-oleoyl-sn-glycero-3-phosphocholine:1-palmitoyl-2-oleoyl-sn-glycero-3-phospho-L-serine** (POPC:POPS, 70:30) and in *Xenopus* oocytes. In both cases the selectivity for monovalent anions relative to monovalent cations had dropped to a value slightly above unity, indicating that the pore formed was only slightly anion selective. Computer simulations were employed as an initial strategy to determine the most promising structures for synthesis and testing. Before those simulations could be conducted, the identity of the pore-forming residues had to be established. The structure of NK_4-M2GlyR-p22 T19R, S22W was analyzed by solution NMR as a monomer in detergent micelles and simulated as five-helix bundles in a membrane environment. Details of helix packing and residue distribution of the pore were analyzed. Results summarized in **Fig. 18a** demonstrate that the pore is mainly lined with A6, R7, L10, T13, T14, T17, T20 and Q21. Note the N- and C-terminal residues, K1-4 and W22, should not be considered as pore lining, even though they are indicated to have high pore-lining probabilities based on their contacts with (bulk) water molecules. The predicted pore-lining interface is largely consistent with the one derived from consideration of amphipathicity. However, the predicted pore-lining interface is broader due to substantial fluctuations of the pore. Participation of residues in helix-helix packing is characterized by calculating the average burial areas of side-chains, shown in **Fig. 18b**. Clearly, most residues with the structured region contribute to helix-helix interactions, except G9, G11, I12, V15 and R19. These residues either lack side chains (G9 and G11) or are fully membrane exposed. (I12, V15, L16 and R19). L10 and Q21 appear to be particularly important for stabilization of the pore assembly with the largest buried surface areas. Ongoing studies are guided by the hypothesis that alterations in one or more of the following parameters-- hydrogen bonding potentials of pore lining residues, electrostatics of pore lining residues, pore length or pore rigidity--will affect anion selectivity. By defining which of these elements increase selectivity we will elucidate how selectivity filters and permeation rates might be modulated so that an optimal sequence to allow for highly-selective Cl^- permeation can be developed. Current experiments are designed to examine the effect of adding the positively charged amino acid L-diaminopropionic acid (DAP; R= CH_2-$^+NH_3$). Computer Modeling studies were performed on both singly and doubly DAP-substituted sequences (**Fig. 19**). Modeling the Potential of Mean Force (PMF) for moving different ions from one side of the channel to the other predicted similar permeabilities through NK_4-M2GlyR-p22 T19R, S22W for both Cl^- and Na^+, while introduction of the cationic DAP residues favored the passage of Cl^-. The double-substituted T13Dap, T20Dap sequence shows the smallest energy wells where Cl^- could become trapped, suggesting that it could be a preferred sequence.

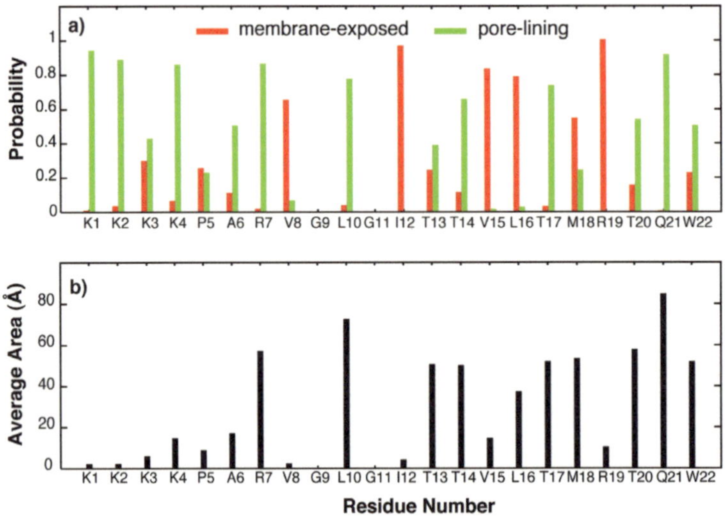

Fig. 18. **a.** Probabilities of a residue being either a pore-lining one or a membrane-exposed one. **b.** Average surface area of burial due to peptide-peptide interactions. The results are calculated from the last 80 ns of 100 ns production simulation of the left-handed channel.

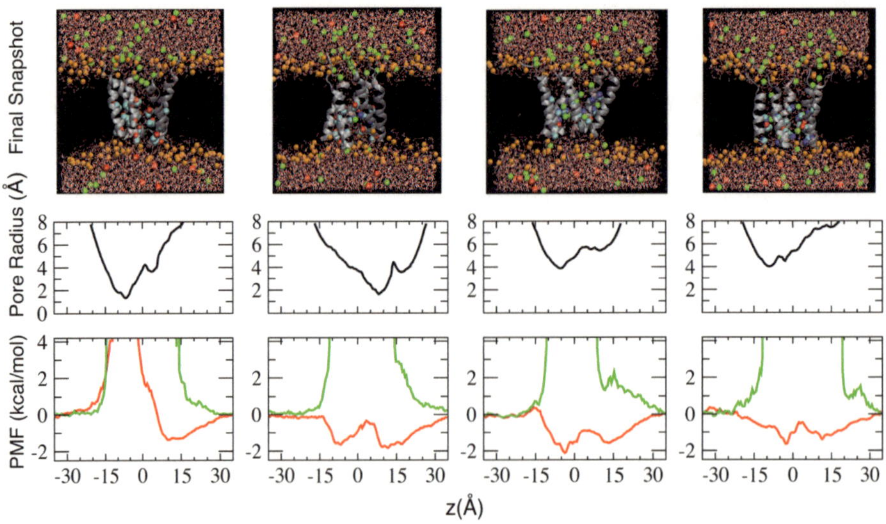

Fig. 19. Summary of the preliminary simulations of NK_4-M2GlyR-p22 T19R, S22W (lane 1) and its several singly (lane 2, T17Dap) and doubly Dap substituted sequences (lane 3, T13Dap,T17Dap; lane 4, T13Dap,T20Dap). The lengths of the simulations are at least 20 ns. The pore profiles were computed using the HOLE program based on the last snapshots shown. The PMFs were computed from equilibrium ion densities. The red line signifies chloride and the green line sodium.

Surprisingly, in generating more cationic channel-forming sequences, assembly, as assessed *in silico*, was not hampered by the presence of inter-peptide charge repulsion between the amino groups on adjacent helical segments. This repulsion appears to be accommodated by a widening of the pore. It might also cause the helices to adopt a staggered registry; however, these modeling studies have not indicated that outcome. Computer modeling of the M2GlyR-p22 T19R, S22W pore predicts the diameter to be about 4-5 Å at the narrowest portion of the channel (position T17). As stated above, modeling indicates that widening of the pore by the introduction of cationic residues results in a shift of the narrowest part of the pore to L10 with about the same pore diameter. The sequences containing multiple DAP residues appear to increase the diameter of the pore to ~8 Å, potentially leading to the passage of larger anions that were previously impermeable (glutamate, isethionate, etc.) and/or increased conductance. Preliminary results indicate that all of the DAP substituted sequences generate ion fluxes both across MDCK monolayers and in *Xenopus* oocytes. Permselectivity, however, remains to be determined.

NK_4-M2GlyR p-22 peptides with both W and R substitutions near the C terminus appear to be optimal structures for ongoing development of a therapeutic agent. These structures exhibited the greatest net ion flux and were among the most potent of the peptides assessed. Importantly, a mucosal immune response was not observed following exposure to these structures. The greatest challenge for ongoing development is the establishment of high anion to cation selectivity. Pore and lipid interfacial side chains have been identified to provide key information that is being used to build new structures in silico. These new structures are now being tested for ion throughput and selectivity. In addition to developing a potentially therapeutic structure, the outcomes of these experiments will provide a wealth of information regarding the contributions of hydrogen bonding, electrostatics, and pore rigidity to ion selectivity.

5. Summary

Nearly seventy-five years have passed since cystic fibrosis of the pancreas was first described as a unique clinical syndrome that was associated with failure to thrive and death in early childhood. The underlying cause of the disease, the absence of an epithelial anion conductance, was determined in the early 1980s and the gene coding for this anion channel was identified by the end of that decade. Even though the underlying cause has been known for more than twenty years, a curative treatment has not been developed, even at the tissue or organ level. Through the years, numerous therapies have been implemented - some with more positive outcomes than others. The commonality of all therapies is their palliative nature - there is no cure for CF although there are promising therapies in the pipeline for some subsets of the patient population (e.g., VX-770 for patients harboring G551D mutations). Supplemental pancreatic enzymes, more potent antibiotics and targeted delivery systems, daily respiratory therapy and the use of anti-inflammatory agents have added years to the typical lifespan and have greatly enhanced the quality of life of those suffering from CF. Nonetheless, additional therapeutic options are needed to address both tissue-specific and generalized disease progression. A synthetic anion-selective channel that can be delivered directly to epithelial cell membranes will provide one such option for improved health.

This line of investigation has as its primary goal to create a therapeutic channel-forming peptide that can be delivered from aqueous solution, insert itself into cell membranes and provide a pathway that is selective for the permeation of anions. The synthetic peptide should be effective at low aqueous concentrations, persistent in the membrane, and should not be antigenic. A particular benefit of this approach is that the therapy could be effective independent of the genetic mutation(s) expressed by each patient.

The development of synthetic channel-forming peptides has progressed through a series of stages including discovery, initial implementation or proof of concept, and optimization for various physical, biochemical and physiological endpoints. The glycine receptor, a naturally occurring anion selective channel, was selected as the simplest chassis from which to start the process. The M2 segment, which constitutes the pore of the pentameric receptor, was used to demonstrate that exogenously applied peptides could support anion movement across an epithelium. This peptide was modified with the addition of lysine residues to increase aqueous solubility and a truncated version was found to be equally effective, which reduced a portion of the burden of peptide synthesis. The truncated version was further modified to establish an anchor at the membrane:water interface. Together, these modifications yielded a peptide that is effective at aqueous concentrations below 50 micromolar and that persists in the epithelium for hours. At various stages in this project, results have shown that the peptides have the desired effects on electrophysiology when tested in murine nasal epithelia and the peptides appear not to induce a mucosal immune response, even when administered with cholera toxin as an adjuvant. Although the underlying mechanism remains to be determined, channel forming peptides were also associated with an increase in glutathione release from CF cells, which also constitutes a therapeutic outcome. Overall, the line of investigation has yielded much new knowledge regarding the design and construction of ion channels. Ongoing studies are focused to modify the ion selectivity of the channel, i.e., to build an anion selective channel for therapeutics and to determine the contribution of structural elements to channel ion selectivity. Clearly, there continues to be a need for new and novel therapies to treat the many aspects of CF. Synthetic anion selective channels constitute a therapeutic modality that has great potential to improve the lives of these patients.

6. Acknowledgements

We thank Gary Radke, Takeo Iwamoto Ph.D., Robert Brandt and Ryan Carlin for their technical assistance. We thank Professor Jianhan Chen for his assistance in redrawing computer simulation figures. This article is contribution no. 12-054-B from the Kansas Agricultural Experiment Station. Manhattan, KS-66506. This study has been supported in part by United States of America PHS grants form the National Institutes of Health to JMT: DK61866, GM43617 and GM074096.

7. References

Accurso, F.J., Rowe, S.M., Clancy, J.P., Boyle, M.P., Dunitz, J.M., Durie, P.R., Sagel, S.D., Hornick, D.B., Konstan, M.W., Donaldson, S.H., Moss, R.B., Pilewski, J.M., Rubenstein, R.C., Uluer, A.Z., Aitken, M.L., Freedman, S.D., Rose, L.M., Mayer-Hamblett, N., Dong, Q., Zha, J., Stone, A.J., Olson, E.R., Ordoñez, C.L., Campbell, P.W., Ashlock, M.A., Ramsey, B.W. (2010) Effect of VX-770 in persons with cystic fibrosis and the G551D-CFTR mutation. *N Engl J Med.* 363(21):1991-2003.

Alexander, C., Ivetac, A., Liu, X., Norimatsu, Y., Serrano, J.R., Landstrom, A., Sansom, M., Dawson, D.C. (2009) Cystic fibrosis transmembrane conductance regulator: using differential reactivity toward channel-permeant and channel-impermeant thiol-reactive probes to test a molecular model for the pore. *Biochemistry*. 2048(42):10078-10088.

Atkuri, K.R., Mantovani, J.J., Herzenberg, L.A., Herzenberg, L.A. (2007) N-Acetylcysteine-a safe antidote for cysteine/glutathione deficiency. *Current Opinion in Pharmacology* 7:355-359.

Baer, M., Sawa, T., Flynn, P., Luehrsen, K., Martinez, D., Wiener-Kronish, J.P., Yarranton, G., Bebbington, C. (2009) An engineered human antibody Fab fragment specific for Pseudomonas aeruginosa PcrV antigen has potent anti-bacterial activity. *Infect Immun*. 77(3):1083-1090.

Beck, E.J., Yang, Y., Yaemsiri, S., Raghuram, V. (2008) Conformational changes in a pore-lining helix coupled to cystic fibrosis transmembrane conductance regulator channel gating. *J Biol Chem*. 283:4957-4966.

Bilton, D., Robinson, P., Cooper, P., Gallagher, C., Kolbe, J., Fox, H., Jaques, A., Charlton, B. (2011) Inhaled dry powder mannitol in cystic fibrosis: An efficacy and safety study. *Eur Respiratory J*. 38(5):1071-1080.

Brady, K.G., Kelley, T.J., Drumm, M.L. (2001) Examining basal chloride transport using the nasal potential. *Am J Physiol Lung Cell Mol Physiol*. 281(5):L1173-1179.

Braun, P., von Heijne, G. (1999) The aromatic residues Trp and Phe have different effects on the positioning of a transmembrane helix in the microsomal membrane. *Biochemistry* 38:9778-9782.

Broughman, J.R., Shank, L.P., Iwamoto, T., Prakash, O., Schultz, B.D., Tomich, J.M., Mitchell, K.E. (2002) Structural implications of placing cationic residues at either the NH2- or COOH- terminus in a pore-forming synthetic peptide. *J Membrane Biol*. 190:93-103.

Broughman, J.R., Shank, L.P., Takeguchi, W., Iwamoto, T., Mitchell, K.E., Schultz, B.D., Tomich, J.M. (2002) Distinct structural elements that direct solution aggregation and membrane assembly in the channel-forming peptide M2GlyR. *Biochemistry* 41:7350-7358.

Broughman, J.R., K. Mitchell, T. Iwamoto, B.D. Schultz, J.M. Tomich. (2001) Amino-terminal modification of a channel forming peptide increases capacity for epithelial anion secretion. *Am. J. Physiol: (Cell Physiol.)* 280:C451-458.

Cheer, S.M., Waugh, J., Noble, S. (2003) Inhaled tobramycin (TOBI): a review of its use in the management of *Pseudomonas aeruginosa* infections in patients with cystic fibrosis. *Drugs* 63:2501-2520.

Chen, X., Kube, D.M., Cooper, M.J., Davis, P.M. (2007) Cell Surface Nucleolin Serves as Receptor for DNA Nanoparticles Composed of Pegylated Polylysine and DNA. *Molecular Therapy* 16:333–342.

Cook, G.A., Prakash, O., Zhang, K., Shank, L.P., Takeguchi, W.A., Robbins, A., Gong, Y.X., Iwamoto, T., Schultz, B.D., Tomich, J.M.. (2004) Activity and structural comparisons of solution associating and monomeric channel-forming peptides derived from the glycine receptor M2 segment. *Biophys J*. 86(3):1424-1435.

Corry, B., Chung, S.H. (2006) Mechanisms of valence selectivity in biological ion channels. *Cell Mol Life Sci*. 63:301-315.

Dawson, D.C., Smith, S.S., Mansoura, M.K. (1999) CFTR: Mechanism of anion conduction. *Physiol Rev*. 79(1 Suppl):S47-75.

de Planque, M.R., Bonev, B.B., Demmers, J.A., Greathouse, D.V., Koeppe, R.E. 2nd, Separovic, F., Watts, A. and Killian, J.A. (2003) Interfacial anchor properties of tryptophan residues in transmembrane peptides can dominate over hydrophobic matching effects in peptide-lipid interactions. *Biochemistry* 42:5341-5348.

Demmers, J.A., van Duijn, E., Haverkamp, J., Greathouse, D.V., Koeppe, R.E. 2nd, Heck, A.J., Killian, J.A. (2001) Interfacial positioning and stability of transmembrane peptides in lipid bilayers studied by combining hydrogen/deuterium exchange and mass spectrometry. *J Biol. Chem.* 276:34501-34508.

Donaldson, S.H., Bennett, W.D., Zeman, K.L., Knowles, M.R., Tarran, R., Boucher, R.C. (2006) Mucus Clearance and Lung Function in Cystic Fibrosis with Hypertonic Saline. *New England Journal of Medicine* 354(3):1848-1851.

Dormer, R.L., Harris, C.M., Clark, Z., Pereira, M.M.C., Doull, I.J.M., Norez, C., Becq F., McPherson, M.A. (2005) Sildenafil (Viagra) corrects ΔF508-CFTR location in nasal epithelial cells from patients with cystic fibrosis. *Thorax* 60:55–59.

Dutzler, R., Campbell, E.B., Cadene, M., Chait, B.T., MacKinnon, R. (2002) X-ray structure of a ClC Cl- channel at 3.0 A reveals the molecular basis of anion selectivity. *Nature* 415(6869):287-294.

Dutzler, R., Campbell, E.B., MacKinnon, R. (2003) Gating the selectivity filter in ClC Cl- channels. *Science* 300:108-112.

Dutzler, R., E.B. Cambell, M. Cadene, B.T. Chait, and R. MacKinnon. (2002) X-ray structure of a ClC chloride channel at 3.0 Å reveals the molecular basis of anion selectivity. *Nature* 415:287-294.

Elkins, M.R., Robinson, M., Rose, B.R., Harbour, C., Moriarty, C.P., Marks, G.B., Belousova, E.G., Xuan, W., Bye, P.T. (2006) A controlled trial of long-term inhaled hypertonic saline in patients with cystic fibrosis. *N Engl J Med.* 354:229-240.

Estévez, R., Jentsch, T. (2002) CLC chloride channels: correlating structure with function. *Current Opinion in Structural Biology* 12:531-539.

Fuchs, H.J., Borowitz, D.S., Christiansen, D.H., Morris, E.M., Nash, M.L., Ramsey, B.W., Rosenstein, B.J., Smith, A.L., Wohl, M.E. (1994) Effect of aerosolized recombinant human DNase on exacerbations of respiratory symptoms and on pulmonary function in patients with cystic fibrosis. *N Engl J Med* 331:637-642.

Freedman, S.D., Katz, M.H., Parker, E.M., Laposata, M., Urman, M.Y., Alvarez, J.G. (1999) A membrane lipid imbalance plays a role in the phenotypic expression of cystic fibrosis in cftr (-/-) mice. *Proc. Natl. Acad. Sci. USA* 96:13995-14000.

Freedman, S.D., Blanco, P.G., Zaman, M.M., Shea, J.C., Ollero, M., Hopper, I.K., Weed, D.A., Gelrud, A., Regan, M.M., Laposata, M., Alvarez, J.G., O'Sullivan, B.P. (2004) Association of cystic fibrosis with abnormalities in fatty acid metabolism. *N Engl J Med.* 350:560-569.

Gao, L., Kim, K.J., Yankaskas, J.R., and Forman, H.J. (1999) Abnormal glutathione transport in cystic fibrosis airway epithelia. *Am J Physiol Lung Cell Mol Physiol* 277:L113–L118.

Gao, L., Broughman, J.R., Iwamoto, T., Tomich, J.M., Venglarik, C.J., Forman, H.J. (2001) Synthetic Cl- channel restores glutathione secretion in airway epithelia. *Am. J. Physiol. (Lung)* 281: L24-L30.

Gibson, R.L., Burns, J.L., Ramsey, B.W. (2003) Pathophysiology and management of pulmonary infections in cystic fibrosis. *Am J Respir Crit Care Med.* 168:918–951.

Granseth, E., von Heijne, G., Elofsson, A. (2005) A study of the membrane-water interface region of membrane proteins. *J Mol. Biol.* 346(1):377-385.

Grasemann, H., Stehling, F., Brunar, H., Widmann, R., Laliberte, T.W., Molina, L., Doring, G., Ratjen, F. (2007) Inhalation of Moli1901 in patients with cystic fibrosis. *Chest* 131:1461–1466.

Gunthorpe, M.J., Lummis, S.C. (2001) Conversion of the ion selectivity of the 5-HT(3a) receptor from cationic to anionic reveals a conserved feature of the ligand-gated ion channel superfamily. *J Biol Chem.* 276:10977-10983.

Harzer, U., Bechinger, B. (2000) Alignment of lysine-anchored membrane peptides under conditions of hydrophobic mismatch: a CD, ^{15}N and ^{31}P solid-state NMR spectroscopy investigation. *Biochemistry* 39:13106-13114.

Herrera, A.I., Al-Rawi, A., Cook G.A., Prakash, O., Tomich, J.M., Chen, J. (2010) Introduction of a C-Terminal Tryptophan in a Pore-Forming Peptide: A Structure/Activity Study. *PROTEINS: Structure, Function, and Genetics* 78(10): 2238-2250.

Hilf, R.J., Dutzler, R. (2008) X-ray structure of a prokaryotic pentameric ligand-gated ion channel. *Nature* 452:375-380.

Hong, H., Park, S., Jiménez, R.H., Rinehart, D., Tamm, L.K. (2007) Role of aromatic side chains in the folding and thermodynamic stability of integral membrane proteins. *J. Am. Chem. Soc.* 129(26):8320-8327.

Ivanov, I., Cheng, X., Sine, S.M., McCammon, J.A. (2007) Barriers to ion translocation in cationic and anionic receptors from the Cys-loop family. *J Am Chem Soc.* 129:8217-8224.

Iwamoto, T., Grove, A., Montal, M. O., Montal, M., Tomich, J. M. (1994) Chemical synthesis and characterization of peptides and oligomeric proteins designed to form transmembrane ion channels. *Int. J. Peptide Protein Res.* 43:597-607.

Jaques, A., Daviskas, E., Turton, J.A., McKay, K., Cooper, P., Stirling, R.G., Robertson, C.F., Bye, P.T., Lesouëf, P.N., Shadbolt, B., Anderson, S.D., Charlton, B. (2008) Inhaled mannitol improves lung function in cystic fibrosis.Chest 133(6):1388–1396.

Jayasinghe, S., Hristova, K., White S.H.(2001) Energetics, stability, and prediction of transmembrane helices. *J Mol Biol.* 312:927-934.

Jensen, M.L., Pedersen, L.N., Timmermann, D.B., Schousboe, A., Ahring, P.K. (2005) Mutational studies using a cation-conducting GABA-A receptor reveal the selectivity determinants of the Cys-loop family of ligand-gated ion channels. *J Neurochem.* 92:962-972.

Jensen, M.L., Schousboe, A., Ahring, P.K. (2005) Charge selectivity of the Cys-loop family of ligand-gated ion channels. *J Neurochem.* 92:217-225.

Kellerman, D., Mospan, R., Engels, J., Schaberg, A., Gorden, J., Smiley, L. (2008) Denufosol: A review of studies with inhaled P2Y(2) agonists that led to phase 3. *Pulm Pharmacol Ther.* 21:600–607.

Keramidasa, A., Moorhousea, A.A., Schofieldb, P.R. and Barry, P.H. (1994) Ligand-gated ion channels: mechanisms underlying ion selectivity. *Progress in Biophysics & Molecular Biology* 86:161–204.

Konstan, M.W., Byard, P.J., Hoppel, C.L., Davis, P.B. (1995) Effect of high-dose ibuprofen in patients with cystic fibrosis. *N Engl J Med.* 332:848–854.

Konstan, M.W., Davis, P.B., Wagener, J.S., Hilliard, K.A., Stern, R.C., Milgram, L.J.H., Kowalczyk, T.H., Hyatt, S.L., Fink, T.L., Gedeon, C.R., Oette, S.M., Payne, J.M., Muhammad, O., Ziady, A.G., Moen, R.C., Cooper, M.J. (2004)Compacted DNA nanoparticles administered to the nasal mucosa of cystic fibrosis subjects are safe and demonstrate partial to complete cystic fibrosis transmembrane regulator reconstitution. *Hum Gene Ther.* 15:1255–1269.

Lazaar, A.L., Sweeney, L.E., MacDonald, A.J., Alexis, N.E., Chen, C., Tal-Singer, R. (2011) SB-656933, a novel CXCR2 selective antagonist, inhibits ex-vivo neutrophil activation and ozone-induced airway inflammation in humans. *British Journal of Clinical Pharmacology.* 72(2):282-293.

Linsdell, P. (2006) Mechanism of chloride permeation in the cystic fibrosis transmembrane conductance regulator chloride channel. *Exp Physiol.* 91:123-129.

Liu, X., Smith, S.S., Sun, F., Dawson, D.C. (2001) CFTR: Covalent modification of cysteine-substituted channels expressed in Xenopus oocytes shows that activation is due to the opening of channels resident in the plasma membrane. *J Gen Physiol.* 118:433-46.

Lobet, S., Dutzler, R. (2006) Ion-binding properties of the ClC chloride selectivity filter. *EMBO J.* 25:24-33.

Lowry, F. (2011) FDA Panel Sends Liprotamase Back to the Drawing Board. Medscape Medical News. http://www.medscape.com/viewarticle/735722

Mall, S., Broadbridge, R., Sharma, R.P., Lee, A.G., East J.M. (2000) Effects of aromatic residues at the ends of transmembrane alpha-helices on helix interactions with lipid bilayers. *Biochemistry* 39:2071-2078.

Mansoura, M.K., Smith, S.S., Choi, A.D., Richards, N.W., Strong, T.V., Drumm, M.L., Collins, F.S., Dawson, D.C. (1998) Cystic fibrosis transmembrane conductance regulator (CFTR) anion binding as a probe of the pore. *Biophys J.* 74:1320-1332.

Marsh, D. (1996) Peptide models for membrane channels. *Biochem J.* 315(Pt 2):345-361.

Mitaku, S., Hirokawa, T., Tsuji T. (2002) Amphiphilicity index of polar amino acids as an aid in the characterization of amino acid preference at membrane-water interfaces. *Bioinformatics* 18:608-616.

Miyazawa, A., Fujiyoshi, Y., Unwin, N. (2003) Structure and gating mechanism of the acetylcholine receptor pore. *Nature* 424:949-955.

Montal, M.O., Reddy, G.L., Iwamoto, T., Tomich, J.M., Montal, M. (1994) Identification of an ion channel-forming motif in the primary structure of CFTR, the Cystic Fibrosis Cl-channel. *Proc. Natl. Acad. Sci. USA* 91:1495-1499.

Mutter, M., Hersperger, R., Gubernator, K., Müller, K. (1989) The construction of new proteins: V. A template-assembled synthetic protein (TASP) containing both a 4-helix bundle and beta-barrel-like structure. *Proteins* 5(1):13-21.

Pettit, R.S. and Johnson, C.E. (2011) Airway-rehydrating agents for the treatment of cystic fibrosis: past, present, and future. *Ann. Pharmacother* 45:49-59.

Pollack, A. (2011) Vertex says trial of Vertex's VX-770, a cystic fibrosis drug, eased breathing - NYTimes.com. The Business of Health Care - Prescriptions Blog - NYTimes.com. http://prescriptions.blogs.nytimes.com/2011/02/23/vertex-says-cystic-fibrosis-drug-helped-patients-breathe-easier/

Ramalho, A.S., Beck, S., Meyer, M., Penque, D., Cutting, G.R., Amaral, M.D. (2002) Five percent of normal cystic fibrosis transmembrane conductance regulator mRNA ameliorates the severity of pulmonary disease in cystic fibrosis. *Am J Respir Cell Mol Biol.* 27:619–627.

Reddy, L.G., Iwamoto, T., Tomich, J.M. and Montal, M. (1993) Synthetic peptides and four-helix bundle proteins as model systems for the pore-forming structure of channel proteins. III. Transmembrane segment M2 of the brain glycine receptor channel is a plausible candidate for the pore-lining structure. *J. Biol. Chem.* 268:14608-14615.

Retsch-Bogart, G. (2011) Role of new therapies in CF lung disease. CF Learning Center http://www.cflearningcenter. com /pdfs/CFLC2011/healthcare/Role_of_New_Therapies_in_CF_Lung_Disease.pdf

Riordan, J.R. (2008) CFTR Function and Prospects for Therapy. *Annu Rev Biochem.* 77:701-726

Saiman, L., Marshall, B.C., Mayer-Hamblett, N., Burns, J.L., Quittner, A.L., Cibene, D.A., Coquillette, S., Fieberg, A.Y., Accurso, F.J., Campbell, P.W. 3rd. (2003) Azithromycin in patients with cystic fibrosis chronically infected with Pseudomonas aeruginosa: a randomized controlled trial. *J A M A* 290:1749–1756.

Sagel, S.D., Sontag, M.K., Anthony, M.M., Emmett, P., Papas, K.A. (2011). Effect of an antioxidant-rich multivitamin supplement in cystic fibrosis. *J Cystic Fibrosis* 10(1):31-36.

Schmieden, V., Grenningloh, G., Schofield, P.R., Betz, H. (1989) Functional expression in Xenopus oocytes of the strychnine binding 48 kd subunit of the glycine receptor. *EMBO J.* 8:695-700.

Sears, H., Gartman, J., Casserly, P. (2011) Treatment options for cystic fibrosis: State of the art and future perspectives. *Reviews on Recent Clinical Trials* 6(2):94-107.

Shank, L.P., Broughman, J.R., Brandt, R.M., Robbins, A.S., Takeguchi, W., Cook, G.A., Hahn, L., Radke, G., Iwamoto, T., Schultz, B.D., Tomich, J.M. (2006) Redesigning channel-forming peptides: amino acid substitutions in channel- forming peptides that enhance rates of supramolecular assembly and raise ion transport activity. *Biophys J.* 90:2138-2150.

Sheridan, C. (2011) First cystic fibrosis drug advances towards approval. *Nature Biotechnology*, 29(6):465-466.

Sine, S.M., Engel, A.G. (2006) Recent advances in cys-loop receptor structure and function. *Nature* 440:448-455.

Smith, S.S., Liu, X., Zhang, Z.R., Sun, F., Kriewall, T.E., McCarty, N.A., Dawson, D.C. (2001) CFTR: Covalent and noncovalent modification suggests a role for fixed charges in anion conduction. *J Gen Physiol.* 118:407-431.

Sunesen, M., de Carvalho, L.P., Dufresne, V., Grailhe, R., Savatier-Duclert, N., Gibor, G., Peretz, A., Attali, B., Changeux, J.P., Paas, Y. (2006) Mechanism of Cl- selection by a glutamate-gated chloride (GluCl) receptor revealed through mutations in the selectivity filter. *J Biol Chem.* 281:14875-14881.

Tang, P., Mandal, P.K., Xu, Y. (2002) NMR structures of the second transmembrane domain of the human glycine receptor alpha(1) subunit: model of pore architecture and channel gating. *Biophys J.* 83:252-262.

Tirouvanziam, R., Conrad, C.K., Bottiglieri, T., Herzenberg, L.A., Moss, R.B. (2006) High-dose oral N-acetylcysteine, a glutathione prodrug, modulates inflammation in cystic fibrosis. *Proc Natl Acad Sci USA* 103:4628–4633.

Tomich, J.M., Wallace, D.P., Henderson, K., Brandt, R., Ambler, C.A., Scott, A.J., Mitchell, K.E., Radke, G., Grantham, J. J. Sullivan, L.P., Iwamoto, T. (1998) Aqueous solubilization of transmembrane peptide sequences with retention of membrane insertion and function. *Biophys J.* 74:256-267.

Unwin, N. (2003) Structure and action of the nicotinic acetylcholine receptor explored by electron microscopy. *FEBS Lett.* 555:91-95.

Unwin, N. (2005) Refined structure of the nicotinic acetylcholine receptor at 4Å resolution. *J Mol Biol.* 346:967-989.

van der Wel, P.C.A., Reed, N.D., Greathouse, D.V., Koeppe, R.E.II (2007) Orientation and motion of tryptophan interfacial anchors in membrane-spanning peptides *Biochemistry* 46(25):7514-7524.

Vogt, B., Ducarme, P., Schinzel, S., Brasseur, R., Bechinger, B. (2000) The topology of lysine-containing amphipathic peptides in bilayers by circular dichroism, solid-state NMR, and molecular modeling. *Biophys J.* 79:2644-2656.

Vogt, B., Ducarme, P., Schinzel, S., Brasseur, R., Bechinger, B. (2000) The topology of lysine-containing amphipathic peptides in bilayers by circular dichroism, solid-state NMR, and molecular modeling. *Biophys J.* 79:2644–2656.

Wallace, D.P., Tomich, J.M., Eppler, J., Iwamoto, T., Grantham, J.J., Sullivan, L.P. (2000) A Channel forming peptide induces Cl^- secretion by T84 cells: Modulation by Ca^{2+}-dependent K^+ channels. *Biochem Biophys Acta* 1464:69-82.

Wallace, D.P., Tomich, J.M., Iwamoto, T., Henderson, K., Grantham, J.J., Sullivan, L.P. (1997) A synthetic peptide derived from the glycine-gated Cl^- channel generates Cl^- and fluid secretion by epithelial monolayers. *Am J Physiol: (Cell Physiol)* 272:C1672-C1679.

Wilschanski, M., Miller, L., Shoseyov, D., Blau, H., Rivlin, J., Aviram, M., Cohen, M., Armoni, S., Yaakov, Y., Pugatch, T., Cohen-Cymberknoh, M., Miller, N.L., Reha, A., Northcutt, V.J., Hirawat, S., Donnelly, K., Elfring, G.L., Ajayi, T., Kerem, E. (2011) Chronic ataluren (PTC124) treatment of nonsense mutation cystic fibrosis. *Eur Respiratory J.* 38(1):59-69.

Wimley W.C., White, S.H. (1996) Experimentally determined hydrophobicity scale for proteins at membrane interfaces. *Nat Struct Biol.* 3:842-848.

Wimley, W.C., White, S.H. (1999) Membrane protein folding and stability: physical principles. *Ann Rev Biomol Struct.* 28:319-365.

Wimley, W.C., White, S.H. (2000) Designing Transmembrane α-Helices That Insert Spontaneously. *Biochemistry* 39:4432-4442.

Yankaskas, J.R., (1993) Papilloma virus immortalized tracheal epithelial cells retain a well-differentiated phenotype. *Am J Physiol Cell Physiol.* 264:C1219–C1230.

Yushmanov, V.E., Mandal, P.K., Liu, Z., Tang, P., Xu, Y. (2003) NMR structure and backbone dynamics of the extended second transmembrane domain of the human neuronal glycine receptor α_1 subunit. *Biochemistry* 42:3989-3995.

Zerhusen, B., Zhao, J., Xie, J., Davis, P.B., Ma, J. (1999) A single conductance pore for Cl- ions formed by two cystic fibrosis transmembrane conductance regulator molecules. *J Biol Chem.* 274:7627-7630.

Zhang, L., Aleksandrov, L.A., Riordan, J.R., Ford, R.C. (2011) Domain location within the cystic fibrosis transmembrane conductance regulator protein investigated by electron microscopy and gold labelling. *Biochim Biophys Acta.* 1808(1):399-404.

Zhang, Z.R., McDonough, S.I., McCarty, N.A. (2000) Interaction between permeation and gating in a putative pore domain mutant in the cystic fibrosis transmembrane conductance regulator. *Biophys J.* 79:298-313.

Zhang, X.D., Li, Y., Yu, W.P., Chen, T.Y. (2006) Roles of K149, G352, and H401 in the channel functions of ClC-0: testing the predictions from theoretical calculations. *J Gen Physiol.* 127:435-447.

Zhou, Z., Hu, S., Hwang, T.C. (2002) Probing an open CFTR pore with organic anion blockers. *J Gen Physiol.* 120:647-662.

14

Improving Cell Surface Functional Expression of ΔF508 CFTR: A Quest for Therapeutic Targets

Yifei Fan, Yeshavanth K. Banasavadi-Siddegowda and Xiaodong Wang
University of Toledo College of Medicine
USA

1. Introduction

Cystic fibrosis (CF) is largely a protein misfolding disease. The deletion of a phenylalanine at residue 508 (ΔF508) in the cystic fibrosis transmembrane conductance regulator (CFTR) accounts for 70% of all disease-causing alleles and is present in at least one copy in 90% of CF patients (Kerem et al., 1989). The ΔF508 mutation impairs the conformational maturation of nascent CFTR (Lukacs et al., 1994), and arrests it in an early folding intermediate (Zhang et al., 1998). As a result, the mutant CFTR is retained in the endoplasmic reticulum (ER) (Cheng et al., 1990) in a chaperone-bound state (Yang et al., 1993), The ER-accumulated mutant CFTR fails to efficiently couple to the coatomer complex II (COPII) ER export machinery (Wang et al., 2004), and is degraded by the ubiquitin proteasome system through the ER-associated degradation (ERAD) pathway (Jensen et al., 1995; Ward et al., 1995), leading to loss of CFTR function at the cell surface.

The folding defect of ΔF508 CFTR appears kinetic in nature (Qu et al., 1997). A small fraction of ΔF508 CFTR is able to exit the ER but the escaped mutant protein is not stable at the cell periphery and is rapidly cleared through lysosomal degradation (Lukacs et al., 1993). This second defect further reduces the cell surface localization of this mutant CFTR. Aside from localization defect, the ΔF508 mutation also impairs the channel gating of CFTR, leading to reduced open probability (Dalemans et al., 1991). The threefold defect of ΔF508 CFTR stems from its defective conformation, and impairs the CFTR functional expression at the cell surface, leading to severe clinical phenotype. Given the autosomal recessive inheritance of the disease, improving plasma membrane functional expression of ΔF508 CFTR will benefit the vast majority of CF patients (Gelman & Kopito, 2002).

Numerous research efforts have been made to improve ΔF508 CFTR cell surface functional expression, including elevating its expression, reducing its degradation, enhancing the efficiency of its maturation, increasing its post-ER stability and improving its channel gating. Restoring ΔF508 CFTR conformation will potentially improve its ER folding, its cell surface stability and its channel gating, leading to efficient ΔF508 CFTR rescue. In this chapter, multiple approaches for ΔF508 CFTR rescue will be reviewed, and their advantages as well as limitations will be discussed.

2. Overview of CFTR biogenesis, quality control and exocytic trafficking

CFTR is a member of the ATP-binding cassette (ABC) transporter family, and is composed of two homologous modules each containing a membrane spanning domain (MSD) followed by a nucleotide-binding domain (NBD) (Riordan et al., 1989) (Fig. 1). CFTR is unique in that it has an unstructured regulatory (R) domain inserted between the two homologous modules (Fig. 1). CFTR has two N-linked glycosylation sites on the fourth extracellular loop (Fig. 1). In the ER, the newly synthesized CFTR acquires core-glycosylation at these two sites. Upon transport to the Golgi, the core-glycosylation is processed into the Golgi-specific complex glycosylation, leading to an up-shift in its apparent molecular weight. This difference in processing provides an important means of discriminating the ER-localized, immature CFTR (band B) and the Golgi-processed, mature form (band C). At the steady state, the majority of CFTR is in its mature form. As ΔF508 CFTR is unable to exit the ER, it largely exists in band B. All the major functional domains of CFTR reside on the cytoplasmic side of membrane. Therefore, chaperone-mediated folding events in the cytoplasm play an important role in CFTR maturation and quality control (Yang et al., 1993; Loo et al., 1998; Meacham et al., 1999; Wang et al., 2006).

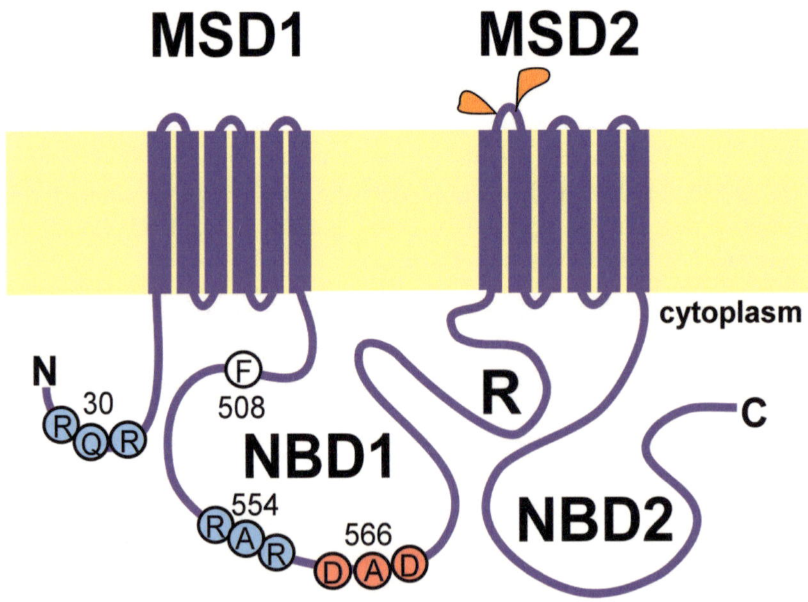

Fig. 1. Domain structure and putative sorting signals of CFTR.

2.1 CFTR de novo folding in the ER

CFTR is synthesized on the ER membrane. Domain folding occurs largely co-translationally (Kleizen et al., 2005). However, further conformational maturation is necessary to form a fully assembled molecule competent for passing the ER quality control and coupling to COPII for ER export (Zhang et al., 1998; Wang et al., 2004). The F508 residue resides in NBD1 (Fig. 1). The ΔF508-induced misfolding of CFTR starts during translation immediately after the NBD1 emerges from the ribosome (Hoelen et al., 2010). This conformational defect originates in NBD1 but spread throughout the whole molecule through domain-domain interactions, leading to a global conformation defect (Du et al., 2005; Du & Lukacs, 2009; Roy et al., 2010). Restoring wild-type-like global conformation is required for ΔF508 CFTR to pass the quality control and egress from the ER (Roy et al., 2010). Second site mutations in NBD1 have been identified that suppress the ΔF508 processing defect (Teem et al., 1993), and at least some of such suppressing mutations can act co-translationally on the NBD1 misfolding (Hoelen et al., 2010). Therefore, the de novo folding of ΔF508 CFTR at both co-translational and post-translational levels can be targeted for its rescue.

2.2 CFTR quality control in the ER

Newly synthesized CFTR undergo quality control before it can exit the ER. ER quality control starts even before CFTR is fully translated (Fig. 2). A membrane-associated ubiquitin ligase complex containing the E3 RMA1, the E2 Ubc6e and Derlin-1 mediates CFTR co-translational quality control (Sun et al., 2006; Younger et al., 2006). BAP31, an integral membrane protein that associates with Derlin-1 as well as the amino terminus of CFTR, promotes ΔF508 CFTR retrotranslocation from the ER and its subsequent degradation by the cytoplasmic 26S proteasome (B. Wang et al., 2008). P97/valosin-containing protein interacts with gp78/autocrine motility factor receptor in coupling CFTR ubiquitination to its retrotranslocation and proteasome degradation (Carlson et al., 2006; Vij et al., 2006). Interestingly, gp78 was found to cooperate with RMA1 in the ERAD of ΔF508 CFTR (Morito et al., 2008). Moreover, ubiquitin C-terminal hydrolase-L1 (UCH-L1) protects CFTR from co-translational ERAD (Henderson et al., 2010). This co-translational quality control of CFTR appears to be regulated by cytoplasmic Hsc70 as DNAJB12 was recently found to cooperate with Hsc70 and RMA1 in ΔF508 CFTR degradation (Grove et al., 2011). Consistent with this, we found that Hsp105, a nucleotide exchange factor (NEF) for Hsc70, promotes co-translational ERAD of CFTR (Saxena et al., 2011a).

A second ER quality control step occurs largely post-translationally, which is mediated through Hsc70 and cochaperone CHIP (Meacham et al., 2001) (Fig. 2). CHIP functions as a scaffold for the formation of multi-subunit E3 ubiquitin ligase for the post-translational ERAD of CFTR, and such degradation activity is also dependent upon Hsc70, Hdj-2 and the E2 UbcH5a (Younger et al., 2004). Interestingly, HspBP1 and BAG-2, two other NEFs for Hsc70, inhibits the CHIP-mediated post-translational ERAD of CFTR (Alberti et al., 2004; Arndt et al., 2005), suggesting a dual role for Hsc70 in regulating co-translational and post-translational ERAD of CFTR.

Nevertheless, inhibiting CFTR ERAD is not sufficient for ΔF508 CFTR to efficiently exit the ER (Jensen et al., 1995; Pagant et al., 2007). Obviously, another quality control system is responsible for the retention of the foldable pool of ΔF508 CFTR in the ER, the mechanism of which is less clear. We recently showed that the ER exit code and domain conformation both contribute significantly to the exportability of CFTR (Roy et al., 2010). Therefore, chaperone association and/or ER exit code presentation might be two important factors for this last checkpoint of the ER quality control of CFTR. A better understanding of its mechanism will lead to much greater improvement in ΔF508 CFTR maturation.

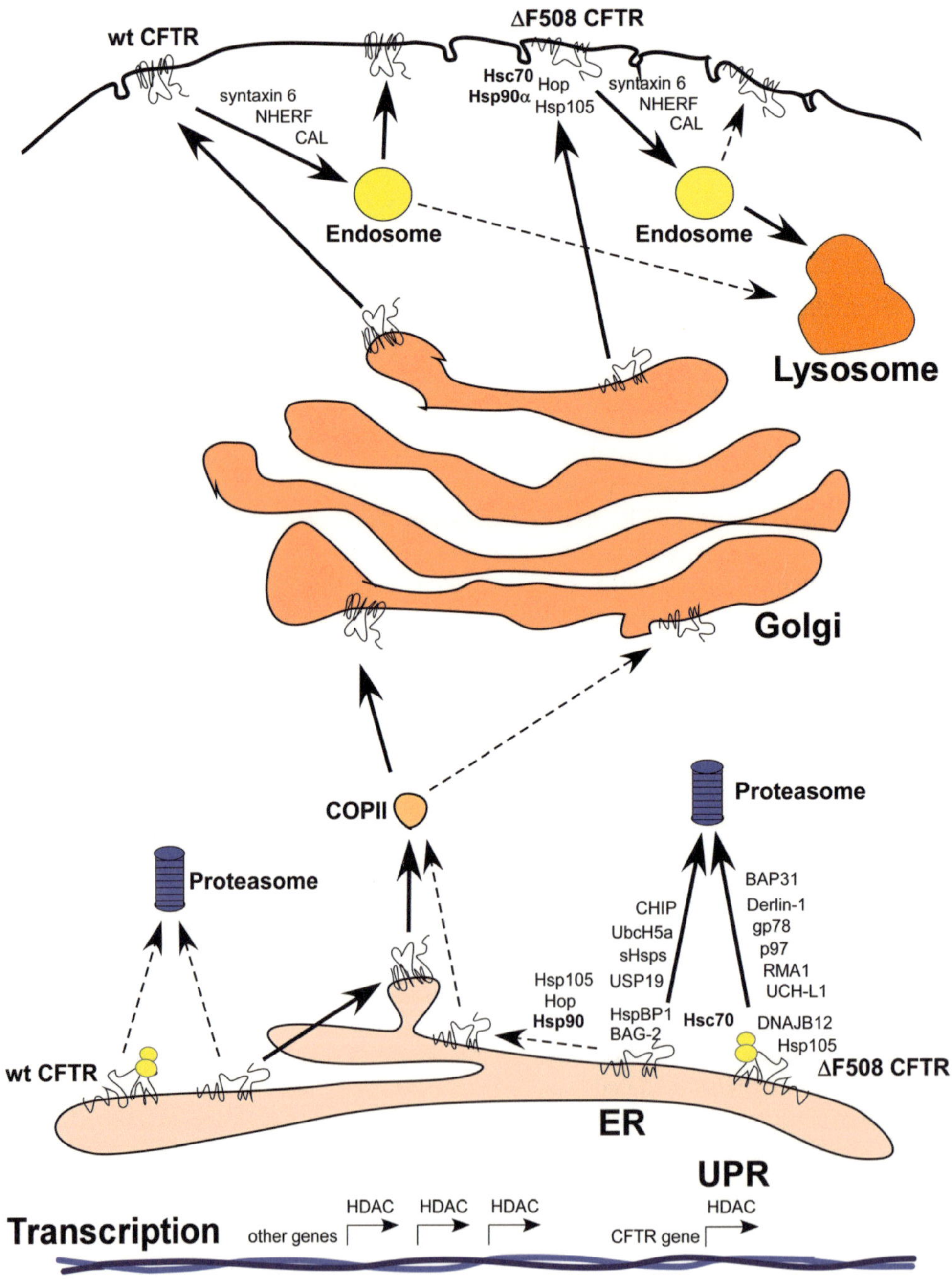

Shown are the transcription, synthesis, folding and quality control of wild-type and ΔF508 CFTR with a great number of regulators at both the ER and peripheral levels, which are potential molecular targets for ΔF508 CFTR rescue. Complete arrows indicate major pathways, and broken arrows denote minor pathways. Enhancement of some of the minor pathways for ΔF508 CFTR can effectively promote its rescue.

Fig. 2. Regulation of CFTR biogenesis and degradation.

2.3 ER-to-Golgi sorting signals within CFTR

Exit of proteins from the ER requires specific sorting signals on the cytoplasmic side of the ER membrane which is recognizable by the cargo selection complex (Sec23/24) of COPII (Aridor et al., 1998; Nishimura et al., 1999; Miller et al., 2002). A di-acidic ER exit motif (DAD) was identified in the NBD1 of CFTR (Fig. 1), and substitution of the second acidic residue (leading to DAA) abolishes CFTR association with Sec24 and dramatically reduces the export efficiency of CFTR (Wang et al., 2004). The ΔF508 mutation also reduces CFTR association with Sec24 (Wang et al., 2004) but the underlying mechanism might be different from the DAA mutant. Using in situ limited proteolysis to probe the domain conformation of CFTR (Zhang et al., 1998), we showed that the DAA mutant has similar domain conformation as wild-type CFTR despite its inability to efficiently exit the ER (Roy et al., 2010). This is in stark contrast to ΔF508 CFTR which displays global conformational defects including NBD1 (Du et al., 2005; Du & Lukacs, 2009; Roy et al., 2010). Furthermore, DAA CFTR displays lower chaperone association and higher post-ER stability when compared with ΔF508 CFTR (Roy et al., 2010). Therefore, the conformational defects in ΔF508 CFTR contribute significantly to its misprocessing.

ER retention/retrieval signals have been found in the cytoplasmic domains of multiple transmembrane cargo proteins (Nilsson et al., 1989; Zerangue et al., 1999). An RXR ER retention/retrieval signal serves as a quality control check point for the assembly of oligomeric cargo proteins in the ER (Zerangue et al., 1999; Margeta-Mitrovic et al., 2000). The RXR signals are exposed in individual subunits or in incompletely assembled oligomers but are concealed only when the proper assembly of the oligomer is achieved. This mechanism prevents the cell surface expression of improperly assembled cargo molecules. Multiple RXR motifs have been identified in the cytoplasmic domains of CFTR (Fig. 1), and the replacement of key arginine residues results in ΔF508 CFTR rescue, suggesting that the RXR motifs might contribute to the ER retention/retrieval of ΔF508 CFTR (Chang et al., 1999). It is proposed that such RXR motifs are shielded by domain-domain interactions in wild-type CFTR but become exposed when the F508 is deleted (Kim Chiaw et al., 2009). In fact, peptides designed to mimic such a sorting motif were found to functionally rescue ΔF508 CFTR (Kim Chiaw et al., 2009). As the key RXR motif in NBD1 contributes significantly to ΔF508 CFTR global conformation (Qu et al., 1997; Hegedus et al., 2006; Roy et al., 2010), it is unclear if the RXR-mimetics rescue ΔF508 CFTR by influencing ΔF508 CFTR conformation. Determining whether the RXR-mimetics are able to bind to the RXR sorting receptor or whether they block the retention/retrieval of other RXR-containing cargo molecules will provide a definitive answer.

3. Defining ΔF508 conformational defects

F508 resides in NBD1 (Fig. 1), and therefore the deletion of this residue should naturally affect the conformation of NBD1. Early in vitro studies using purified NBD1 revealed a kinetic folding defect in ΔF508 NBD1 (Qu & Thomas, 1996; Qu et al., 1997). However, the crystal structure of ΔF508 NBD1 revealed no major conformational change from the wild-type domain (Lewis et al., 2005). In the mean time, it was found that ΔF508 mutation causes major conformation changes in NBD2 (Du et al., 2005), highlighting the importance of domain-domain interactions in ΔF508 misfolding. This notion was strengthened by the finding that F508 side chain contributes significantly to NBD1 folding in the context of full-length CFTR (Thibodeau et al., 2005), and by the finding that F508 residue mediates the contact between NBD1 and cytoplasmic loop 4 (CL4) in MSD2 (Serohijos et al., 2008a). Therefore, deletion of F508 triggers a global conformational change in CFTR, leading to misprocessing (Du & Lukacs, 2009).

The apparent lack of a detectable NBD1 conformational change as a result of the ΔF508 mutation remains an enigma as how can the ΔF508 mutation trigger such a profound global conformational change without significantly impacting NBD1 conformation in the first place? The finding that some of the solubilization mutations included in ΔF508 NBD1 for crystallography studies actually rescue the ΔF508 processing defect in the context of full-length CFTR reopened this question (Pissarra et al., 2008). Another twist in our understanding of the impact of F508 deletion on NBD1 conformation came from the finding that the removal of the regulatory insert (RI), a 32-residue segment within NBD1 that is unique to CFTR but not shared by the NBD1's of other ABC transporters, renders ΔF508 NBD1 soluble, dimer-forming and displaying wild-type-like conformation (Atwell et al., 2010). Another study shows that, in the context of full-length CFTR protein, removal of the RI restores maturation, stability and function of ΔF508 CFTR, suggesting that the RI contributes significantly to ΔF508 misfolding in NBD1(Aleksandrov et al., 2010).

Using in situ limited proteolysis, we identified a definite conformational change within NBD1 as a result of ΔF508 mutation (Roy et al., 2010). The ΔF508 NBD1 conformation, like the conformation of other domains of ΔF508 CFTR, resembles the conformation of an earlier folding intermediate of wild-type CFTR (Zhang et al., 1998; Roy et al., 2010). Furthermore, rescue of ΔF508 CFTR using low temperature or R555K substitution leads to NBD1 as well as global conformational reversion, suggesting that conformational correction is prerequisite for the rescue of the folding and export defects of ΔF508 CFTR (Roy et al., 2010). Using crystallography and hydrogen/deuterium exchange mass spectrometry, Lewis, et al. showed that ΔF508 mutation increases the exposure of the 509-511 loop and increases the dynamics in its vicinity (Lewis et al., 2010). Consistent with the above, a conformational change in ΔF508 NBD1 was observed using a cysteine-labelling technique, and such conformational change is reversed by second site mutations in NBD1 (He et al., 2010). Interestingly, the second site mutations also restore the interactions between NBD1 and its contacting domains (He et al., 2010). Combination of G550E, R553M and R555K suppressor mutations in NBD1 produces a dramatic increase in ΔF508 CFTR processing, and this is accompanied by the enhanced folding of ΔF508 NBD1 both in isolation and in the context of full-length CFTR (Thibodeau et al., 2010). An interesting finding is that while NBD2 is not required for CFTR processing (Pollet et al., 2000), it contributes to ΔF508 CFTR rescue by second site mutations as well as by low temperature (Du & Lukacs, 2009; Cheng et al., 2010). Furthermore, the rescue of ΔF508 CFTR by suppressor mutations requires a continuous full-length CFTR peptide (Cheng et al., 2010), suggesting a role for peptide backbone tension in ΔF508 CFTR rescue (Thibodeau et al., 2005).

Taken together, ΔF508 mutation causes increased exposure of the 509-511 loop in NBD1 and increases its dynamics. These changes not only alter the conformation of NBD1, but through NBD1's interface with CL4 and NBD2, alter the conformation of other domains, leading to global conformational change. Second site mutations within NBD1 can partially correct the

ΔF508 NBD1 conformational defect, which spread to other domains through domain-domain interactions, leading to partial restoration of global conformation as well as processing. Conformation repair is at the heart of ΔF508 correction.

4. Elevating ΔF508 CFTR expression

The severe reduction in ΔF508 CFTR cell surface functional expression results from its defective export, reduced peripheral stability, and subnormal channel gating. Nevertheless, a small fraction of the mutant CFTR can leak from the ER and make its way to cell surface. One simple approach to enhance ΔF508 CFTR cell surface localization is to increase its expression. This can be achieved in cells heterologously expressing ΔF508 CFTR under the control of metallothionein promoter by treatment with sodium butyrate (Cheng et al., 1995). In CF airway epithelial cells, 4-phenylburyrate, a histone deacetylase (HDAC) inhibitor dramatically increases the expression of ΔF508 CFTR at the protein level (Rubenstein et al., 1997). Recently, a group of other HDAC inhibitors including Trichostatin A, suberoylanilide hydroxamic acid (SAHA) and Scriptaid were found to potently increase ΔF508 CFTR transcription in CFBE41o- cells (Hutt et al., 2010).

Interestingly, over-accumulation of ΔF508 CFTR in the ER induces the unfolded protein response (UPR) (Gomes-Alves et al., 2010), and induction of UPR inhibits CFTR endogenous transcription (Rab et al., 2007). The UPR-induced CFTR transcriptional repression is mediated through the transcription factor ATF6, and both DNA methylation and histone deacetylation contribute to this process (Bartoszewski et al., 2008). Therefore, there is a limit to which the transcription of endogenous ΔF508 CFTR can be increased but HDAC inhibitors may potentially alleviate the UPR-induced CFTR transcriptional repression (Fig. 2).

The expression of ΔF508 CFTR can also be regulated at the post-transcriptional level. A recent study revealed that the synonymous codon change of I507 in the ΔF508 allele can cause mRNA misfolding, leading to reduced rate of translation and/or impaired co-translational folding of ΔF508 CFTR (Bartoszewski et al., 2010). Therefore, codon-dependent mRNA folding represents a new mechanism by which ΔF508 CFTR expression can be regulated. Although it is not realistic to change the nucleotide sequence of ΔF508 CFTR in CF patients, identification of this novel mechanism opens up new opportunities for therapeutic intervention at the level of mRNA processing, folding, and stability.

5. Reducing ΔF508 CFTR ERAD

The vast majority of ΔF508 CFTR synthesized in the cells is degraded through the ERAD pathway (Jensen et al., 1995; Ward et al., 1995). Inhibition of ERAD will certainly increase the steady state level of ΔF508 CFTR in the ER and subsequently increase its cell surface localization (Fig. 2). Significant advance in understanding the mechanism of ERAD of ΔF508 CFTR has been achieved during the past 16 years. Hsc70 has been found to regulate both the co-translational and post-translational ERAD of ΔF508 CFTR with two distinct sets of cochaperones (Meacham et al., 2001; Zhang et al., 2001; Alberti et al., 2004; Arndt et al., 2005; Grove et al., 2011; Saxena et al., 2011a). While the functional relationship between the two remains unclear, multiple cochaperones, such as CHIP (Meacham et al., 2001), HspBP1

(Alberti et al., 2004), BAG-2 (Arndt et al., 2005), Hdj-2 (Younger et al., 2004), DNAJB12 (Grove et al., 2011) and Hsp105 (Saxena et al., 2011a) may be targeted for increasing the steady state levels of ΔF508 CFTR. Moreover, 4-phenylbutyrate, which rescues ΔF508 CFTR (Rubenstein et al., 1997), was found to reduce the expression level of Hsc70, subsequently decreases its association with ΔF508 CFTR, and therefore inhibits the ERAD of ΔF508 CFTR (Rubenstein & Zeitlin, 2000). More recently, a soluble sulfogalactosyl ceramide mimic that inhibits the Hsp40-activated Hsc70 ATPase activity, promotes the rescue of ΔF508 CFTR from ERAD (Park et al., 2009). In addition to Hsc70, small heat-shock proteins (sHsps) preferentially associate with ΔF508 CFTR and promote its ERAD (Ahner et al., 2007). It is believed that small heat-shock proteins bind to misfolded ΔF508 CFTR, prevent its aggregation and maintain its solubility during the ERAD (Ahner et al., 2007).

ERAD components such as RMA1 (Younger et al., 2006), gp78 (Morito et al., 2008), Derlin-1 (Sun et al., 2006; Younger et al., 2006), BAP31(B. Wang et al., 2008) and p97 (Carlson et al., 2006; Vij et al., 2006) can also be targeted. Although not essential for ERAD of CFTR (Carlson et al., 2006), interference of p97 expression in CF airway epithelial cells increases the steady state levels of ΔF508 CFTR in bands B and C, and enhances the CFTR-mediated chloride conductance across the plasma membrane (Vij et al., 2006). Interestingly, this effect is accompanied by reduction in interleukin-8 level which might alleviate the CF-associated airway inflammation (Vij et al., 2006). Other regulators of the p97-gp78 complex have been identified, which also influence the steady state level of ΔF508 CFTR (Nagahama et al., 2009; Ballar et al., 2010). Recently, ubiquitin-specific protease 19 (USP19), an ER-localized, membrane-anchored deubiquitinating enzyme, was shown to rescue ΔF508 CFTR from ERAD (Hassink et al., 2009), suggesting that deubiquitinating enzymes are another class of viable targets for rescuing ΔF508 CFTR (Fig. 2).

6. Enhancing ΔF508 CFTR maturation

Despite its obvious importance in rescuing ΔF508 CFTR, relatively little is known concerning how to improve the maturation of ΔF508 CFTR in the ER. The major reason is that ΔF508 CFTR hardly matures if at all at physiological temperature. However, at reduced temperature, ΔF508 CFTR does achieve conformational maturation much more efficiently, leading to greatly enhanced functional expression at the cell surface (Denning et al., 1992). Interestingly, such a temperature-sensitive phenotype is cell-dependent, suggesting that cellular machinery plays an essential role in the process (X. Wang et al., 2008). We found that the increased conformational stability provided by low temperature combines with chaperone actions in facilitating ΔF508 CFTR maturation at reduced temperature (Roy et al., 2010). Therefore, the temperature-dependent maturation of ΔF508 CFTR serves as an excellent model system in understanding the role of the cellular chaperone machinery in the forward folding of ΔF508 CFTR.

Mild heat shock greatly potentiates the temperature rescue of ΔF508 CFTR, and this is dependent upon transcription, suggesting that the upregulation of heat inducible chaperones promotes ΔF508 CFTR maturation (X. Wang et al., 2008). Using a series of chaperone- or cochaperone-deficient cell lines, we demonstrate that an Hsp70-Hsp90 chaperone network operates on the cytoplasmic face of the ER membrane facilitating the maturation of ΔF508 CFTR at reduced temperature. Cochaperone Hop, which physically and functionally links Hsp70 and Hsp90 through its multiple tetratricopeptide repeat (TPR) domains, is essential for the temperature-dependent maturation of ΔF508 CFTR, and Hsp105 is an integral player in the system (Saxena et al., 2011b). We also found that Hsc70, Hsp90β, Hop, Hsp105 and Hdj-2 are functionally linked during the temperature rescue of ΔF508 CFTR. Depletion of Hsp90β, Hop or Hsp105 also reciprocally reduces some or all of other chaperone components (Saxena et al., 2011b). It is highly likely that these folding components, and perhaps other yet unidentified chaperones or cochaperones, form a functionally organized chaperone network on the cytoplasmic side of the ER membrane, facilitating the conformational maturation of ΔF508 CFTR at reduced temperature. Given a clear role for Hsp90 in wild-type CFTR maturation at physiological temperature (Loo et al., 1998), we believe such a cytoplasmic chaperone network functions in the cell under physiological conditions. While its effect on ΔF508 CFTR maturation is more pronounced at reduced temperature, it should also impact ΔF508 CFTR maturation at the physiological temperature. Consistent with this prediction, overexpressing Hsp105 promotes ΔF508 CFTR processing at both the reduced and physiological temperatures (Saxena et al., 2011a). An in-depth analysis of this process will reveal novel molecular targets that promote the maturation of ΔF508 CFTR (Fig. 2).

Another approach to enhance ΔF508 CFTR maturation is through transcomplementation (Cormet-Boyaka et al., 2004). Such rescue requires co-expression of a sizeable segment of CFTR that contains wild-type sequence corresponding to the region where F508 is located. Such transcomplementation does not result in changes in Hsc70 association but is believed to improve ΔF508 CFTR forward folding through intra- and/or inter-molecular domain-domain interactions. A related but distinct approach to promote ΔF508 CFTR maturation is to co-express a fragment of ΔF508 CFTR containing NBD1 and R domains (Sun et al., 2008). This mutant fragment of CFTR can actually sequester key chaperone components from the endogenous ΔF508 CFTR and lead to its rescue. Moreover, co-expressing an N-terminal truncated CFTR mutant (Δ264) can not only transcomplement ΔF508 CFTR but also dramatically increases the protein expression levels of both wild-type and ΔF508 CFTR (Cebotaru et al., 2008). As the Δ264 mutant CFTR associates with VCP and HDAC6, two components involved in retrotranslocation of proteins from the ER, and is more efficiently degraded by the proteasome than ΔF508 CFTR, high level expression of this mutant may interfere with ΔF508 CFTR ERAD and hence increase its steady state level. Taken together, co-expression of CFTR fragments might rescue ΔF508 CFTR by improving its folding, helping it escape ER quality control and protecting it from ERAD. As these fragments have much lower molecular weight than full-length CFTR, they can be used as potential agents for CF gene therapy.

7. Increasing ΔF508 CFTR peripheral stability

The ΔF508 CFTR has reduced conformational stability in post-ER compartments and therefore turns over rapidly at the cell periphery (Lukacs et al., 1993; Sharma et al., 2001; Sharma et al., 2004). Increasing ΔF508 CFTR half-life at cell periphery is an important strategy for effective rescue of ΔF508 CFTR. CAL, a Golgi-associated, PDZ domain-containing protein that binds to the C-terminus of CFTR, reduces the half-life of CFTR at the cell surface (Cheng et al., 2002). RNA interference of endogenous CAL in CF airway epithelial cells increases plasma membrane expression of ΔF508 CFTR and enhances transepithelial chloride current (Wolde et al., 2007). The Na^+/H^+ exchanger regulatory factor (NHERF), a subplasma membrane PDZ domain protein, competes with CAL in associating with CFTR and promotes its plasma membrane localization (Cheng et al., 2002). Knockdown of NHERF1 promotes the degradation of temperature-rescued ΔF508 CFTR at the cell surface of human airway epithelial cells (Kwon et al., 2007). Expression of dominant-negative dynamin 2 mutant K44A increases CFTR cell surface expression, and counteracts the effect of CAL overexpression on CFTR cell surface stability (Cheng et al., 2004). SNARE protein syntaxin 6 binds to CAL and reduces CFTR cell surface stability in a CAL-dependent manner (Cheng et al., 2010). Therefore, CAL and its functional partners are viable molecular targets for increasing cell surface stability of ΔF508 CFTR (Fig. 2).

Cytoplasmic chaperone Hsc70 was shown to mediate the uncoating of clathrin-coated vesicles (Schmid & Rothman, 1985; Chappell et al., 1986) and hence regulates the peripheral trafficking of membrane bound cargo proteins such as CFTR. Recently, a more direct role for cytoplasmic Hsp70-Hsp90 chaperone network in regulating ΔF508 CFTR peripheral quality control was revealed, where Hsc70, Hsp90α, Hop and other chaperone components collaborate with the ubiquitin system in promoting the cell surface degradation of this mutant CFTR (Okiyoneda et al., 2010). This finding uncovers a great number of new potential chaperone targets for regulating cell surface stability of ΔF508 CFTR. However, as the cytoplasmic Hsp70-Hsp90 chaperone network also facilitates the maturation of CFTR in the ER (Loo et al., 1998; Meacham et al., 1999; Wang et al., 2006), a critical balance must be maintained between the two seemingly opposing effects of the Hsp70-Hsp90 chaperone network at the ER and the peripheral levels in order to effectively rescue ΔF508 CFTR (Fig. 2).

Of particular interest, we found that Hsp105 is involved in both processes. At the ER level, Hsp105 facilitates the Hsp70-Hsp90-mediated maturation of ΔF508 CFTR at reduced temperature (Saxena et al., 2011b). At the peripheral level, Hsp105 preferentially associates with the rescued ΔF508 CFTR, and stabilizes it in post-ER compartments (Saxena et al., 2011a). It is currently unclear whether Hsp105 functionally relates to Hsc70, Hop and Hsp90α at the cell periphery or it act on its own. While Hsp105 acts in the same direction as the cytoplasmic Hsp70-Hsp90 network at the ER level, it acts in opposite direction to Hsc70, Hop and Hsp90α at the cell periphery. Understanding these aspects is critical to the effective enhancement of ΔF508 CFTR cell surface functional expression by modulating cytoplasmic chaperone machinery.

8. Improving ΔF508 CFTR channel gating: Potentiator or corrector?

Although the primary defect in ΔF508 CFTR is impaired export (Cheng et al., 1990), it has aberrant channel gating as reflected in reduced channel open probability (Dalemans et al., 1991). Correcting such a defect will also improve the overall cell surface functional expression of ΔF508 CFTR. The G551D substitution in CFTR, a mutation causing severe CF, does not impact its export to plasma membrane but primarily impairs its channel opening (Tsui, 1995; Li et al., 1996). VX-770, a small molecule potentiator (improving channel gating) developed for G551D CFTR by the Vertex Pharmaceuticals Inc., also increases the channel open probability of ΔF508 CFTR (Van Goor et al., 2009). Interestingly, small molecule compound VRT-532 display both corrector (improving maturation) and potentiator activities for ΔF508 CFTR by binding directly to the mutant protein (Wellhauser et al., 2009). Recently, a fragment of a phenylglycine-type potentiator was successfully linked to a fragment of a bithiazole corrector to form a "hybrid" potentiator-corrector molecule, the cleavage of which by intestinal enzymes is able to release separate potentiator and corrector for ΔF508 rescue in vivo (Mills et al., 2010). Using high-throughput screen, multiple small molecules with independent potentiator and corrector activities for ΔF508 CFTR were also identified (Phuan et al., 2011). Using the above approaches, more efficient rescue of ΔF508 CFTR can be achieved.

9. Conformational repair: One stone and three birds

Given that the root cause of CF in the majority of patients lies in the conformational defects of ΔF508 CFTR, repairing its conformational defects will potentially lead to improved export, stability (both in the ER and at the cell periphery) and channel gating. Effective development of novel approaches in conformational repair relies on a thorough understanding of the conformational defects of ΔF508 CFTR and their correction. Given that F508 residue resides in NBD1, NBD1 is a central domain for the understanding of ΔF508 conformational repair. In addition, as domain-domain interactions within CFTR play an important role in altering or maintaining CFTR global conformation (Du et al., 2005; Du & Lukacs, 2009), key interfaces between different domains are also important in CFTR conformational repair (Serohijos et al., 2008a).

An excellent attempt was made early on in screening for suppressor mutations in NBD1 which restores the export of ΔF508 CFTR (Teem et al., 1993). This was made possible by swapping a portion of CFTR NBD1 into yeast *STE6* gene encoding an ABC transporter that delivers α-factor out of the cell which is necessary for mating. When ΔF508 mutation is included into the *STE6*-CFTR chimera, the yeast fails to transport α-factor. Using this system, second site mutations within the CFTR NBD1 portion were identified that rescue ΔF508 CFTR (Teem et al., 1993; Teem et al., 1996). Interestingly, R555K, one of such ΔF508 suppressor mutations, causes a global conformational reversion in ΔF508 CFTR, leading to increased export and enhanced post-ER stability (Roy et al., 2010). R555K, when combined with other rescue subsitutions, improves ΔF508 CFTR conformation and processing (Chang et al., 1999; Hegedus et al., 2006), and significantly increases the open probability of ΔF508 CFTR (Roxo-Rosa et al., 2006). These data support the notion that conformational repair is a highly effective approach for enhancing ΔF508 CFTR cell surface functional expression, ameliorating all three facets of ΔF508 defect.

Another approach for designing NBD1 conformational repair employs molecular dynamics simulation. Molecular dynamics has the advantage over structural biology in that it reveals information on folding kinetics and dynamics. Using this approach, key differences in the distribution of meta-stable intermediates have been identified between wild-type and ΔF508 NBD1, and additional rescue mutations can be designed (Serohijos et al., 2008b). These rescue mutations, if validated experimentally, will significantly advance our understanding of NBD1 folding both alone and in the context of full-length CFTR.

High resolution crystal structure of full-length CFTR is currently unavailable. However, the crystal structures of multiple ABC transporters including the p-glycoprotein have been solved (Locher et al., 2002; Dawson & Locher, 2006; Aller et al., 2009). Attempts to use these structures as bases for modeling full-length CFTR have provided new insights into the role of F508 residue in domain-domain interactions (Jordan et al., 2008; Loo et al., 2008; Serohijos et al., 2008a; Mornon et al., 2009). These studies, when backed up by biochemical analyses, are an excellent start point to probe ΔF508 global conformational defects and their repair.

10. Large-scale target identification for the rescue of ΔF508 CFTR

Aside from the above mechanism-based identification of therapeutic targets for ΔF508 rescue, several large-scale target identification regimes have been quite successful. The functional follow-up of these studies has yielded and will yield many novel molecular targets.

The first such attempt was to use proteomics to identify CFTR-interacting proteins between wild-type and ΔF508 CFTR (Wang et al., 2006), which revealed, among others, an ER-associated chaperone network facilitating CFTR biogenesis and quality control. In an attempt to gain information on the potential mechanism of ΔF508 chemical rescue by 4-phenylbutyrate, a pharmacoproteomic approach was used to identify changes in protein expression in CF airway epithelial cells in response to 4-phenylbutyrate treatment (Singh et al., 2006). This approach was then followed by a comparison of ΔF508 CFTR-interacting proteins between the chemically rescued (by 4-phenylbutyrate) and genetically repaired (by introducing wild-type CFTR) CF airway epithelial cells (Singh et al., 2008). Protein targets involved in the ERAD, protein folding and inflammatory response have been identified, and proteins that were modulated in the ER as well as on the plasma membrane have been isolated (Singh et al., 2008).

Recently, a high-throughput functional screen was designed to identify proteins that promote the rescue of ΔF508 CFTR (Trzcinska-Daneluti et al., 2009). In this study, 450 different proteins were fused to a chloride-senstive yellow fluorescent protein and were expressed in a ΔF508 CFTR-expressing stable cell line. The cells were screened for their ability to rescue the ΔF508 functional defect at the plasma membrane. Several proteins that are known to rescue ΔF508 CFTR as well as novel target proteins have been identified. Further functional characterization will reveal their usefulness as potential therapeutic targets.

Another excellent approach worth noting is the use of functional small interfering RNA screen to identify proteins that are involved in peripheral quality control of ΔF508 CFTR (Okiyoneda et al., 2010). This approach took advantage of a well developed cell surface ELISA assay measuring CFTR plasma membrane localization, where three HA-tags have been engineered in an extracellular domain of CFTR. The siRNAs targeting a great number of ubiquitin E3 ligases, ESCRT proteins, E2 enzymes and chaperone/cochaperones were introduced into the above cells, and the plasma membrane stability of the rescued ΔF508 CFTR-3HA was quantified. This study led to the identification of an Hsp70-Hsp90 chaperone network facilitating the peripheral quality control of ΔF508 CFTR. Functional followup of these chaperone proteins will not only reveal critical mechanistic information but also uncover yet unidentified molecular targets.

11. Small molecule modulators for ΔF508 CFTR

One of the major strategies for developing effective therapeutics for CF is to identify small molecule compounds that can improve ΔF508 CFTR cell surface functional expression. Using cell-based functional assay for CFTR-mediated chloride conductance combined with high-throughput screening of small molecule compound libraries, multiple CFTR modulators have been identified, affecting ΔF508 CFTR trafficking and/or channel function (Van Goor et al., 2006; Verkman et al., 2006). Once promising scafolds have been identified, structural optimization can be performed to enhance their biological activities, pharmacokinetics, and safety. In fact several of the above compounds are currently in clinical trial for treating CF.

While the functional screening as mentioned above has the benefit of identifying small molecule compounds that improve the aggregate endpoint readout on ΔF508 CFTR cell surface functional expression, the mechanisms by which these compounds do so are unknown. The compounds can either bind directly to CFTR to affect its folding and/or channel gating, or they can bind to other cellular proteins that regulate CFTR biogenesis, cell surface protein-protein interactions, or its degradation. Understanding these mechanistic aspects of a specific CFTR modulator will lead to the design and identification of additional molecular targets and CFTR modulators. This is especially important as only a limited number of efficacious CFTR modulators have been identified through the functional screen. In order to obtain an FDA-approved drug for CF, more of such compounds are desparately needed to feed into the CF drug discovery pipeline.

Recently, new screening strategies have been designed to improve the variety of workable lead compounds. These compounds might not have been identified during the functional screen because they do not provide the above-the-threshold functional readouts. However, if they have special properties that can enhance certain key aspects of ΔF508 CFTR rescue, such compounds can be further engineered or optimized to produce a much greater efficacy in terms of functional rescue of ΔF508 CFTR. A new strategry has been developed where small molecule compound libraries were screened by their ability to improve the plasma membrane localization of ΔF508 CFTR (Carlile et al., 2007).

A conformation-based virtual screen for ΔF508 CFTR modulators represents one step further as it aims at the core defect of ΔF508 CFTR (i.e. abberrant conformation). Recently, one attempt was made by the EPIX Pharmaceuticals Ltd to identify small molecule correctors for ΔF508 CFTR (Kalid et al., 2010). In this study, a total of three potential small molecule binding cavities were identified at a number of domain-domain interfaces of CFTR, and small molecule compounds were screened in silico for their ability to bind to these cavities. The initial hits derived from the virtual screen were then subjected to functional screen, which yielded a ten-fold increase in hit rate as compared to conventional screen regimes.

An alternative to the above high-throughput screening approach is to explore the possibility of using FDA-approved drugs for other conditions or other small molecule compounds that are safe for human use for rescuing ΔF508 CFTR. Sodium 4-phenylbutyrate is approved for clinical use in patients with urea cycle disorders. 4-Phenylbutyrate, like sodium butyrate, is also a transcriptional regulator that inhibits HDAC (Jung, 2001). 4-Phenylbutyrate was shown to rescue ΔF508 CFTR through a number of mechanisms including biosynthesis, folding and transport (Rubenstein et al., 1997; Rubenstein & Zeitlin, 2000; Choo-Kang & Zeitlin, 2001; Wright et al., 2004; Singh et al., 2006). More recently, SAHA (Vorinostat), an HDAC inhibitor approved by FDA for the treatment of cutaneous T cell lymphoma through epigenetic pathways (Monneret, 2007), was shown to restore cell surface functional expression of ΔF508 CFTR to 28% of wild-type level (Hutt et al., 2010). Doxorubicin (Adriamycin), a cancer chemotherapy agent, increases cell surface functional expression of ΔF508 CFTR through increasing its folding, promoting its chaperone dissociation and inhibiting its ubiquitination (Maitra et al., 2001; Maitra & Hamilton, 2007). Sildenafil (Viagra) was also shown to promote ΔF508 CFTR apical trafficking by unknown mechanism (Dormer et al., 2005). S-Nitrosoglutathione (GSNO), an endogenous bronchodilator (Gaston et al., 1993), was found to increase the expression and maturation of ΔF508 CFTR in airway epithelial cells (Zaman et al., 2006). Interestingly, GSNO was recently found to function at least in part through inhibiting Hop expression (Marozkina et al., 2010), suggesting that small molecules compound can promote ΔF508 CFTR rescue through modulating chaperone machinery.

12. Chaperone environment: A critical but complex part of the equation

Cellular chaperone machinery plays an important role in the synthesis, maturation, quality control of CFTR (Fig. 2). Due to misfolding, ΔF508 CFTR has more extensive association with molecular chaperones (Yang et al., 1993; Jiang et al., 1998; Meacham et al., 1999; Wang et al., 2006; Sun et al., 2008; Roy et al., 2010). Therefore, the impact of chaperone machinery on ΔF508 CFTR is greater than on wild-type CFTR. This notion is further underscored by the recent finding that cytoplasmic Hsp70-Hsp90 chaperone network promotes the peripheral quality control of ΔF508 CFTR (Okiyoneda et al., 2010). Modulating chaperone environment can not only impact the quality control of ΔF508 CFTR at either the ER or the peripheral level but also can dramatically influence its maturation (Loo et al., 1998; Zhang et al., 2002; Saxena et al., 2007; Saxena et al., 2011b).

Heat shock response is a transcriptional program by which cells upregulate the expression of an array of genes including those encoding molecular chaperones to cope with the massive need for protein folding and degradation as a result of elevated temperature or toxic agents (Morimoto et al., 1990). Therefore, conditions or agents that induce heat shock response will up-regulate the cellular chaperone machinery to enhance folding and ERAD of ΔF508 CFTR. Consistent with this finding, mild heat shock dramatically potentiates the temperature-rescue of ΔF508 CFTR (X. Wang et al., 2008). Another cellular response that up-regulate the cellular chaperone machinery is the unfolded protein response (UPR) (Sidrauski et al., 1998). This is particularly relevant to ΔF508 CFTR as over accumulation of this mutant protein in the ER induces such a response, leading to downregulation of CFTR endogenous transcription (Rab et al., 2007; Bartoszewski et al., 2008). Aside from the above two, the inherent variation in the cellular chaperone machinery among different tissues or cell types will also significantly affect the cell surface functional expression of ΔF508 CFTR (Varga et al., 2004; X. Wang et al., 2008; Rowe et al., 2010). Therefore, understanding the functional organization of the chaperone machinery in airway epithelial cells is highly relevant to the development of effective rescue strategies for ΔF508 CFTR.

Certain chemicals such as celastrol can globally influence the cellular chaperone machinery through inducing the heat shock response (Westerheide et al., 2004). Other epigentic modulators can also influence the expression of mutliple molecular chaperones (Wright et al., 2004; Hutt et al., 2010). Interfering with ER lumenal chaperone activities by depleting the ER calcium stores promotes the escape of ΔF508 CFTR from the ER quality control and enhances its cell surface expression (Egan et al., 2002). Certain small molecule compounds directly modulate the expression or activity of molecular chaperones (Jiang et al., 1998; Loo et al., 1998; Marozkina et al., 2010). Furthermore, small molecule compound can act as chemical chaperones to stabilize the conformation of ΔF508 CFTR, enhancing its cell surface functional expression (Brown et al., 1996; Fischer et al., 2001).

13. Conclusion

The ΔF508 mutation is present in over 90% of CF patients. This mutation impairs the conformational maturation of CFTR leading to defective export, reduced stability and abberrant channel gating. Improving the cell surface functional expression of this mutant CFTR will benefit the vast majority of CF patients. While many approaches can be taken toward this goal, conformational rescue is the most effective, postitively impacting all three molecular defects of ΔF508 CFTR. The ΔF508 CFTR molecule is the most important target for the development of therapeutics. A clear understanding of its biogenesis, quality control and conformation is fundamental. In the cell, the synthesis, folding, quality control, trafficking and degradation of CFTR is dependent upon its interactions with multiple cellular machineries (Fig. 2). Such interactions provide additional opportunites for therapeutic interventions. The cellular protein homeostasis as regulated by the chapeorone machinery provides an important chemical environment for ΔF508 CFTR. Such an enironment is regulated by multiple cellular responses or epigenetic modulators. Understanding the relationship between such cellular environment and ΔF508 CFTR cell surface functional expression will provide additional molecular targets for intervention.

14. Acknowledgment

We thank the Cystic Fibrosis Foundation, the American Heart Association and the University of Toledo Health Science Campus for support.

15. References

Ahner, A., Nakatsukasa, K., Zhang, H., Frizzell, R. A. & Brodsky, J. L. (2007). Small heat-shock proteins select deltaF508-CFTR for endoplasmic reticulum-associated degradation. *Mol Biol Cell* Vol.18, No.3, (Mar 2007), pp.806-14

Alberti, S., Bohse, K., Arndt, V., Schmitz, A. & Hohfeld, J. (2004). The cochaperone HspBP1 inhibits the CHIP ubiquitin ligase and stimulates the maturation of the cystic fibrosis transmembrane conductance regulator. *Mol Biol Cell* Vol.15, No.9, (Sep 2004), pp.4003-10

Aleksandrov, A. A., Kota, P., Aleksandrov, L. A., He, L., Jensen, T., Cui, L., Gentzsch, M., Dokholyan, N. V. & Riordan, J. R. (2010). Regulatory insertion removal restores maturation, stability and function of DeltaF508 CFTR. *J Mol Biol* Vol.401, No.2, (Aug 13 2010), pp.194-210

Aller, S. G., Yu, J., Ward, A., Weng, Y., Chittaboina, S., Zhuo, R., Harrell, P. M., Trinh, Y. T., Zhang, Q., Urbatsch, I. L. & Chang, G. (2009). Structure of P-glycoprotein reveals a molecular basis for poly-specific drug binding. *Science* Vol.323, No.5922, (Mar 27 2009), pp.1718-22

Aridor, M., Weissman, J., Bannykh, S., Nuoffer, C. & Balch, W. E. (1998). Cargo selection by the COPII budding machinery during export from the ER. *J Cell Biol* Vol.141, No.1, (Apr 6 1998), pp.61-70

Arndt, V., Daniel, C., Nastainczyk, W., Alberti, S. & Hohfeld, J. (2005). BAG-2 Acts as an Inhibitor of the Chaperone-associated Ubiquitin Ligase CHIP. *Mol Biol Cell* Vol.16, No.12, (Dec 2005), pp.5891-900

Atwell, S., Brouillette, C. G., Conners, K., Emtage, S., Gheyi, T., Guggino, W. B., Hendle, J., Hunt, J. F., Lewis, H. A., Lu, F., Protasevich, II, Rodgers, L. A., Romero, R., Wasserman, S. R., Weber, P. C., Wetmore, D., Zhang, F. F. & Zhao, X. (2010). Structures of a minimal human CFTR first nucleotide-binding domain as a monomer, head-to-tail homodimer, and pathogenic mutant. *Protein Eng Des Sel* Vol.23, No.5, (May 2010), pp.375-84

Ballar, P., Ors, A. U., Yang, H. & Fang, S. (2010). Differential regulation of CFTRDeltaF508 degradation by ubiquitin ligases gp78 and Hrd1. *Int J Biochem Cell Biol* Vol.42, No.1, (Jan 2010), pp.167-73

Bartoszewski, R., Rab, A., Twitty, G., Stevenson, L., Fortenberry, J., Piotrowski, A., Dumanski, J. P. & Bebok, Z. (2008). The mechanism of cystic fibrosis transmembrane conductance regulator transcriptional repression during the unfolded protein response. *J Biol Chem* Vol.283, No.18, (May 2 2008), pp.12154-65

Bartoszewski, R. A., Jablonsky, M., Bartoszewska, S., Stevenson, L., Dai, Q., Kappes, J., Collawn, J. F. & Bebok, Z. (2010). A synonymous single nucleotide polymorphism in DeltaF508 CFTR alters the secondary structure of the mRNA and the expression of the mutant protein. *J Biol Chem* Vol.285, No.37, (Sep 10 2010), pp.28741-8

Brown, C. R., Hong-Brown, L. Q., Biwersi, J., Verkman, A. S. & Welch, W. J. (1996). Chemical chaperones correct the mutant phenotype of the delta F508 cystic fibrosis transmembrane conductance regulator protein. *Cell Stress Chaperones* Vol.1, No.2, (Jun 1996), pp.117-25

Carlile, G. W., Robert, R., Zhang, D., Teske, K. A., Luo, Y., Hanrahan, J. W. & Thomas, D. Y. (2007). Correctors of protein trafficking defects identified by a novel high-throughput screening assay. *Chembiochem* Vol.8, No.9, (Jun 18 2007), pp.1012-20

Carlson, E. J., Pitonzo, D. & Skach, W. R. (2006). p97 functions as an auxiliary factor to facilitate TM domain extraction during CFTR ER-associated degradation. *Embo J* Vol.25, No.19, (Oct 4 2006), pp.4557-66

Cebotaru, L., Vij, N., Ciobanu, I., Wright, J., Flotte, T. & Guggino, W. B. (2008). Cystic fibrosis transmembrane regulator missing the first four transmembrane segments increases wild type and DeltaF508 processing. *J Biol Chem* Vol.283, No.32, (Aug 8 2008), pp.21926-33

Chang, X. B., Cui, L., Hou, Y. X., Jensen, T. J., Aleksandrov, A. A., Mengos, A. & Riordan, J. R. (1999). Removal of multiple arginine-framed trafficking signals overcomes misprocessing of delta F508 CFTR present in most patients with cystic fibrosis. *Mol Cell* Vol.4, No.1, (Jul 1999), pp.137-42

Chappell, T. G., Welch, W. J., Schlossman, D. M., Palter, K. B., Schlesinger, M. J. & Rothman, J. E. (1986). Uncoating ATPase is a member of the 70 kilodalton family of stress proteins. *Cell* Vol.45, No.1, (Apr 11 1986), pp.3-13

Cheng, J., Cebotaru, V., Cebotaru, L. & Guggino, W. B. (2010). Syntaxin 6 and CAL mediate the degradation of the cystic fibrosis transmembrane conductance regulator. *Mol Biol Cell* Vol.21, No.7, (Apr 1 2010), pp.1178-87

Cheng, J., Moyer, B. D., Milewski, M., Loffing, J., Ikeda, M., Mickle, J. E., Cutting, G. R., Li, M., Stanton, B. A. & Guggino, W. B. (2002). A Golgi-associated PDZ domain protein modulates cystic fibrosis transmembrane regulator plasma membrane expression. *J Biol Chem* Vol.277, No.5, (Feb 1 2002), pp.3520-9

Cheng, J., Wang, H. & Guggino, W. B. (2004). Modulation of mature cystic fibrosis transmembrane regulator protein by the PDZ domain protein CAL. *J Biol Chem* Vol.279, No.3, (Jan 16 2004), pp.1892-8

Cheng, S. H., Fang, S. L., Zabner, J., Marshall, J., Piraino, S., Schiavi, S. C., Jefferson, D. M., Welsh, M. J. & Smith, A. E. (1995). Functional activation of the cystic fibrosis trafficking mutant delta F508-CFTR by overexpression. *Am J Physiol* Vol.268, No.4 Pt 1, (Apr 1995), pp.L615-24

Cheng, S. H., Gregory, R. J., Marshall, J., Paul, S., Souza, D. W., White, G. A., O'Riordan, C. R. & Smith, A. E. (1990). Defective intracellular transport and processing of CFTR is the molecular basis of most cystic fibrosis. *Cell* Vol.63, No.4, (Nov 16 1990), pp.827-34

Choo-Kang, L. R. & Zeitlin, P. L. (2001). Induction of HSP70 promotes DeltaF508 CFTR trafficking. *Am J Physiol Lung Cell Mol Physiol* Vol.281, No.1, (Jul 2001), pp.L58-68

Cormet-Boyaka, E., Jablonsky, M., Naren, A. P., Jackson, P. L., Muccio, D. D. & Kirk, K. L. (2004). Rescuing cystic fibrosis transmembrane conductance regulator (CFTR)-processing mutants by transcomplementation. *Proc Natl Acad Sci U S A* Vol.101, No.21, (May 25 2004), pp.8221-6

Dalemans, W., Barbry, P., Champigny, G., Jallat, S., Dott, K., Dreyer, D., Crystal, R. G., Pavirani, A., Lecocq, J. P. & Lazdunski, M. (1991). Altered chloride ion channel kinetics associated with the delta F508 cystic fibrosis mutation. *Nature* Vol.354, No.6354, (Dec 19-26 1991), pp.526-8

Dawson, R. J. & Locher, K. P. (2006). Structure of a bacterial multidrug ABC transporter. *Nature* Vol.443, No.7108, (Sep 14 2006), pp.180-5

Denning, G. M., Anderson, M. P., Amara, J. F., Marshall, J., Smith, A. E. & Welsh, M. J. (1992). Processing of mutant cystic fibrosis transmembrane conductance regulator is temperature-sensitive. *Nature* Vol.358, No.6389, (Aug 27 1992), pp.761-4

Dormer, R. L., Harris, C. M., Clark, Z., Pereira, M. M., Doull, I. J., Norez, C., Becq, F. & McPherson, M. A. (2005). Sildenafil (Viagra) corrects DeltaF508-CFTR location in nasal epithelial cells from patients with cystic fibrosis. *Thorax* Vol.60, No.1, (Jan 2005), pp.55-9

Du, K. & Lukacs, G. L. (2009). Cooperative assembly and misfolding of CFTR domains in vivo. *Mol Biol Cell* Vol.20, No.7, (Apr 2009), pp.1903-15

Du, K., Sharma, M. & Lukacs, G. L. (2005). The DeltaF508 cystic fibrosis mutation impairs domain-domain interactions and arrests post-translational folding of CFTR. *Nat Struct Mol Biol* Vol.12, No.1, (Jan 2005), pp.17-25

Egan, M. E., Glockner-Pagel, J., Ambrose, C., Cahill, P. A., Pappoe, L., Balamuth, N., Cho, E., Canny, S., Wagner, C. A., Geibel, J. & Caplan, M. J. (2002). Calcium-pump inhibitors induce functional surface expression of Delta F508-CFTR protein in cystic fibrosis epithelial cells. *Nat Med* Vol.8, No.5, (May 2002), pp.485-92

Fischer, H., Fukuda, N., Barbry, P., Illek, B., Sartori, C. & Matthay, M. A. (2001). Partial restoration of defective chloride conductance in DeltaF508 CF mice by trimethylamine oxide. *Am J Physiol Lung Cell Mol Physiol* Vol.281, No.1, (Jul 2001), pp.L52-7

Gaston, B., Reilly, J., Drazen, J. M., Fackler, J., Ramdev, P., Arnelle, D., Mullins, M. E., Sugarbaker, D. J., Chee, C., Singel, D. J. & et al. (1993). Endogenous nitrogen oxides and bronchodilator S-nitrosothiols in human airways. *Proc Natl Acad Sci U S A* Vol.90, No.23, (Dec 1 1993), pp.10957-61

Gelman, M. S. & Kopito, R. R. (2002). Rescuing protein conformation: prospects for pharmacological therapy in cystic fibrosis. *J Clin Invest* Vol.110, No.11, (Dec 2002), pp.1591-7

Gomes-Alves, P., Couto, F., Pesquita, C., Coelho, A. V. & Penque, D. (2010). Rescue of F508del-CFTR by RXR motif inactivation triggers proteome modulation associated with the unfolded protein response. *Biochim Biophys Acta* Vol.1804, No.4, (Apr 2010), pp.856-65

Grove, D. E., Fan, C. Y., Ren, H. Y. & Cyr, D. M. (2011). The endoplasmic reticulum-associated Hsp40 DNAJB12 and Hsc70 cooperate to facilitate RMA1 E3-dependent degradation of nascent CFTRDeltaF508. *Mol Biol Cell* Vol.22, No.3, (Feb 2011), pp.301-14

Hassink, G. C., Zhao, B., Sompallae, R., Altun, M., Gastaldello, S., Zinin, N. V., Masucci, M. G. & Lindsten, K. (2009). The ER-resident ubiquitin-specific protease 19 participates in the UPR and rescues ERAD substrates. *EMBO Rep* Vol.10, No.7, (Jul 2009), pp.755-61

He, L., Aleksandrov, L. A., Cui, L., Jensen, T. J., Nesbitt, K. L. & Riordan, J. R. (2010). Restoration of domain folding and interdomain assembly by second-site suppressors of the DeltaF508 mutation in CFTR. *Faseb J* Vol.24, No.8, (Aug 2010), pp.3103-12

Hegedus, T., Aleksandrov, A., Cui, L., Gentzsch, M., Chang, X. B. & Riordan, J. R. (2006). F508del CFTR with two altered RXR motifs escapes from ER quality control but its channel activity is thermally sensitive. *Biochim Biophys Acta* Vol.1758, No.5, (May 2006), pp.565-72

Henderson, M. J., Vij, N. & Zeitlin, P. L. (2010). Ubiquitin C-terminal hydrolase-L1 protects cystic fibrosis transmembrane conductance regulator from early stages of proteasomal degradation. *J Biol Chem* Vol.285, No.15, (Apr 9 2010), pp.11314-25

Hoelen, H., Kleizen, B., Schmidt, A., Richardson, J., Charitou, P., Thomas, P. J. & Braakman, I. (2010). The primary folding defect and rescue of DeltaF508 CFTR emerge during translation of the mutant domain. *PLoS One* Vol.5, No.11, (Nov 2010), pp.e15458

Hutt, D. M., Herman, D., Rodrigues, A. P., Noel, S., Pilewski, J. M., Matteson, J., Hoch, B., Kellner, W., Kelly, J. W., Schmidt, A., Thomas, P. J., Matsumura, Y., Skach, W. R., Gentzsch, M., Riordan, J. R., Sorscher, E. J., Okiyoneda, T., Yates, J. R., 3rd, Lukacs, G. L., Frizzell, R. A., Manning, G., Gottesfeld, J. M. & Balch, W. E. (2010). Reduced histone deacetylase 7 activity restores function to misfolded CFTR in cystic fibrosis. *Nat Chem Biol* Vol.6, No.1, (Jan 2010), pp.25-33

Jensen, T. J., Loo, M. A., Pind, S., Williams, D. B., Goldberg, A. L. & Riordan, J. R. (1995). Multiple proteolytic systems, including the proteasome, contribute to CFTR processing. *Cell* Vol.83, No.1, (Oct 6 1995), pp.129-35

Jiang, C., Fang, S. L., Xiao, Y. F., O'Connor, S. P., Nadler, S. G., Lee, D. W., Jefferson, D. M., Kaplan, J. M., Smith, A. E. & Cheng, S. H. (1998). Partial restoration of cAMP-stimulated CFTR chloride channel activity in DeltaF508 cells by deoxyspergualin. *Am J Physiol* Vol.275, No.1 Pt 1, (Jul 1998), pp.C171-8

Jordan, I. K., Kota, K. C., Cui, G., Thompson, C. H. & McCarty, N. A. (2008). Evolutionary and functional divergence between the cystic fibrosis transmembrane conductance regulator and related ATP-binding cassette transporters. *Proc Natl Acad Sci U S A* Vol.105, No.48, (Dec 2 2008), pp.18865-70

Jung, M. (2001). Inhibitors of histone deacetylase as new anticancer agents. *Curr Med Chem* Vol.8, No.12, (Oct 2001), pp.1505-11

Kalid, O., Mense, M., Fischman, S., Shitrit, A., Bihler, H., Ben-Zeev, E., Schutz, N., Pedemonte, N., Thomas, P. J., Bridges, R. J., Wetmore, D. R., Marantz, Y. & Senderowitz, H. (2010). Small molecule correctors of F508del-CFTR discovered by structure-based virtual screening. *J Comput Aided Mol Des* Vol.24, No.12, (Dec 2010), pp.971-91

Kerem, B., Rommens, J. M., Buchanan, J. A., Markiewicz, D., Cox, T. K., Chakravarti, A., Buchwald, M. & Tsui, L. C. (1989). Identification of the cystic fibrosis gene: genetic analysis. *Science* Vol.245, No.4922, (Sep 8 1989), pp.1073-80

Kim Chiaw, P., Huan, L. J., Gagnon, S., Ly, D., Sweezey, N., Rotin, D., Deber, C. M. & Bear, C. E. (2009). Functional rescue of DeltaF508-CFTR by peptides designed to mimic sorting motifs. *Chem Biol* Vol.16, No.5, (May 29 2009), pp.520-30

Kleizen, B., van Vlijmen, T., de Jonge, H. R. & Braakman, I. (2005). Folding of CFTR Is Predominantly Cotranslational. *Mol Cell* Vol.20, No.2, (Oct 28 2005), pp.277-87

Kwon, S. H., Pollard, H. & Guggino, W. B. (2007). Knockdown of NHERF1 enhances degradation of temperature rescued DeltaF508 CFTR from the cell surface of human airway cells. *Cell Physiol Biochem* Vol.20, No.62007), pp.763-72

Lewis, H. A., Wang, C., Zhao, X., Hamuro, Y., Conners, K., Kearins, M. C., Lu, F., Sauder, J. M., Molnar, K. S., Coales, S. J., Maloney, P. C., Guggino, W. B., Wetmore, D. R., Weber, P. C. & Hunt, J. F. (2010). Structure and dynamics of NBD1 from CFTR characterized using crystallography and hydrogen/deuterium exchange mass spectrometry. *J Mol Biol* Vol.396, No.2, (Feb 19 2010), pp.406-30

Lewis, H. A., Zhao, X., Wang, C., Sauder, J. M., Rooney, I., Noland, B. W., Lorimer, D., Kearins, M. C., Conners, K., Condon, B., Maloney, P. C., Guggino, W. B., Hunt, J. F. & Emtage, S. (2005). Impact of the deltaF508 mutation in first nucleotide-binding domain of human cystic fibrosis transmembrane conductance regulator on domain folding and structure. *J Biol Chem* Vol.280, No.2, (Jan 14 2005), pp.1346-53

Li, C., Ramjeesingh, M., Wang, W., Garami, E., Hewryk, M., Lee, D., Rommens, J. M., Galley, K. & Bear, C. E. (1996). ATPase activity of the cystic fibrosis transmembrane conductance regulator. *J Biol Chem* Vol.271, No.45, (Nov 8 1996), pp.28463-8

Locher, K. P., Lee, A. T. & Rees, D. C. (2002). The E. coli BtuCD structure: a framework for ABC transporter architecture and mechanism. *Science* Vol.296, No.5570, (May 10 2002), pp.1091-8

Loo, M. A., Jensen, T. J., Cui, L., Hou, Y., Chang, X. B. & Riordan, J. R. (1998). Perturbation of Hsp90 interaction with nascent CFTR prevents its maturation and accelerates its degradation by the proteasome. *Embo J* Vol.17, No.23, (Dec 1 1998), pp.6879-87

Loo, T. W., Bartlett, M. C. & Clarke, D. M. (2008). Processing mutations disrupt interactions between the nucleotide binding and transmembrane domains of P-glycoprotein and the cystic fibrosis transmembrane conductance regulator (CFTR). *J Biol Chem* Vol.283, No.42, (Oct 17 2008), pp.28190-7

Lukacs, G. L., Chang, X. B., Bear, C., Kartner, N., Mohamed, A., Riordan, J. R. & Grinstein, S. (1993). The delta F508 mutation decreases the stability of cystic fibrosis transmembrane conductance regulator in the plasma membrane. Determination of functional half-lives on transfected cells. *J Biol Chem* Vol.268, No.29, (Oct 15 1993), pp.21592-8

Lukacs, G. L., Mohamed, A., Kartner, N., Chang, X. B., Riordan, J. R. & Grinstein, S. (1994). Conformational maturation of CFTR but not its mutant counterpart (delta F508) occurs in the endoplasmic reticulum and requires ATP. *Embo J* Vol.13, No.24, (Dec 15 1994), pp.6076-86

Maitra, R. & Hamilton, J. W. (2007). Altered biogenesis of deltaF508-CFTR following treatment with doxorubicin. *Cell Physiol Biochem* Vol.20, No.52007), pp.465-72

Maitra, R., Shaw, C. M., Stanton, B. A. & Hamilton, J. W. (2001). Increased functional cell surface expression of CFTR and DeltaF508-CFTR by the anthracycline doxorubicin. *Am J Physiol Cell Physiol* Vol.280, No.5, (May 2001), pp.C1031-7

Margeta-Mitrovic, M., Jan, Y. N. & Jan, L. Y. (2000). A trafficking checkpoint controls GABA(B) receptor heterodimerization. *Neuron* Vol.27, No.1, (Jul 2000), pp.97-106

Marozkina, N. V., Yemen, S., Borowitz, M., Liu, L., Plapp, M., Sun, F., Islam, R., Erdmann-Gilmore, P., Townsend, R. R., Lichti, C. F., Mantri, S., Clapp, P. W., Randell, S. H., Gaston, B. & Zaman, K. (2010). Hsp 70/Hsp 90 organizing protein as a nitrosylation target in cystic fibrosis therapy. *Proc Natl Acad Sci U S A* Vol.107, No.25, (Jun 22 2010), pp.11393-8

Meacham, G. C., Lu, Z., King, S., Sorscher, E., Tousson, A. & Cyr, D. M. (1999). The Hdj-2/Hsc70 chaperone pair facilitates early steps in CFTR biogenesis. *Embo J* Vol.18, No.6, (Mar 15 1999), pp.1492-505

Meacham, G. C., Patterson, C., Zhang, W., Younger, J. M. & Cyr, D. M. (2001). The Hsc70 co-chaperone CHIP targets immature CFTR for proteasomal degradation. *Nat Cell Biol* Vol.3, No.1, (Jan 2001), pp.100-5

Miller, E., Antonny, B., Hamamoto, S. & Schekman, R. (2002). Cargo selection into COPII vesicles is driven by the Sec24p subunit. *Embo J* Vol.21, No.22, (Nov 15 2002), pp.6105-13

Mills, A. D., Yoo, C., Butler, J. D., Yang, B., Verkman, A. S. & Kurth, M. J. (2010). Design and synthesis of a hybrid potentiator-corrector agonist of the cystic fibrosis mutant protein DeltaF508-CFTR. *Bioorg Med Chem Lett* Vol.20, No.1, (Jan 1 2010), pp.87-91

Monneret, C. (2007). Histone deacetylase inhibitors for epigenetic therapy of cancer. *Anticancer Drugs* Vol.18, No.4, (Apr 2007), pp.363-70

Morimoto, R. I., Tissières, A., Georgopoulos, C. & Cold Spring Harbor Laboratory. (1990). *Stress proteins in biology and medicine*, Cold Spring Harbor Laboratory Press, 0879693371, Cold Spring Harbor, N.Y.

Morito, D., Hirao, K., Oda, Y., Hosokawa, N., Tokunaga, F., Cyr, D. M., Tanaka, K., Iwai, K. & Nagata, K. (2008). Gp78 cooperates with RMA1 in endoplasmic reticulum-associated degradation of CFTRDeltaF508. *Mol Biol Cell* Vol.19, No.4, (Apr 2008), pp.1328-36

Mornon, J. P., Lehn, P. & Callebaut, I. (2009). Molecular models of the open and closed states of the whole human CFTR protein. *Cell Mol Life Sci* Vol.66, No.21, (Nov 2009), pp.3469-86

Nagahama, M., Ohnishi, M., Kawate, Y., Matsui, T., Miyake, H., Yuasa, K., Tani, K., Tagaya, M. & Tsuji, A. (2009). UBXD1 is a VCP-interacting protein that is involved in ER-associated degradation. *Biochem Biophys Res Commun* Vol.382, No.2, (May 1 2009), pp.303-8

Nilsson, T., Jackson, M. & Peterson, P. A. (1989). Short cytoplasmic sequences serve as retention signals for transmembrane proteins in the endoplasmic reticulum. *Cell* Vol.58, No.4, (Aug 25 1989), pp.707-18

Nishimura, N., Bannykh, S., Slabough, S., Matteson, J., Altschuler, Y., Hahn, K. & Balch, W. E. (1999). A di-acidic (DXE) code directs concentration of cargo during export from the endoplasmic reticulum. *J Biol Chem* Vol.274, No.22, (May 28 1999), pp.15937-46

Okiyoneda, T., Barriere, H., Bagdany, M., Rabeh, W. M., Du, K., Hohfeld, J., Young, J. C. & Lukacs, G. L. (2010). Peripheral protein quality control removes unfolded CFTR from the plasma membrane. *Science* Vol.329, No.5993, (Aug 13 2010), pp.805-10

Pagant, S., Kung, L., Dorrington, M., Lee, M. C. & Miller, E. A. (2007). Inhibiting endoplasmic reticulum (ER)-associated degradation of misfolded Yor1p does not permit ER export despite the presence of a diacidic sorting signal. *Mol Biol Cell* Vol.18, No.9, (Sep 2007), pp.3398-413

Park, H. J., Mylvaganum, M., McPherson, A., Fewell, S. W., Brodsky, J. L. & Lingwood, C. A. (2009). A soluble sulfogalactosyl ceramide mimic promotes Delta F508 CFTR escape from endoplasmic reticulum associated degradation. *Chem Biol* Vol.16, No.4, (Apr 24 2009), pp.461-70

Phuan, P. W., Yang, B., Knapp, J., Wood, A., Lukacs, G. L., Kurth, M. J. & Verkman, A. S. (2011). Cyanoquinolines with Independent Corrector and Potentiator Activities Restore Δphe508-Cystic Fibrosis Transmembrane Conductance Regulator Chloride Channel Function in Cystic Fibrosis. *Mol Pharmacol* Vol.80, No.4, (Oct 2011), pp683-93

Pissarra, L. S., Farinha, C. M., Xu, Z., Schmidt, A., Thibodeau, P. H., Cai, Z., Thomas, P. J., Sheppard, D. N. & Amaral, M. D. (2008). Solubilizing Mutations Used to Crystallize One CFTR Domain Attenuate the Trafficking and Channel Defects Caused by the Major Cystic Fibrosis Mutation. *Chem Biol* Vol.15, No.1, (Jan 2008), pp.62-9

Pollet, J. F., Van Geffel, J., Van Stevens, E., Van Geffel, R., Beauwens, R., Bollen, A. & Jacobs, P. (2000). Expression and intracellular processing of chimeric and mutant CFTR molecules. *Biochim Biophys Acta* Vol.1500, No.1, (Jan 3 2000), pp.59-69

Qu, B. H., Strickland, E. H. & Thomas, P. J. (1997). Localization and suppression of a kinetic defect in cystic fibrosis transmembrane conductance regulator folding. *J Biol Chem* Vol.272, No.25, (Jun 20 1997), pp.15739-44

Qu, B. H. & Thomas, P. J. (1996). Alteration of the cystic fibrosis transmembrane conductance regulator folding pathway. *J Biol Chem* Vol.271, No.13, (Mar 29 1996), pp.7261-4

Rab, A., Bartoszewski, R., Jurkuvenaite, A., Wakefield, J., Collawn, J. F. & Bebok, Z. (2007). Endoplasmic reticulum stress and the unfolded protein response regulate genomic cystic fibrosis transmembrane conductance regulator expression. *Am J Physiol Cell Physiol* Vol.292, No.2, (Feb 2007), pp.C756-66

Riordan, J. R., Rommens, J. M., Kerem, B., Alon, N., Rozmahel, R., Grzelczak, Z., Zielenski, J., Lok, S., Plavsic, N., Chou, J. L., Drumm, M. L., Iannuzzi, M. C., Collins, F. S. & Tsui, L. C. (1989). Identification of the cystic fibrosis gene: cloning and characterization of complementary DNA. *Science* Vol.245, No.4922, (Sep 8 1989), pp.1066-73

Rowe, S. M., Pyle, L. C., Jurkevante, A., Varga, K., Collawn, J., Sloane, P. A., Woodworth, B., Mazur, M., Fulton, J., Fan, L., Li, Y., Fortenberry, J., Sorscher, E. J. & Clancy, J. P. (2010). DeltaF508 CFTR processing correction and activity in polarized airway and non-airway cell monolayers. *Pulm Pharmacol Ther* Vol.23, No.4, (Aug 2010), pp.268-78

Roxo-Rosa, M., Xu, Z., Schmidt, A., Neto, M., Cai, Z., Soares, C. M., Sheppard, D. N. & Amaral, M. D. (2006). Revertant mutants G550E and 4RK rescue cystic fibrosis mutants in the first nucleotide-binding domain of CFTR by different mechanisms. *Proc Natl Acad Sci U S A* Vol.103, No.47, (Nov 21 2006), pp.17891-6

Roy, G., Chalfin, E. M., Saxena, A. & Wang, X. (2010). Interplay between ER exit code and domain conformation in CFTR misprocessing and rescue. *Mol Biol Cell* Vol.21, No.4, (Feb 2010), pp.597-609

Rubenstein, R. C., Egan, M. E. & Zeitlin, P. L. (1997). In vitro pharmacologic restoration of CFTR-mediated chloride transport with sodium 4-phenylbutyrate in cystic fibrosis epithelial cells containing delta F508-CFTR. *J Clin Invest* Vol.100, No.10, (Nov 15 1997), pp.2457-65

Rubenstein, R. C. & Zeitlin, P. L. (2000). Sodium 4-phenylbutyrate downregulates Hsc70: implications for intracellular trafficking of DeltaF508-CFTR. *Am J Physiol Cell Physiol* Vol.278, No.2, (Feb 2000), pp.C259-67

Saxena, A., Banasavadi-Siddegowda, Y. K., Fan, Y., Bhattacharya, S., Liao, Y., Giovannucci, D. R., Frizzell, R. A. & Wang, X. (2011a). Hsp105 regulates CFTR biogenesis and quality control at multiple levels. *Pediatric Pulmonology* Vol.46, No.S34, (Oct 2011), pp.215-215

Saxena, A., Bhattacharya, S., Fan, Y., Banasavadi-Siddegowda, Y. K., Chalfin, E. M., Roy, G., Mai, J., Sanchez, E. R. & Wang, X. (2011b). Cochaperones Hop and Hsp105 functionally link Hsp70 and Hsp90 during DeltaF508 CFTR maturation at low temperature. *Pediatric Pulmonology* Vol.46, No.S34, (Oct 2011), pp.215-215

Saxena, A., Chalfin, E. M., Roy, G. & Wang, X. (2007). HSP105 reveals distinct conformational maturation pathways for wild-type and Delta F508 CFTR at reduced temperature. *Pediatric Pulmonology*, Vol.42, No.S30, (Aug 2007), pp.212-212

Schmid, S. L. & Rothman, J. E. (1985). Two classes of binding sites for uncoating protein in clathrin triskelions. *J Biol Chem* Vol.260, No.18, (Aug 25 1985), pp.10050-6

Serohijos, A. W., Hegedus, T., Aleksandrov, A. A., He, L., Cui, L., Dokholyan, N. V. & Riordan, J. R. (2008a). Phenylalanine-508 mediates a cytoplasmic-membrane domain contact in the CFTR 3D structure crucial to assembly and channel function. *Proc Natl Acad Sci U S A* Vol.105, No.9, (Mar 4 2008a), pp.3256-61

Serohijos, A. W., Hegedus, T., Riordan, J. R. & Dokholyan, N. V. (2008b). Diminished self-chaperoning activity of the DeltaF508 mutant of CFTR results in protein misfolding. *PLoS Comput Biol* Vol.4, No.2, (Feb 2008b), pp.e1000008

Sharma, M., Benharouga, M., Hu, W. & Lukacs, G. L. (2001). Conformational and temperature-sensitive stability defects of the delta F508 cystic fibrosis transmembrane conductance regulator in post-endoplasmic reticulum compartments. *J Biol Chem* Vol.276, No.12, (Mar 23 2001), pp.8942-50

Sharma, M., Pampinella, F., Nemes, C., Benharouga, M., So, J., Du, K., Bache, K. G., Papsin, B., Zerangue, N., Stenmark, H. & Lukacs, G. L. (2004). Misfolding diverts CFTR from recycling to degradation: quality control at early endosomes. *J Cell Biol* Vol.164, No.6, (Mar 15 2004), pp.923-33

Sidrauski, C., Chapman, R. & Walter, P. (1998). The unfolded protein response: an intracellular signalling pathway with many surprising features. *Trends Cell Biol* Vol.8, No.6, (Jun 1998), pp.245-9

Singh, O. V., Pollard, H. B. & Zeitlin, P. L. (2008). Chemical rescue of deltaF508-CFTR mimics genetic repair in cystic fibrosis bronchial epithelial cells. *Mol Cell Proteomics* Vol.7, No.6, (Jun 2008), pp.1099-110

Singh, O. V., Vij, N., Mogayzel, P. J., Jr., Jozwik, C., Pollard, H. B. & Zeitlin, P. L. (2006). Pharmacoproteomics of 4-phenylbutyrate-treated IB3-1 cystic fibrosis bronchial epithelial cells. *J Proteome Res* Vol.5, No.3, (Mar 2006), pp.562-71

Sun, F., Mi, Z., Condliffe, S. B., Bertrand, C. A., Gong, X., Lu, X., Zhang, R., Latoche, J. D., Pilewski, J. M., Robbins, P. D. & Frizzell, R. A. (2008). Chaperone displacement from mutant cystic fibrosis transmembrane conductance regulator restores its function in human airway epithelia. *Faseb J* Vol.22, No.9, (Sep 2008), pp.3255-63

Sun, F., Zhang, R., Gong, X., Geng, X., Drain, P. F. & Frizzell, R. A. (2006). Derlin-1 promotes the efficient degradation of the cystic fibrosis transmembrane conductance regulator (CFTR) and CFTR folding mutants. *J Biol Chem* Vol.281, No.48, (Dec 1 2006), pp.36856-63

Teem, J. L., Berger, H. A., Ostedgaard, L. S., Rich, D. P., Tsui, L. C. & Welsh, M. J. (1993). Identification of revertants for the cystic fibrosis delta F508 mutation using STE6-CFTR chimeras in yeast. *Cell* Vol.73, No.2, (Apr 23 1993), pp.335-46

Teem, J. L., Carson, M. R. & Welsh, M. J. (1996). Mutation of R555 in CFTR-delta F508 enhances function and partially corrects defective processing. *Receptors Channels* Vol.4, No.11996), pp.63-72

Thibodeau, P. H., Brautigam, C. A., Machius, M. & Thomas, P. J. (2005). Side chain and backbone contributions of Phe508 to CFTR folding. *Nat Struct Mol Biol* Vol.12, No.1, (Jan 2005), pp.10-6

Thibodeau, P. H., Richardson, J. M., 3rd, Wang, W., Millen, L., Watson, J., Mendoza, J. L., Du, K., Fischman, S., Senderowitz, H., Lukacs, G. L., Kirk, K. & Thomas, P. J. (2010). The cystic fibrosis-causing mutation deltaF508 affects multiple steps in cystic fibrosis transmembrane conductance regulator biogenesis. *J Biol Chem* Vol.285, No.46, (Nov 12 2010), pp.35825-35

Trzcinska-Daneluti, A. M., Ly, D., Huynh, L., Jiang, C., Fladd, C. & Rotin, D. (2009). High-content functional screen to identify proteins that correct F508del-CFTR function. *Mol Cell Proteomics* Vol.8, No.4, (Apr 2009), pp.780-90

Tsui, L. C. (1995). The cystic fibrosis transmembrane conductance regulator gene. *Am J Respir Crit Care Med* Vol.151, No.3 Pt 2, (Mar 1995), pp.S47-53

Van Goor, F., Hadida, S., Grootenhuis, P. D., Burton, B., Cao, D., Neuberger, T., Turnbull, A., Singh, A., Joubran, J., Hazlewood, A., Zhou, J., McCartney, J., Arumugam, V., Decker, C., Yang, J., Young, C., Olson, E. R., Wine, J. J., Frizzell, R. A., Ashlock, M. & Negulescu, P. (2009). Rescue of CF airway epithelial cell function in vitro by a CFTR potentiator, VX-770. *Proc Natl Acad Sci U S A* Vol.106, No.44, (Nov 3 2009), pp.18825-30

Van Goor, F., Straley, K. S., Cao, D., Gonzalez, J., Hadida, S., Hazlewood, A., Joubran, J., Knapp, T., Makings, L. R., Miller, M., Neuberger, T., Olson, E., Panchenko, V., Rader, J., Singh, A., Stack, J. H., Tung, R., Grootenhuis, P. D. & Negulescu, P. (2006). Rescue of ΔF508-CFTR trafficking and gating in human cystic fibrosis airway primary cultures by small molecules. *Am J Physiol Lung Cell Mol Physiol* Vol.290, No.6, (Jun 2006), pp.L1117-30

Varga, K., Jurkuvenaite, A., Wakefield, J., Hong, J. S., Guimbellot, J. S., Venglarik, C. J., Niraj, A., Mazur, M., Sorscher, E. J., Collawn, J. F. & Bebok, Z. (2004). Efficient intracellular processing of the endogenous cystic fibrosis transmembrane conductance regulator in epithelial cell lines. *J Biol Chem* Vol.279, No.21, (May 21 2004), pp.22578-84

Verkman, A. S., Lukacs, G. L. & Galietta, L. J. (2006). CFTR chloride channel drug discovery--inhibitors as antidiarrheals and activators for therapy of cystic fibrosis. *Curr Pharm Des* Vol.12, No.182006), pp.2235-47

Vij, N., Fang, S. & Zeitlin, P. L. (2006). Selective inhibition of endoplasmic reticulum-associated degradation rescues DeltaF508-cystic fibrosis transmembrane regulator and suppresses interleukin-8 levels: therapeutic implications. *J Biol Chem* Vol.281, No.25, (Jun 23 2006), pp.17369-78

Wang, B., Heath-Engel, H., Zhang, D., Nguyen, N., Thomas, D. Y., Hanrahan, J. W. & Shore, G. C. (2008). BAP31 interacts with Sec61 translocons and promotes retrotranslocation of CFTRDeltaF508 via the derlin-1 complex. *Cell* Vol.133, No.6, (Jun 13 2008), pp.1080-92

Wang, X., Koulov, A. V., Kellner, W. A., Riordan, J. R. & Balch, W. E. (2008). Chemical and biological folding contribute to temperature-sensitive DeltaF508 CFTR trafficking. *Traffic* Vol.9, No.11, (Nov 2008), pp.1878-93

Wang, X., Matteson, J., An, Y., Moyer, B., Yoo, J. S., Bannykh, S., Wilson, I. A., Riordan, J. R. & Balch, W. E. (2004). COPII-dependent export of cystic fibrosis transmembrane conductance regulator from the ER uses a di-acidic exit code. *J Cell Biol* Vol.167, No.1, (Oct 11 2004), pp.65-74

Wang, X., Venable, J., LaPointe, P., Hutt, D. M., Koulov, A. V., Coppinger, J., Gurkan, C., Kellner, W., Matteson, J., Plutner, H., Riordan, J. R., Kelly, J. W., Yates, J. R., 3rd & Balch, W. E. (2006). Hsp90 cochaperone Aha1 downregulation rescues misfolding of CFTR in cystic fibrosis. *Cell* Vol.127, No.4, (Nov 17 2006), pp.803-15

Ward, C. L., Omura, S. & Kopito, R. R. (1995). Degradation of CFTR by the ubiquitin-proteasome pathway. *Cell* Vol.83, No.1, (Oct 6 1995), pp.121-7

Wellhauser, L., Kim Chiaw, P., Pasyk, S., Li, C., Ramjeesingh, M. & Bear, C. E. (2009). A small-molecule modulator interacts directly with deltaPhe508-CFTR to modify its ATPase activity and conformational stability. *Mol Pharmacol* Vol.75, No.6, (Jun 2009), pp.1430-8

Westerheide, S. D., Bosman, J. D., Mbadugha, B. N., Kawahara, T. L., Matsumoto, G., Kim, S., Gu, W., Devlin, J. P., Silverman, R. B. & Morimoto, R. I. (2004). Celastrols as inducers of the heat shock response and cytoprotection. *J Biol Chem* Vol.279, No.53, (Dec 31 2004), pp.56053-60

Wolde, M., Fellows, A., Cheng, J., Kivenson, A., Coutermarsh, B., Talebian, L., Karlson, K., Piserchio, A., Mierke, D. F., Stanton, B. A., Guggino, W. B. & Madden, D. R. (2007). Targeting CAL as a negative regulator of DeltaF508-CFTR cell-surface expression: an RNA interference and structure-based mutagenetic approach. *J Biol Chem* Vol.282, No.11, (Mar 16 2007), pp.8099-109

Wright, J. M., Zeitlin, P. L., Cebotaru, L., Guggino, S. E. & Guggino, W. B. (2004). Gene expression profile analysis of 4-phenylbutyrate treatment of IB3-1 bronchial epithelial cell line demonstrates a major influence on heat-shock proteins. *Physiol Genomics* Vol.16, No.2, (Jan 15 2004), pp.204-11

Yang, Y., Janich, S., Cohn, J. A. & Wilson, J. M. (1993). The common variant of cystic fibrosis transmembrane conductance regulator is recognized by hsp70 and degraded in a pre-Golgi nonlysosomal compartment. *Proc Natl Acad Sci U S A* Vol.90, No.20, (Oct 15 1993), pp.9480-4

Younger, J. M., Chen, L., Ren, H. Y., Rosser, M. F., Turnbull, E. L., Fan, C. Y., Patterson, C. & Cyr, D. M. (2006). Sequential quality-control checkpoints triage misfolded cystic fibrosis transmembrane conductance regulator. *Cell* Vol.126, No.3, (Aug 11 2006), pp.571-82

Younger, J. M., Ren, H. Y., Chen, L., Fan, C. Y., Fields, A., Patterson, C. & Cyr, D. M. (2004). A foldable CFTRΔF508 biogenic intermediate accumulates upon inhibition of the Hsc70-CHIP E3 ubiquitin ligase. *J Cell Biol* Vol.167, No.6, (Dec 20 2004), pp.1075-85

Zaman, K., Carraro, S., Doherty, J., Henderson, E. M., Lendermon, E., Liu, L., Verghese, G., Zigler, M., Ross, M., Park, E., Palmer, L. A., Doctor, A., Stamler, J. S. & Gaston, B. (2006). S-nitrosylating agents: a novel class of compounds that increase cystic fibrosis transmembrane conductance regulator expression and maturation in epithelial cells. *Mol Pharmacol* Vol.70, No.4, (Oct 2006), pp.1435-42

Zerangue, N., Schwappach, B., Jan, Y. N. & Jan, L. Y. (1999). A new ER trafficking signal regulates the subunit stoichiometry of plasma membrane K(ATP) channels. *Neuron* Vol.22, No.3, (Mar 1999), pp.537-48

Zhang, F., Kartner, N. & Lukacs, G. L. (1998). Limited proteolysis as a probe for arrested conformational maturation of delta F508 CFTR. *Nat Struct Biol* Vol.5, No.3, (Mar 1998), pp.180-3

Zhang, H., Peters, K. W., Sun, F., Marino, C. R., Lang, J., Burgoyne, R. D. & Frizzell, R. A. (2002). Cysteine string protein interacts with and modulates the maturation of the cystic fibrosis transmembrane conductance regulator. *J Biol Chem* Vol.277, No.32, (Aug 9 2002), pp.28948-58

Zhang, Y., Nijbroek, G., Sullivan, M. L., McCracken, A. A., Watkins, S. C., Michaelis, S. & Brodsky, J. L. (2001). Hsp70 molecular chaperone facilitates endoplasmic reticulum-associated protein degradation of cystic fibrosis transmembrane conductance regulator in yeast. *Mol Biol Cell* Vol.12, No.5, (May 2001), pp.1303-14

15

Fine Tuning of CFTR Traffic and Function by PDZ Scaffolding Proteins

Florian Bossard[1], Emilie Silantieff[2] and Chantal Gauthier[2]
[1]*Department of Physiology; McGill University, Montreal, Quebec,*
[2]*L'Institut du Thorax, INSERM UMR 1087, CNRL UMR 6291,*
Université de Nantes; Nantes
[1]*Canada*
[2]*France*

1. Introduction

Cystic fibrosis (CF) is the most common lethal genetic disorder in Caucasian population (Welsh et al., 1995). This pathology is due to mutations in the CF transmembrane conductance regulator (CFTR) encoding gene leading to alterations or loss of function of this channel (Kerem et al., 1989; Riordan et al., 1989; Rommens et al., 1989). CF affects several organs such as sweat glands, reproductive system and gastrointestinal tract, but the first cause of morbidity and mortality is respiratory system affections. While gene therapy for replacement of CFTR was a promising curative approach since the discovery of the CFTR gene, it turned to be more difficult than initially thought and no cure has arisen so far. Protein-protein interactions are powerful regulators of both protein trafficking and function, and can be enhanced or prevented by small molecules and short peptides (Zhang et al., 2011). Modulating these protein interactions are becoming a hopeful approach to develop new treatments for various diseases, including CF.

2. CFTR protein localization, structure and functions

CFTR protein is a chloride channel expressed at the apical membrane of polarized cells (Dalemans et al., 1992) and randomly expressed at the plasma membrane of non-polarized cells (Cheng et al., 1990). Moreover, CFTR protein has been also localized at the membrane of organelles such as endoplasmic reticulum (ER) where it is inserted upon biosynthesis (Pasyk & Foskett, 1995), Trans-Golgi network where it matures, endosomes where it interchanges with plasma membrane (Lukacs et al., 1992) and lysosomes where it is degraded (Barasch et al., 1991). CFTR is the only chloride channel of the adenosine triphosphate (ATP) Binding Cassette (ABC) transporters family. As several ABC transporters, CFTR protein is composed of two transmembrane domains (TMD) and two nucleotide binding domains (NBD). Unlike the other ABC transporters, CFTR also possesses a regulatory (R) domain. CFTR gating is controlled by two simultaneous phenomena: (i) the fixation and the hydrolysis of ATP on NBD domains (Anderson et al., 1991) and (ii) the phosphorylation of specific residues on the R domain by different kinases such as the 3′-5′ cyclic adenosine monophosphate (cAMP) dependant protein kinase (PKA) (Berger et al., 1991; Tabcharani et al., 1991). In addition to be a chloride channel, CFTR also regulates other transmembrane proteins. Thereby, in several epithelial cells, CFTR expression decreases the epithelial Na^+ channel (ENaC) (Stutts et al., 1995) and Ca^{2+}-dependent Cl^- channel (CaCC) (Kunzelmann et al., 1997; Wei et al., 1999) activities; and increases the function of the outwardly rectifying Cl^- channel (ORCC) (Egan et al., 1992; Gabriel et al., 1993), the $Cl^-/HCO3^+$ exchangers of SLC26 family (Ko et al., 2002), the Renal Outer Medullary K^+ channel (ROMK) (Loussouarn et al., 1996) and some aquaporins (AQP) (Schreiber et al., 1997; Schreiber et al., 1999). Consequently, CFTR loss of function is responsible of a general dysregulation of ion transports in cells. Moreover, the regulation of most of these ion channels by CFTR occurs through interactions with Postsynaptic density-95/ Disc large/ Zonula occludens-1 (PDZ) scaffolding proteins (Lohi et al., 2003; Mohler et al., 1999; Pietrement et al., 2008; Yoo et al., 2004).

3. CFTR interacts with PDZ proteins through its C-terminus tail

PDZ domains are highly conserved sequences of about 80-90 amino acids known to be the most abundant protein-protein interaction modules in the human genome. Their three-dimensional structure is composed of 6 β sheets and 2 α helixes forming a cavity able to receive a protein motif of 3 to 7 amino acids, generally expressed at the C-terminus cytosolic tail of the target proteins (Bezprozvanny & Maximov, 2001; Fanning & Anderson, 1999; Harris & Lim, 2001; Hung & Sheng, 2002). However, intra-protein motifs able to bind PDZ domains have also been described (Hillier et al., 1999; Paasche et al., 2005; Slattery et al., 2011). A single PDZ domain can bind several target proteins with variable affinities. Moreover, a single PDZ motif can be recognized by different PDZ domains. To date, four types of PDZ motifs have been reported (Table 1).

PDZ domain	Protein motif
Type I	S/T-x-Φ
Type II	Φ-x-Φ
Type III	Ψ-x-Φ
Type IV	D-x-V

x: any amino-acid; Φ: hydrophobic amino-acid; Ψ: hydrophilic amino-acid

Table 1. Consensus sequences linking the different PDZ domains.

A PDZ protein can have several PDZ domains and so can interact simultaneously with several partner proteins. In addition, PDZ proteins can also form homo- or hetero multimeric structure (Fouassier et al., 2000; Lalonde & Bretscher, 2009; Lau & Hall, 2001; Shenolikar et al., 2001) thus forming wide submembrane docking networks for multiple transmembrane proteins where they can interact with each other and with anchored cytosolic regulatory proteins. Therefore, PDZ proteins play an important role in protein stability at the plasma membrane (i.e. endocytosis and recycling) and function. Some PDZ proteins are ubiquitous and others have a cell type-specific expression. Considering the organ or the tissue, PDZ proteins can be implicated in cellular morphology, cellular polarity, intercellular contacts, cell migration and cell growth (Altschuler et al., 2003; Hall et al., 1998; Kocher et al., 1999; C. Li et al., 2005; 2007; Naren et al., 2003; Pietrement et al., 2008; Seidler et al., 2009; Short et al., 1998; Singh et al., 2009; Wang et al., 1998; 2000; Yoo et al., 2004). CFTR possesses at its C-terminus a consensus motif, (D/E)-T-(R/K)-L, which belongs to the type I class of PDZ domain-binding motifs and is conserved across species (Table 2).

Species	CFTR C-terminal sequence
Human	SSKCKSKPQIAALKEETEEEVQ**DTRL**
Frog	SSKRKSRPQISALQEETEEEVQ**DTRL**
Rat	SSKQKPRTQITAVKEETEEEVQ**ETRL**
Mouse	SSKHKPRTQITALKEETEEEVQ**ETRL**
Dogfish	SSKRKTRPKISALQEEAEEDLQ**ETRL**
Sheep	SSRQRSRANIAALKEETEEEVQ**ETKL**
Bovine	SSRQRSRSNIAALKEETEEEVQ**ETKL**
Rabbit	SSKHKSRPQITALKEEAEEEVQ**GTRL**

Table 2. C-terminal sequence of CFTR protein from various species.

3.1 Role of CFTR C-terminus

Patients harbouring a C-terminal truncation of CFTR such as the deletion of the 26 last amino acids (CFTR-S1455X) have a mild CF phenotype. A first study described that a mother and her daughter, both heterozygous for CFTR-S1455X and deletion of exon 14a (del14a) mutations, exhibited no CF phenotype but only an increase in sweat Cl^- concentration, while a second daughter homozygous for del14a mutant had a severe CF phenotype (Mickle et al., 1998). A second study described two sisters heterozygous for F508del, the most common CF mutation, and CFTR-S1455X with also no CF phenotype and an elevated sweat Cl^- secretion (Salvatore et al., 2005). Those studies suggest that deletion of CFTR C-terminus has no major incidence on the phenotype of patients. The role of CFTR C-terminus was also studied *in vitro* using plasmid constructs where CFTR's PDZ binding motif was deleted (ΔTRL-CFTR). The resulting phenotype of ΔTRL-CFTR in polarized and non-polarized cells is controversial. In type I MDCK cells, Moyer and colleagues have demonstrated that PDZ binding motif is an apical polarization signal and its deletion decreases CFTR activity (Moyer et al., 1999; 2000). On the opposite, several teams have described that deletion of the PDZ binding motif of CFTR has no effect on its apical membrane localization nor its function in numerous cells such as BHK-21, COS-1, type II MDCK, CaCo-2, PANC-1 and primary human airway epithelial cells (Benharouga et al., 2003; Milewski et al., 2005; Ostedgaard et al., 2003). The discrepancy between these studies can be explained by additional sorting motifs (Milewski et al., 2005), but also by the use of MDCK type I cells as the unique polarized cell line by Moyer et al., whereas different non polarized cell models were used by the other groups. Indeed, MDCK type I and II cells exhibit different polarized sorting (Svennevig et al., 1995). Accordingly, CFTR polarized expression would be differentially regulated depending on the type or the origin of the cells. The role in this process of the six PDZ proteins described so far to interact with CFTR is not clearly established, but they indubitably have different functions in CFTR polarized expression.

3.2 Na^+/H^+ exchanger regulatory factor family proteins

Na^+/H^+ Exchanger Regulatory Factor (NHERF) family proteins possess multiple PDZ domains. NHERF1 (also called EBP50 for Ezrin-radixin-moesin Binding Phosphoprotein of 50 kDa), the most studied member of the NHERF family, is the first protein evoked to interact with CFTR through its PDZ domain (Hall et al., 1998; Short et al., 1998; Wang et al., 1998). The NHERF family comprises four members: NHERF1 and NHERF2 (also called E3KARP for Na^+/H^+ Exchanger 3 Kinase A Regulatory Protein) have two PDZ domains while NHERF3 (also called PDZK1, CAP70 or NaPi CAP-1) and NHERF4 (also called PDZK2, IKEPP or NaPi CAP-2) have 4 PDZ domains (Fig.1). In addition, NHERF1 and NHERF2 have in their C-terminus tail a consensus sequence for ezrin binding, allowing their anchor to the actin cytoskeleton (Reczek et al., 1997).

NHERF1 and NHERF2 have similar functions but their cell expression is generally mutually exclusive *in vivo* (Ingraffea et al., 2002). In human lungs, NHERF1 is expressed in epithelial cells while NHERF2 is expressed in alveolar cells (Ingraffea et al., 2002). However, it seems not to be the case in cell lines. The affinity of CFTR C-terminus for PDZ domains varies across NHERF family members Indeed, CFTR C-terminus tail interacts preferentially with PDZ1 domain of NHERF1 (Wang et al., 1998) but with PDZ2 domain of NHERF2 (Hall et al., 1998; Sun et al., 2000). NHERF1 C-terminus tail interacts with its own PDZ2 domain preventing NHERF1 binding to ezrin. This auto-inhibition of NHERF1 is abolished by PKC phosphorylation (J. Li et al., 2007), which promotes macromolecular complex formation. In addition, both NHERF1 and NHERF2 have been shown to form homo- and heterodimers (Lau & Hall, 2001; Shenolikar et al., 2001).

CFTR C-terminus tail can interact with three out of four PDZ domains of NHERF3 (Wang et al., 2000). To date, only one team has demonstrated an interaction between CFTR and NHERF4 in transfected sf9 insect cells (Hegedüs et al., 2003). On the opposite of NHERF1 and NHERF2, NHERF3 and NHERF4 cannot anchor CFTR to the actin network. However, as NHERF3 is able to bind NHERF1, it can indirectly link CFTR to the cytoskeleton (Lalonde & Bretscher, 2009).

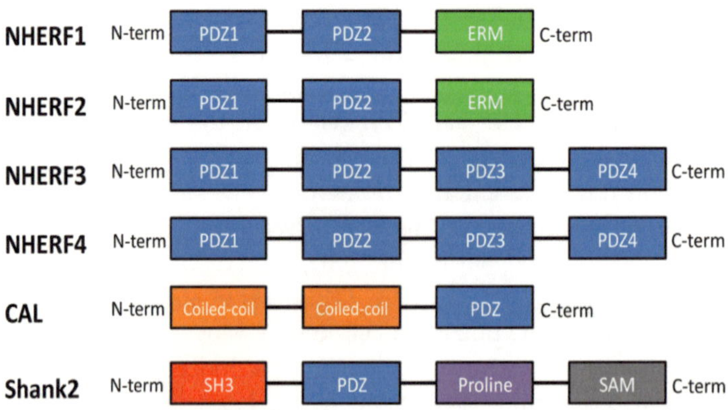

NHERF: Na^+/H^+ exchanger Regulatory Factor; CAL: CFTR Associated Ligand; ERM: Ezrin-Radixin-Moesin domain; PDZ: Postsynaptic density-95/ Disc large/ Zonula occludens-1; SAM: sterile Alpha Motif; SH3: Src Homology 3 domain; C-term: C-terminal; N-term: N-terminal.

Fig. 1. PDZ domain containing proteins interacting with CFTR C-terminus tail.

3.3 CFTR-associated ligand

CFTR-Associated Ligand (CAL, also called Golgi-associated PDZ and coiled-coil motif containing protein, GOPC, or PDZ Protein Interacting Specifically with TC10, PIST) is a protein of approximately 50 kDa containing a single PDZ domain and two coiled-coil domains (Fig.1). CAL can form homodimers independently of its single PDZ domain but through its N-terminal portion (Cheng et al., 2002; Cushing et al., 2008; Neudauer et al., 2001). CAL is ubiquitously expressed in the Golgi apparatus of human tissues. Although it has no transmembrane domain, CAL is associated with membranes by interacting with resident proteins from the Trans-Golgi network *via* its coiled-coil domain (Cheng et al., 2002). CAL can interact with CFTR C-terminus tail through its PDZ domain as determined by yeast two-hybrid assay and co-immunoprecipiation (Cheng et al., 2002).

3.4 Shank2

Shank2 (also known as Cortactin-binding protein 1, CortBP1; or Proline-rich synapse-associated protein 1, ProSAP1) contains a single PDZ domain and other sites for protein–protein interaction, including an SH3 domain, a long proline-rich region, and a sterile alpha motif (SAM) domain (Fig.1). The SAM domain is able to self-associate to form dimers (Gisler et al., 2001). Shank2 is expressed abundantly in brain as well as in kidney, liver, intestine, and pancreas. In this last tissue, it is localized to the luminal pole in pancreatic duct cells and luminal area of colonic epithelia (Du et al., 1998; Kim et al., 2004; Lee et al., 2007; Lim et al., 1999). Shank2 has been shown to be associated with CFTR through its PDZ domain in the yeast two-hybrid system and in mammalian cells (Kim et al., 2004).

4. PDZ interactions regulate CFTR trafficking

4.1 NHERF family proteins form a subapical network for CFTR plasma membrane docking

NHERF1, NHERF2 and NHERF3 can auto-assemble in a regulated fashion and form a subapical network serving as a cytoskeleton-anchored platform for the docking of multiple regulatory and transmembrane proteins. CFTR binding to this station is PDZ-dependent and results in increased stability at the plasma membrane. Indeed, a CFTR mutant truncated for its C-terminal PDZ interacting motif is highly mobile at the plasma membrane, whereas intact CFTR exhibits a greater immobile fraction or a more confined diffusion (Bates et al., 2006; Haggie et al., 2004; 2006). Moreover, C-terminal truncation of CFTR alters its endocytic/recycling dynamics. While CFTR endocytosis from the apical plasma membrane seems to be unaffected in polarized MDCK type I cells, C-terminal deletion decreases its recycling efficiency (Swiatecka-Urban et al., 2002). Despite the reported decrease in the half-life of ΔTRL-CFTR at the apical plasma membrane, the same group observed that its degradation rate was not accelerated. Albeit this should lead to an intracellular accumulation of ΔTRL-CFTR, it is not the case (Benharouga et al., 2003; Milewski et al., 2005; Ostedgaard et al., 2003), because other trafficking mechanisms may compensate for the recycling defect of ΔTRL-CFTR in order to ensure its observed apical localization. Recently, preliminary results from Bossard et al. (2010) reconcile this discrepancy by reporting a new intracellular trafficking pathway for CFTR polarized sorting. Indeed, apically endocytosed

CFTR is efficiently recycled back to the apical plasma membrane but a significant fraction is constitutively trafficked to the basolateral plasma membrane. This mistargeted pool is transiently localized at the basolateral cell surface, as it is rapidly rerouted to the apical plasma membrane. This transcytotic pathway occurs in various polarized cell lines such as canine kidney (MDCK type II), human airway (CFBE41o-) and pig kidney (LLC-PK1) epithelia (Bossard et al., 2010). When comparing wt- and ΔTRL-CFTR dynamics in CFBE epithelia, both proteins exhibit similar half-life and apical surface stability. However, ΔTRL-CFTR undergoes a faster endocytosis from the apical plasma membrane, a slower recycling to the apical membrane and a more intense transcytotic pathway (Fig.2). Those characteristics could compensate for ΔTRL-CFTR recycling defect and explain the comparable half-life and apical stability with its wt counterpart (Bossard et al., 2010). This new insight into CFTR intracellular trafficking uncovers a novel role of PDZ adaptors in protein sorting, and raises further questions about the cause of the mild CF phenotype observed in patients with C-terminally truncated CFTR mutants.

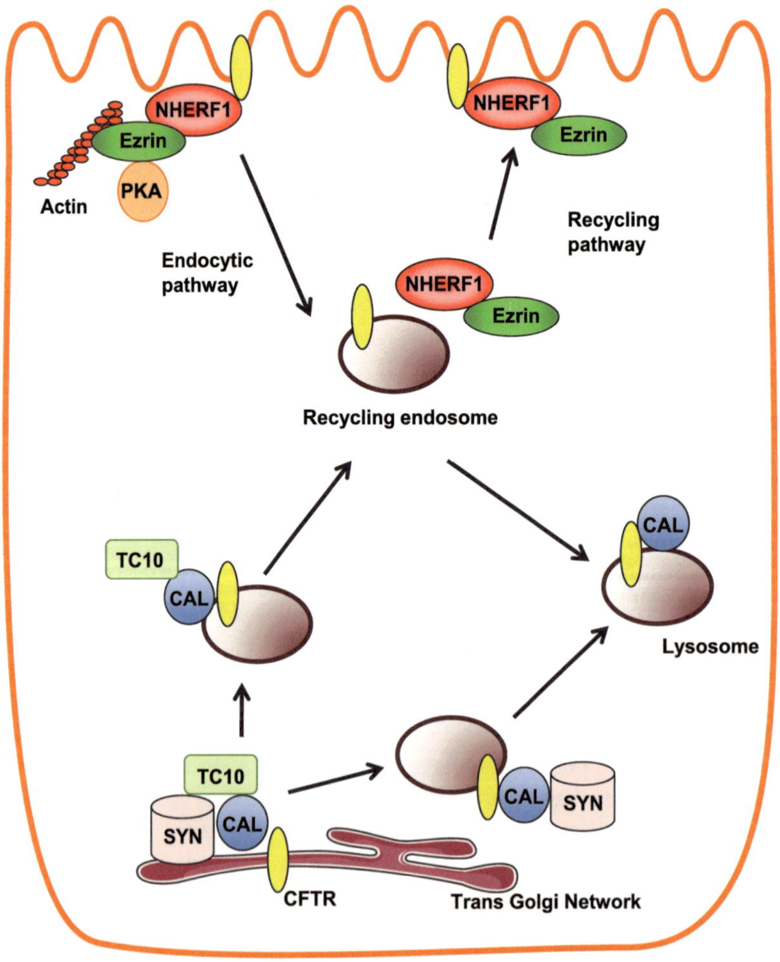

Fig. 2. Regulation of intracellular traffic of CFTR by interaction with several proteins with PDZ domains. SYN: synthaxine 6.

4.2 CAL targets CFTR to lysosomal degradation

PDZ interaction of CAL with CFTR occurs at the endosomal level and targets CFTR to lysosomal degradation (Cheng et al., 2004). This CAL-dependent sorting of CFTR is counteracted by NHERF1 binding (Cheng et al., 2002). Comparable to CFTR, both the beta1-adrenergic receptor and cadherin 23 interact with CAL, leading to their intracellular accumulation and/or degradation (Fig.2); these interactions can be competitively counteracted by binding with other PDZ domain-containing proteins (He et al., 2004; Xu et al., 2010). Likewise, CAL is an intracellular retention partner for the somatostatin receptor subtype 5 and the metabotropic glutamate receptor subtypes 1a (Wente et al., 2005; Zhang et al., 2008).

Accordingly, both inhibition of CAL protein expression and NHERF1 overexpression are efficient in promoting the cell surface expression and function of the most common disease-associated mutant, F508del-CFTR (Bossard et al., 2007; Guerra et al., 2005; Wolde et al., 2007). Interestingly, the conformational and molecular interactions between CFTR and CAL differ from those between CFTR and NHERF1, indicating that PDZ-selective inhibitors can be designed to improve CFTR mutant expression (Amacher et al., 2011; Cushing et al., 2010; Piserchio et al., 2005). CAL/CFTR interaction is modulated by the Rho family small GTPase, TC10. Its activation redistributes CAL to the plasma membrane and reverses CAL-mediated CFTR degradation (Cheng et al., 2005). Thus, CAL can play opposite roles on CFTR trafficking depending on the activation of TC10, which is a molecular switch between the degradation and exocytosis pathways. Moreover, the Q-SNARE [Q-soluble N-ethylmaleimide-sensitive fusion protein (NSF) attachment protein receptor] protein syntaxin 6 interacts with both CAL and CFTR (Charest et al., 2001; Cheng et al., 2010). Syntaxin 6 binds the N-terminal half of CFTR after its interaction with CAL, and this binding mediates CFTR lysosomal degradation (Cheng et al., 2010).

4.3 Do Shank2 and NHERF4 regulate CFTR trafficking?

Only one study reports the modulation of CFTR membrane expression by Shank2. Shank2 overexpression tends to increase CFTR membrane expression and stability (Kim et al., 2004).

Since the first study showing a CFTR/NHERF4 interaction (Hegedüs et al., 2003), no more data were published. This could be explained, in part, by the fact that NHERF4 is not expressed in lungs. Its expression is restricted to the gastrointestinal tract and kidney in mouse (Gisler et al., 2001; Scott et al., 2002; Watanabe et al., 2006) without data in human. In particular, NHERF4 is localized close to or at the apical plasma membrane (Gisler et al., 2001; Scott et al., 2002; Van De Graaf et al., 2006; Watanabe et al., 2006), consistent with CFTR localization.

5. PDZ interactions regulate CFTR function

As a phosphorylation-regulated chloride channel, CFTR physical and functional proximity to kinases and phosphodiesterases has fundamental importance. NHERF1, NHERF2 and NHERF3 have all been reported to link CFTR to PKA. Indeed, NHERF1 and NHERF2 both interact with ezrin, a well known A kinase anchoring protein (AKAP) (Fig.2) (Reczek et al.,

1997; Sun et al., 2000). Likewise, NHERF3 is able to bind the dual-specific A-kinase anchoring protein 2 (D-AKAP2) with higher affinity than NHERF1 (Gisler et al., 2003). Moreover, AKAPs are also anchors for phosphodiesterases (PDE) (Dodge-Kafka et al., 2005; Willoughby et al., 2006), allowing local fine tuning of cAMP concentration for proper regulation of CFTR channel activity. The PDE4D is the most abundant PDE in airway epithelia and forms a cAMP diffusion barrier at the apical confinement where CFTR is localized (Barnes et al., 2005). As Shank2 is associated with PDE4D, thus reducing local cAMP availability, this could explain the observed inhibition of CFTR chloride activity (Lee et al., 2007).

CFTR activation by PKA is potentiated by PKC (Winpenny et al., 1995). As NHERF1 binds the Receptor for Activated C Kinase (RACK1) through PDZ1 interaction, this interaction could anchor PKC epsilon isoform in the vicinity of CFTR and facilitate its activation (Liedtke et al., 2002; 2004).

Besides anchoring cytosolic regulatory proteins, the apical docking station formed by PDZ proteins brings other transmembrane proteins closer to CFTR for reciprocal regulation. Likewise, CFTR and the ENaC display cross-functional regulation (Jiang et al., 2000). This regulation involves NHERF1 that binds the Yes-associated protein 65 (YAP65) through its PDZ2 domain and CFTR C-terminus through PDZ1 (Mohler et al., 1999). YAP65 is an anchoring protein for the cytosolic tyrosine kinase c-Yes, a member of the Src family, which has been reported to inhibit ENaC (Gilmore et al., 2001; Mohler et al., 1999). Furthermore, NHERF1 allows the adrenergic regulation of CFTR by bridging it with the beta2-adrenoceptor at the apical plasma membrane (Naren et al., 2003; Taouil et al., 2003). NHERF2 can form a molecular bond connecting CFTR to the lysophosphatidic acid type 2 receptor or the Na^+/H^+ exchanger isoform 3. The activation of those latter proteins is able to inhibit CFTR chloride current (Bagorda et al., 2002; Favia et al., 2006; C. Li et al., 2005). Moreover, NHERF3 connects CFTR to the cAMP transporter multidrug resistance protein 4 (MRP4), which enhances CFTR function (C. Li et al., 2007).

An additional mechanism for PDZ proteins to regulate CFTR activity is their ability to form CFTR homodimers as detected in the plasma membrane of mammalian cells (Ramjeesingh et al., 2003). The formation of CFTR dimers is triggered by NHERF1, NHERF2 and NHERF3 leading to an increase in CFTR channel activity (Li et al., 2004; J. Li et al., 2005; Wang et al., 2000).

The PDZ protein CAL has not been reported to have direct influence on CFTR chloride current. However, CAL-mediated lysosomal degradation of CFTR indirectly decreases CFTR channel activity by reducing its apical plasma membrane density.

Some studies have reported that annexin A5 (AnxA5) could be involved in the traffic of CFTR. Recently, in oocytes, AnxA5 inhibited CFTR-mediated whole-cell membrane conductance presumably by a mechanism independent of PDZ-binding domain at the C-terminus of CFTR but PKC-dependent and resulted from either endocytosis activation and/or exocytosis block. In contrast, in human cells, co-expression of AnxA5 augmented CFTR whole-cell currents, an effect that was independent of CFTR PDZ-binding domain. Those results suggest that AnxA5 has multiple effects on CFTR, but the effect observed is cell system-dependent (Faria et al., 2011).

6. Are PDZ proteins potential targets for drug therapy in CF?

Because PDZ proteins regulate CFTR membrane expression and/or function, several studies have investigated the potential therapeutic effectiveness of these proteins. To date, only the potential therapeutic role of NHERF1 overexpression or CAL silencing has been investigated.

6.1 NHERF1 overexpression restores F508del-CFTR plasma membrane expression

In 2005, Guerra and colleagues observed that mouse NHERF1 but not NHERF2 overexpression increased F508del-CFTR plasma membrane expression and activity in human bronchial epithelial cell line endogenously expressing F508del-CFTR (CFBE41o-) (Guerra et al., 2005) (Fig.2). Four years later, our team demonstrated in A549 and type II MDCK cells microinjected with F508del-CFTR plasmid that human NHERF1 overexpression restored F508del-CFTR apical plasma membrane expression and chloride channel activity (Bossard et al., 2007). This effect was abolished in the presence of a sense oligonucleotide complementary to NHERF1 mRNA sequence attesting that this mechanism is specific to NHERF1 overexpression (Bossard et al., 2007). Moreover, in type II MDCK cells microinjected with a CFTR double mutant: F508del and K1468X (deletion of the 12 last C-terminus amino acids, thus avoiding PDZ-based interaction), NHERF1 overexpression had no effect on F508del-K1468X-CFTR expression and activity certifying that an interaction between F508del-CFTR and NHERF1 is required (Bossard et al., 2007). Immunostaining experiments confirmed these results by demonstrating a colocalization of F508del-CFTR and NHERF1 at the apical plasma membrane (Bossard et al., 2007). Furthermore, it is important to note that NHERF1 overexpression was not a nonspecific global rescue of ER-retained proteins because it did not restore the plasma membrane expression of an unrelated trafficking defective mutant potassium channel, KCNQ1 [mutant P117L highlighted by Dahimene et al. (2006)] (Bossard et al., 2007).

Thereby, we are currently investigating the effects of NHERF1 overexpression on F508del-CFTR expression and activity *in vivo* by non viral gene transfer using block copolymers in homozygous F508del-CFTR mice (Desigaux et al., 2005).

6.2 CAL silencing restores F508del-CFTR plasma membrane expression

RNA interference targeting endogenous CAL specifically increases cell surface expression of the F508del-CFTR mutant and thus enhances transepithelial chloride currents in polarized CFBE41o- cells overexpressing F508del-CFTR (Wolde et al., 2007) (Fig.3).

Recently, it has been demonstrated that CAL interaction with F508del-CFTR can be avoided by using a blocking peptide, iCAL36 (ANSRWPTSII), which specifically targets CAL but not NHERF1, NHERF2 or NHERF3 PDZ domain (Cushing et al., 2010). The presence of iCAL36 extends F508del-CFTR half-life at the plasma membrane in the human bronchial epithelial cell line CFBE41o- (Cushing et al., 2010) (Fig.3). It is important to mention that this blocking peptide needs a delivery agent to allow its entry into the cells, thereby limiting its potential therapeutic use.

Syntaxin 6 acts at the Trans-Golgi Network where its silencing enhances the protein expression of the rescued, post-ER F508del-CFTR mutant, but not of the non-rescued, ER-trapped F508del-CFTR (Cheng et al., 2010). Thus, impairing CAL interaction with F508del-CFTR or other CFTR mutants as well as the inhibition of CAL/Syntaxin 6 interaction could represent new therapeutic tools for CF (Fig.3).

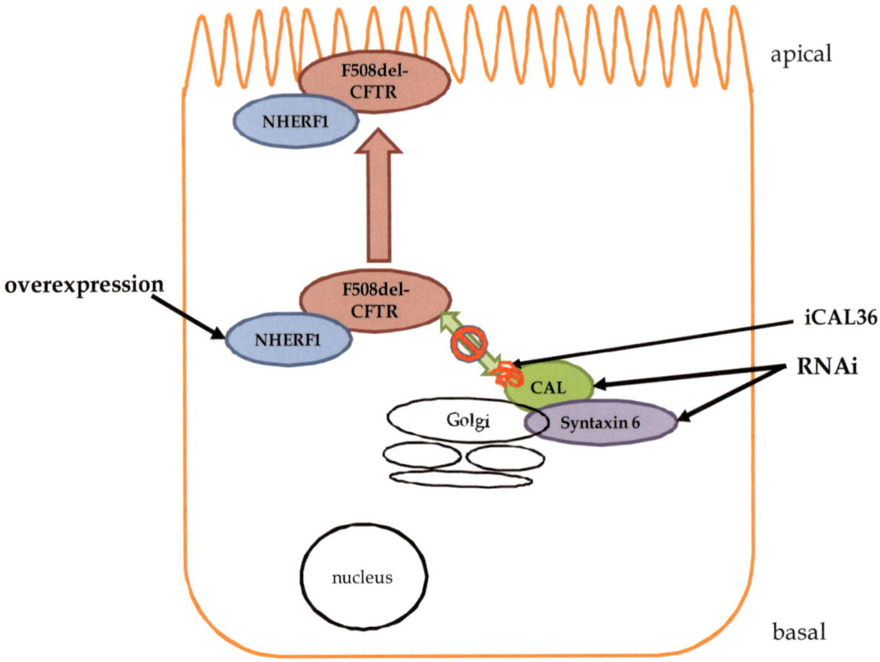

Fig. 3. Strategies for modulation of F508del-CFTR interactions with NHERF1 and CAL to enhance its apical plasma membrane expression.

6.3 Are PDZ interactions a potential drug target for CF treatment?

Since several decades, drug research has focused on finding compounds targeting receptors, ion channels, metabolic transporters and enzymes. More recently, the comprehension of the interrelated omics (genomics, proteomics, transcriptomics, metabonomics, interactomics, signalomics…) suggests that the protein-protein interactions could play a virtually universal role. Among them, PDZ-based interactions are a ubiquitous mechanism to modulate complex cellular processes. Therefore, the inhibition of a single protein-protein interaction should be highly selective in order to avoid undesirable effects.

Besides its conformational-related trafficking defect, the most frequent CFTR mutant, F508del-CFTR, also exhibits an intrinsic functional deficiency, suggesting that its potent rescue to the apical membrane might not be sufficient to restore a healthy phenotype. Consequently, PDZ protein-targeted drugs acting as a corrector treatment should be complemented with a potentiator treatment for effective therapeutic outcome. Moreover, drug or peptide candidates targeting PDZ interaction act exclusively as inhibitors, whereas PDZ interaction reinforcement (e.g. with NHERF1, NHERF2 and NHERF3) would also be suitable for CF treatment. Selective inhibition of interaction between CFTR and PDZ proteins, should likely target CAL and Shank2, which are inhibitors of CFTR expression and/or function. The physical properties of small molecule inhibitors - i.e. cell permeability, good oral bioavailability and high affinity - make them better candidates than peptidic inhibitors (including antibodies) which usually are rapidly degraded and have poor pharmacokinetics. Synthetic inhibitors can target the C-terminus (or sometimes internal)

PDZ motif or the PDZ domain of the PDZ adaptor, rendering either one unavailable for interaction. Taking CFTR as an example target, the inhibitor should avoid CFTR interaction with CAL but not with NHERF1, NHERF2 or NHERF3. This could be accomplished by competitive inhibition (i) if the small molecule inhibitor can block an interaction interface specific to CAL but not to NHERF1, NHERF2 or NHERF3, or (ii) if the affinity of CFTR C-terminus for the small molecule is similar to that for CAL, and lower than that for NHERF1, NHERF2 or NHERF3 which has already been reported (Cushing et al., 2008). It is important that the small molecules that bind CAL to inhibit CAL/CFTR interaction, should not interfere with CAL's other partners in order to prevent any possible adverse effect. In any case, the crystal structure of both interacting partners and especially the geometry of the protein-protein interaction interface can help to rationally design small molecules inhibitors. Moreover, the targeted interaction could only be material in specific organs, tissues, cell types and subcellular compartments, hence complicating the task to achieve targeted drug delivery and selective effects. Although, small molecule inhibitors of PDZ-based interactions are of great interest as research tools for understanding the involvement of these scaffolding proteins in protein trafficking and function, their usefulness as therapeutic agents is still elusive and needs further investigations.

7. Conclusion

In conclusion, PDZ domains containing proteins have a fundamental role in the regulation of CFTR trafficking and chloride channel activity. The modulation of their selective interaction with CFTR using gene therapy and/or drug treatments is an auspicious approach for the treatment of patients harboring CFTR trafficking defect mutations such as F508del, but it remains to be intensively and carefully investigated in order to assess their specificity and possible side effects.

8. Acknowledgment

Our work was supported by the Association "Vaincre la mucoviscidose".

9. References

Altschuler, Y.; Hodson, C. & Milgram, S. L. (2003). The Apical Compartment: Trafficking Pathways, Regulators and Scaffolding Proteins. *Current Opinion in Cell Biology*, 15, 4, pp. 423-429.

Amacher, J. F.; Cushing, P. R.; Weiner, J. A. & Madden, D. R. (2011). Crystallization and Preliminary Diffraction Analysis of the Cal Pdz Domain in Complex with a Selective Peptide Inhibitor. *Acta crystallographica*, 67, Pt 5, pp. 600-603.

Anderson, M. P.; Berger, H. A.; Rich, D. P.; Gregory, R. J.; Smith, A. E. & Welsh, M. J. (1991). Nucleoside Triphosphates Are Required to Open the Cftr Chloride Channel. *Cell*, 67, 4, pp. 775-784.

Bagorda, A.; Guerra, L.; Di Sole, F.; Hemle-Kolb, C.; Cardone, R. A.; Fanelli, T.; Reshkin, S. J.; Gisler, S. M.; Murer, H. & Casavola, V. (2002). Reciprocal Protein Kinase a Regulatory Interactions between Cystic Fibrosis Transmembrane Conductance Regulator and Na+/H+ Exchanger Isoform 3 in a Renal Polarized Epithelial Cell Model. *The Journal of Biological Chemistry*, 277, 24, pp. 21480-21488.

Barasch, J.; Kiss, B.; Prince, A.; Saiman, L.; Gruenert, D. & Al-Awqati, Q. (1991). Defective Acidification of Intracellular Organelles in Cystic Fibrosis. *Nature*, 352, 6330, pp. 70-73.

Barnes, A. P.; Livera, G.; Huang, P.; Sun, C.; O'neal, W. K.; Conti, M.; Stutts, M. J. & Milgram, S. L. (2005). Phosphodiesterase 4d Forms a Camp Diffusion Barrier at the Apical Membrane of the Airway Epithelium. *The Journal of Biological Chemistry*, 280, 9, pp. 7997-8003.

Bates, I. R.; Hebert, B.; Luo, Y.; Liao, J.; Bachir, A. I.; Kolin, D. L.; Wiseman, P. W. & Hanrahan, J. W. (2006). Membrane Lateral Diffusion and Capture of Cftr within Transient Confinement Zones. *Biophysical Journal*, 91, 3, pp. 1046-1058.

Benharouga, M.; Sharma, M.; So, J.; Haardt, M.; Drzymala, L.; Popov, M.; Schwapach, B.; Grinstein, S.; Du, K. & Lukacs, G. L. (2003). The Role of the C Terminus and Na+/H+ Exchanger Regulatory Factor in the Functional Expression of Cystic Fibrosis Transmembrane Conductance Regulator in Nonpolarized Cells and Epithelia. *The Journal of Biological Chemistry*, 278, 24, pp. 22079-22089.

Berger, H. A.; Anderson, M. P.; Gregory, R. J.; Thompson, S.; Howard, P. W.; Maurer, R. A.; Mulligan, R.; Smith, A. E. & Welsh, M. J. (1991). Identification and Regulation of the Cystic Fibrosis Transmembrane Conductance Regulator-Generated Chloride Channel. *The Journal of Clinical Investigation*, 88, 4, pp. 1422-1431.

Bezprozvanny, I. & Maximov, A. (2001). Pdz Domains: More Than Just a Glue. *Proceedings of the National Academy of Sciences of the United States of America*, 98, 3, pp. 787-789.

Bossard, F.; Robay, A.; Toumaniantz, G.; Dahimene, S.; Becq, F.; Merot, J. & Gauthier, C. (2007). Nhe-Rf1 Protein Rescues Deltaf508-Cftr Function. *American Journal of Physiology - Lung Cellular and Molecular Physiology*, 292, 5, pp. L1085-1094.

Bossard, F.; Veit, G.; Borot, F.; Barrière, H. & Lukacs, G. L. (2010). Cellular Mechanism of Cftr Polarized Expression in Epithelia. *Proceedings of 50th annual meeting of the American Society for Cell Biology*, Philadelphia, PA, USA, December 2010. In: *Molecular Biology of the Cell*, 21, pp. 4299.

Charest, A.; Lane, K.; Mcmahon, K. & Housman, D. E. (2001). Association of a Novel Pdz Domain-Containing Peripheral Golgi Protein with the Q-Snare (Q-Soluble N-Ethylmaleimide-Sensitive Fusion Protein (Nsf) Attachment Protein Receptor) Protein Syntaxin 6. *The Journal of Biological Chemistry*, 276, 31, pp. 29456-29465.

Cheng, J.; Moyer, B. D.; Milewski, M. I.; Loffing, J.; Ikeda, M.; Mickle, J. E.; Cutting, G. R.; Li, M.; Stanton, B. A. & Guggino, W. B. (2002). A Golgi-Associated Pdz Domain Protein Modulates Cystic Fibrosis Transmembrane Regulator Plasma Membrane Expression. *The Journal of Biological Chemistry*, 277, 5, pp. 3520-3529.

Cheng, J.; Wang, H. & Guggino, W. B. (2004). Modulation of Mature Cystic Fibrosis Transmembrane Regulator Protein by the Pdz Domain Protein Cal. *The Journal of Biological Chemistry*, 279, 3, pp. 1892-1898.

Cheng, J.; Wang, H. & Guggino, W. B. (2005). Regulation of Cystic Fibrosis Transmembrane Regulator Trafficking and Protein Expression by a Rho Family Small Gtpase Tc10. *The Journal of Biological Chemistry*, 280, 5, pp. 3731-3739.

Cheng, J.; Cebotaru, V.; Cebotaru, L. & Guggino, W. B. (2010). Syntaxin 6 and Cal Mediate the Degradation of the Cystic Fibrosis Transmembrane Conductance Regulator. *Molecular Biology of the Cell*, 21, 7, pp. 1178-1187.

Cheng, S. H.; Gregory, R. J.; Marshall, J.; Paul, S.; Souza, D. W.; White, G. A.; O'riordan, C. R. & Smith, A. E. (1990). Defective Intracellular Transport and Processing of Cftr Is the Molecular Basis of Most Cystic Fibrosis. *Cell*, 63, 4, pp. 827-834.

Cushing, P. R.; Fellows, A.; Villone, D.; BoisgueRin, P. & Madden, D. R. (2008). The Relative Binding Affinities of Pdz Partners for Cftr: A Biochemical Basis for Efficient Endocytic Recycling†. *Biochemistry*, 47, 38, pp. 10084-10098.

Cushing, P. R.; Vouilleme, L.; Pellegrini, M.; Boisguerin, P. & Madden, D. R. (2010). A Stabilizing Influence: Cal Pdz Inhibition Extends the Half-Life of Deltaf508-Cftr. *Angewandte Chemie International Edition in English*, 49, 51, pp. 9907-9911.

Dahimene, S.; Alcolea, S.; Naud, P.; Jourdon, P.; Escande, D.; Brasseur, R.; Thomas, A.; Baro, I. & Merot, J. (2006). The N-Terminal Juxtamembranous Domain of Kcnq1 Is Critical for Channel Surface Expression: Implications in the Romano-Ward Lqt1 Syndrome. *Circulation Research*, 99, 10, pp. 1076-1083.

Dalemans, W.; Hinnrasky, J.; Slos, P.; Dreyer, D.; Fuchey, C.; Pavirani, A. & Puchelle, E. (1992). Immunocytochemical Analysis Reveals Differences between the Subcellular Localization of Normal and Delta Phe508 Recombinant Cystic Fibrosis Transmembrane Conductance Regulator. *Experimental Cell Research*, 201, 1, pp. 235-240.

Desigaux, L.; Gourden, C.; Bello-Roufaï, M.; Richard, P.; Oudrhiri, N.; Lehn, P.; Escande, D.; Pollard, H. & Pitard, B. (2005). Nonionic Amphiphilic Block Copolymers Promote Gene Transfer to the Lung. *Human Gene Therapy*, 16, 7, pp. 821-829.

Dodge-Kafka, K. L.; Soughayer, J.; Pare, G. C.; Carlisle Michel, J. J.; Langeberg, L. K.; Kapiloff, M. S. & Scott, J. D. (2005). The Protein Kinase a Anchoring Protein Makap Coordinates Two Integrated Camp Effector Pathways. *Nature*, 437, 7058, pp. 574-578.

Du, Y.; Weed, S. A.; Xiong, W. C.; Marshall, T. D. & Parsons, J. T. (1998). Identification of a Novel Cortactin Sh3 Domain-Binding Protein and Its Localization to Growth Cones of Cultured Neurons. *Molecular and Cellular Biology*, 18, 10, pp. 5838-5851.

Egan, M.; Flotte, T.; Afione, S.; Solow, R.; Zeitlin, P. L.; Carter, B. J. & Guggino, W. B. (1992). Defective Regulation of Outwardly Rectifying Cl- Channels by Protein Kinase a Corrected by Insertion of Cftr. *Nature*, 358, 6387, pp. 581-584.

Fanning, A. S. & Anderson, J. M. (1999). Protein Modules as Organizers of Membrane Structure. *Current Opinion in Cell Biology*, 11, 4, pp. 432-439.

Faria D., Dahimène S., Alessio L., Scott-Ward T., Schreiber R., Kunzelmann K., Amaral M.D. Effect of Annexin A5 on CFTR: regulated traffic or scaffolding? *Molecular Membrane Biology*, 28(1), pp. 14-29

Favia, M.; Fanelli, T.; Bagorda, A.; Di Sole, F.; Reshkin, S. J.; Suh, P. G.; Guerra, L. & Casavola, V. (2006). Nhe3 Inhibits Pka-Dependent Functional Expression of Cftr by Nherf2 Pdz Interactions. *Biochemical and Biophysical Research Communications*, 347, 2, pp. 452-459.

Fouassier, L.; Yun, C. C.; Fitz, J. G. & Doctor, R. B. (2000). Evidence for Ezrin-Radixin-Moesin-Binding Phosphoprotein 50 (Ebp50) Self-Association through Pdz-Pdz Interactions. *The Journal of Biological Chemistry*, 275, 32, pp. 25039-25045.

Gabriel, S. E.; Clarke, L. L.; Boucher, R. C. & Stutts, M. J. (1993). Cftr and Outward Rectifying Chloride Channels Are Distinct Proteins with a Regulatory Relationship. *Nature*, 363, 6426, pp. 263-268.

Gilmore, E. S.; Stutts, M. J. & Milgram, S. L. (2001). Src Family Kinases Mediate Epithelial Na+ Channel Inhibition by Endothelin. *The Journal of Biological Chemistry*, 276, 45, pp. 42610-42617.

Gisler, S. M.; Stagljar, I.; Traebert, M.; Bacic, D.; Biber, J. R. & Murer, H. (2001). Interaction of the Type Iia Na/Pi Cotransporter with Pdz Proteins. *The Journal of Biological Chemistry*, 276, 12, pp. 9206-9213.

Gisler, S. M.; Madjdpour, C.; Bacic, D.; Pribanic, S.; Taylor, S. S.; Biber, J. & Murer, H. (2003). Pdzk1: Ii. An Anchoring Site for the Pka-Binding Protein D-Akap2 in Renal Proximal Tubular Cells. *Kidney International*, 64, 5, pp. 1746-1754.

Guerra, L.; Fanelli, T.; Favia, M.; Riccardi, S. M.; Busco, G.; Cardone, R. A.; Carrabino, S.; Weinman, E. J.; Reshkin, S. J.; Conese, M. & Casavola, V. (2005). Na+/H+ Exchanger Regulatory Factor Isoform 1 Overexpression Modulates Cystic Fibrosis Transmembrane Conductance Regulator (Cftr) Expression and Activity in Human Airway 16hbe14o- Cells and Rescues Deltaf508 Cftr Functional Expression in Cystic Fibrosis Cells. *The Journal of Biological Chemistry*, 280, 49, pp. 40925-40933.

Haggie, P. M.; Stanton, B. A. & Verkman, A. S. (2004). Increased Diffusional Mobility of Cftr at the Plasma Membrane after Deletion of Its C-Terminal Pdz Binding Motif. *The Journal of biological chemistry*, 279, 7, pp. 5494-5500.

Haggie, P. M.; Kim, J. K.; Lukacs, G. L. & Verkman, A. S. (2006). Tracking of Quantum Dot-Labeled Cftr Shows near Immobilization by C-Terminal Pdz Interactions. *Molecular Biology of the Cell*, 17, 12, pp. 4937-4945.

Hall, R. A.; Ostedgaard, L. S.; Premont, R. T.; Blitzer, J. T.; Rahman, N.; Welsh, M. J. & Lefkowitz, R. J. (1998). A C-Terminal Motif Found in the Beta2-Adrenergic Receptor, P2y1 Receptor and Cystic Fibrosis Transmembrane Conductance Regulator Determines Binding to the Na+/H+ Exchanger Regulatory Factor Family of Pdz Proteins. *Proceedings of the National Academy of Sciences of the United States of America*, 95, 15, pp. 8496-8501.

Harris, B. Z. & Lim, W. A. (2001). Mechanism and Role of Pdz Domains in Signaling Complex Assembly. *Journal of Cell Science*, 114, Pt 18, pp. 3219-3231.

He, J.; Bellini, M.; Xu, J.; Castleberry, A. M. & Hall, R. A. (2004). Interaction with Cystic Fibrosis Transmembrane Conductance Regulator-Associated Ligand (Cal) Inhibits Beta1-Adrenergic Receptor Surface Expression. *The Journal of Biological Chemistry*, 279, 48, pp. 50190-50196.

Hegedüs, T.; Sessler, T.; Scott, R.; Thelin, W.; Bakos, É.; Váradi, A.; Szabó, K.; Homolya, L.; Milgram, S. L. & Sarkadi, B. (2003). C-Terminal Phosphorylation of Mrp2 Modulates Its Interaction with Pdz Proteins. *Biochemical and Biophysical Research Communications*, 302, 3, pp. 454-461.

Hillier, B. J.; Christopherson, K. S.; Prehoda, K. E.; Bredt, D. S. & Lim, W. A. (1999). Unexpected Modes of Pdz Domain Scaffolding Revealed by Structure of Nnos-Syntrophin Complex. *Science*, 284, 5415, pp. 812-815.

Hung, A. Y. & Sheng, M. (2002). Pdz Domains: Structural Modules for Protein Complex Assembly. *The Journal of Biological Chemistry*, 277, 8, pp. 5699-5702.

Ingraffea, J.; Reczek, D. & Bretscher, A. (2002). Distinct Cell Type-Specific Expression of Scaffolding Proteins Ebp50 and E3karp: Ebp50 Is Generally Expressed with Ezrin in Specific Epithelia, Whereas E3karp Is Not. *European Journal of Cell Biology*, 81, 2, pp. 61-68.

Jiang, Q.; Li, J.; Dubroff, R.; Ahn, Y. J.; Foskett, J. K.; Engelhardt, J. & Kleyman, T. R. (2000). Epithelial Sodium Channels Regulate Cystic Fibrosis Transmembrane Conductance Regulator Chloride Channels in Xenopusoocytes. *The Journal of Biological Chemistry*, 275, 18, pp. 13266-13274.

Kerem, B.; Rommens, J. M.; Buchanan, J. A.; Markiewicz, D.; Cox, T. K.; Chakravarti, A.; Buchwald, M. & Tsui, L. C. (1989). Identification of the Cystic Fibrosis Gene: Genetic Analysis. *Science*, 245, 4922, pp. 1073-1080.

Kim, J. Y.; Han, W.; Namkung, W.; Lee, J. H.; Kim, K. H.; Shin, H.; Kim, E. & Lee, M. G. (2004). Inhibitory Regulation of Cystic Fibrosis Transmembrane Conductance Regulator Anion-Transporting Activities by Shank2. *The Journal of Biological Chemistry*, 279, 11, pp. 10389-10396.

Ko, S. B.; Shcheynikov, N.; Choi, J. Y.; Luo, X.; Ishibashi, K.; Thomas, P. J.; Kim, J. Y.; Kim, K. H.; Lee, M. G.; Naruse, S. & Muallem, S. (2002). A Molecular Mechanism for Aberrant Cftr-Dependent Hco(3)(-) Transport in Cystic Fibrosis. *EMBO Journal*, 21, 21, pp. 5662-5672.

Kocher, O.; Comella, N.; Gilchrist, A.; Pal, R.; Tognazzi, K.; Brown, L. F. & Knoll, J. H. (1999). Pdzk1, a Novel Pdz Domain-Containing Protein up-Regulated in Carcinomas and Mapped to Chromosome 1q21, Interacts with Cmoat (Mrp2), the Multidrug Resistance-Associated Protein. *Laboratory Investigation*, 79, 9, pp. 1161-1170.

Kunzelmann, K.; Kiser, G. L.; Schreiber, R. & Riordan, J. R. (1997). Inhibition of Epithelial Na+ Currents by Intracellular Domains of the Cystic Fibrosis Transmembrane Conductance Regulator. *FEBS Letters*, 400, 3, pp. 341-344.

Lalonde, D. P. & Bretscher, A. (2009). The Scaffold Protein Pdzk1 Undergoes a Head-to-Tail Intramolecular Association That Negatively Regulates Its Interaction with Ebp50. *Biochemistry*, 48, 10, pp. 2261-2271.

Lau, A. G. & Hall, R. A. (2001). Oligomerization of Nherf-1 and Nherf-2 Pdz Domains: Differential Regulation by Association with Receptor Carboxyl-Termini and by Phosphorylation. *Biochemistry*, 40, 29, pp. 8572-8580.

Lee, J. H.; Richter, W.; Namkung, W.; Kim, K. H.; Kim, E.; Conti, M. & Lee, M. G. (2007). Dynamic Regulation of Cystic Fibrosis Transmembrane Conductance Regulator by Competitive Interactions of Molecular Adaptors. *The Journal of Biological Chemistry*, 282, 14, pp. 10414-10422.

Li, C.; Roy, K.; Dandridge, K. & Naren, A. P. (2004). Molecular Assembly of Cystic Fibrosis Transmembrane Conductance Regulator in Plasma Membrane. *The Journal of Biological Chemistry*, 279, 23, pp. 24673-24684.

Li, C.; Dandridge, K. S.; Di, A.; Marrs, K. L.; Harris, E. L.; Roy, K.; Jackson, J. S.; Makarova, N. V.; Fujiwara, Y.; Farrar, P. L.; Nelson, D. J.; Tigyi, G. J. & Naren, A. P. (2005). Lysophosphatidic Acid Inhibits Cholera Toxin-Induced Secretory Diarrhea through Cftr-Dependent Protein Interactions. *The Journal of Experimental Medicine*, 202, 7, pp. 975-986.

Li, C.; Krishnamurthy, P. C.; Penmatsa, H.; Marrs, K. L.; Wang, X. Q.; Zaccolo, M.; Jalink, K.; Li, M.; Nelson, D. J.; Schuetz, J. D. & Naren, A. P. (2007). Spatiotemporal Coupling of Camp Transporter to Cftr Chloride Channel Function in the Gut Epithelia. *Cell*, 131, 5, pp. 940-951.

Li, J.; Dai, Z.; Jana, D.; Callaway, D. J. E. & Bu, Z. (2005). Ezrin Controls the Macromolecular Complexes Formed between an Adapter Protein Na+/H+ Exchanger Regulatory

Factor and the Cystic Fibrosis Transmembrane Conductance Regulator. *The Journal of Biological Chemistry*, 280, 45, pp. 37634-37643.

Li, J.; Poulikakos, P. I.; Dai, Z.; Testa, J. R.; Callaway, D. J. & Bu, Z. (2007). Protein Kinase C Phosphorylation Disrupts Na+/H+ Exchanger Regulatory Factor 1 Autoinhibition and Promotes Cystic Fibrosis Transmembrane Conductance Regulator Macromolecular Assembly. *The Journal of Biological Chemistry*, 282, 37, pp. 27086-27099.

Liedtke, C. M.; Yun, C. H. C.; Kyle, N. & Wang, D. (2002). Protein Kinase C(Epsilon)-Dependent Regulation of Cystic Fibrosis Transmembrane Regulator Involves Binding to a Receptor for Activated C Kinase (Rack1) and Rack1 Binding to Na+/H+ Exchange Regulatory Factor. *The Journal of Biological Chemistry*, 277, 25, pp. 22925-22933.

Liedtke, C. M.; Raghuram, V.; Yun, C. C. & Wang, X. (2004). Role of a Pdz1 Domain of Nherf1 in the Binding of Airway Epithelial Rack1 to Nherf1. *American Journal of Physiology - Cell Physiology*, 286, 5, pp. C1037-1044.

Lim, S.; Naisbitt, S.; Yoon, J.; Hwang, J. I.; Suh, P. G.; Sheng, M. & Kim, E. (1999). Characterization of the Shank Family of Synaptic Proteins. Multiple Genes, Alternative Splicing, and Differential Expression in Brain and Development. *The Journal of Biological Chemistry*, 274, 41, pp. 29510-29518.

Lohi, H.; Lamprecht, G.; Markovich, D.; Heil, A.; Kujala, M.; Seidler, U. & Kere, J. (2003). Isoforms of Slc26a6 Mediate Anion Transport and Have Functional Pdz Interaction Domains. *American Journal of Physiology - Cell Physiology*, 284, 3, pp. C769-779.

Loussouarn, G.; Demolombe, S.; Mohammad-Panah, R.; Escande, D. & Baro, I. (1996). Expression of Cftr Controls Camp-Dependent Activation of Epithelial K+ Currents. *American Journal of Physiology*, 271, 5 Pt 1, pp. C1565-1573.

Lukacs, G. L.; Chang, X. B.; Kartner, N.; Rotstein, O. D.; Riordan, J. R. & Grinstein, S. (1992). The Cystic Fibrosis Transmembrane Regulator Is Present and Functional in Endosomes. Role as a Determinant of Endosomal Ph. *The Journal of Biological Chemistry*, 267, 21, pp. 14568-14572.

Mickle, J. E.; Macek, M., Jr.; Fulmer-Smentek, S. B.; Egan, M. M.; Schwiebert, E.; Guggino, W.; Moss, R. & Cutting, G. R. (1998). A Mutation in the Cystic Fibrosis Transmembrane Conductance Regulator Gene Associated with Elevated Sweat Chloride Concentrations in the Absence of Cystic Fibrosis. *Human Molecular Genetics*, 7, 4, pp. 729-735.

Milewski, M. I.; Lopez, A.; Jurkowska, M.; Larusch, J. & Cutting, G. R. (2005). Pdz-Binding Motifs Are Unable to Ensure Correct Polarized Protein Distribution in the Absence of Additional Localization Signals. *FEBS letters*, 579, 2, pp. 483-487.

Mohler, P. J.; Kreda, S. M.; Boucher, R. C.; Sudol, M.; Stutts, M. J. & Milgram, S. L. (1999). Yes-Associated Protein 65 Localizes P62(C-Yes) to the Apical Compartment of Airway Epithelia by Association with Ebp50. *The Journal of Cell Biology*, 147, 4, pp. 879-890.

Moyer, B. D.; Denton, J.; Karlson, K. H.; Reynolds, D.; Wang, S.; Mickle, J. E.; Milewski, M.; Cutting, G. R.; Guggino, W. B.; Li, M. & Stanton, B. A. (1999). A Pdz-Interacting Domain in Cftr Is an Apical Membrane Polarization Signal. *The Journal of Clinical Investigation*, 104, 10, pp. 1353-1361.

Moyer, B. D.; Duhaime, M.; Shaw, C.; Denton, J.; Reynolds, D.; Karlson, K. H.; Pfeiffer, J.; Wang, S.; Mickle, J. E.; Milewski, M.; Cutting, G. R.; Guggino, W. B.; Li, M. & Stanton, B. A. (2000). The Pdz-Interacting Domain of Cystic Fibrosis Transmembrane Conductance Regulator Is Required for Functional Expression in the Apical Plasma Membrane. *The Journal of Biological Chemistry*, 275, 35, pp. 27069-27074.

Naren, A. P.; Cobb, B.; Li, C.; Roy, K.; Nelson, D.; Heda, G. D.; Liao, J.; Kirk, K. L.; Sorscher, E. J.; Hanrahan, J. & Clancy, J. P. (2003). A Macromolecular Complex of Beta 2 Adrenergic Receptor, Cftr, and Ezrin/Radixin/Moesin-Binding Phosphoprotein 50 Is Regulated by Pka. *Proceedings of the National Academy of Sciences of the United States of America*, 100, 1, pp. 342-346.

Neudauer, C. L.; Joberty, G. & Macara, I. G. (2001). Pist: A Novel Pdz/Coiled-Coil Domain Binding Partner for the Rho-Family Gtpase Tc10. *Biochemical and Biophysical Research Communications*, 280, 2, pp. 541-547.

Ostedgaard, L. S.; Randak, C.; Rokhlina, T.; Karp, P.; Vermeer, D.; Ashbourne Excoffon, K. J. & Welsh, M. J. (2003). Effects of C-Terminal Deletions on Cystic Fibrosis Transmembrane Conductance Regulator Function in Cystic Fibrosis Airway Epithelia. *Proceedings of the National Academy of Sciences of the United States of America*, 100, 4, pp. 1937-1942.

Paasche, J. D.; Attramadal, T.; Kristiansen, K.; Oksvold, M. P.; Johansen, H. K.; Huitfeldt, H. S.; Dahl, S. G. & Attramadal, H. (2005). Subtype-Specific Sorting of the Eta Endothelin Receptor by a Novel Endocytic Recycling Signal for G Protein-Coupled Receptors. *Molecular Pharmacology*, 67, 5, pp. 1581-1590.

Pasyk, E. A. & Foskett, J. K. (1995). Mutant (Delta F508) Cystic Fibrosis Transmembrane Conductance Regulator Cl- Channel Is Functional When Retained in Endoplasmic Reticulum of Mammalian Cells. *The Journal of Biological Chemistry*, 270, 21, pp. 12347-12350.

Pietrement, C.; Da Silva, N.; Silberstein, C.; James, M.; Marsolais, M.; Van Hoek, A.; Brown, D.; Pastor-Soler, N.; Ameen, N.; Laprade, R.; Ramesh, V. & Breton, S. (2008). Role of Nherf1, Cystic Fibrosis Transmembrane Conductance Regulator, and Camp in the Regulation of Aquaporin 9. *The Journal of Biological Chemistry*, 283, 5, pp. 2986-2996.

Piserchio, A.; Fellows, A.; Madden, D. R. & Mierke, D. F. (2005). Association of the Cystic Fibrosis Transmembrane Regulator with Cal: Structural Features and Molecular Dynamics. *Biochemistry*, 44, 49, pp. 16158-16166.

Ramjeesingh, M.; Kidd, J. F.; Huan, L. J.; Wang, Y. & Bear, C. E. (2003). Dimeric Cystic Fibrosis Transmembrane Conductance Regulator Exists in the Plasma Membrane. *Biochemical Journal*, 374, 3, pp. 793-797.

Reczek, D.; Berryman, M. & Bretscher, A. (1997). Identification of Ebp50: A Pdz-Containing Phosphoprotein That Associates with Members of the Ezrin-Radixin-Moesin Family. *The Journal of Cell Biology*, 139, 1, pp. 169-179.

Riordan, J. R.; Rommens, J. M.; Kerem, B.; Alon, N.; Rozmahel, R.; Grzelczak, Z.; Zielenski, J.; Lok, S.; Plavsic, N.; Chou, J. L. & Et Al. (1989). Identification of the Cystic Fibrosis Gene: Cloning and Characterization of Complementary DNA. *Science*, 245, 4922, pp. 1066-1073.

Rommens, J. M.; Iannuzzi, M. C.; Kerem, B.; Drumm, M. L.; Melmer, G.; Dean, M.; Rozmahel, R.; Cole, J. L.; Kennedy, D.; Hidaka, N. & Et Al. (1989). Identification of the Cystic Fibrosis Gene: Chromosome Walking and Jumping. *Science*, 245, 4922, pp. 1059-1065.

Salvatore, D.; Tomaiuolo, R.; Vanacore, B.; Elce, A.; Castaldo, G. & Salvatore, F. (2005). Isolated Elevated Sweat Chloride Concentrations in the Presence of the Rare Mutation S1455x: An Extremely Mild Form of Cftr Dysfunction. *American Journal of Medical Genetics*, 133A, 2, pp. 207-208.

Schreiber, R.; Greger, R.; Nitschke, R. & Kunzelmann, K. (1997). Cystic Fibrosis Transmembrane Conductance Regulator Activates Water Conductance in Xenopus Oocytes. *Pflügers Archiv European Journal of Physiology*, 434, 6, pp. 841-847.

Schreiber, R.; Nitschke, R.; Greger, R. & Kunzelmann, K. (1999). The Cystic Fibrosis Transmembrane Conductance Regulator Activates Aquaporin 3 in Airway Epithelial Cells. *The Journal of Biological Chemistry*, 274, 17, pp. 11811-11816.

Scott, R. O.; Thelin, W. R. & Milgram, S. L. (2002). A Novel Pdz Protein Regulates the Activity of Guanylyl Cyclase C, the Heat-Stable Enterotoxin Receptor. *The Journal of Biological Chemistry*, 277, 25, pp. 22934-22941.

Seidler, U.; Singh, A. K.; Cinar, A.; Chen, M.; Hillesheim, J.; Hogema, B. & Riederer, B. (2009). The Role of the Nherf Family of Pdz Scaffolding Proteins in the Regulation of Salt and Water Transport. *Annals of the New York Academy of Sciences*, 1165, pp. 249-260.

Shenolikar, S.; Minkoff, C. M.; Steplock, D. A.; Evangelista, C.; Liu, M. & Weinman, E. J. (2001). N-Terminal Pdz Domain Is Required for Nherf Dimerization. *FEBS letters*, 489, 2-3, pp. 233-236.

Short, D. B.; Trotter, K. W.; Reczek, D.; Kreda, S. M.; Bretscher, A.; Boucher, R. C.; Stutts, M. J. & Milgram, S. L. (1998). An Apical Pdz Protein Anchors the Cystic Fibrosis Transmembrane Conductance Regulator to the Cytoskeleton. *The Journal of Biological Chemistry*, 273, 31, pp. 19797-19801.

Singh, A. K.; Riederer, B.; Krabbenhã¶Ft, A.; Rausch, B.; Bonhagen, J.; Lehmann, U.; De Jonge, H. R.; Donowitz, M.; Yun, C.; Weinman, E. J.; Kocher, O.; Hogema, B. M. & Seidler, U. (2009). Differential Roles of Nherf1, Nherf2, and Pdzk1 in Regulating Cftr-Mediated Intestinal Anion Secretion in Mice. *The Journal of Clinical Investigation*, 119, 3, pp. 540-550.

Slattery, C.; Jenkin, K. A.; Lee, A.; Simcocks, A. C.; Mcainch, A. J.; Poronnik, P. & Hryciw, D. H. (2011). Na+-H+ Exchanger Regulatory Factor 1 (Nherf1) Pdz Scaffold Binds an Internal Binding Site in the Scavenger Receptor Megalin. *Cellular Physiology and Biochemistry*, 27, 2, pp. 171-178.

Stutts, M.; Canessa, C.; Olsen, J.; Hamrick, M.; Cohn, J.; Rossier, B. & Boucher, R. (1995). Cftr as a Camp-Dependent Regulator of Sodium Channels. *Science*, 269, 5225, pp. 847-850.

Sun, F.; Hug, M. J.; Lewarchik, C. M.; Yun, C. H.; Bradbury, N. A. & Frizzell, R. A. (2000). E3karp Mediates the Association of Ezrin and Protein Kinase a with the Cystic Fibrosis Transmembrane Conductance Regulator in Airway Cells. *The Journal of Biological Chemistry*, 275, 38, pp. 29539-29546.

Svennevig, K.; Prydz, K. & Kolset, S. O. (1995). Proteoglycans in Polarized Epithelial Madin-Darby Canine Kidney Cells. *Biochemical Journal*, 311 (Pt 3), pp. 881-888.

Swiatecka-Urban, A.; Duhaime, M.; Coutermarsh, B.; Karlson, K. H.; Collawn, J.; Milewski, M.; Cutting, G. R.; Guggino, W. B.; Langford, G. & Stanton, B. A. (2002). Pdz Domain

Interaction Controls the Endocytic Recycling of the Cystic Fibrosis Transmembrane Conductance Regulator. *The Journal of Biological Chemistry*, 277, 42, pp. 40099-40105.

Tabcharani, J. A.; Chang, X. B.; Riordan, J. R. & Hanrahan, J. W. (1991). Phosphorylation-Regulated Cl- Channel in Cho Cells Stably Expressing the Cystic Fibrosis Gene. *Nature*, 352, 6336, pp. 628-631.

Taouil, K.; Hinnrasky, J.; Hologne, C.; Corlieu, P.; Klossek, J.-M. & Puchelle, E. (2003). Stimulation of Î^{2}2-Adrenergic Receptor Increases Cystic Fibrosis Transmembrane Conductance Regulator Expression in Human Airway Epithelial Cells through a Camp/Protein Kinase a-Independent Pathway. *The Journal of Biological Chemistry*, 278, 19, pp. 17320-17327.

Van De Graaf, S.; Hoenderop, J.; Van Der Kemp, A.; Gisler, S. & Bindels, R. (2006). Interaction of the Epithelial Ca≪Sup≫2+≪/Sup≫ Channels Trpv5 and Trpv6 with the Intestine- and Kidney-Enriched Pdz Protein Nherf4. *Pflügers Archiv European Journal of Physiology*, 452, 4, pp. 407-417.

Wang, S.; Raab, R. W.; Schatz, P. J.; Guggino, W. B. & Li, M. (1998). Peptide Binding Consensus of the Nhe-Rf-Pdz1 Domain Matches the C-Terminal Sequence of Cystic Fibrosis Transmembrane Conductance Regulator (Cftr). *FEBS letters*, 427, 1, pp. 103-108.

Wang, S.; Yue, H.; Derin, R. B.; Guggino, W. B. & Li, M. (2000). Accessory Protein Facilitated Cftr-Cftr Interaction, a Molecular Mechanism to Potentiate the Chloride Channel Activity. *Cell*, 103, 1, pp. 169-179.

Watanabe, C.; Kato, Y.; Sugiura, T.; Kubo, Y.; Wakayama, T.; Iseki, S. & Tsuji, A. (2006). Pdz Adaptor Protein Pdzk2 Stimulates Transport Activity of Organic Cation/Carnitine Transporter Octn2 by Modulating Cell Surface Expression. *Drug Metabolism and Disposition*, 34, 11, pp. 1927-1934.

Wei, L.; Vankeerberghen, A.; Cuppens, H.; Eggermont, J.; Cassiman, J. J.; Droogmans, G. & Nilius, B. (1999). Interaction between Calcium-Activated Chloride Channels and the Cystic Fibrosis Transmembrane Conductance Regulator. *Pflügers Archiv European Journal of Physiology*, 438, 5, pp. 635-641.

Welsh, M. J.; Tsui, L. C.; Boat, T. M. & Beaudet, A. L. (1995). Cystic Fibrosis, In: *The Metabolic and Molecular Bases of Inherited Disease.*, Scriver, C. R., Beaudet, A. L., Sly, W. S. & Valle, D., pp. 3799-3876, McGraw-Hill, New-York, NY.

Wente, W.; Stroh, T.; Beaudet, A.; Richter, D. & Kreienkamp, H.-J. R. (2005). Interactions with Pdz Domain Proteins Pist/Gopc and Pdzk1 Regulate Intracellular Sorting of the Somatostatin Receptor Subtype 5. *The Journal of Biological Chemistry*, 280, 37, pp. 32419-32425.

Willoughby, D.; Wong, W.; Schaack, J.; Scott, J. D. & Cooper, D. M. F. (2006). An Anchored Pka and Pde4 Complex Regulates Subplasmalemmal Camp Dynamics. *EMBO Journal*, 25, 10, pp. 2051-2061.

Winpenny, J. P.; Mcalroy, H. L.; Gray, M. A. & Argent, B. E. (1995). Protein Kinase C Regulates the Magnitude and Stability of Cftr Currents in Pancreatic Duct Cells. *American Journal of Physiology - Cell Physiology*, 268, 4, pp. C823-C828.

Wolde, M.; Fellows, A.; Cheng, J.; Kivenson, A.; Coutermarsh, B.; Talebian, L.; Karlson, K.; Piserchio, A.; Mierke, D. F.; Stanton, B. A.; Guggino, W. B. & Madden, D. R. (2007). Targeting Cal as a Negative Regulator of Deltaf508-Cftr Cell-Surface Expression: An Rna Interference and Structure-Based Mutagenetic Approach. *The Journal of Biological Chemistry*, 282, 11, pp. 8099-8109.

Xu, Z.; Oshima, K. & Heller, S. (2010). Pist Regulates the Intracellular Trafficking and Plasma Membrane Expression of Cadherin 23. *BMC cell biology*, 11, pp. 80.

Yoo, D.; Flagg, T. P.; Olsen, O.; Raghuram, V.; Foskett, J. K. & Welling, P. A. (2004). Assembly and Trafficking of a Multiprotein Romk (Kir 1.1) Channel Complex by Pdz Interactions. *The Journal of Biological Chemistry*, 279, 8, pp. 6863-6873.

Zhang, J.; Cheng, S.; Xiong, Y.; Ma, Y.; Luo, D.; Jeromin, A.; Zhang, H. & He, J. (2008). A Novel Association of Mglur1a with the Pdz Scaffold Protein Cal Modulates Receptor Activity. *FEBS Letters*, 582, 30, pp. 4117-4124.

Zhang W., Penmatsa H., Ren A., Punchihewa C., Lemoff A., Yan B., Fujii N., Naren A.P. (2011). Functional regulation of cystic fibrosis transmembrane conductance regulator-containing macromolecular complexes: a small-molecule inhibitor approach. *Biochemical Journal*, 435(2), pp. 451-62.

16

CFTR Gene Transfer and Tracking the CFTR Protein in the Airway Epithelium

Gaëlle Gonzalez, Pierre Boulanger and Saw-See Hong
University of Lyon 1
France

1. Introduction

Cystic fibrosis (CF) is an autosomal recessive genetic disease caused by mutations in a single gene, the *cystic fibrosis transmembrane conductance regulator (CFTR)* gene. This disease primarily involves epithelial cells of the respiratory system, intestine, pancreas, gall bladder, and sweat glands. Although several organs are affected, the main cause of CF mortality and morbidity is due to pulmonary complications associated with impaired clearance and obstruction by viscous mucus secretions, which makes the lung epithelial cells the principle target for CF treatment. A monogenic disease such as CF was *a priori* an ideal candidate for gene therapy, as treatment of the disease was thought to be feasible with the introduction of the normal alleles of the *CFTR* gene into the airway epithelial cells to code for the functional protein.

2. CFTR gene transfer to the airway epithelium

The lung can be divided anatomically and physiologically into two regions, (i) the airways, consisting of the trachea, bronchi and bronchioles which brings air to the peripheral lung and (ii) the alveoli where the exchange of gas takes place. The airway epithelium is normally covered by a thin layer of mucus and acts as a natural barrier against foreign particles, including pathogens. In CF individuals, the airways are filled with sputum consisting of inflammatory cells, cell debris, highly viscous mucus and DNA, causing obstruction of the airways, constituting the major barrier for gene transfer as it prevents the cellular uptake of the vectors by the airway epithelial cells (Griesenbach, Alton et al., 2009; Hida et al., 2011).

The main target tissue for CF gene therapy is believed to be the airway epithelium, which exhibits all ion transport functions of CFTR and is easily accessible. However, the nature of the cells which are the best target for CF gene therapy is still debatable. The transfer of genes to the airway results in gene expression primarily in lung epithelial cells, and the transgene is localised to the lung without much systemic distribution. The highest level of CFTR gene expression is found in the bronchial submucosal gland cells (Merten et al., 1996; Kammouni et al., 1999; Chow et al., 2000) and it was suggested that these glandular cells may be better reached by vasculature and systemic application of the vector rather than by the airways (Boucher, 1999 ; Kolb et al., 2006).

There are several ways of introducing therapeutic genes into human cells but the most efficient method of gene transfer into human cells is by the use of viral vectors. Viruses have evolved and developed natural strategies to enter, transfer their genetic material and reproduce in specific tissues of their hosts, making them highly adapted as vectors to transfer genes into their natural target cells. Since 1989, twenty-nine clinical trials for CF have been carried out using adenovirus or adeno-associated virus vectors and non-viral vectors. In these gene therapy protocols, the major site of vector administration was the respiratory airways such as the nasal and lung epithelium. Unfortunately, the somewhat disappointing results of these clinical trials showed that CF gene therapy was more difficult than originally anticipated. The viral and non-viral vectors used in these trials revealed their limitations and inefficacy in gene transfer to the human airway epithelium.

2.1 Adenovirus (Ad) vector

The adenovirus as a gene transfer vector has several advantages over other vectors : (i) its capacity to incorporate large transgenes; (ii) its ease for genetic manipulation (Hong et al., 2003; Magnusson et al., 2007; Magnusson et al., 2001); and (iii) its facility to be produced to high titres. The efficiency of Ad vectors in gene transfer has been demonstrated in numerous systems (Henning et al., 2002; Gaden et al., 2004; Toh et al., 2005) and the functional analysis of transgenes expressed by Ad can be tested *in vitro* in cell lines, *ex vivo* in tissues and *in vivo* in animal models. *In vitro* studies demonstrated that recombinant Ad vectors can express CFTR in cultured CF airway epithelial cells and correct the Cl^- transport defect (Zabner et al., 1993). Following this, a number of *in vivo* studies in animals and in tracheal explants showed that Ad vectors can express CFTR as well as reporter genes in the airway epithelia (Rosenfeld et al., 1992; Harvey et al., 1999; Scaria et al., 1998).

Ten CF clinical trials involving Ad vectors were conducted during the period 1993-2001 (available in Clinical Trials website : http://www.wiley.com//legacy/wileychi/genmed/clinical/). The first Ad vector used in CF gene therapy trials involving CF patients was a serotype 2 (Ad2) vector, genetically modified in the E1 region to carry the CFTR cDNA, under the E1a promoter and had the same polyadenylation addition site as the E1b and pIX transcripts (Zabner et al., 1993). The results obtained from the early clinical trials with Ad vector administration in the nasal and pulmonary tissues showed that the Ad vectors were well-tolerated at low to intermediate doses in humans, and partially corrected the chloride transport (Zabner et al., 1993, Crystal, 1995; Welsh et al., 1995;).

One major difficulty which was revealed from the clinical trials was the inefficient *CFTR* gene transfer to the airway epithelium of CF patients (Perricone et al., 2001). It is known today that several factors were responsible for the low efficiency of *CFTR* gene transfer (Crystal, 1995): (*i*) the nonspecific inflammatory reactions (Otake et al., 1998) and immune response to the Ad-CFTR vector (Gahery-Segard et al., 1998 ; Piedra et al., 1998); (*ii*) the airway epithelial cells lack high affinity receptors for Ad (Zabner et al., 1997), as these receptors have a basolateral localization, which makes them inaccessible to Ad-CFTR vectors (Walters et al., 1999); (*iii*) mechanical factors, like bronchial mucus (Arcasoy et al., 1997 ; Perricone et al., 2000; Hida et al., 2011), or local bacterial infections, can negatively influence the effective binding of Ad vectors to the surface of epithelial cells, and the subsequent delivery of the therapeutic gene; (*iv*) a combination of the above different mechanisms, or/and intrinsic properties of differentiated airway epithelial cells (Gaden et al., 2002). Another hurdle encountered with Ad vectors was that gene transfer to the airway epithelia was transient and the use of recombinant adenovirus vectors would require repeated administration. The requirement for repeated vector administration is a major concern as this will generate neutralizing antibodies against the vector in gene therapy recipients which would subsequently reduce gene transfer efficacy.

2.2 Adeno-associated virus (AAV) vector

AAV gene transfer vectors have attracted much interest due to their good safety profile (no known pathology has been found to be associated with AAV in humans), broad tissue tropism and more importantly prolonged gene expression due to the integration of their DNA into the cellular genome. These vectors are thought to exhibit less inflammatory and immune reactions than the adenovirus. However, there are still technical problems concerning the small cloning capacity which could barely accommodate the *CFTR* gene (4.7 kb), and the difficulty in achieving high titers during AAV vector production.

Six CF gene therapy clinical trials using AAV vectors were carried out from 1999 - 2007 (Clinical Trials website : http://www.wiley.com//legacy/wileychi/genmed/clinical/). The first AAV-CFTR vector used showed physiological correction of chloride transport in nasal epithelial cells in gene therapy recipients, even in those with low CFTR mRNA expression (Wagner JA et al, 1999). The more recent clinical trials used the AAV vector, TgAAV-CFTR, developed by Targeted Genetics Corp, which carried the weak AAV long terminal repeat (LTR) promoter to drive CFTR gene expression (Griesenbach et al., 2009). The clinical data showed that repeated doses of aerosolised AAV-CFTR vector treatment did not result in significant therapeutic improvement (Moss et al., 2007). The reasons for these disappointing results could likely be that (i) AAV was inefficient in transducing airway epithelial cells via the apical membrane, (ii) the LTR promoter used to drive CFTR expression was too weak, or (iii) repeated administration of AAV to the lung resulted in the development of an anti-viral immune response (Griesenbach et al., 2009). In brief, the vector was well tolerated but there are still concerns about the toxicity and immunological responses related to the repeated administration of this vector. In addition, it was reported recently that insertional mutagenesis was observed in neonatal mice models treated with recombinant AAV vectors : the mice developed hepatocellular carcinoma which was associated with AAV vector integration (Dosante et al., 2007).

2.3 Non-viral vectors

Nine CF gene therapy clinical trials have been carried out using non-viral or synthetic vectors from 1995-2004 (Clinical Trials website : http://www.wiley.com//legacy /wileychi/genmed/clinical/). There are three main non-viral vector systems : cationic liposomes, DNA-polymer conjugates and naked DNA. Non-viral vectors have their limitations such as (i) low efficiency in gene transfer as compared to viral vectors, and (ii) loss of efficacy with repeated administrations. However, the major advantage of these vectors is that they are less immunogenic compared to Ad and AAV vectors. Their inefficacy is mainly due to intracellular barriers such as endosomal sequestration and cytoplasmic degradation, where Ca^{2+}-sensitive cytosolic nucleases restrict the half-life of DNA to 50-90 mins (Pollard et al., 2001). The nuclear membrane of non-dividing, airway epithelial cells constitutes another intracellular barrier as the nuclear entry of exogenous DNA occurs only in cells that are actively dividing (Ferrari et al., 2002).

To date, only cationic liposome-based systems have been tested in CF clinical trials. The first cationic liposome vector used was DC-Chol (3β{*N*-[*N'*,*N'*-dimethylaminoethane]carbamoyl} cholesterol) mixed with DOPE (dioleoylphosphatidyl ethanolamine), complexed to CFTR plasmid DNA, and administered to patients via the nose. Cationic liposomes facilitate gene transfer by their interaction with DNA via their positively charged side chains and enhancing fusion with the host cell membrane via the hydrophobic lipid portion. The results obtained were encouraging as partial restoration of CFTR function was observed. However, the transfection efficiency and the duration of expression would need to be increased for therapeutic benefit (Caplen et al., 1995). Improvements to non-viral vector gene transfer efficiency to the lung have been proposed by using DNA condensed to molecular conjugates carrying a 17 amino acid peptide ligand which targets the serpin-enzyme complex receptor expressed on the apical surface of airway epithelial cells (Ziady et al., 2002).

Recently, three non-viral gene transfer agents : (i) cationic liposome (GL67A), (ii) compacted DNA nanoparticle with polyethyleneglycol-substituted lysine 30-mer (NP) and, (iii) 25kDa-branched polyethyeneimine (PEI) were evaluated *in vivo* in a sheep lung model. The efficacy profile of these agents to deliver a plasmid carrying the CFTR cDNA to the ovine airway epithelium by aerosol administration was compared. The results showed that GL67A was overall the best gene transfer agent for aerosol delivery to the sheep lung, and was selected for clinical trials in CF patients (McLachlan et al., 2011). In an ongoing clinical trial by the UK CF Gene Therapy Consortium and funded by the CF Trust, CF patients were given a single dose of a plasmid carrying the CFTR cDNA, complexed to the cationic lipid GL67A. This initial single-dose clinical trial will assess the safety and duration of CFTR expression in patients. Another clinical trial is planned for to determine whether repeated non-viral CFTR gene transfer (12 doses over 12 months) will improve CF lung disease (Sinn et al., 2011).

3. Tracking the CFTR in cells using GFP-CFTR fusion protein

The green fluorescent protein (GFP) is a 27-kDa protein from the jellyfish *Aequorea victoria*, discovered by Shimomura and co-workers in the 1960's and was shown to emit bright green fluorescence under UV light (Shimomura et al., 1962). It took another 30 years before this protein was cloned and its functionality demonstrated in different organisms (Prasher et al., 1994 ; Chalfie et al. 1994; Inouye and Tsuji 1994 ; Tsien, 1998). The GFP is widely used today as a biological marker in cell biology and gene transfer technology. The GFP can be detected in living cells without selection or staining, and be genetically fused to other proteins to produce fluorescent chimeras and generally does not alter the function or cellular localization of the fusion protein (Gerdes and Kaether, 1996 ; Lippincott-Schwartz and Smith, 1997). It is used as a reporter protein for studying complex biological processes such as organelle dynamics and protein trafficking. In gene transfer experiments, the GFP serves an *in vivo* marker, allowing for the determination of gene transfer efficiency and for selection of cells positive for the transgene. Other applications of GFP in gene therapy involve the use of GFP-tagged therapeutic proteins to determine the site, level and duration of expression, or for the correlation between gene transfer efficiency and therapeutic outcome (Wahlfors et al., 2001).

3.1 Construction and *in vitro* applications of GFP-CFTR

The CFTR protein is a 1,480 residue glycosylated molecule with 12 transmembrane domains and 3 intracytoplasmic domains (Figure 1). The protein is highly glycosylated at two asparagine residues on the extracellular loop 4, in both the immature and mature-glycosylated forms (Sheppard and Welsh, 1999). The immature CFTR has a high content of oligosaccharides of the mannoside type, and exists in the endoplasmic reticulum as a precursor before its transit to the trans-Golgi network. During the transit, the CFTR is processed into its mature form with the addition of complex carbohydrate chains containing polylactosaminoglycan sequences (O'Riordan et al., 2000). A functional CFTR requires the protein to be fully glycosylated, and its function as a chloride channel in epithelial cells is dependent on its cellular trafficking and transport to the apical membrane.

The first direct visualization of the CFTR protein within cells was made possible by the genetic fusion of the green fluorescent protein (GFP) to the N-terminus of the CFTR protein. The choice of adding the GFP-tag at the N-terminus (Figure 1) was such that it would have minimal interference with the membrane-targeting signal thought to be encoded in the C-terminus of the protein (Milewski et al., 2001; Moyer et al., 1998). Functional and cell trafficking studies of the CFTR protein and its mutants were made possible with the expression of the GFP-fused protein in different cell lines, using expression plasmids (Moyer et al., 1999; Loffing-Cueni et al., 2001; Haggie, Stanton, and Verkman, 2002). The GFP-CFTR fusion construct displayed functionality in terms of apical membrane localisation in Madin-Darby Canine Kidney (MDCK) cells. Short circuit current measurements showed that the protein mediated cAMP-activated transepithelial chloride transport across monolayers of stably transfected MDCK cells (Moyer et al., 1998). Studies of the dynamics of CFTR protein responses to bacterial infections, the manner by which the CFTR protein responds to, interacts with, and mediates translocation of *P. aeruginosa* and serovar *S. typhi* from the cell surface into the cell were also done using a GFP-CFTR fused protein (Gerçeker et al., 2000).

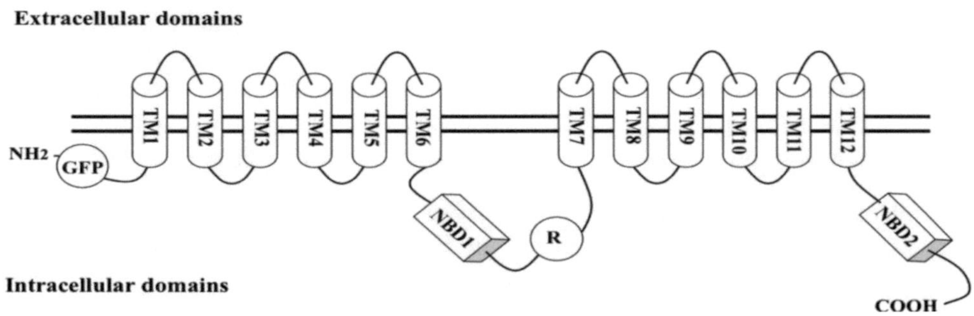

Fig. 1. Schematic representation of the GFP-CFTR fusion protein and the topology of the different domains. The GFP is located on the N-terminus of the CFTR protein. GFP, green fluorescent protein ; TM, transmembrane domain ; NBD1, nucleotide binding domain 1 ; NBD2, nucleotide binding domain 2 ; R, regulatory domain ; NH2, protein aminoterminus ; COOH, protein carboxyterminus.

3.2 *Ex vivo* applications of GFP-CFTR

The GFP-CFTR fusion constructs have also been inserted into viral vectors such as Adenovirus (Vais, 2004; Granio et al., 2007; Granio et al., 2010) and Sendai virus (Ban et al., 2007) to facilitate the detection and direct tracking of the protein after gene transfer. When the Ad vectors, Ad5-GFP-CFTR and Ad5-GFP-CFTRΔF508, were used to transduce reconstituted airway epithelium from ΔF508 CF patients, the biologically active GFP-CFTR and the mutant GFP-CFTRΔF508 proteins could be directly tracked in the epithelial cells by confocal fluorescence microscopy due to their GFP-tag (Granio et al., 2007 ; see Figure 2, A and B). The GFP-CFTR protein (green) was observed to be located on the apical membrane of the reconstituted airway epithelium, at the same plane as the ZO-1 protein (red) which is the marker for tight junctions at the apical membrane. The nuclei of the cells were stained blue with DAPI (Figure 2, A and B). In epithelial cells infected with the Ad5 expressing the GFP-CFTRΔF508, the fluorescence was observed in the central and basal areas of the cytoplasm and none expressed at the apical surface (Figures 2, B and D). This was the first report showing the direct localization of an exogenous GFP-tagged CFTR protein on reconstituted human epithelial cells after Ad-mediated gene transfer (Granio et al., 2007).

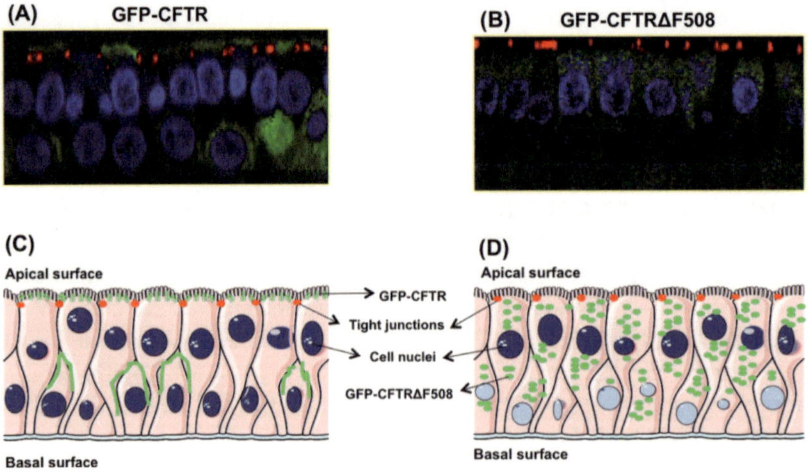

Fig. 2. Cellular localisation of the GFP-CFTR and GFP-CFTRΔF508 protein in *ex vivo* reconstituted human airway epithelium after gene transfer with Ad5-GFP-CFTR (A) and Ad5-GFP-CFTRΔF508 (B). (A), (B) : reconstructed images of sagittal sections of transduced epithelia generated from the z-stack images obtained in confocal fluorescence microscopy. (C), (D) : schematic representation of the images shown in (A) and (B), respectively.

The availability of appropriate cell receptors at the apical surface of airway epithelial cells is a crucial factor for the efficient uptake of viral vectors. A majority of viral vectors such as Adenovirus, AAV, Measles virus and pseudotyped retroviruses can only infect airway epithelial cells via the basal membrane (Kremer et al., 2007; Sinn et al., 2002; Teramoto et al., 1998; Zabner et al., 1997). Airway epithelial cells are not easily transduced by Ad5-based vectors as the Coxsackie-Adenovirus Receptor (CAR), a high affinity receptor for Ad5 and many other Ad serotypes vectors are mainly localised in the tight junctions and not at the apical surface (Walters et al., 1999), and thus not accessible to Ad vectors. One strategy of overcoming this physical barrier was to design an Ad vector which will recognise a receptor expressed on the apical surface of airway epithelium. The Ad serotype 35 (Ad35) or a chimeric Ad5F35 vector (a serotype 5 capsid carrying serotype 35 fibers), which both recognise CD46 as receptor, a molecule found on the apical surface of human airway epithelium (Gaggar, Shayakhmetov, and Lieber, 2003; Sinn et al., 2002; Corjon et al., 2011) would be capable of directly infecting the airway epithelia from the apical membrane .

The demonstration was recently made with a chimeric Ad5F35 vector expressing GFP-CFTR. This chimeric vector transduced efficiently well-differentiated human airway epithelium via the apical membrane and showed stable expression of the GFP-CFTR protein. Measurements of transepithelial ion transport showed the correction of the chloride channel function at relatively low vector doses in ΔF508 CF airway epithelial cells (Granio et al., 2010). This is a successful example of a viral vector which was genetically modified to target a receptor on the apical surface of the airway epithelial cells for efficient gene transduction. In a separate study using an *in vivo* mice model, the Ad5F35 vector was found to preferentially target the lungs of CD46-transgenic mice after systemic administration of the vector (Greig et al., 2009). The chimeric Ad5F35 vector therefore shows promise as an efficient lung targeted gene transfer vector for CF.

3.3 *In vivo* applications of GFP-CFTR

A study was conducted to determine whether a GFP-CFTR fusion protein was functional as a transgene when expressed *in vivo*, in colonic and airway epithelial cells of CF mice, and had the capacity to correct the CF defect. To assess the *in vivo* function of the GFP-CFTR, bitransgenic mice *cftr ~Ss1D/~551D KI8-GFP-CFTR +/-* were obtained by breeding K 18-GFP-CFTR mice to *cftr c551D/c551D* CF mice. The analysis of transcripts, protein and electrolyte transport in the colon and airways indicated that the K18-GFP-CFTR was expressed and partially restored the ion transport in the G551D CF mice model. Thus, it appeared that *in vivo*, the GFP-CFTR fusion protein was capable of supporting the complex interactions required to regulate epithelial chloride transport (Oceandy et al., 2003).

4. Development of new vectors for CFTR transfer

4.1 Human parainfluenza virus

The human parainfluenza virus type 3 (PIV3) can infect the human airway epithelium and specifically targets ciliated epithelial cells (Zhang et al., 2005). *In vitro* studies using PIV3-based vectors for *CFTR* gene transfer to CF epithelial cells resulted in the complete reversal of the CF phenotype, with the transepithelial ion transport, airway surface liquid volume regulation and mucus transport, restored to levels observed in non-CF epithelial cells (Zhang et al., 2009). *In vivo* administration of a PIV3 vector carrying a transgene coding for the rhesus α-fetoprotein (rhAFP) to the nasal epithelium of the rhesus macaque (*Macaca mulatta*) showed expression and secretion of the rhAFP in the mucosal and serosal compartments. The transgene expression was transient and paralleled vector persistance, suggesting that as PIV3 was cleared, rhAFP expression was lost (Zhang et al., 2010). The specificity of the PIV3 vectors for the airways make them particularly interesting as gene transfer vectors for CF therapy.

4.2 Respiratory syncytial virus

The respiratory syncytial virus (RSV) can infect the lungs of CF patients, despite the physical barriers of the respiratory tract, such as the sticky and mucus-rich environment of the CF lung. In addition, this virus has a natural tropism for the luminal ciliated cells of the airways (Zhang et al., 2002). It was suggested that since RSV has the capacity for reinfections, repeated administrations of an RSV-based vector would be possible. Recently, it was demonstrated that a RSV vector carrying the *CFTR* gene can infect both non-CF and CF airway epithelium, and in particular the ciliated cells. In CF cells, the CFTR was expressed at the apical surface and showed correction of chloride channel activity which was equivalent in level observed in normal human airway epithelial cultures. Further studies in animal models are needed to determine the immune response to this vector, as well as its persistence in single and repeated administration (Kwilas et al., 2010).

4.3. Integrative vectors

The major goal of gene therapy is to have the delivered transgene safely and stably maintained in replicating cells. One approach to achieve genetic stability is via integration of the transgene into the host cell genome, using integrating vectors such as retrovirus and AAV vectors. The main dangers of integrative vectors are their uncontrolled or random integration which can cause (i) transgene silencing if the insertion occurs in condensed heterochromatin, or (ii) insertional mutagenesis if the integration event occurs near growth-promoting genes leading to oncogenesis. The latter was encountered with lentivirus and AAV vectors, in animal models as well as in human clinical trials (Donsante et al., 2007; Hacein-Bey-Abina S, 2003).

Just as for Ad vectors, lentiviral gene transfer to the human airway epithelium is inefficient due to the lack of receptors. The strategy of ''pseudotyping'' or substitution of the lentivirus envelope with the envelope protein of another virus, such as Ebola virus (Kobinger et al., 2003), baculovirus (Sinn et al., 2008) or Sendai virus (Mitomo et al., 2010) have demonstrated increase in gene transfer efficiency to the airway epithelium. Before the application of lentiviral vectors for pulmonary gene transfer, preclinical studies in large animal models will need to be carried out to carefully assess their efficacy and safety.

4.4 Episomal vectors

Extrachromosomal or episomal vectors are gene transfer agents which has the capacity of persisting in the nucleus of transduced cells without integrating into the host genome. Due to their nonintegrative nature, there is theoretically no risk of the physical disruption of the cell genome. In addition, episomal vectors can persist in multiple copies per cell, resulting in high expression of the therapeutic gene (Lufino, Edser, and Wade-Martins, 2009). Many of the episomal systems which has been developed are based on sequences derived from viruses such as the Epstein-Barr and Polyoma viruses, which have certain phases of their viral life cycle maintained episomally. The two major requirements of episomal vectors are the presence of a viral origin of replication and the expression of a virally encoded protein which is necessary for vector replication and its repartition into the daughter cells upon cell division.

4.4.1 Polyoma-derived episomal vectors

The first stable episomal plasmid vector described in the literature contained sequences derived from the BK virus which belongs to the polyomavirus family. This episomal vector which carried most of the BK viral genome could persist at a stable copy number of 20–120 copies/cell, depending on the cell line used, and showed low percentage of integration events (Milanesi et al., 1984). Its replication depended on the presence of the BK-derived origin of replication and a *trans*activating factor, a viral protein called large T antigen, which is responsible for binding to the viral origin of replication and mediating the vector replication. Replicating vectors based on Simian Vacuolating virus 40 (SV40) were among the first viral-based episomal systems to be developed. SV40 is a nonenveloped DNA virus with a double-stranded genome belonging to the family of polyomaviruses (Vera and Fortes, 2004). The SV40-derived vectors are composed of a *cis*-acting elements, essentially the SV40 origin of replication, and the sequence encoding for the SV40 T antigen.

4.4.2 Epstein-Barr-derived episomal vector

The major progress toward the development of an efficient episomal gene transfer vector came from plasmids based on the Epstein-Barr virus (EBV), a member of the family of herpesviruses. The EBV is capable of life-long persistence as an extrachromosomal, circular multicopy plasmid carried by B-lymphocytes in a latent state (Lindahl et al., 1976). The origin of replication (*oriP,* origin of plasmid replication) of EBV requires the *trans*-acting factor EBV Nuclear Antigen-1 (EBNA-1) for replication (Rawlins et al., 1985; Yates, Warren, and Sugden, 1985). The EBNA-1 binds to metaphase chromosomes and interphase chromatin, and this interaction facilitates the partition of *oriP* plasmids into daughter cells during mitosis (Ito et al., 2002). Plasmid constructs containing EBV episomal elements have been tested in pre-clinical animal models for treatment of diseases such as hemophilia and diabetes. The delivery of the EBV-based episomes were made by injections to the target tissues. Although the efficacy of transduction was less efficient *in vivo* compared to viral vectors, long term expression of the therapeutic gene was obtained (Mei et al., 2006 ; Yoo et al., 2006).

4.4.3 Adeno-EBV hybrid episomal vector

A hybrid Adenovirus-EBV (Ad-EBV) episomal vector has a major interest as it exploits the advantages of both vectors, combining the efficiency of gene transfer of the Ad vector with the episomal replicative nature of the EBV vector. Helper-dependent adenovirus (HD-Ad) vectors which are deleted of all viral coding regions, also known as gutless Ad, (Kochanek et al., 1996 ; Parks et al., 1996), are also interesting vectors as they are less immunogenic. The use of HD-Ad vectors for the development of episomal Ad-EBV vector brings further advantage to these vectors for their use in gene therapy.

Circular replicating Ad-EBV vectors can be obtained by co-infecting an adenovirus carrying EBNA-1 and *oriP* elements with a *loxP* site at both ends, with a second adenovirus encoding Cre recombinase, whose expression will result in the circularisation of the first virus (Dorigo et al., 2004; Gallaher et al., 2009). Another strategy described for obtaining circular Ad episomes which does not rely on the expression of a viral protein such as EBNA-1, was based on the human origin of replication derived from the *lamin B2* locus with the site-specific FLPe recombinase and *Frt* recognition sites. This vector system produces circular episomes free of viral coding or bacterial DNA sequences (Kreppel and Kochanek, 2004). A more recent study described the development of an HD-Ad-EBV vector in which Cre recombinase is transiently expressed from a hepatocyte-specific promoter such that the vector generation and transgene expression are tissue specific. The results obtained using this strategy were highly promising as long-term persistence of the circularized vector DNA and stable transgene expression in hepatocytes was observed in immunocompetent mice (Gil et al., 2010).

5. Conclusions

Profitable lessons have been drawn from the past two decades of CF gene therapy trials using different transfer vectors. The numerous difficulties and problems encoutered have helped in the improvement and design of future gene transfer vectors. New viral vectors such as RSV and PIV which specifically targets cilliated lung epithelial cells have been developed for pulmonary gene transfer. Significant improvement have been made for high-density Ad episomal vectors to achieve efficiency and specificity of transduction, coupled to long-term vector persistance and stable transgene expression. In parallel, the GFP has served as a very useful *in vivo* marker for the evaluation of gene transfer vectors. The visualization of CFTR protein *in situ* by means of the GFP fluorescent tag has contributed towards a better comprehension of CFTR multiple functions such as its cellular trafficking and the dynamics of its interactions with intracellular as well as extracellular partners.

6. Acknowledgments

The authors are grateful to the French Cystic Fibrosis Foundation (Vaincre la Mucoviscidose, VLM) and the University of Lyon 1 for their support. GG is financially supported by a doctoral fellowship from VLM. SSH is an INSERM Research Associate. PB is Emeritus Professor of the University of Lyon 1.

7. References

Arcasoy, S.M., Latoche, J., Gondor, M., Watkins, S. C., Henderson, A., Hughey, R., Finn, O.J., & Pilewski, J.M. (1997). MUC1 and other sialoglycoconjugates inhibit adenovirus-mediated gene transfer to epithelial cells. *Am. J. Respir. Cell Mol. Biol.* 17, 422-435.

Ban, H., Inoue, M., Griesenbach, U., Munkonge, F., Chan, M., Iida, A., Alton, E.W.F. W., & Hasegawa, M. (2007). Expression and maturation of Sendai virus vector-derived CFTR protein: functional and biochemical evidence using a GFP-CFTR fusion protein. *Gene Ther.* 14, 1688-1694.

Boucher, R. C. (1999). Status of gene therapy for cystic fibrosis lung disease. *J. Clin. Invest.* 103, 441-445.

Caplen, N.J., Alton, E.W., Middleton, P.G., Dorin, J.R., Stevenson, B.J., Gao, X., Durham, S.R., Jeffery, P.K., Hodson, M.E., Coutelle, C., Huang, L., Porteous, D.J., Williamson,

R., & Geddes, D.M. (1995). Liposome-mediated CFTR gene transfer to the nasal epithelium of patients with cystic fibrosis. *Nat. Med.* 1, 39–46

Chalfie, M., Tu, Y., Euskirchen, G., Ward, W.W. & Prasher, D.C. (1994). Green fluorescent protein as a marker for gene expression. *Science* 263, 802-805.

Chow, Y.H., Plumb, J., Wen, Y., Steer, B.M., Lu, Z., Buchwald, M., & Hu, J. (2000). Targeting transgene expression to airway epithelia and submucosal glands, prominent sites of human CFTR expression. *Mol. Ther.* 2, 359-367.

Corjon, S., Gonzalez, G., Henning, P., Grichine, A., Lindholm, L., Boulanger, P., Fender, P. & Hong, S.S. (2011). Cell entry and trafficking of human adenovirus bound to blood factor X is determined by the fiber serotype and not hexon:heparan sulfate interaction. *PLoS One*, 6, e18205.

Crystal, R. G. (1995). Transfer of genes to humans: early lessons and obstacles to success. *Science* 270, 404-410.

Donsante, A., Miller, D.G., Li, Y., Vogler, C., Brunt, E. M., Russell, D.W., & Sands, M.S. (2007). AAV vector integration sites in mouse hepatocellular carcinoma. *Science* 317, 477.

Dorigo, O., Gil, J. S., Gallaher, S.D., Tan, B.T., Castro, M.G., Lowenstein, P.R., Calos, M. P., & Berk, A.J. (2004). Development of a novel helper-dependent adenovirus-Epstein-Barr virus hybrid system for the stable transformation of mammalian cells. *J. Virol.* 78, 6556-6566.

Ferrari, S., Geddes, D.M., & Alton, E.W.F.W. (2002). Barriers to and new approaches for gene therapy and gene delivery in cystic fibrosis. *Adv. Drug Deliv. Rev.* 54, 1373-1393.

Gaden, F., Franqueville, L., Hong, S.S., Legrand, V., Figarella, C., & Boulanger, P. (2002). Mechanism of restriction of normal and cystic fibrosis transmembrane conductance regulator-deficient human tracheal gland cells to adenovirus infection and ad-mediated gene transfer. *Am. J. Respir. Cell Mol. Biol.* 27, 628-640.

Gaden, F., Franqueville, L., Magnusson, M.K., Hong, S.S., Merten, M.D., Lindholm, L., & Boulanger, P. (2004). Gene transduction and cell entry pathway of fiber-modified adenovirus type 5 vectors carrying novel endocytic peptide ligands selected on human tracheal glandular cells. *J. Virol.* 78, 7227-7247.

Gaggar, A., Shayakhmetiv, D.M., & Lieber, A. (2003). CD46 is a cellular receptor for group B adenoviruses. *Nat. Med.* 9, 1408-1412.

Gahery-Segard, H., Farace, F., Godfrin, D., Gaston, J., Lengagne, R., Tursz, T., Boulanger, P., & Guillet, J. G. (1998). Immune response to recombinant capsid proteins of adenovirus in humans: antifiber and anti-penton base antibodies have a synergistic effect on neutralizing activity. *J. Virol.* 72, 2388-2397.

Gallaher, S.D., Gil, J.S., Dorigo, O., & Berk, A.J. (2009). Robust in vivo transduction of a genetically stable Epstein-Barr virus episome to hepatocytes in mice by a hybrid viral vector. *J. Virol.* 83, 3249-3257.

Gerçeker, A.A., Zaidi, T., Marks, P., Golan, D.E., & Pier, G.B. (2000). Impact of heterogeneity within cultured cells on bacterial invasion: analysis of *Pseudomonas aeruginosa* and *Salmonella enterica* Serovar Typhi entry into MDCK cells by using green fluorescent protein-labelled cystic fibrosis transmembrane conductance regulator receptor. *Infect. Immun.* 68, 861-870.

Gerdes, H.H., & Kaether, C. (1996). Green fluorescent protein: applications in cell biology. *FEBS Lett.* 389, 44-47.

Gil, J.S., Gallaher, S.D., & Berk, A.J. (2010). Delivery of an EBV episome by a self-circularizing helper-dependent adenovirus: long-term transgene expression in immunocompetent mice. *Gene Ther.* 17, 1288-1293.

Granio, O., Ashbourne Excoffon, K.J.D., Henning, P., Melin, P., Norez, C., Gonzalez, G., Karp, P.H., Magnusson, M.K., Habib, N., Lindholm, L., Becq, F., Boulanger, P., Zabner, J., & Hong, S.S. (2010). Adenovirus 5-fiber 35 chimeric vector mediates efficient apical correction of the cystic fibrosis transmembrane conductance regulator defect in cystic fibrosis primary airway epithelia. *Hum. Gene Ther.* 21, 251-269.

Granio, O., Norez, C., Ashbourne Excoffon, K.J.D., Karp, P.H., Lusky, M., Becq, F., Boulanger, P., Zabner, J., & Hong, S.S. (2007). Cellular localization and activity of Ad-delivered GFP-CFTR in airway epithelial and tracheal cells. *Am. J. Respir. Cell Mol. Biol.* 37, 631-639.

Greig, J.A., Buckley, S.M., Waddington, S.N., Parker, A.L., Bhella, D., Pink, R., Rahim, A.A., Morita, T., Nicklin, S.A., McVey, J.H., & Baker, A.H. (2009). Influence of coagulation factor X on in vitro and in vivo gene delivery by adenovirus (Ad) 5, Ad35, and chimeric Ad5/Ad35 vectors. *Mol. Ther.* 17, 1683-1691.

Griesenbach, U., Alton, E.W.F.W., & Consortium., o. b. o. t. U. C. F. G. T. (2009). Gene transfer to the lung: Lessons learned from more than 2 decades of CF gene therapy. *Adv. Drug Del. Rev.* 61, 128-139.

Griesenbach, U., Geddes, D.M., & Alton, E.W.F.W. (2004). Gene therapy for cystic fibrosis: an example for lung gene therapy. *Gene Therapy* 11, S43-S50.

Hacein-Bey-Abina, S., Von Kalle C., Schmidt, M., McCormack, M.P., Wulffraat, N., Leboulch, P., Lim, A., Osborne, C.S., Pawliuk, R., Morillon, E., Sorensen, R., Forster, A., Fraser, P., Cohen, J.I., de Saint Basile, G., Alexander, I., Wintergerst, U., Frebourg, T., Aurias, A., Stoppa-Lyonnet, D., Romana, S., Radford-Weiss, I., Gross, F., Valensi, F., Delabesse, E., Macintyre, E., Sigaux, F., Soulier, J., Leiva, L.E., Wissler, M., Prinz, C., Rabbitts, T.H., Le Deist, F., Fischer, A., & Cavazzana-Calvo, M. (2003). LMO2-associated clonal T cell proliferation in two patients after gene therapy for SCID-X1. *Science* 302, 415-419.

Haggie, P.M., Stanton, B.A., & Verkman, A.S. (2002). Diffusional mobility of the cystic fibrosis transmembrane conductance regulator mutant, dF508-CFTR, in the endoplasmic reticulum measured by photobleaching of GFP-CFTR chimeras. *J. Biol. Chem.* 277, 16419-16425.

Harvey, B.G., Leopold, P.L., Hackett, N.R., Grasso, T.M., Williams, P.M., Tucker, A.L., Kaner, R.J., Ferris, B., Gonda, I., Sweeney, T.D., Ramalingam, R., Kovesdi, I., Shak, S., & Crystal, R.G. (1999). Airway epithelual CFTR mRNA expression in cystic fibrosis patients after repetitive administration of a recombinant adenovirus. *J. Clin. Invest.* 104, 1245-1255.

Henning, P., Magnusson, M.K., Gunneriusson, E., Hong, S.S., Boulanger, P., Nygren, P. A., & Lindholm, L. (2002). Genetic modification of Ad5 tropism by a novel class of ligands based on a three-helix bundle scaffold derived from staphylococcal protein A. *Hum. Gene Ther.* 13, 1427-1439.

Hida, K., Lai, S. K., Suk, J.S., Won, S.Y., Boyle, M.P., & Hanes, J. (2011). Common gene therapy viral vectors do not efficiently penetrate sputum from cystic fibrosis patients. *PLoS One* 6(5), e19919.

Hong, S.S., Magnusson, M.K., Henning, P., Lindholm, L., & Boulanger, P. (2003). Adenovirus (Ad) stripping: a novel method to generate liganded Ad vectors with new cell target specificity. *Mol. Ther.* 7, 692-699.

Inouye, S. & Tsuji, F.I. (1994). *Aequorea* green fluorescent protein. Expression of the gene and fluorescence characteristics of the recombinant protein. *FEBS Lett.* 341, 277-280.

Ito, S., Gotoh, E., Ozawa, S., & Yanagi, K. (2002). Epstein-Barr virus nuclear antigen-1 is highly colocalized with interphase chromatin and its newly replicated regions in particular. *J. Gen. Virol.* 83, 2377-2383.

Kammouni, W., Moreau, B., Becq, F., Saleh, A., Pavirani, A., Figarella, C., & Merten, M.D. (1999). A cystic fibrosis tracheal gland cell line, CF-KM4. Correction by adenovirus-mediated CFTR gene transfer. *Am. J. Respir. Cell Mol. Biol.* 20, 684-691.

Kobinger, G.P., Schumer, G.P., Medina, M.F., Weiner, D.J. & Wilson, J.M. (2003). Stable and efficient gene transfer in airway of non-human primates with HIV vector pseudotyped with deletion mutant of the Ebola envelope glycoproteins. *Pediatr. Pulmonol. Suppl.* 25, 256.

Kochanek, S., Clemens, P.R., Mitani, K., Chen, H.H., Chan, S., & Caskey, C.T. (1996). A new adenoviral vector: replacement of all viral coding sequences with 28 kb of DNA independently expressing both full-length dystrophin and beta-galactosidase. *Proc. Natl. Acad. Sci. USA* 93, 5731-5736.

Kolb, M., Martin, G., Medina, M., Ask, K., & Gauldie, J. (2006). Gene therapy for pulmonary diseases. *Chest* 130, 879-884.

Kremer, K.L., Dunning, K.R., Parsons, D.W., & Anson, D.S. (2007). Gene delivery to airway epithelial cells in vivo: a direct comparison of apical and basolateral transduction strategies using pseudotyped lentivirus vectors. *J. Gene Med.* 9, 362-368.

Kreppel, F., & Kochanek, S. (2004). Long-term transgene expression in proliferating cells mediated by episomally maintained high-capacity adenovirus vectors. *J. Virol.* 78, 9-22.

Kwilas, A.R., Yednak, M.A., Zhang, L., Liesman, R., Collins, P.L., Pickles, R.J. & Peeples, M.E. (2010). Respiratory syncytial virus engineered to express the cystic fibrosis transmembrane conductance regulator corrects the bioelectric phenotype of human cystic fibrosis airway epithelium *in vitro*. *J. Virol.* 84, 7770-7781.

Lindahl, T., Adams, A., Bjursell, G., Bornkamm, G.W., Kasch-Dierich, C., & Jehn, U. (1976). Covalently closed circular duplex DNA of Epstein-Barr virus in a human lymphoid cell line. *J. Mol. Biol.* 102, 511-530.

Lippincott-Schwartz, J., & Smith, C.L. (1997). Insights into secretory and endocytic membrane traffic using fluorescent protein chimeras. *Curr. Opin. Neurobiol.* 7, 631-639.

Loffing-Cueni, D., Loffing, J., Shaw, C., Taplin, A.M., Govindan, M., Stanton, C.A., & Stanton, B.A. (2001). Trafficking of GFP-tagged dF508-CFTR to the plasma membrane in a polarized epithelial cell line. *Am. J. Physiol. Cell Physiol.* 281, C1889-C1897.

Lufino, M.M.P., Edser, P.A.H., & Wade-Martins, R. (2009). Advances in high-capacity extrachromosomal vector technology: episomal maintenance, vector delivery and transgene expression. *Mol. Ther.* 16, 1525-1538.

Magnusson, M.K., Henning, P., Myhre, S., Wikman, M., Uil, T. G., Friedman, M., Andersson, K.M.E., Hong, S.S., Hoeben, R.C., Habib, N.A., Stahl, S., Boulanger, P., & Lindholm, L. (2007). An Ad5 vector genetically re-targeted by an AffibodyTM molecule with specificity for tumor antigen HER2/neu. *Cancer Gene Ther.* 14, 468-479.

Magnusson, M.K., Hong, S.S., Boulanger, P., & Lindholm, L. (2001). Genetic re-targeting of adenovirus: a novel strategy employing 'de-knobbing' of the fiber. *J. Virol.* 75, 7280-7289.

McLachlan, G., Davidson, H., Holder, E., Davies, L.A., Pringle, I.A., Sumner-Jones, S.G., Baker, A., Tennant, P., Gordon, C., Vrettou, C., Blundell, R., Hyndman, L., Stevenson, B., Wilson, A., Doherty, A., Shaw, D.J., Coles, R.L., Painter, H., Cheng, S.H., Scheule, R.K., Davies, J.C., Innes, J.A., Hyde, S.C., Griesenbach, U., Alton, E.W., Boyd, A.C., Porteous, D.J., Gill, D.R., & Collie, D.D. Pre-clinical evaluation of three non-viral gene transfer agents for cystic fibrosis after aerosol delivery to the ovine lung. (2011). *Gene Ther.* Epub ahead of print, doi:10.1038/gt.2011.55

Mei, W. H., Qian, G. X., Zhang, X. Q., Zhang, P., and Lu, J. (2006). Sustainied expression of Epstein-Barr virus episomal vector mediated factor VIII in vivo following muscle electroporation. *Haemophilia* 12, 271-279.

Merten, M.D., Kammouni, W., Renaud, W., Birg, F., Mattei, M.G., & Figarella, C. (1996). A transformed human tracheal gland cell line, MM-39, that retains serous secretory functions. *Am. J. Respir. Cell Mol. Biol.* 15, 520-528.

Milanesi, G., Barbanti-Brodano, G., Negrini, M., Lee, D., Corallini, A., Caputo, A., Grossi, M.P., & Ricciardi, R.P. (1984). BK virus-plasmid expression vector that persists episomally in human cells and shuttles into Escherichia coli. *Mol. Cell Biol.* 4, 1551-1560.

Milewski, M.I., Mickle, J.E., Forrest, J.K., Stafford, D.M., Moyer, B.D., Cheng, J., Guggino, W.B., Stanton, B.A., & Cutting, G.R. (2001). A PDZ-binding motif is essential but not sufficient to localize the C terminus of CFTR to the apical membrane. *J. Cell Sci.* 114, 719-726.

Mitomo, K., Griesenbach, U., Inoue, M., Somerton, L., Meng, C., Akiba, E., Tabata, T., Ueda, Y., Frankel, G.M., Farley, R., Singh, C., Chan, M., Munkonge, F., Brum, A., Xenariou, S., Escudero-Garcia, S., Hasegawa, M., & Alton, E.W. (2010). Toward gene therapy for cystic fibrosis using a lentivirus pseudotyped with Sendai virus envelopes. *Mol. Ther.,* 18, 1173–1182.

Moss, R.B., Milla, C., Colomba, J., Accurso, F., Zeitlin, P.L., Clancy, J.P., Spencer, L.T., Pilewski, J., Waltz, D.A., Dorkin, H.L., Ferkol, T., Pian, M., Ramsey, B., Carter, B.J., Martin, D.B., & Heald, A.E. (2007). Repeated aerosolized AAV-CFTR for treatment of cystic fibrosis: a randomised placebo-controlled phase 2B trial. *Hum. Gene Ther.* 18, 726-732.

Moyer, B.D., Loffing, J., Schwiebert, E.M., Loffing-Cueni, D., Halpin, P.A., Karlson, K.H., Ismailov, I.I., Guggino, W.B., Langford, G.M., & Stanton, B.A. (1998). Membrane trafficking of the cystic fibrosis gene product, cystic fibrosis transmembrance conductance regulator, tagged with green fluorescent protein in Madin-Darby canine kidney cells. *J. Biol. Chem.* 273, 21759-21768.

Moyer, B.D., Loffing-Cueni, D., Loffing, J., Reynolds, D., & Stanton, B.A. (1999). Butyrate increases apical membrane CFTR but reduces chloride secretion in MDCK cells. *Am. J. Physiol. Renal Physiol.* 277, F271-276.

O'Riordan, C.R., Lachapelle, A.L., Marshall, J., Higgins, E.A., & Cheng, S.H. (2000). Characterization of the oligosaccharide conductance regulator. *Glycobiology* 10, 1225-1233.

Oceandy, D., McMorran, B., Schreiber, R., Wainwright, B.J., & Kunzelmann, K. (2003). GFP-tagged CFTR transgene is functional in the G551D cystic fibrosis mouse colon. *J. Membrane Biol.* 192, 159-167.

Otake, K., Ennist, D.L., Harrod, K., & Trapnell, B.C. (1998). Nonspecific inflammation inhibits adenovirus-mediated pulmonary gene transfer and expression independent of specific acquired immune responses. *Hum. Gene Ther.* 9, 2207-2222.

Parks, R.J., Chen, L., Anton, M., Sankar, U., Rudnicki, M.A., & Graham, F.L. (1996). A helper-dependent adenovirus vector system: removal of helper virus by Cre-mediated excision of the viral packaging signal. *Proc. Natl. Acad. Sci. USA* 93, 13565-13570.

Perricone, M.A., Morris, J.E., Pavelka, K., Plog, M.S., O'Sullivan, B.P., Joseph, P.M., Dorkin, H., Lapey, A., Balfour, R., Meeker, D.P., Smith, A.E., Wadsworth, S.C., & St George, J.A. (2001). Aerosol and lobar administration of a recombinant adenovirus to individuals with cystic fibrosis. ii. transfection efficiency in airway epithelium. *Hum. Gene Ther.* 12, 1383-1394.

Perricone, M.A., Rees, D.D., Sacks, C.R., Smith, K.A., Kaplan, J.M., & St George, J.A. (2000). Inhibitory effect of cystic fibrosis sputum on adenovirus-mediated gene transfer in cultured epithelial cells. *Hum. Gene Ther.* 11, 1997-2008.

Piedra, P.A., Poveda, G.A., Ramsey, B., McCoy, K., & Hiatt, P.W. (1998). Incidence and prevalence of neutralizing antibodies to the common adenoviruses in children with cystic fibrosis: implication for gene therapy with adenovirus vectors. *Pediatrics* 101, 1013-1019.

Pollard, H., Toumaniantz, G., Amos, J.L., Avet-Loiseau, H., Guihard, G., Behr, J.P. & Escande, D. (2001). Ca^{2+}-sensitive cytosolic nucleases prevent efficient delivery to the nucleus of injected plasmids. *J. Gene Med.* 3, 153-164.

Prasher, D.C., Eckenrode, V.K., Ward, W.W., Prendergast, F.G. & Cormier, M.J. (1992). Primary structure of the *Aequorea victoria* green-fluorescent protein. *Gene* 111, 229-233.

Rawlins, D.R., Milman, G., Hayward, S.D., & Hayward, G.S. (1985). Sequence-specific DNA binding of the Epstein-Barr virus nuclear antigen (EBNA-1) to clustered sites in the plasmid maintenance region. *Cell* 42, 859-868.

Rosenfeld, M.A., Yoshimura, K., Trapnell, B.C., Yoneyama, K., Rosenthal, E.R., Dalemans, W., Fukayama, M., Bargon, J., Stier, L.E., Stratford-Perricaudet, L., Perricaudet, M., Guggino, W.B., Pavirani, A., Lecocq, J.-P., & Crystal, R.G. (1992). In vivo transfer of the human cystic fibrosis transmembrane conductance regulator gene to the airway epithelium. *Cell* 68, 143-155.

Scaria, A., St George, J.A., Jiang, C., Kaplan, J.M., Wadsworth, S.C., & Gregory, R.J. (1998). Adenovirus-mediated persistent cystic fibrosis transmembrane conductance regulator expression in mouse airway epithelium. *J. Virol.* 72, 7302-7309.

Sheppard, D., & Welsh, M.J. (1999). Structure and function of the CFTR chloride channel. *Physiol. Rev.* 79, S23-S45.

Shimomura, O., Johnson, F.H., & Saiga, Y. (1962). Extraction, purification and properties of aequorin, a bioluminescent protein from the luminous hydromedusan, *Aequorea. J. Cell Comp. Physiol.* 59, 223-239.

Sinn, P.L., Williams, G., Vongpunsawad, S., Cattaneo, R., & McCray Jr, P.B. (2002). Measles virus preferentially transduces the basolateral surface of well-differentiated human airway epithelia. *J. Virol.* 76, 2403-2409.

Sinn, P.L., Arias, A.C., Brogden, K.A. & McCray, P.B. Jr (2008). Lentivirus vector can be readministered to nasal epithelia without blocking immune responses. *J. Virol.*, 82, 10684–10692.

Sinn, P.L., Reshma, M.A., & McCray Jr, P.B. (2011). Genetic therapies for cystic fibrosis lung disease. *Human Mol. Genetics,* 20, R79-R86.

Teramoto, S., Bartlett, J.S., McCarty, D., Xiao, X., Samulski, R.J., & Boucher, R.C. (1998). Factors influencing adeno-associated virus-mediated gene transfer to human cystic fibrosis airway epithelial cells: comparison with adenovirus vectors. *J. Virol.* 72, 8904-8912.

Toh, M.L., Hong, S.S., van de Loo, F., Franqueville, L., Lindholm, L., van den Berg, W., Boulanger, P., & Miossec, P. (2005). Enhancement of Ad-mediated gene delivery to rheumatoid arthritis synoviocytes and synovium by fiber modifications: role of RGD and non-RGD-binding integrins. *J. Immunol.* 175, 7687-7698.

Tsien, R.Y. (1998). The green fluorescent protein. *Ann. Rev. Biochem.* 67, 509-544.

Vais, H., Gao, G.P., Yang, M., Tran, P., Louboutin, J.P., Somanathan, S., Wilson, J.M., & Reenstra, W.W. (2004). Novel adenoviral vectors coding for GFP-tagged wtCFTR and deltaCFTR: characterization of expression and electrophysiological properties in A549 cells. *Pflugers Arch.*, 449, 278-287.

Vera, M., & Fortes, P. (2004). Simian virus-40 as a gene therapy vector. *DNA Cell Biol.* 23, 271-282.

Wagner, J.A., Messner, A.H., Moran, M.L., Daifuku, R., Kouyama, K., Desch, J.K., Manley, S., Norbash, A.M., Conrad, C.K., Friborg, S., Reynolds, T., Guggino, W.B., Moss, R.B., Carter, B.J., Wine, J.J., Flotte, T.R., & Gardner, P. (1999). Safety and biological efficacy of an adeno-associated virus vector-cystic fibrosis transmembrane regulator (AAV-CFTR) in the cystic fibrosis maxillary sinus. *Laryngoscope* 109, 266-274.

Wahlfors, J., Loimas, S., Pasanen, T., & Hakkarainen, T. (2001). Green fluorescent protein (GFP) fusion constructs in gene therapy research. *Histochem. Cell Biol.* 115, 59-65.

Walters, R.W., Grunst, T., Bergelson, J.M., Finberg, W., Welsh, M.J., & Zabner, J. (1999). Basolateral localization of fiber receptors limits adenovirus infection from the apical surface of airway epithelia. *J. Biol. Chem.* 274, 10219-10226.

Welsh, M.J., Zabner, J., Graham, S.M., Smith, A.E., Moscicki, R.A., & Wadsworth, S.C. (1995). Adenovirus-mediated gene transfer for cystic fibrosis. Part A. Safety of dose and repeat administration in the nasal epithelium. Part B. Clinical efficacy in the maxillary sinus. *Hum. Gene Ther.* 6, 205-218.

Yates, J.L., Warren, N., & Sugden, B. (1985). Stable replication of plasmids derived from Epstein-Barr virus in various mammalian cells. *Nature* 313, 812-815.

Yoo, H. S., Mazda, O., Lee, H. Y., Kim, J. C., Kwon, S. M., Lee, J. E., Kwon, I. C., Jeong, H., Jeong, Y. S., and Jeong, S. Y. (2006). In vivo gene therapy of type I diabetic mellitus using a cationic emulsion containing an Epstein-Barr virus-based plasmid vector. *J. Control Release* 112, 139-144.

Zabner, J., Couture, L.A., Gregory, R.J., Graham, S.M., Smith, A.E., & Welsh, M.J. (1993). Adenovirus-mediated gene transfer transiently corrects the chloride transport defect in nasal epithelia of patients with cystic fibrosis. *Cell* 75, 207-216.

Zabner, J., Freimuth, P., Puga, A., Fabrega, A., & Welsh, M.J. (1997). Lack of high affinity fiber receptor activity explains the resistance of ciliated airway epithelia to adenovirus infection. *J. Clin. Invest.* 100, 1144-1149.

Ziady, A.G., Kelley, T.J., Milliken, E., Ferkol, T., & Davis, P.B. (2002). Functional evidence of CFTR gene transfer in nasal epithelium of cystic fibrosis mice *in vivo* following luminal application of DNA complexes targeted to the serpin-enzyme complex receptor. *Mol. Ther.* 5, 413-419.

Zhang, L., Peeples, M.E., Boucher, R.C., Collins, P.L., & R. J. Pickles. (2002). Respiratory syncytial virus infection of human airway epithelial cells is polarized, specific to ciliated cells, and without obvious cytopathology. *J. Virol.* 76, 5654–5666.

Zhang, L., Bukreyev, A., Thompson, C.I., Watson, B., Peeples, M.E., Collins, P.L., & Pickles, R.J. (2005). Infection of ciliated cells by human parainfluenza virus type 3 in an in vitro model of human airway epithelium. *J. Virol.* 79, 1113–1124.

Zhang, L., Button, B., Gabriel, S.E., Burkett, S., Yan, Y., Skiadopoulos, M.H., Dang, Y.L., Vogel, L.N., McKay, T., Mengos, A., Boucher, R.C., Collins, P.L., & Pickles, R.J. (2009). CFTR delivery to 25% of surface epithelial cells restores normal rates of mucus transport to human cystic fibrosis airway epithelium. *PLoS Biol.* 7, e1000155.

Zhang, L., Limberis, M.P., Thompson, C., Antunes, M.B., Luongo, C., Wilson J.M., Collins, P.L. & Pickles, R.J. (2010). α-fetoprotein gene delivery to the nasal epithelium of nonhuman primates by human parainfluenza viral vectors. *Hum. Gene Ther.* 21, 1657-1664.

17

VIP as a Corrector of CFTR Trafficking and Membrane Stability

Valerie Chappe[1] and Sami I. Said[2]
[1]*Dalhousie University,*
[2]*SUNY-Stony Brook University*
[1]*Canada,*
[2]*USA*

1. Introduction

Cystic Fibrosis (CF) is a fatal autosomal recessive disease characterized by abnormal ion transport across epithelia, viscous mucus secretions, chronic bacterial infections, and inflammation in the airways that result from misprocessed or nonfunctional CFTR (Cystic Fibrosis Transmembrane conductance Regulator) chloride channels, normally located at the apical membrane of epithelial cells in exocrine tissues. CFTR activity is regulated by the Vasoactive Intestinal Peptide (VIP), a neuropeptide with potent anti-inflammatory, bronchodilatory and immunomodulatory functions. In airway sub-mucosal glands and other exocrine tissues, VIP is the major physiological activator for CFTR-dependent secretions, which contribute to local innate defense. When CFTR is defective or absent from the apical membrane of epithelial cells, due to mutations in the CFTR gene, airway glands no longer secrete in response to VIP stimulation and synergy with acetylcholine is lost. Although it is thought that VIP receptors are not altered in CF epithelial tissues, early studies have demonstrated that innervations by VIP-containing nerve fibers of the skin sweat glands, nasal and intestinal mucosa of CF patients is almost absent compared to healthy individuals, suggesting that absence of VIP stimulation could play a central role in the development of CF pathology.

Our group has recently demonstrated that VIP regulates CFTR membrane stability via activation of the $VPAC_1$ receptor and the $G_{\alpha i/q}$ signaling cascade in a PKCε-dependent manner. We also found that prolonged VIP exposure can rescue trafficking to the cell membrane and function of ΔF508-CFTR channels; the most commonly found mutation in CF. Our most recent *in vivo* studies using VIP knock-out (KO) mice provides clear evidence of the importance of VIP in maintaining healthy exocrine tissues, and the molecular link, between the absence of VIP stimulation and the development of a CF-like phenotype. We also observed a corrective effect with exogenous VIP administration, which restored normal trafficking and stabilized functional CFTR channels at the apical membrane of epithelial cells of the lung and small intestine (Fig. 1&2).

This mini-review summarizes recent and past findings on the role VIP in CFTR regulation and how it relates to the development of CF.

2. VIP historical background: Discovery as a vasodilator peptide in lung and intestine and rediscovery as a neuropeptide

First discovered as a smooth-muscle-relaxant, vasodilator peptide in the lung (Said, 1969), VIP was soon thereafter isolated from porcine intestine (Said and Mutt, 1970), chemically characterized (Mutt and Said, 1974), and synthesized (Bodanszky *et al*, 1973).

A 28 amino-acid residue peptide, VIP is structurally related to several other peptides, said to make up a "family," including pituitary adenylate cyclase-activating peptides (PACAP) 27 & 38, secretin, glucagon, helodermin, sauvagine, urotensin I, and gastric inhibitory peptide (glucose-dependent insulinotropic peptide) (Said, 2006).

With the aid of specific radioimmunoassay and immunofluorescence techniques, VIP immunoreactivity was detected in normal tissues and organs outside of the gastrointestinal tract, and found at high concentrations, as well as in certain neurogenic and endocrine tumors associated with excessive VIP secretion and high plasma levels (Said and Faloona, 1975). Eventually, the peptide was "rediscovered" in normal brain and peripheral nerves (Said and Rosenberg, 1976), and its true identity was recognized as a neuropeptide with neurotransmitter or neuromodulator properties. VIP is now considered to have physiologic regulatory influences on multiple organ systems, to be involved in the pathogenesis of several human disorders, and to have potential therapeutic benefit in a variety of disorders (Said, 1991b).

3. Role of VIP in exocrine secretion

As a neuropeptide, VIP was found to richly innervate all exocrine glands, including the pancreas, sweat, salivary, lachrymal, bronchial, and intestinal glands. Investigators learned that VIP worked in unison with cholinergic nerves, serving primarily to promote blood flow, and together with acetylcholine, to regulate and coordinate exocrine function (Lundberg *et al*, 1980). Evidence was accumulating that VIP, acting via receptors on these glands (Heinz-Erian *et al*, 1986), stimulated water and chloride transport across intestinal and tracheobronchial mucosa, $HCO3^-$ secretion by pancreatic acini, and promoted the movement of water and chloride across other epithelial surfaces (Heinz-Erian *et al*, 1985).

4. Is there a link to CF?

The above observations suggested that VIP exerted a regulatory influence on exocrine function, that appeared to run opposite to the observed defects in CF. With my associates (Said & colleagues), therefore, we postulated that the exocrine abnormalities of CF might be caused by a deficiency of VIP innervation. Accordingly, we examined the presence, distribution, and density of VIP-immunoreactive nerves supplying the sweat glands of normal subjects and CF patients. We selected sweat glands because: a) they express one of the cardinal functional abnormalities of the disease; b) unlike other exocrine organs involved in the disease, such as the lungs, sweat glands remain free of infection or morphologic changes; and c) they are easily accessible through skin biopsy (Heinz-Erian *et al*, 1985).

4.1 Deficient VIP – Containing nerves in CF exocrine tissues

Normal skin showed a rich network of VIP-immunoreactive nerves around secretory sweat gland acini, and a moderate innervation of the reabsorptive ducts. Individual VIP-positive nerve fibers were closely associated with basement membrane of both acini and duct cells. VIP innervation in CF samples, by contrast, was either absent or minimal both in the acini and in the ducts (Heinz-Erian *et al*, 1985).

Other than the skin, VIPergic neurons are also present in other sites of important CF manifestation such as the mucosa of the small intestinal, the pancreas and the respiratory epithelium. As observed in the skin, a deficiency, specifically in VIP-immunoreactive nerves, was observed in the nasal and intestinal mucosa of CF patients (Wattchow *et al*, 1988) while other types of nerve fibers were still present. The loss of VIP-immunoreactive nerve fibers was not however generalized and normal innervation was observed in intestinal muscles.

These findings, later confirmed by other investigators (Savage *et al*, 1990), raised the questions: 1) Is the decreased VIP innervation of CF glands and ducts causally related to the chloride ion abnormality in CF? and 2) what is the role of VIP, if any, in the pathogenesis, or correction, of CF pathology? Both questions remained unanswered for many years to follow.

4.2 Changes in CF submucosal glands

In response to VIP stimulation, normal human submucosal glands, in which CFTR is highly expressed, secrete low level of mucus which participates in the airways innate defense noteworthy by enabling mucociliary clearance (Wine, 2007). In CF glands, however, mucous secretion in response to VIP or cAMP elevation is altered (Joo *et al*, 2002). Mucus becomes more acidic (Song *et al*, 2006) and more viscous (Jayaraman *et al*, 2001) compared to normal. The same dysfunction is observed in CFTR-KO mice (Ianowski *et al*, 2007). VIP and cholinergic agonists synergistically induce mucous secretion from healthy human and pig glands but this synergy is absent in CF tissues (Choi *et al*, 2007). However, the secretion of large amounts of mucus in response to acute stimulation, primarily under the vagal pathway[1], and cholinergic stimulation are still present although altered (Wine, 2007).

5. Recent confirmation of a link, from studies of VIP and VIP-KO mice

We have recently used VIP knockout C57/Bl6 mice to demonstrate *in vivo* the central role of VIP in CFTR regulation and exocrine epithelial tissue integrity. These mice have been proven to be a very good model for airways diseases such as bronchial asthma (Szema *et al*, 2006; Hamidi *et al*, 2006; Said, 2009). They display airways inflammation and hyper-responsiveness to methacholine. They also present moderate pulmonary hypertension, right ventricular hypertrophy, and thickened pulmonary arteries (Said et al, 2007). We have used H&E staining for pathological assessment of the lung, small intestine and pancreas (Fig. 1). Interestingly, changes observed resembled those seen in CF. VIP-KO intestinal tissues had a significant increase in goblet and inflammatory cells. In the lung, we observed lymphocyte aggregation, increased airway secretion, alveolar thickening and edema. The pancreas presented increased secretion and increased infiltration with inflammatory cells surrounding ducts. These pathological changes could be reversed, closed to a wild-type phenotype, by VIP treatment consisting of intra-peritoneal injections of VIP (15μg) every other day for 3 weeks (Fig. 1) (Alcolado, 2010).

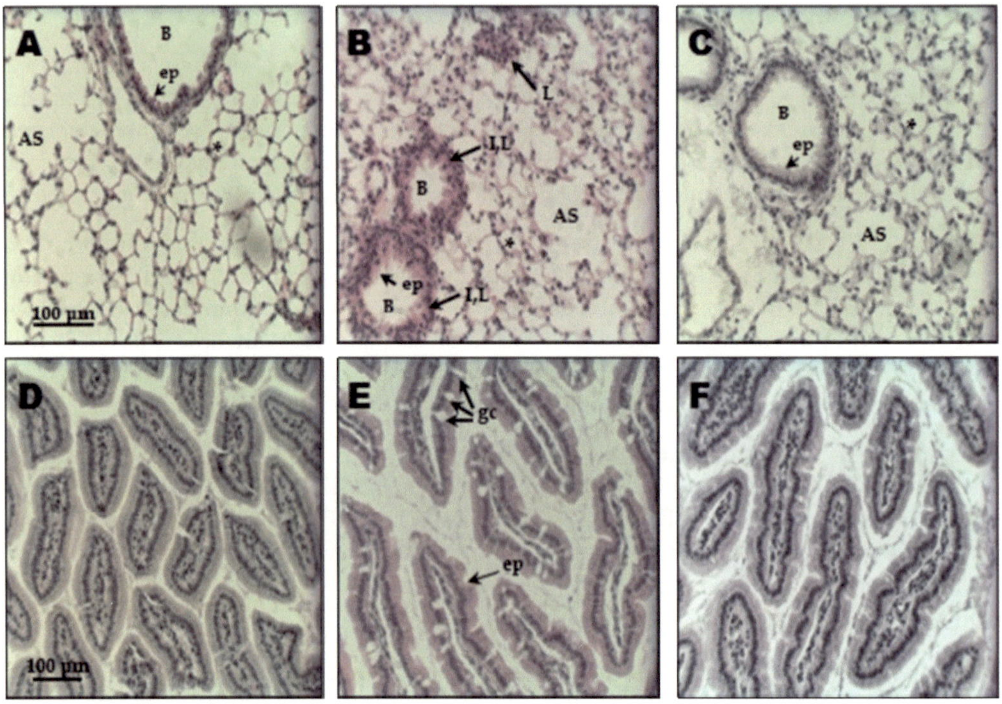

Histology sections of lung (upper panels) and duodenum (lower panels) from wild-type (**A** & **D**), VIP-KO (**B** & **E**) and VIP-KO treated (**C** & **F**) mice. Samples were embedded in paraffin before sectioning. 5 µm thick sections were mounted onto microscopy slides before hematoxylin and eosin (H & E) staining. Images were taken with a light microscope at 20X magnification. Compared to normal tissue, VIP-KO lungs show signs of inflammation (I) and lymphocyte aggregation (dark blue staining), thickening of the mucosa around bronchiolar space, thickening of the alveolar walls and the presence of inflammatory cells. The bronchiolar epithelium (ep) is also damaged. All these pathological signs are reversed to normal after VIP treatment (**C**). In the duodenum, transversal sections show increased amount of goblet cells and epithelium damage in the upper villi of VIP-KO mice tissues. As for the lung, these pathological signs are reversed by VIP treatment.
AS= alveolar sac, B = bronchioles, ep=epithelium, gc = goblet cells, I = inflammation, L = lymphocytes aggregation, * alveoli.

Fig. 1. VIP-KO mice lung and duodenum present pathological signs reversible by VIP treatment (adapted from Alcolado, 2010).

VIP binds to class II seven transmembrane spanning domain G protein-coupled receptors (GPCR) on the basolateral membrane of epithelial cells (Laburthe *et al*, 2007, 2002; Dickson *et al*, 2006; Chastre *et al*, 1989). VIP can bind to 3 receptors: $VPAC_1$, $VPAC_2$ and PAC_1. The highest affinity is for $VPAC_1$ (EC_{50} < 0.1nM) followed by $VPAC_2$ (EC_{50} =10 nM) and very little affinity for PAC_1 (EC_{50} ~40 nM). The PAC_1 receptor has a much greater affinity for Pituitary Adenylate Cyclase-Activating Polypeptide (EC_{50} ~0.2 nM) (Dickson and Finlayson, 2009). Other members of this peptide family, such as secretin and helodermin, can also bind to VPAC receptors although with much lower affinity than VIP (Laburthe *et al*, 2007) . Although VIP innervating fibres were found to be absent from CF intestinal mucosa (Wattchow *et al*, 1988), a study on CF foetuses revealed the presence of VIP receptors with unaltered pharmacology in the small intestine (Chastre *et al*, 1989).

In the VIP-KO mice model, we confirmed the expression of $VPAC_1$, $VPAC_2$ and PAC_1 by RT-PCR. Immunoblotting of lung and duodenum tissue lysates revealed unchanged PAC_1 expression in VIP-KO mice tissues compared to wild-type (WT), whereas VPAC 1 and 2 were found to be more abundant in VIP-KO tissues. These 2 receptors expression level remained up-regulated after VIP treatment (Conrad, 2011). CFTR localization was examined by immunostaining followed by confocal microscopy (Fig. 2). WT tissues showed CFTR predominantly at the apical membrane of epithelial cells in contrast to VIP-KO tissues, where CFTR distribution was mainly observed intracellularly. No changes in CFTR protein abundance or maturation were observed in immunoblots. Interestingly, VIP treatment restored strong CFTR membrane localization (Fig. 2), confirming the important role of VIP chronic exposure to maintain CFTR channels at the membrane, where it can exert its function, and for exocrine epithelial tissues integrity. Inflammation and damage observed in VIP-KO tissues can be attributed, at least in part, to the lack of CFTR-dependent secretions which ultimately depend on VIP stimulation both for acute and long-term regulation of CFTR function. These observations provide evidence of the molecular link between early observations of deficient VIP-containing fibers innervation of epithelial layers of exocrine organs in CF tissues and the absence of CFTR-dependent secretions.

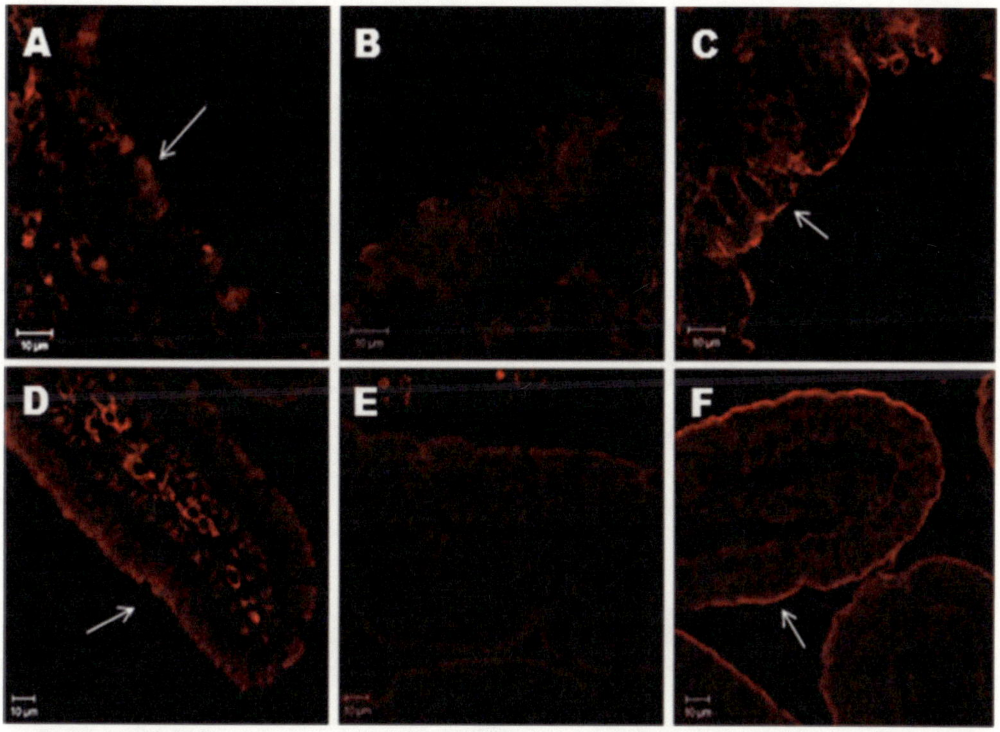

Paraffin embedded tissues (lung: upper panels, duodenum: lower panels) were sliced into 5 µm sections and mounted onto microscopy slides before immunostaining with the monoclonal anti-CFTR antibody MAB1660 (1:100). Arrows indicate apical CFTR signal. A & D: wild-type, B & E: VIP-KO, C & F: VIP-KO treated mice.

Fig. 2. CFTR localization at the apical membrane of epithelial cells is lost in VIP-KO tissues and restored by VIP treatment (adapted from Alcolado, 2010).

6. Molecular role of VIP in CFTR regulation

6.1 Regulation of CFTR activation by VIP acute stimulation

CFTR is activated mainly by protein kinase A (PKA)-dependent phosphorylation, with protein kinase C (PKC) stimulation playing an enhancing and permissive role to subsequent responsiveness to PKA (Chappe *et al*, 2008; Jia *et al*, 1997), in part through direct phosphorylation of conserved consensus sequences in CFTR Regulatory (R) domain (Chappe *et al*, 2003; Chappe *et al*, 2004). Hormones and neurotransmitters, such as VIP, which raise cellular cyclic AMP level, can stimulate acute CFTR channel activity. VIP is the most abundant peptide in the airways and the $VPAC_1$ receptor has been shown to stimulate CFTR-dependent chloride secretion upon VIP binding through activation of both PKA- and PKC-dependent signaling pathways in airway submucosal glands epithelial cell line Calu-3 (Chappe *et al*, 2008; Derand *et al*, 2004). Although class II GPCR are generally coupled to $G_{\alpha s}{}^2$ and adenylate cyclase activation to increase intracellular cAMP content, numerous reports have demonstrated that VIP receptors can couple to alternate G proteins and elicit signaling cascades cross-talk involving $G_{\alpha i/q}{}^2$, PKC and calcium release on top of the conventional $G_{\alpha s}$ and cAMP cascade (Derand *et al*, 2004; Bewley *et al*, 2006; Chappe *et al*, 2008; Sreedharan *et al*, 1994; Xia *et al*, 1996; Shreeve *et al*, 2000; Rafferty *et al*, 2009) (Fig. 3).

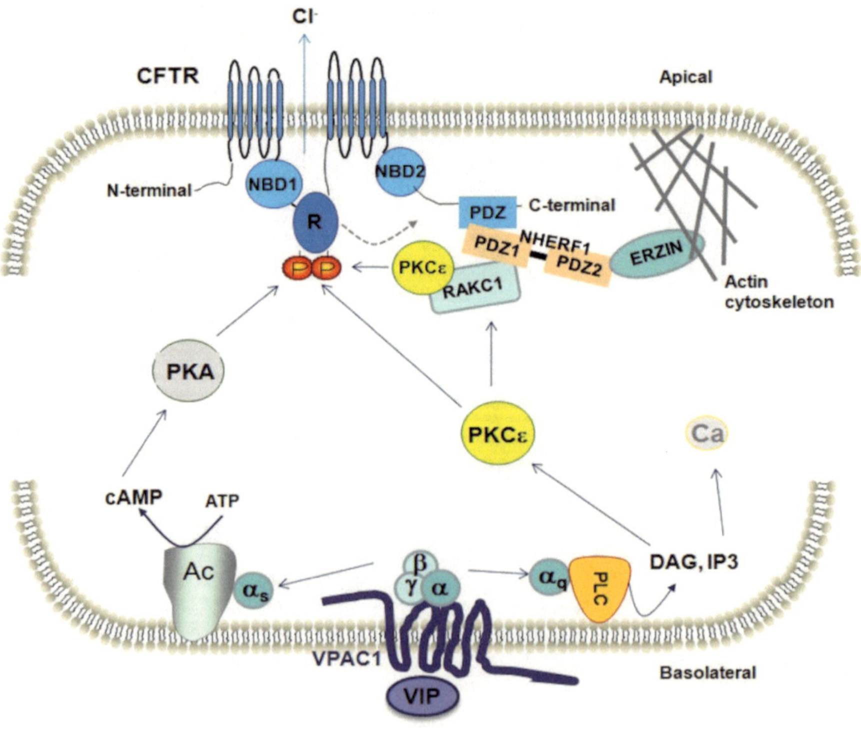

Fig. 3. CFTR regulation by VIP.

After binding to the $VPAC_1$ receptor, on the basolateral membrane, VIP induces the activation of both PKA and PKC signalling cascades. On the right end side of this cartoon is displayed the PKCε cascade of activation, as observed in our experiments and by others. The $G\alpha_q$ protein activates phospholipase C (PLC) which produces inositol tri-phosphate (IP3) and diacylglycerol (DAG). IP3 induces calcium release whereas DAG stimulates PKCε. PKCε can directly phosphorylate membrane CFTR on specific sites in the Regulatory domain. The activated PKCε also binds to the receptor for active kinase C (RAKC1) and translocate to the plasma membrane where RAKC1 binds to the PDZ domain 1 of NHERF1 (Na+/H+ Exchanger Regulatory Factor-1). This complex interacts with CFTR C-terminal, on a PDZ motif, and to ERZIN which anchors the whole complex to the actin cytoskeleton. This regulation maintains CFTR at the membrane and reduces its endocytosis. The co-localization of PKCε and CFTR is thought to maintain CFTR phosphorylation which contributes to its activation. We observed that the phosphorylated R domain relocates from its initial position, close to the Nucleotide Binding domains (NBD), to a new position with increased binding strength. We hypothesize here that re-binding of the phosphorylated R domain will further increase CFTR stability at the membrane through interaction with the PKCε-RAKC1-NHERF1 complex. In parallel (see left side), the $VPAC_1$ receptor can activate the PKA signalling cascade by associating with the $G\alpha_s$ protein which activates Adenylyl cyclase (Ac) to produce intracellular cAMP. This second messenger stimulates PKA. Direct phosphorylation of the CFTR R domain by PKA activates the channel gating. CFTR gating is further enhanced by PKC phosphorylation.

6.2 Role of VIP in CFTR membrane insertion and stability

Control of CFTR recycling is an important mechanism for the regulation of CFTR-dependent secretions. Adapters and proteins involved in CFTR endocytosis have been studied in detail (Ameen et al, 2007; Okiyoneda and Lukacs, 2007), but its regulation by physiological agonists is far less well understood and seems to be cell-type specific. Although CFTR function as a chloride channel requires apical membrane localization to participate in the regulation of exocrine secretions, it is mostly present in recycling endosomes, forming an important submembranar pool of mature proteins (Bradbury *et al*, 1994; Bradbury and Bridges, 1994; Webster *et al*, 1994). CFTR has a relatively long half-life: 16-24 hrs and a rapid turnover, although variable among cell lines: 2-16% per minute (Chappe *et al*, 2008; Lukacs *et al*, 1993; Swiatecka-Urban *et al*, 2005). CFTR is internalized by clathrin coated vesicles due to the presence of a dileucine and tyrosine endocytotic signals in its C-terminal. The tyrosine based motif interacts with the clathrin adapter complex AP-2 to enter into clathrin coated pits. CFTR also interacts with actin-binding proteins like myosin VI and to N-SWAP to recycle back to the plasma membrane via recycling endosomes (Okiyoneda and Lukacs, 2007; Swiatecka-Urban *et al*, 2004; Ganeshan *et al*, 2006). Conflicting results exist regarding the role of cAMP or other second messengers in CFTR recycling probably due to disparity in epithelial cells studied or the use of over-expressing systems which might saturate the normal pathway for CFTR trafficking. Both PKA and PKC-dependent mechanisms have been reported.

6.2.1 In intact tissues

Spiny dogfish shark (*Squalus acanthias)* rectal glands highly regulate salt secretion upon hormonal signals. These glands express a CFTR ortholog with 72% identity to the human CFTR. Acute VIP stimulation of these glands produces an increase in CFTR-mediated chloride secretions. Immunofluorescence labeling also revealed a redistribution of CFTR from intracellular to apical membrane localization following VIP stimulation (Lehrich *et al*, 1998).

In rats, a subpopulation of epithelial cells found in the small intestinal villi was identified as CFTR High Expresser cells (CHE) (Ameen *et al*, 1995). In response to VIP stimulation, CFTR present in sub-apical vesicular pool redistributed to the apical membrane but returned to the intracellular pool after removal of VIP (Ameen *et al*, 1999; Ameen *et al*, 2000).

6.2.2 In cell lines

Our lab has established that prolonged VIP stimulation of polarized airway epithelial cells stabilizes CFTR at the cell surface by reducing its internalization rate by more than 50%. The consequence of this regulation is an increase in CFTR-mediated chloride secretion. This was demonstrated initially in Calu-3 cells, a widely used model for submucosal gland serous cells, which express $VPAC_1$ receptors on their basolateral membrane and wild-type CFTR at the apical surface. Analysis of surface proteins by biotinylation and streptavidin extraction methods, revealed a large increase in apical CFTR after VIP exposure which was significant after 10 min and maximal within 2 hrs of VIP treatment. No changes in total CFTR or the proportion of fully glycosylated CFTR were measured in any tested condition, confirming that the VIP regulation was on mature CFTR recycling and did not affect its trafficking. Interestingly, the signaling cascade involved in this mechanism was $VPAC_1$ and $G_{\alpha i}$ mediated and involved the activation of PKC (Chappe *et al*, 2008). Direct activation of PKC by phorbol esters could mimic VIP effect with more than 2 fold increase in apical CFTR after 2 hrs of treatment. Functional evidence of increased membrane CFTR density after PKC stimulation were also reported in the human colon cell line HT29 together with increased mucus secretion (Bajnath *et al*, 1995). Contrary to previous observations in intestinal epithelial cells (Ameen *et al*, 2003; Bradbury and Bridges, 1992), raising intracellular cAMP by forskolin had no effect on the amount of CFTR at the apical membrane of Calu-3 cells. It is thus evident that VIP effect on CFTR membrane insertion is coupled to different signaling pathways in airways and intestinal cells, with the latter having more complex regulation possibly depending on the cellular model considered.

6.2.3 Rescue of ΔF508-CFTR maturation and membrane stability

The most common mutation in CF is the deletion of a phenylalanine residue at position 508 (ΔF508) that causes improper folding of the CFTR protein, resulting in its retention in the endoplasmic reticulum and proteosomal degradation of the majority of the newly synthesized CFTR proteins (Cheng *et al*, 1990; Kartner *et al*, 1992; Penque *et al*, 2000). However, part of the ΔF508-CFTR protein can still mature and reach the cell membrane where it retains some chloride channel function (Bronsveld *et al*, 2000; Penque *et al*, 2000; Kopito, 1999). Many efforts on CF research are devoted to attempt to rescue ΔF508-CFTR defective trafficking to restore normal epithelial function. Interestingly, ΔF508-CFTR retains some chloride channel activity when rescued from degradation by low temperature, chemical chaperones or other correctors. However, the half-life of the mutant protein is considerably shorter than that of the wild-type CFTR, mainly due to instability at the apical membrane (Lukacs *et al*, 1993; Denning *et al*, 1992; Dormer *et al*, 2001; Sharma *et al*, 2001).

We have investigated the potential rescue and stability at the cell membrane of ΔF508-CFTR by VIP treatment in the human nasal epithelial cells JME/CF15, derived from a ΔF508 homozygous patient (Jefferson *et al*, 1990). Immunostaining experiments with specific anti-

CFTR antibodies, followed by confocal microscopy confirmed intracellular localization of ΔF508-CFTR under control conditions, at 37°C, whereas membrane localization was observed in cells cultured at 27°C for 48hrs (Rafferty *et al*, 2009). The important finding of this study was that when JME/CF15 cells, maintained at physiological temperature (37°C), were treated with VIP (300 nM) for 1 or 2 hrs, mature ΔF508-CFTR proteins were observed in western blot experiments and immunostaining confirmed localization at the cell membrane. Functional assays confirmed the presence of CFTR-dependent chloride secretion after VIP treatment at 37°C. In these nasal cells, which express the $VPAC_1$ receptor, we found that VIP-dependent rescue of ΔF508-CFTR trafficking was mediated by the PKA-dependent signaling cascade (Fig. 4). We also found that ΔF508-CFTR membrane insertion obtained at low temperature could be enhanced by prolonged VIP treatment (1 to 2 hrs) which induced a large increase in ΔF508-CFTR function. As previously observed for wild-type CFTR, this regulation involved the $G_{\alpha q}$ and PKC signaling cascade but not the $G_{\alpha s}$ - PKA cascade (Fig. 4).

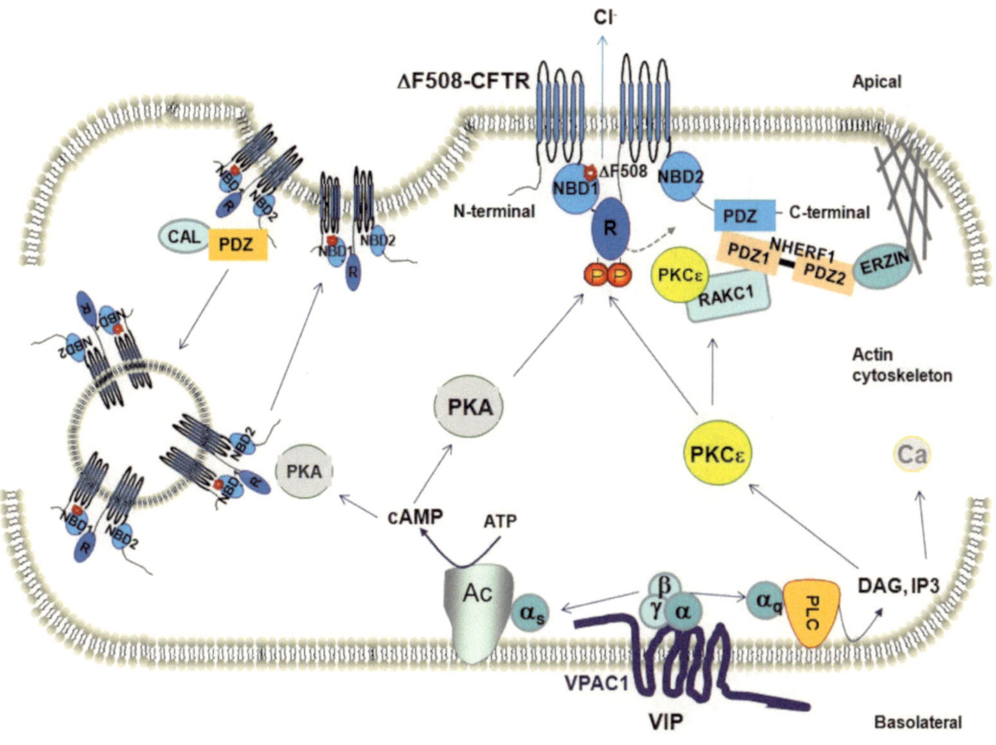

Fig. 4. Regulation of ΔF508-CFTR by VIP.

After binding to the $VPAC_1$ receptor, on the basolateral membrane, VIP induces the activation of both PKA and PKC signalling cascades. On the right side of this cartoon is displayed the PKCε cascade of activation, as observed in our experiments and by others. The $G\alpha_q$ protein activates phospholipase C (PLC) which produces inositol tri-phosphate (IP3) and diacylglycerol (DAG). IP3 induces calcium release whereas DAG stimulates PKCε. PKCε can directly phosphorylate membrane CFTR on specific sites in the Regulatory domain. The activated PKCε also binds to the receptor for active kinase C (RAKC1) and translocates to the plasma membrane where RAKC1 binds to the PDZ domain 1 of NHERF1. This complex interacts with CFTR C-terminal, on a PDZ motif, and to ERZIN which anchors the whole complex to the actin cytoskeleton. This regulation maintains CFTR at the membrane and reduces its endocytosis. The co-localization of PKCε and CFTR is thought to maintain CFTR phosphorylation which contributes to its activation. We observed that the phosphorylated R domain relocates from its initial position, close to the Nucleotide Binding domains (NBD), to a new unidentified position with increased binding strenght. We hypothesize here that re-binding of the phosphorylated R domain will further increase CFTR stability at the membrane through interaction with the PKCε-RAKC1-NHERF1 complex. In parallel (see left side), the $VPAC_1$ receptor can activate the PKA signalling cascade by associating with the $G\alpha_s$ protein which activates Adenylyl cyclase (Ac) to produce intracellular cAMP. This second messenger stimulates PKA. Direct phosphorylation of the CFTR R domain by PKA activates the channel and is further enhanced by PKC phosphorylation. We also observed that the activated PKA contributes to ΔF508-CFTR trafficking and insertion to the plasma membrane. We hypothesize that PKA effect counteracts the action of the CFTR Associated Ligand (CAL) which had been shown to bind to CFTR C-terminal PDZ motif, and compete with NHERF1, to retain CFTR in endosomes and target ΔF508-CFTR to lysosomal degradation.

Evidence from airway cells thus demonstrates that VIP mechanism of regulation of CFTR activity involves both PKA and PKC signaling in a synergistic manner to rescue defective trafficking of mutant CFTR, activate CFTR gating through direct phosphorylation of its regulatory domain, and most importantly, stabilize CFTR channels at the cell surface by reducing their internalization rate, thus optimizing CFTR-dependent secretions.

6.2.4 Role of PKCε

In both recombinant and native systems, we have investigated the role of PKC on VIP-dependent CFTR membrane stability. PKC isoforms comprise calcium-dependent (α, β_1, β_2, γ) and calcium-independent novel isoforms (δ, ε, η, θ). All necessitate diacyl glycerol to be activated (Reyland, 2009; Dempsey *et al*, 2000; Gallegos and Newton, 2008). With specific inhibitors and siRNA treatments we found that only PKCε, a novel calcium-independent isoform, mediated VIP-dependent increase in CFTR membrane stability in the JME/CF15 epithelial nasal cells and also in the recombinant BHK cells stably expressing wild-type or ΔF508-CFTR (Alcolado *et al*, 2011). This is not surprising as PKCε was previously reported to co-localize with CFTR at the apical membrane of airway epithelial cells and to play a permissive role on CFTR-dependent chloride secretion (Liedtke and Cole, 1998; Liedtke *et al*, 2001; Liedtke *et al*, 2002). The C-terminal of CFTR interacts with either CAL or NHERF1. These two scaffolding proteins regulate CFTR membrane density in an opposite manner. While CAL, which is mostly found in the trans-golgi network, promotes CFTR targeting to lysosomal degradation, NHERF1, which is localized at the cell apical membrane, rather participate in maintaining CFTR at the membrane by tethering it to the actin cytoskeleton (Cheng, J., 2002, 2004). Structural studies indicate that CAL and NEHRF1 might compete for the same binding site in CFTR C-terminal, and their differential interaction with CFTR is thought to regulate the steady-state level of mature CFTR present at the apical membrane of epithelial cells (Ladias ,

2003; Wolde, 2007). Part of this regulation involves activated PKCε which binds to RACK1 and translocates to the plasma membrane. RACK1 interacts directly with NHERF1 by PDZ domain interaction at the apical membrane of epithelial cells. It is hypothesized that the complex composed of PKCε - RACK1-NHERF1 interacts with CFTR to regulate its membrane stability (Fig. 3 & 4).

7. Conclusions

Although VIP binding to the $VPAC_2$ receptor plays an important role in the relaxation of smooth muscles and is a matter of intense study for respiratory diseases such as bronchial asthma (Hamidi *et al*, 2006; Alessandrini *et al*, 1993; Groneberg *et al*, 2001; Groneberg *et al*, 2006; Jaeger *et al*, 1996; Onoue *et al*, 2004; Said, 1991a), our recent studies have highlighted the important role of the $VPAC_1$ receptor and differential activation of the PKA or PKC signalling pathways in airway epithelial cells to regulate CFTR-dependent secretions. *In vivo* data set VIP, or its analogs, as a potential candidate for the treatment of CF as it corrects many features of this disease including the molecular basis. Further investigation of VIP potential to rescue exocrine epithelial secretions should be conducted to uncover the large potential of this peptide in the treatment of respiratory diseases, which are the third cause of hospitalization and death in North America.

8. Footnotes

1. Airway defense in response to acute stress such as intense exercise is under the control of the vagal nerve pathway (see Kubin, 2006 and Wine, 2007 for review).
2. G proteins are composed of 3 subunits: α, β and γ. They mediate signaling cascades initiated by ligand binding to membrane receptors of the G protein coupled receptors (GPCR) family. Once activated, the α subunit dissociates from βγ and translocates to a target effector: cellular enzymes and ion channels. The α subunits, which mediate most of the known signals, comprise 4 different types which will initiate specific signaling cascades: α_s, α_q, α_i, $\alpha_{12/13}$. The α_s subunit's effector is the adenylyl cylcase and it initiates the cAMP signaling cascade. The α_q subunit rather activates phospolipase C and initiates the calcium and PKC signaling cascades (for review see Musnier, 2010).

9. Acknowledgments

The authors thank all lab members and collaborators involved in this research: Nicole Alcolado, Dustin Conrad, Frederic Chappe, Dr.Younes Anini, Dr. Zaholin Xu. We also thank Cystic Fibrosis Canada, Nova Scotia Health Research Foundation, Canadian Institutes of Health Research, Canadian Foundation for Innovation, The National Science and Engineering Research Council of Canada and The National Institutes of Health for funding.

10. References

Alcolado N, Conrad DJ, Rafferty S, Chappe FG, Chappe VM. (2011). VIP-dependent increase in F508del-CFTR membrane localization is mediated by PKCε. *Am J Physiol Cell Physiol* ; 301(1): C56-65.

Alcolado N. (2010). Regulation of CFTR membrane localization by Vasoactive Intestinal Peptide (VIP). *Dalhousie University, Master of Science-Physiology* .

Alessandrini F, Thakkar M, Foda HD, Said SI, Lodi R, Pakbaz H, et al. (1993). Vasoactive intestinal peptide enhances lung preservation. *Transplantation* 56, 964-73.

Ameen N, Silvis M, Bradbury NA. (2007). Endocytic trafficking of CFTR in health and disease. *J Cyst Fibros* 6, 1-14.

Ameen NA, Ardito T, Kashgarian M, Marino CR. (1995). A unique subset of rat and human intestinal villus cells express the cystic fibrosis transmembrane conductance regulator. *Gastroenterology* 108, 1016-23.

Ameen NA, Marino C, Salas PJ. (2003). cAMP-dependent exocytosis and vesicle traffic regulate CFTR and fluid transport in rat jejunum in vivo. *Am J Physiol Cell Physiol* 284, C429-38.

Ameen NA, Martensson B, Bourguinon L, Marino C, Isenberg J, McLaughlin GE. (1999). CFTR channel insertion to the apical surface in rat duodenal villus epithelial cells is upregulated by VIP in vivo. *J Cell Sci* 112 (Pt 6), 887-94.

Ameen NA, van Donselaar E, Posthuma G, de Jonge H, McLaughlin G, Geuze HJ, et al. (2000). Subcellular distribution of CFTR in rat intestine supports a physiologic role for CFTR regulation by vesicle traffic. *Histochem Cell Biol* 114, 219-28.

Bajnath RB, Dekker K, De Jonge HR, Groot JA. (1995). Chloride secretion induced by phorbol dibutyrate and forskolin in the human colonic carcinoma cell line HT-29Cl.19A is regulated by different mechanisms. *Pflugers Arch* 430, 705-12.

Bewley MS, Pena JT, Plesch FN, Decker SE, Weber GJ, Forrest JN,Jr. (2006). Shark rectal gland vasoactive intestinal peptide receptor: Cloning, functional expression, and regulation of CFTR chloride channels. *Am J Physiol Regul Integr Comp Physiol* 291, R1157-64.

Bodanszky M, Klausner YS, Said SI. (1973). Biological activities of synthetic peptides corresponding to fragments of and to the entire sequence of the vasoactive intestinal peptide. *Proc Natl Acad Sci U S A* 70, 382-4.

Bradbury NA. (1999). Intracellular CFTR: Localization and function. *Physiol Rev* 79, S175-91.

Bradbury NA, Bridges RJ. (1994). Role of membrane trafficking in plasma membrane solute transport. *Am J Physiol* 267, C1-24.

Bradbury NA, Bridges RJ. (1992). Endocytosis is regulated by protein kinase A, but not protein kinase C in a secretory epithelial cell line. *Biochem Biophys Res Commun* 184, 1173-80.

Bradbury NA, Cohn JA, Venglarik CJ, Bridges RJ. (1994). Biochemical and biophysical identification of cystic fibrosis transmembrane conductance regulator chloride channels as components of endocytic clathrin-coated vesicles. *J Biol Chem* 269, 8296-302.

Bronsveld I, Mekus F, Bijman J, Ballmann M, Greipel J, Hundrieser J, et al. (2000). Residual chloride secretion in intestinal tissue of deltaF508 homozygous twins and siblings with cystic fibrosis. the european CF twin and sibling study consortium. *Gastroenterology* 119, 32-40.

Chappe FG, Loewen ME, Hanrahan JW, Chappe VM. (2008). VIP increases CFTR levels in the apical membrane of calu-3 cells through a PKC-dependent mechanism. *J Pharmacol Exp Ther* 327, 226-38.

Chappe V, Hinkson DA, Howell LD, Evagelidis A, Liao J, Chang XB, et al. (2004). Stimulatory and inhibitory protein kinase C consensus sequences regulate the cystic fibrosis transmembrane conductance regulator. *Proc Natl Acad Sci U S A* 101, 390-5.

Chappe V, Hinkson DA, Zhu T, Chang XB, Riordan JR, Hanrahan JW. (2003). Phosphorylation of protein kinase C sites in NBD1 and the R domain control CFTR channel activation by PKA. *J Physiol* 548, 39-52.

Chastre E, Bawab W, Faure C, Emami S, Muller F, Boue A, et al. (1989). Vasoactive intestinal peptide and its receptors in fetuses with cystic fibrosis. *Am J Physiol* 257, G561-9.

Cheng J, Moyer BD, Milewski M, Loffing J, Ikeda M, Mickle JE, et al. (2002). A golgi-associated PDZ domain protein modulates cystic fibrosis transmembrane regulator plasma membrane expression. *J Biol Chem* 277, 3520-9.

Cheng J, Wang H, Guggino WB. (2004). Modulation of mature cystic fibrosis transmembrane regulator protein by the PDZ domain protein CAL. *J Biol Chem* 279, 1892-8.

Cheng SH, Gregory RJ, Marshall J, Paul S, Souza DW, White GA, et al. (1990). Defective intracellular transport and processing of CFTR is the molecular basis of most cystic fibrosis. *Cell* 63, 827-34.

Choi JY, Joo NS, Krouse ME, Wu JV, Robbins RC, Ianowski JP, et al. (2007). Synergistic airway gland mucus secretion in response to vasoactive intestinal peptide and carbachol is lost in cystic fibrosis. *J Clin Invest* 117, 3118-27.

Conrad DJ. (2011). Increased VIP receptors expression mediates CFTR membrane localization in response to VIP treatment in VIP knockout mice. *Dalhousie University, Master of Science-Physiology* .

Denning GM, Anderson MP, Amara JF, Marshall J, Smith AE, Welsh MJ. (1992). Processing of mutant cystic fibrosis transmembrane conductance regulator is temperature-sensitive. *Nature* 358, 761-4.

Derand R, Montoni A, Bulteau-Pignoux L, Janet T, Moreau B, Muller JM, et al. (2004). Activation of VPAC1 receptors by VIP and PACAP-27 in human bronchial epithelial cells induces CFTR-dependent chloride secretion. *Br J Pharmacol* 141, 698-708.

Dickson L, Aramori I, McCulloch J, Sharkey J, Finlayson K. (2006). A systematic comparison of intracellular cyclic AMP and calcium signalling highlights complexities in human VPAC/PAC receptor pharmacology. *Neuropharmacology* 51, 1086-98.

Dickson L, Finlayson K. (2009). VPAC and PAC receptors: From ligands to function. *Pharmacol Ther* 121, 294-316.

Dormer RL, Derand R, McNeilly CM, Mettey Y, Bulteau-Pignoux L, Metaye T, et al. (2001). Correction of delF508-CFTR activity with benzo(c)quinolizinium compounds through facilitation of its processing in cystic fibrosis airway cells. *J Cell Sci* 114, 4073-81.

Ganeshan R, Nowotarski K, Di A, Nelson DJ, Kirk KL. (2006). CFTR surface expression and chloride currents are decreased by inhibitors of N-WASP and actin polymerization. *Biochim Biophys Acta* ; DOI: S0167-4889(06)00313-2 [pii]; 10.1016/j.bbamcr.2006.09.031 [doi].

Groneberg DA, Hartmann P, Dinh QT, Fischer A. (2001). Expression and distribution of vasoactive intestinal polypeptide receptor VPAC(2) mRNA in human airways. *Lab Invest* 81, 749-55.

Groneberg DA, Rabe KF, Fischer A. (2006). Novel concepts of neuropeptide-based drug therapy: Vasoactive intestinal polypeptide and its receptors. *Eur J Pharmacol* 533, 182-94.

Groneberg DA, Springer J, Fischer A. (2001). Vasoactive intestinal polypeptide as mediator of asthma. *Pulm Pharmacol Ther* 14, 391-401.

Hamidi SA, Szema AM, Lyubsky S, Dickman KG, Degene A, Mathew SM, et al. (2006). Clues to VIP function from knockout mice. *Ann N Y Acad Sci* 1070, 5-9.

Heinz-Erian P, Dey RD, Flux M, Said SI. (1985). Deficient vasoactive intestinal peptide innervation in the sweat glands of cystic fibrosis patients. *Science* 229, 1407-8.

Heinz-Erian P, Paul S, Said SI. (1986). Receptors for vasoactive intestinal peptide on isolated human sweat glands. *Peptides* 7 Suppl 1, 151-4.

Ianowski JP, Choi JY, Wine JJ, Hanrahan JW. (2007). Mucus secretion by single tracheal submucosal glands from normal and cystic fibrosis transmembrane conductance regulator knockout mice. *J Physiol* 580, 301-14.

Jaeger E, Bauer S, Joyce MW, Foda HD, Berisha HI, Said SI. (1996). Structure-activity studies on VIP: IV. the synthetic agonist helodermin-fragment-(1-28)-amide is a potent VIP-agonist with prolonged duration of tracheal relaxant activity. *Ann N Y Acad Sci* 805, 499-504.

Jayaraman S, Joo NS, Reitz B, Wine JJ, Verkman AS. (2001). Submucosal gland secretions in airways from cystic fibrosis patients have normal [na(+)] and pH but elevated viscosity. *Proc Natl Acad Sci U S A* 98, 8119-23.

Jefferson DM, Valentich JD, Marini FC, Grubman SA, Iannuzzi MC, Dorkin HL, et al. (1990). Expression of normal and cystic fibrosis phenotypes by continuous airway epithelial cell lines. *Am J Physiol* 259, L496-505.

Jia Y, Mathews CJ, Hanrahan JW. (1997). Phosphorylation by protein kinase C is required for acute activation of cystic fibrosis transmembrane conductance regulator by protein kinase A. *J Biol Chem* 272, 4978-84.

Joo NS, Irokawa T, Wu JV, Robbins RC, Whyte RI, Wine JJ. (2002). Absent secretion to vasoactive intestinal peptide in cystic fibrosis airway glands. *J Biol Chem* 277, 50710-5.

Kartner N, Augustinas O, Jensen TJ, Naismith AL, Riordan JR. (1992). Mislocalization of delta F508 CFTR in cystic fibrosis sweat gland. *Nat Genet* 1, 321-7.

Kopito RR. (1999). Biosynthesis and degradation of CFTR. *Physiol Rev* 79, S167-73.

Kubin L, Alheid GF, Zuperku EJ, McCrimmon DR. (2006). Central pathways of pulmonary and lower airway vagal afferents. *J Appl Physiol* 101, 618-27.

Laburthe M, Couvineau A, Marie JC. (2002). VPAC receptors for VIP and PACAP. *Receptors Channels* 8, 137-53.

Laburthe M, Couvineau A, Tan V. (2007). Class II G protein-coupled receptors for VIP and PACAP: Structure, models of activation and pharmacology. *Peptides* 28, 1631-9.

Ladias JA. (2003). Structural insights into the CFTR-NHERF interaction. *J Membr Biol* 192, 79-88.

Lehrich RW, Aller SG, Webster P, Marino CR, Forrest JN,Jr. (1998). Vasoactive intestinal peptide, forskolin, and genistein increase apical CFTR trafficking in the rectal gland of the spiny dogfish, squalus acanthias. acute regulation of CFTR trafficking in an intact epithelium. *J Clin Invest* 101, 737-45.

Liedtke CM, Cole TS. Antisense oligonucleotide to PKC-epsilon alters cAMP-dependent stimulation of CFTR in calu-3 cells. Am J Physiol. 1998 Nov;275(5 Pt 1):C1357-64.

Liedtke CM, Cody D, Cole TS. Differential regulation of Cl- transport proteins by PKC in Calu-3 cells. Am J Physiol Lung Cell Mol Physiol. 2001 Apr;280(4):L739-47.

Liedtke CM, Yun CH, Kyle N, Wang D. Protein kinase C epsilon-dependent regulation of cystic fibrosis transmembrane regulator involves binding to a receptor for activated C kinase (RACK1) and RACK1 binding to Na+/H+ exchange regulatory factor. J Biol Chem. 2002 Jun 21;277(25):22925-33.

Lukacs GL, Chang XB, Bear C, Kartner N, Mohamed A, Riordan JR, et al. (1993). The delta F508 mutation decreases the stability of cystic fibrosis transmembrane conductance regulator in the plasma membrane. determination of functional half-lives on transfected cells. *J Biol Chem* 268, 21592-8.

Lundberg JM, Anggard A, Fahrenkrug J, Hokfelt T, Mutt V. (1980). Vasoactive intestinal polypeptide in cholinergic neurons of exocrine glands: Functional significance of coexisting transmitters for vasodilation and secretion. *Proc Natl Acad Sci U S A* 77, 1651-5.

Musnier A, Blanchot B, Reiter E, Crepieux P. (2010). GPCR signalling to the translation machinery. *Cell Signal* 22, 707-16.

Mutt V, Said SI. (1974). Structure of the porcine vasoactive intestinal octacosapeptide. the amino-acid sequence. use of kallikrein in its determination. *Eur J Biochem* 42, 581-9.

Okiyoneda T, Lukacs GL. (2007). Cell surface dynamics of CFTR: The ins and outs. *Biochim Biophys Acta* 1773, 476-9.

Onoue S, Endo K, Ohmori Y, Yamada S, Kimura R, Yajima T, et al. (2004). Long-acting analogue of vasoactive intestinal peptide, [R15, 20, 21, L17]-VIP-GRR (IK312532), protects rat alveolar L2 cells from the cytotoxicity of cigarette smoke. *Regul Pept* 123, 193-9.

Penque D, Mendes F, Beck S, Farinha C, Pacheco P, Nogueira P, et al. (2000). Cystic fibrosis F508del patients have apically localized CFTR in a reduced number of airway cells. *Lab Invest* 80, 857-68.

Rafferty S, Alcolado N, Norez C, Chappe F, Pelzer S, Becq F, et al. (2009). Rescue of functional F508del-CFTR by VIP in the human nasal epithelial cell line JME/CF15. *J Pharmacol Exp Ther* 331(1), 2-13.

Said SI. (2006). Vasoactive intestinal peptide. In *Encyclopedia of Respiratory Medicine,* ed. Laurent GJ SS. pp. 517-520. Elsevier.

Said SI, Hamidi SA, Dickman KG, Szema AM, Lyubsky S, Lin RZ etal. (2007). Moderate Pulmonary Arterial Hypertension in Male Mice Lacking the Vasoactive Intestinal Peptide Gene. *Ciculation* 115:1260-1268

Said SI. (1969). A peptide fraction from lung tissue with prolonged peripheral vasodilator activity. *Scandinavian journal of clinical laboratory investigation.Supplement* 107, 51-6.

Said SI. (2009). Animal models of airway hyperresponsiveness. *Eur Respir J* 33, 217-8.

Said SI. (1991a). Vasoactive intestinal polypeptide (VIP) in asthma. *Ann N Y Acad Sci* 629, 305-18.

Said SI. (1991b). Vasoactive intestinal polypeptide biologic role in health and disease. *Trends Endocrinol Metab* 2, 107-12.

Said SI, Faloona GR. (1975). Elevated plasma and tissue levels of vasoactive intestinal polypeptide in the watery-diarrhea syndrome due to pancreatic, bronchogenic and other tumors. *N Engl J Med* 293, 155-60.

Said SI, Mutt V. (1970). Polypeptide with broad biological activity: Isolation from small intestine. *Science* 169, 1217-8.

Said SI, Rosenberg RN. (1976). Vasoactive intestinal polypeptide: Abundant immunoreactivity in neural cell lines and normal nervous tissue. *Science* 192, 907-8.

Savage MV, Brengelmann GL, Buchan AM, Freund PR. (1990). Cystic fibrosis, vasoactive intestinal polypeptide, and active cutaneous vasodilation. *J Appl Physiol* 69, 2149-54.

Sharma M, Benharouga M, Hu W, Lukacs GL. (2001). Conformational and temperature-sensitive stability defects of the delta F508 cystic fibrosis transmembrane conductance regulator in post-endoplasmic reticulum compartments. *J Biol Chem* 276, 8942-50.

Shreeve SM, Sreedharan SP, Hacker MP, Gannon DE, Morgan MJ. (2000). VIP activates G(s) and G(i3) in rat alveolar macrophages and G(s) in HEK293 cells transfected with the human VPAC(1) receptor. *Biochem Biophys Res Commun* 272, 922-8.

Song Y, Salinas D, Nielson DW, Verkman AS. (2006). Hyperacidity of secreted fluid from submucosal glands in early cystic fibrosis. *Am J Physiol Cell Physiol* 290, C741-9.

Sreedharan SP, Patel DR, Xia M, Ichikawa S, Goetzl EJ. (1994). Human vasoactive intestinal peptide1 receptors expressed by stable transfectants couple to two distinct signaling pathways. *Biochem Biophys Res Commun* 203, 141-8.

Swiatecka-Urban A, Boyd C, Coutermarsh B, Karlson KH, Barnaby R, Aschenbrenner L, et al. (2004). Myosin VI regulates endocytosis of the cystic fibrosis transmembrane conductance regulator. *J Biol Chem* 279, 38025-31.

Swiatecka-Urban A, Brown A, Moreau-Marquis S, Renuka J, Coutermarsh B, Barnaby R, et al. (2005). The short apical membrane half-life of rescued {delta}F508-cystic fibrosis transmembrane conductance regulator (CFTR) results from accelerated endocytosis of {delta}F508-CFTR in polarized human airway epithelial cells. *J Biol Chem* 280, 36762-72.

Szema AM, Hamidi SA, Lyubsky S, Dickman KG, Mathew S, Abdel-Razek T, et al. (2006). Mice lacking the VIP gene show airway hyperresponsiveness and airway inflammation, partially reversible by VIP. *Am J Physiol Lung Cell Mol Physiol* 291, L880-6.

Wattchow DA, Furness JB, Costa M. (1988). Distribution and coexistence of peptides in nerve fibers of the external muscle of the human gastrointestinal tract. *Gastroenterology* 95, 32-41.

Webster P, Vanacore L, Nairn AC, Marino CR. (1994). Subcellular localization of CFTR to endosomes in a ductal epithelium. *Am J Physiol* 267, C340-8.

Wine JJ. (2007). Parasympathetic control of airway submucosal glands: Central reflexes and the airway intrinsic nervous system. *Auton Neurosci* 133, 35-54.

Wolde M, Fellows A, Cheng J, Kivenson A, Coutermarsh B, Talebian L, Karlson,K.; Piserchio,A.; Mierke,D.F.; Stanton,B.A.; Guggino,W.B.; Madden,D.R. (2007). Targeting CAL as a negative regulator of DeltaF508-CFTR cell-surface expression: An RNA interference and structure-based mutagenetic approach. *J Biol Chem* 282, 8099-109.

Xia M, Sreedharan SP, Goetzl EJ. (1996). Predominant expression of type II vasoactive intestinal peptide receptors by human T lymphoblastoma cells: Transduction of both Ca2+ and cyclic AMP signals. *J Clin Immunol* 16, 21-30.

18

Pharmacological Potential of PDE5 Inhibitors for the Treatment of Cystic Fibrosis

Bob Lubamba, Barbara Dhooghe, Sabrina Noël and Teresinha Leal
Louvain Centre for Toxicology and Applied Pharmacology,
Université Catholique de Louvain, Brussels,
Belgium

1. Introduction

Recent basic research has aroused great interest in the therapeutic potential of phosphodiesterase type 5 (PDE5) inhibitors, such as sildenafil, vardenafil and taladafil, for the treatment of cystic fibrosis (CF). CF is the most common, life-threatening, recessively inherited disease in Caucasian populations. An estimated 1 in 2,500 Caucasian live births are affected and approximately 80,000 people in the world are diagnosed with CF. Due to mutation in the CF transmembrane conductance regulator (*CFTR*) gene [1,2], which encodes the main chloride channel expressed in epithelia, CF causes abnormal mucociliary clearance mainly in the lungs, leading to a vicious cycle of obstruction/infection/inflammation that progressively and irreversibly damages the lung tissue and architecture. Although many organs are affected in CF, pulmonary disease is the major cause of morbidity and mortality [3,4]. Despite more than two decades of intensive investigation of the genetics [1,2], pathophysiology and clinical phenotypes of CF [3,4], there is still no cure for CF. As a matter of fact, therapies have been limited to alleviating clinical manifestations. Although life expectancy and quality of life have progressively improved, CF continues to inflict major burdens and to shorten lives.

The most common disease allele, p.Phe508del (F508del), corresponding to deletion of a single phenylalanine residue at position 508 of a single polypeptide chain of 1480 amino acids, interferes with CFTR function because the mutant protein does not efficiently fold into the native protein structure. Although the mutant F508del is correctly translated, it is held back in the endoplasmic reticulum; the misfolded protein is directed towards proteosomal degradation and fails to reach the apical membrane of many epithelial cells [5]. An effective candidate drug to treat F508del-CF patients should be able to correct the localization of CFTR protein by increasing its expression at the apical membrane of epithelial cells. Indeed, it has been recognized that rescuing F508del-CFTR to the plasma membrane is followed by an improved efflux of chloride ions across the epithelium related to some residual channel activity of the mutant protein [6]. Therefore, finding a compound that promotes CFTR channel activity would be of great benefit. Searching for such compounds, we and others have demonstrated the potential of PDE5 inhibitors for the treatment of CF. Indeed, basic studies have provided evidence that PDE5 inhibitors, already in clinical use for the treatment of erectile dysfunction and/or of pulmonary arterial hypertension, rescue F508del-CFTR trafficking [7,8] and improve its channel activity [9,10].

PDE are enzymes that regulate the intracellular levels of the second messengers, such as cyclic AMP and GMP, by controlling their rate of degradation. The enzymes catalyze the hydrolysis of the 3′ cyclic phosphate bonds of adenosine (Figure 1) and/or guanosine 3′5′ cyclic monophosphate.

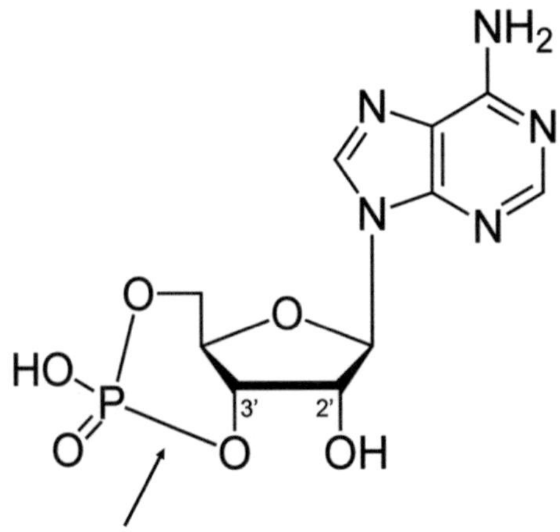

Fig. 1. **Structure of cyclic AMP.** Arrow indicates the site of hydrolyses by phosphodiesterases: the 3′ cyclic phosphate bond.

Many of the early studies on cyclic nucleotides were directed toward understanding PDE activity since at that time it was much easier to measure PDE activity than either cAMP or cGMP themselves or the enzymes that catalyzed their synthesis. More recently, it became clear that there were likely to be multiple isoforms of PDEs with different kinetic and regulatory properties. They are characterized by their specificity and sensitivity to calcium-calmodulin and by their affinity for cAMP or cGMP [11]. PDEs were classified on the basis of their amino acid sequences, substrate specificities, pharmacological properties and tissue distributions.

2. Cyclic nucleotide phosphodiesterases

2.1 Isoforms of phosphodiesterases

It is now very clear that any single cell type can express several different PDE isoforms and also that the nature and localization of these PDEs are likely to be major regulators of the local concentrations of cAMP or cGMP in the cell. Eleven cyclic PDE families with varying selectivities for cAMP and/or cGMP have been identified in mammalian tissues [12-16] (Table 1).

PDEs are therefore important regulators of diverse biochemical mechanisms mediated by cAMP and /or cGMP. Despite this heterogeneity, there is a surprising degree of homology within their catalytic domains; however, slight structural differences in these domains determine whether a PDE is cAMP-specific (PDE4, PDE7, PDE8), cGMPspecific (PDE5, PDE6, PDE9) or has dual substrate specificity (PDE1, PDE2, PDE3, PDE10, PDE11) [17-18].

PDE isoenzyme	Substrate	Km (μM) cAMP	Km (μM) GMP	Tissue expression	Specific inhibitors
1	Ca^{2+}/calmodulin stimulated	80	3	Heart, brain, lung, smooth muscle, T lymphocytes, sperm	KS505a, bepril, Vinpocetine, Flunarizine and Amiodarone
2	cGMP-stimulated	30	10	Adrenal gland, heart, lung, liver, platelets	EHNA, BAY 60-7550, Oxindole and PDP
3	cGMP-inhibited cAMP-selective	0.4	0.3	Heart, lung, liver, platelets, Kidney, T lymphocytes, adipocytes, inflammatory cells	Cilostamide, Enoxamone, Milrinone, Siguazodan
4	cAMP-specific	4		Sertoli cells, kidney, brain, liver, lung, inflammatory cells	Rolipram, Roflumilast, Cilomilast, Drotaverine, ibudilast
5	cGMP-specific	150	1	Lung, platelets, vascular, smooth muscle	Sildenafil, Vardenafil, Tadalafil, Zaprinast
6	cGMP-specific		60	Photoreceptor	Dipyridamole
7	cAMP-specific, high-affinity	700	15	Skeletal muscle, heart, kidney, Brain, pancreas, T lymphocytes	BRL-50481, BC30
8	cAMP-selective	0.06		Testes, eye, liver, skeletal muscle, Heart, kidney, ovary, brain, T lymphocytes	PF-04957325
9	cGMP-specific	230	0.2	Kidney, liver, lung, brain	BAY 73-6691
10	cGMP-sensitive, cAMP-selective	0.2	13	Testes, brain	None
11	cGMP-sensitive, dual specificity	0.7	0.6	Skeletal muscle, prostate, kidney, liver, pituitary, testes and salivary glands	None

Table 1. Phosphodiesterase families and specific inhibitors

PDE1s are calcium dependent activators or regulators: they have been shown to activate cyclic nucleotide PDE in a calcium-dependent manner. PDE1s are present in many tissues and are abundant mainly in the central nervous system, heart, skeletal muscle and kidney [19-21].

PDE2 metabolizes both cGMP and cAMP although its affinity for cGMP is slightly higher than for cAMP [22]. High PDE2 activity can be found in heart [23] and brain. Lower expression of PDE2 was found in lung, placenta, liver, skeletal muscle, kidney and pancreas [24].

PDE3s are characterized by their high affinity and their ability to metabolize both cAMP and cGMP. They are also distinguished by their ability to be activated by several phosphorylation pathways including the PKA and PI3K/PKB pathways. PDE3s are moderately expressed in platelets as well as in vascular smooth muscle [25] and oocytes.

PDE4s have a higher affinity for cAMP, they are expressed in inflammatory cells such as T cells, B cells, eosinophils, neutrophils, airway epithelial cells and endothelial cells [26-28], cardiovascular tissues and smooth muscles. Differential expression of PDE4s can be modulated by inflammatory factors and expressed in lung macrophages from patients with chronic obstructive pulmonary disease (COPD).

PDE5 has a higher affinity for cGMP and was identified, isolated and characterized in rat platelets [29,30] and rat lung [31,32]. PDE5 is widely expressed in pulmonary vascular smooth muscle of pulmonary arteries and veins, bronchial blood vessels and airway smooth muscle [33]. Recent data show that PDE5 may modulate pulmonary arterial pressure induced by cardiac hypertrophy and fibrosis ([34].

PDE6s are phosphodiesterases characterized by their affinity for cGMP and are expressed in the photoreceptor outer segments of the mammalian retina, in which they mediate transduction of the light signal into an electrical response [35].

PDE7 are characterized by their high affinity and selectivity for cAMP as substrate. PDE7 protein expression is largest in T cell lines, blood T cells, epithelial cell lines, airway and vascular smooth muscle cells, lung fibroblasts and eosinophils and in neutrophils [36].

PDE8s are cAMP specific and have a very high affinity for cAMP as a substrate. PDE8s are distributed in various human tissues and are abundant in testis [37-40]. Functionally, PDE8s have been reported to be involved in regulation of T-cell activation [41], chemotaxis of activated lymphocytes [42], modulation of testosterone production in Leydig cells [43], and possibly potentiation of biphasic insulin response to glucose [44].

PDE9 is one of the more recently discovered PDE families. It is perhaps most notable as the PDE family having the highest affinity for cGMP. Further, compared with other cGMP-specific PDEs, PDE9 apparently lacks the non catalytic cGMP-binding domain, which is present in PDE5, PDE6, and also PDE2. The mRNA encoding PDE9 is well expressed in many examined human tissues, including spleen, small intestine, and brain [45,46].

PDE10 was isolated and characterized as a dual-substrate gene family in 1999 from mouse [47] as well as from human fetal lung [48] and fetal brain [49]. This PDE family was recently shown to be associated to the progressive neurodegenerative Huntington's disease (HD) since PDE10 mRNA decreases prior to the onset of motor symptoms in transgenic HD mice expressing exon 1 of the human Huntington gene [50].

PDE11 are characterized by their high affinity for both cAMP and cGMP, although kinetic characteristics for the variants are different [51-53]. PDE 11 mRNA occurs at higher levels in skeletal muscle, prostate, kidney, liver, pituitary and salivary glands, and testis.

3. PDE inhibitors as pharmacological tools in the treatment of diseases

The principle that inhibition of PDE activity could be a valid therapeutic tool is now well accepted. It is commonly accepted that concentrations of cAMP and cGMP in most cells are typically <1 to 10μM [54]. This means that a competitive inhibitor would not need to compete with very high levels of endogenous substrate in order to be effective.

The history of the PDE starts with the work of Henry Hyde Salter in 1887. It has been shown that caffeine has a bronchodilatator effect and that it was a non selective inhibitor of PDE activity. The caffeine and other xanthines have been used as therapeutic agents in respiratory diseases [55].

Inhibition of cyclic nucleotide PDEs allow cAMP/cGMP concentrations to increase within cells. Therefore, inhibition of PDE is a useful way of causing a variety of cellular effects and can influence various physiological mechanisms. Many PDE inhibitors are recognized as pharmacological agents. In fact, some compounds such as theophylline have been used as drugs in medical practice long before they were identified as PDE inhibitors. Currently, both non selective and selective PDE inhibitors are explored as therapeutic agents.

3.1 Non selective PDE inhibitors

Non selective inhibitors of the PDE such as theophylline, caffeine and papaverin have been used for more than 70 years in the western world for treatment of various diseases [56-59] and were identified as PDE inhibitors, i.e. as compounds that specifically inhibit the activity of PDE and not of other phosphohydrolases. During the last 10 years, a better understanding of physiological roles, cellular expression, specific inhibitors of the PDE isoforms, as well as of their clinical indications has been acquired. These non selective PDE inhibitors inhibit PDE competitively with low affinity and do not discriminate between PDE isozymes; both cAMP and cGMP–PDE activities are inhibited. Theophylline and other methylxantines are potent antagonists of adenosine receptors [60]. Theophylline had been prescribed for the first time in 1937 for the treatment of asthma; it is also perceived to be an orally active anti-inflammatory agent for use in asthma or COPD [57,61]. Paraxanthine, the primary metabolite of caffeine, acts through the ryanodine receptor to elevate intracellular calcium concentration and increases viability of neuronal cells in culture [62]. 3-isobutyl-1-methylxanthine (IBMX) was synthesized by Wells et al (1975), it has a much higher affinity for PDEs and at low concentrations, it preferentially inhibits cGMP-PDE over cAMP-PDE [63].

3.2 Selective PDE inhibitors

3.2.1 Inhibitors without therapeutic action

PDE2 is involved in a variety of physiological processes. The availability of PDE selective inhibitors has greatly facilitated the elucidation of PDE2 function in various tissues. One of the first specific inhibitors for PDE2 was erythro 9-(2 hydroxy-3-nonyl) adenine (EHNA) which potentiates the effects of NMDA (N-methyl-D-aspartate) activated receptors in cGMP, but has no effect on cAMP concentration [64]. EHNA is also a potent inhibitor of adenosine deaminase (ADA); it exerts a concentration dependent inhibition of the cGMP-stimulated PDE2 but does not inhibit other PDEs [65]. The strong expression of PDE2 in neurons of the hippocampus and cortex [66] suggests that this enzyme may control intraneuronal second messenger concentrations in these areas. Bayer (Germany) has developed a selective PDE2 inhibitor, the Bay 60-7550, which enhances long-term potentiation of synaptic transmission without altering basal synaptic transmission. BAY 60-7550 can improve memory functions by enhancing neural plasticity [67,68].

3.2.2 Inhibitors with therapeutic action

Some selective PDE inhibitors act directly on the catalytic site of PDE1s, such as vinpocetine. This PDE inhibitor has been used in memory loss [69] and in treating detrusor instabilities and urgency incontinence [70]. PDE inhibitor can improve neural plasticity or restore this function in different neurological conditions [71,72]. Vinpocetine treatment was also shown to revert the effects of early alcohol exposure in learning performance in the water maze [73]. It was recently demonstrated that vinpocetine has a strong anti-inflammatory effect [74]. This new action of vinpocetine, combined with its potential to enhance neuronal plasticity suggest that this drug may have beneficial effects in conditions such as Alzheimer and Parkinson diseases where inflammation and poor neuronal plasticity are present [75].

There are a relatively large number of PDE3 selective inhibitors including milrinone, cilostamide and cilostazol, which were identified as potential therapeutic tools in cardiovascular disease and asthma. Inhibition of PDE3 activity increase L-type Ca^{2+} currents in cardiomyocytes isolated from human, rat and frog heart, an effect that contributes to the positive inotropic effects of these inhibitors [76]. Milrinone has an inotropic and vasodilator effect for "wet and cold" heart failure [77], a case of heart failure with congestion and hypoperfusion [78]. It has been reported that the combination of inhaled and intravenous milrinone could be an effective treatment of secondary pulmonary hypertension in high-risk cardiac valve surgery patients [79].

PDE4 inhibitors have been developed for the treatment of asthma and COPD, diseases characterised by inflammatory and immune responses [80]. Rolipram is a highly selective first generation PDE4 inhibitor that has been used for many years as a research tool to investigate the role of PDE4. Several studies have shown that rolipram inhibits neutrophilic and eosinophilic inflammation [81]; it proved to be an effective antidepressant, but side effects such as nausea and gastro-intestinal disturbance terminated its clinical development [82]. Roflumilast was beneficial, as assessed by improvement in lung function, even when added to a long acting β_2 agonist or a long acting inhaled antimuscarinic [83].

The use of inhibitors of PDE5 (sildenafil (Viagra; Pfizer Inc, US), vardenafil (Levitra; GlaxoSmithKline, UK) and tadalafil (Cialis; Eli Lilly, US)) in the treatment of male erectile dysfunction is the first commercial success for PDE inhibitors. Sildenafil (under the tradename Revatio) and tadalafil (under the tradename Adcirca) have also been approved for the treatment of pulmonary arterial hypertension (PAH). PDE5 is a cGMP-specific phosphodiesterase encoded by a single gene. Recent data show that PDE5 may modulate pressure-induced cardiac hypertrophy and fibrosis [34]. Although sildenafil has an acceptable degree of selectivity, increased specificity for PDE5, particularly over PDE1 and PDE6 will reduce or eliminate the incidence of visual disturbances associated with the flushing and headaches that are observed with sildenafil [84]. In the case of all the other PDE5 inhibitors that have been described in the peer-reviewed literature, improvements in selectivity were determined empirically, and compounds were optimized on the basis of structure- activity explorations of the chemical series in question. PDE5 is abundantly expressed in lung tissue and appears to be up regulated in PAH [85,86]. PDE5 is involved in endothelial dysfunction by inactivating cGMP, the second messenger of the nitric oxide (NO) pathway in the pulmonary vasculature [85-87]. It has been reported that sildenafil and vardenafil raise hippocampal cGMP levels and improve memory in aged rats [88] and mice [89].

The PDE7 family is composed of two genes coding for high-affinity, rolipram-insensitive, cAMP-specific enzymes. The presence of high concentrations of PDE7 mRNA in the human striatum and dentate gyrus suggests that selective inhibitors could be used to increase cAMP concentration in these areas without some of the side effects associated with PDE4 inhibition [40,90,91]. Several distinct PDE7 inhibitors have been reported [92,93]; however, their effects on central nervous system (CNS) function have yet to be described. It has been shown that selective inhibition of PDE7 or dual PDE4/7 inhibition may provide a novel therapeutic approach for the treatment of chronic lymphocytic leukemia (CLL) by enhancing killing and increasing specificity for CLL cells [94].

The company Pfizer reported on a small molecule called PF-04957325 that selectively inhibits PDE8 with an *in vitro* IC50 of 0.7nM against PDE8A, of 0.2nM against PDE8B, and >1.5µM against all other PDE isoforms [95]. PDE8-selective inhibitors might be used to correct adrenal insufficiency, and a PDE8 activator might be used to treat Cushing's syndrome [96].

4. Pharmacological potential of PDE inhibitors for the treatment of cystic fibrosis

As an important second messenger signaling molecule, cAMP controls a wide variety of eukaryotic and prokaryotic responses to extracellular cues [97]. For cAMP-dependent signaling pathways to be effective, the intracellular cAMP concentration is tightly controlled at the level of both of synthesis and degradation. CF is characterized by defective cAMP-dependent chloride conductance in epithelial cells and is caused by a defect in the targeting of the chloride channel CFTR.

4.1 Non selective PDE inhibitors

Non specific inhibitors of the PDE such as IBMX, theophylline and DPMX (7-methyl-1,3 dipropyl xanthine) have been shown to activate normal and mutated CFTR chloride channels in epithelia [98]. It is well known that the methylxanthines, found naturally in tea, coffee and cocoa, stimulate the central nervous system, relax bronchial smooth muscle, and stimulate cardiac muscle. These purine derivatives function as adenosine receptor antagonists and as PDE inhibitors. Due to impact on the cAMP pathway and activity at low concentrations, studies have been done looking at their effect on the cAMP activated CFTR channel. The PDE inhibitor, IBMX also functions as an adenosine receptor antagonist. It has been reported that IBMX increases the CFTR chloride current in Xenopus oocytes expressing the F508del-CFTR [99]. In 1993, when studying CF nasal bronchial epithelial tissues with F508del-CFTR, Grubb et al. found that IBMX (5 mM) associated to forskolin (0.01 mM) did not stimulate chloride efflux *in vitro* [100]. Haws et al. studied the effect of IBMX and 8-cyclopentyl-1,3-dipropylxanthine (CPX), another non specific PDE and an A1 adenosine receptor antagonist, on stably transfected cells with F508del-CFTR [101]. In this study, both IBMX (5 mM) and CPX potentiated the effect of forskolin on CFTR-mediated efflux of ^{125}I by 2.5-fold. There was a 7-fold increase in cAMP levels associated with IBMX treatment, but not CPX treatment. A potentiation by IBMX of prostaglandin E (PGE2)-induced HCO_3^- secretion has been reported in the rat duodenum *in vivo* [102,103].

4.2 Selective PDE inhibitors

PDE inhibitors increase cAMP by inhibiting one or more enzymes involved in cAMP degradation. Cyclic AMP-activated PKA mediates phosphorylation of CFTR and increases the open probability of the CFTR channel. Drugs in this class include amrinone and milrinone. These drugs also cause vasodilation, which may be beneficial for the CF airways. In 1991, Drumm et al. showed that inhibiting PDE had a larger effect on CFTR activation than have adenylate cyclase stimulants [99]. Using airway epithelial cell lines expressing wild-type CFTR, Calu-3 and 16HBE cells, it has been found that, at 100μM concentrations, PDE 3 inhibitors (milrinone, amrinone) without adenylate cyclase activators, stimulate chloride efflux 13.7-fold [104]. They found no effect on chloride efflux by IBMX, a non specific PDE, by rolipram, a PDE4 inhibitor or by dipyridamole, a PDE5 inhibitor. The increase of channel efflux by the type 3 PDE inhibitor was not associated with a significant rise in cAMP concentrations but it was inhibited by protein kinase A inhibitors (H-8 and Rp-cAMPS), suggesting that it might work through a more distal signal. Kelley et al. also looked at endogenous CFTR in transformed nasal polyp tissue of patients homozygous for F508del (CF-T43) [105]. They found that, when administered in the presence of a β-agonist (isoproterenol) and protein kinase A activator, milrinone and amrinone, at 100μM concentrations, increased chloride efflux by 19-61% from baseline. Mice homozygous for F508del Cftr were administered with a combination of milrinone (100 μM) and forskolin (10 μM) [106]. This combination of drugs resulted in an increased magnitude of the murine nasal potential difference (PD). The implications of this study are exciting; but the effect has not been confirmed by others [107].

It has been shown that CFTR has a major role in the regulation of duodenal HCO_3^- secretion [108]. Furthermore, O'Grady et al. [109] showed that both PDE1 and PDE3 are involved in the activation of CFTR in T84 cells and human colonic epithelial cells. In 2007, Hayashi M et al. [110] suggested that PDE1 and PDE3 are involved in the regulation of duodenal HCO_3^- secretion and that the response to PGE2 is associated with both PDE1 and PDE3, while the response to NO is mainly modulated by PDE1 [110]. McPherson et al. showed that a selective cyclic nucleotide PDE5 inhibitor partially corrected defective L-adrenergic stimulation of mucin secretion in CFTR antibody-inhibited submandibular cells. The PDE5 inhibitor did not increase cAMP levels, nor did it potentiate isoproterenol-induced cAMP rise [111]. Of note, Dormer et al. (2005) demonstrated that the PDE5 inhibitor sildenafil (Viagra) also acts as a pharmacological chaperone. Because sildenafil is approved for clinical use, they speculated that their data might speed up the development of new therapies for CF [7].

5. The clinical pharmacokinetics of PDE5 inhibitors

Lung tissue is a rich source of PDE, including PDE5, the major function of which is acceleration of the decay of cGMP [112].

5.1 Sildenafil

Sildenafil citrate was the first selective PDE5 inhibitor approved for the treatment of erectile dysfunction. Sildenafil, however, is only approximately 10-fold as potent for PDE5 as for PDE6, which is found in the photoreceptors of the human retina. This lower selectivity toward PDE6 is presumed to be the cause for color vision abnormalities observed with high doses or plasma levels of sildenafil.

Sildenafil is relatively lipophilic with a weakly basic center in the piperazine tertiary amine, resulting in only partial ionization at physiological pH. Following oral administration, sildenafil is rapidly absorbed, reaching peak plasma concentrations within 1 hour (range, 0.5-2 hours). The first-order absorption rate constant was estimated as 2.6 hours^{-1} based on population pharmacokinetic data in patients with erectile dysfunction [113]. Administration of sildenafil after a high-fat meal caused reductions in the rate of absorption and extent of systemic exposure. The time-to-peak (t_{max}) was delayed by approximately 1 hour, and maximum concentration (C_{max}) was reduced by 29%. The systemic exposure of sildenafil after a high-fat meal was reduced by 11% [114].

Sildenafil is highly bound to plasma proteins, and the protein binding is independent of drug concentrations. After intravenous administration, the mean steady-state volume of distribution of sildenafil is 105 L, which substantially exceeds the total volume of body water (approximately 42 L), indicating distribution into tissues and possibly binding to extravascular proteins. Sildenafil is extensively metabolized, without unchanged sildenafil being detected in either urine or feces. After an oral dose, metabolites are predominantly excreted into the feces (73%-88%) and to a lesser extent into the urine (6%-15%) [115]. Plasma concentrations of sildenafil was reported to decline biexponentially, with a mean terminal half-life of 3 to 5 hours, independent of the route of administration [114]. Sildenafil is primarily metabolized by the cytochrome P-450 (CYP) isoenzyme CYP3A4 and to a lesser extent CYP2C9 [116]. Sildenafil is extensively metabolized, with more than 12 metabolites identified.

The principal routes of metabolism are N-demethylation, oxidation, and aliphatic hydroxylation [115]. Plasma concentrations of N-demethylation are approximately 40% that of sildenafil, so that the metabolite accounts for approximately 20% of the pharmacological effects of sildenafil. The metabolite profile is qualitatively similar after intravenous and oral administration, but higher concentrations of N-desmethyl sildenafil after oral administration indicate the important role of first-pass metabolism in the metabolite formation.

5.2 Vardenafil

Vardenafil hydrochloride was the first second generation PDE5 inhibitor approved for the treatment of erectile dysfunction. Vardenafil has a high selectivity for the inhibition of PDE5 compared with the other known phosphodiesterases [117,118]. Unlike sildenafil and tadalafil, vardenafil was developed from the outset specifically to treat erectile dysfunction.

Vardenafil is rapidly absorbed, with plasma concentrations being detected in all subjects within 8 to 15 minutes after oral administration.

Peak plasma concentrations were observed 0.25 to 3 hours after administration, with a median of 0.7 hours for the 20 and 40 mg dose level, and slightly later, with 0.9 hours for the 10 mg dose level [117,119]. The absolute bioavailability of vardenafil was described as approximately 15%. Vardenafil pharmacokinetics is largely unaffected by food containing moderate amounts of fat. Minimal changes (<15%) in mean vardenafil C_{max} and no change in median t_{max} were observed when vardenafil was administered with a moderate-fat evening meal compared to dosing on an empty stomach. When 20mg oral vardenafil was administered immediately after consumption of a high-fat breakfast, the mean C_{max} was 18% lower and the median t_{max} was delayed by 1 hour.

Based on *in vitro* investigations in human plasma, approximately 93% to 95% of the drug is bound to plasma proteins, approximately 80% to albumin, and 11% to α1-acid glycoprotein [120]. It was also demonstrated that the binding to plasma proteins was fully reversible in all the tested species and was concentration independent. The major metabolite of vardenafil has similar protein-binding properties as the parent drug, with a bound fraction of 93% to 95%. The volume of distribution estimate for vardenafil after intravenous administration is relatively high, 208 L, implying extensive drug distribution into tissues.

Vardenafil is extensively metabolized, with more than 14 metabolites identified. The major metabolite, M1, and 2 minor metabolites, M4 and M5, as well as their respective glucuronides, are all a result of the degradation of vardenafil's piperazine ring. M1 is N-desethyl vardenafil, M4 is reduced by a 2-carbon fragment of the piperazine ring of vardenafil, and M5 is the N-desethyl derivative of M4. Metabolism is predominantly mediated by CYP3A4 and to a smaller extent by CYP3A5 and CYP2C isoforms. All 3 metabolites have pharmacologic activity. The major circulating metabolite, M1, has 28% of vardenafil's potency for PDE5 inhibition, while M4 and M5 possess 5.6% and 4.9%, respectively [120].

5.3 Tadalafil

Tadalafil is a selective and potent inhibitor of PDE5 with an IC50 of 0.94 nM. It exhibits high selectivity toward PDE5 compared to other PDEs. Tadalafil is structurally different from both sildenafil and vardenafil, and the different structures are reflected in distinct differences in the clinical pharmacology profiles of these drugs [121]. Like sildenafil, tadalafil was developed initially for use in cardiovascular disease and was subsequently used for the treatment of erectile dysfunction [122]. Tadalafil was the last of the 3 PDE5 inhibitors approved for erectile dysfunction.

Tadalafil is rapidly absorbed after oral administration with a median time to reach peak plasma concentration of 2 hours (range, 0.5-6 hours) [118,121]. Absolute bioavailability of tadalafil following oral dosing has not been reported, but at least 36% of the dose is absorbed from an oral solution. The time course of oral absorption could successfully be modeled by a rapid first-order process. Population estimates of the first-order absorption rate constant from phase II and phase III studies are 1.75 and 1.86 hours^{-1}, respectively [123]. The absorption and pharmacodynamic properties of tadalafil are not affected by either food or alcohol, and thus the drug can be administered without regard for food or alcohol consumption [124]. Smoking and body mass index had a weak effect on the pharmacokinetics of tadalafil. It has been reported that the clinical response to tadalafil may be evident as early as 16 minutes and may persist for up to 24 to 36 hours post dose [124,125]

Tadalafil has an apparent volume of distribution of 60 to 70 L, with an interindividual variability of 40% to 50%. This indicates that tadalafil is distributed into tissues. Plasma protein binding was reported as 94%, with α1-acid glycoprotein and albumin as principal binding proteins. A population pharmacokinetic analysis in patients taking tadalafil suggests a body weight dependency of the volume of distribution at steady state.

Tadalafil is excreted primarily as inactive metabolites, mainly in the feces and to a lesser extent in urine. The mean elimination half-life for tadalafil was 17.5 hours, and the mean apparent oral clearance was 2.5 L/h in healthy subjects [126]. The nearly exclusive elimination via hepatic metabolism and the relatively low value for oral clearance indicate that tadalafil has a low intrinsic clearance with regard to hepatic metabolism and can be classified as a drug with low hepatic extraction ratio.

Tadalafil is primarily metabolized by CYP3A4 to a catechol metabolite, which further undergoes extensive methylation and glucuronidation to form methylcatechol and methylcatechol glucuronide metabolites. This was confirmed by interaction studies with rifampin as potent CYP3A inducer and

ketoconazole as a potent CYP3A inhibitor. The main circulating metabolite in plasma is methylcatechol glucuronide, which has a ≥ 10 000-fold less affinity for PDE5 than the analogue drug, tadalafil, and is thus expected to be clinically inactive at observed metabolite concentrations [126]. Several other inactive metabolites have also been identified in plasma, urine, or feces.

5.4 Comparison of PDE5 inhibitors

Although the 3 currently available PDE5 inhibitors, sildenafil, vardenafil, and tadalafil, have all shown to be effective in the treatment of erectile dysfunction, there are distinct differences between the compounds regarding their selectivity and specificity for PDE inhibition with consequences especially for the safety profile but also biopharmaceutic and pharmacokinetic disparities that largely affect the efficacy profile of these compounds. Sildenafil and vardenafil are very similar in terms of their chemical structure, whereas tadalafil with a methyldione structure differs markedly from sildenafil and vardenafil (Figure 2). These chemical similarities and differences are also reflected in similarities and dissimilarities of their clinical pharmacokinetics.

All 3 PDE5 inhibitors are rapidly absorbed after oral administration, with peak concentrations reached slightly earlier for vardenafil compared to sildenafil and tadalafil. Although no clear concentration-effect relationships have been established for any of the 3 PDE5 inhibitors, rapid absorption is considered an essential for a rapid onset of efficacy. Administration of a high-fat meal had no significant effect on the rate and extent of absorption of tadalafil but decreased the rate of absorption for sildenafil and vardenafil. All 3 drugs are lipophilic and have a volume of distribution larger than the volume of total body water, indicating tissue uptake and binding. Furthermore, all 3 compounds are highly protein bound, with free plasma concentration fractions of only 4% to 6%.

The major route of elimination for all PDE5 inhibitors is hepatic metabolism, with renal excretion of unchanged drug accounting for 1% or less of the elimination pathways. Based on their relatively high systemic clearance after intravenous administration, sildenafil and vardenafil can be classified as non restrictively cleared drugs with intermediate to high hepatic extraction ratio. The relatively comparable distribution volumes together with the substantial differences in systemic clearance among the PDE5 inhibitors result in distinct differences of the elimination half-life, 3 to 5 hours for sildenafil and vardenafil compared to 17.5 hours for tadalafil. Tadalafil, however, has been detected in plasma even 5 days after oral administration due to its long half-life. This suggests the possibility of accumulation if taken regularly and in short intervals, which may result in an increased risk of side effects with the excessive use of this PDE5 inhibitor.

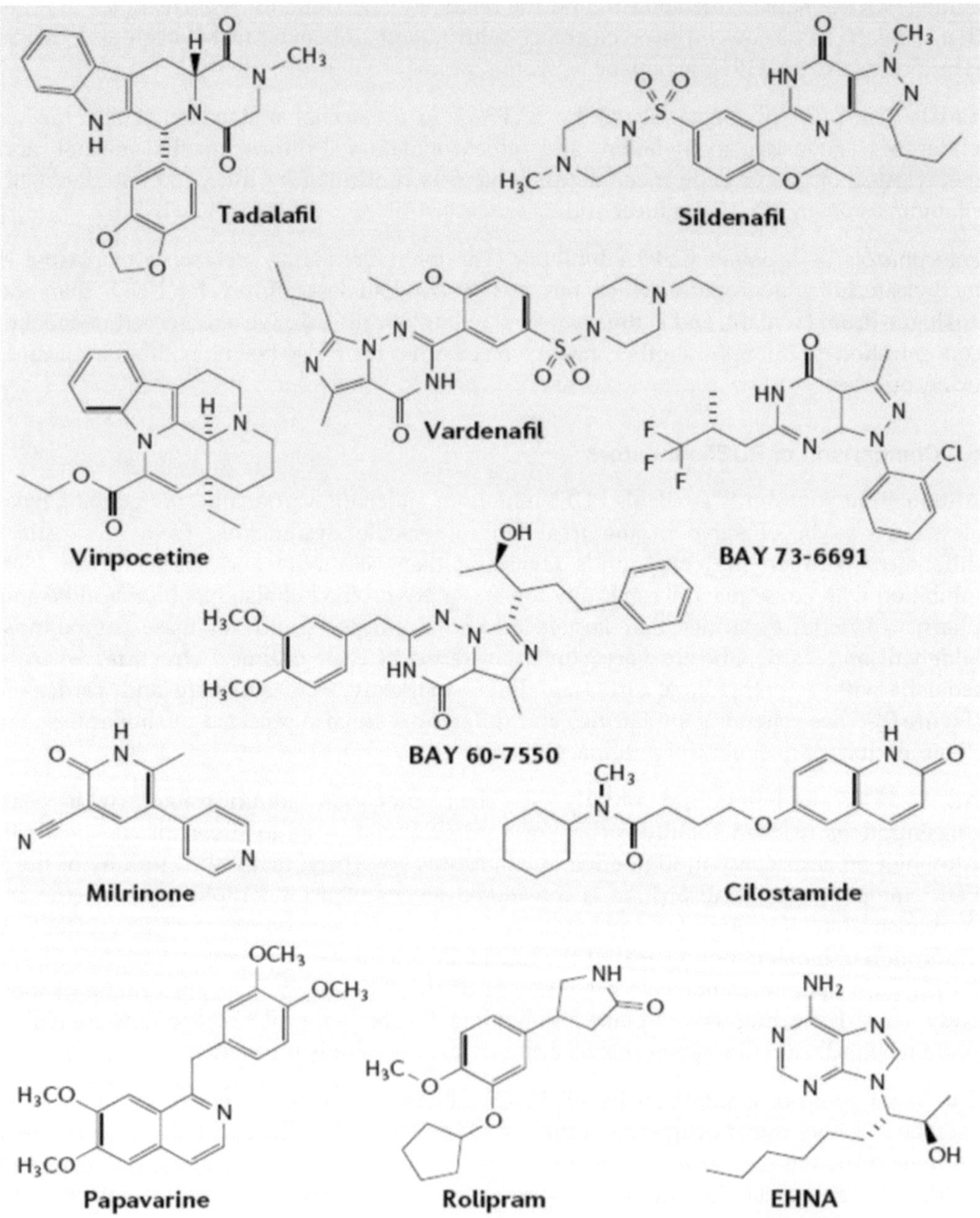

Fig. 2. **Structures of selected examples of phosphodiesterase inhibitors.** The figure shows various selective phosphodiesterase (PDE) inhibitors mentioned in this chapter. Of these, the PDE5 inhibitors sildenafil, vardenafil and tadalafil have been approved for treatment of erectile dysfunction. Sildenafil and vardenafil have also recently been approved as a treatment for pulmonary hypertension.

6. Administration of PDE5 inhibitors at clinical doses activates defective chloride transport in CF

At present, many efforts are focused on CFTR pharmacotherapy which corrects the abnormal protein pharmacologically by various approaches such as the direct correction of stop codon mutations, CFTR channel activation, or correction of CFTR trafficking defects.

High-throughput screening (HTS) has been used to identify molecules that increase F508del-CFTR activity [127,129]. Such molecules have been categorized according to whether they alleviate the folding/cellular processing defect (correctors) or increase the responsiveness of F508del-CFTR channels already present in the membrane to cAMP activation (potentiators). Sildenafil has also been shown to correct F508del-CFTR processing when used at high micromolar concentrations [7].

To test the hypothesis that PDE5 inhibitors (sildenafil, vardenafil and taladafil) are able to restore transepithelial ion transport abnormalities of the F508del-CFTR protein, we have conducted experimental studies [9,10] in CF mice homozygous for the F508del mutation [130] and in their corresponding wild-type homozygous normal mice. The F508del-Cftr mouse model has been chosen because F508del is the most common and one of the most severe CF mutation and because the mouse model recapitulates, at different levels, the human disease. Epithelia of the F508del-CF mouse model are characterized by defective electrolyte transport, and *Pseudomonas aeruginosa* lipopolysaccharide (LPS) exposure mimics several aspects of CF airway epithelial inflammation such as increased pro-inflammatory cytokines, most notably interleukin (IL)-8, IL-6, and Tumor Necrosis Factor (TNF)-α, and neutrophil infiltrate cells.

In our protocols, CFTR function has been assessed *in vivo* by measuring the transepithelial nasal PD, a delicate technique that has been increasingly used as an index of therapeutic efficacy in novel fundamental therapies, either in animal models [9,10,131] or in CF patients [132]. Our results provide clear evidence that intraperitoneal injection of PDE5 inhibitors (Figure 3), at clinical doses, to F508del-CF mice interact with CFTR, propping open the mutant protein to allow a normal flow of chloride ions across the epithelium of nasal mucosa, thereby completely restoring the decreased or even abolished CFTR-dependent chloride transport [9]. In F508del mice, but not in *Cftr* knockout mice, the chloride conductance, evaluated by perfusing the nasal mucosa with a chloride-free solution in the presence of amiloride and with forskolin, is corrected 1 h after sildenafil administration. A more prolonged effect, persisting for at least 24 h, is observed with vardenafil. Moreover, vardenafil, but not sildenafil, is able to stimulate chloride transport associated with normal wild-type Cftr protein [9]. The forskolin response is increased after treatment with sildenafil or vardenafil in wild-type and in F508del mutant animals. In F508del mice, the chloride conductance in the presence of 200 μM DIDS (4-4′-diisothiocyanostilbene-2,2′-disulphonic acid), an inhibitor of alternative chloride channels, was much higher after sildenafil injection than following placebo treatment (Figure 4). No effect on the sodium conductance was detected in any group of animals. Altogether, these data provide preclinical evidence that sildenafil and vardenafil stimulate, by a direct and not a by-pass effect, chloride transport activity of F508del-CFTR protein.

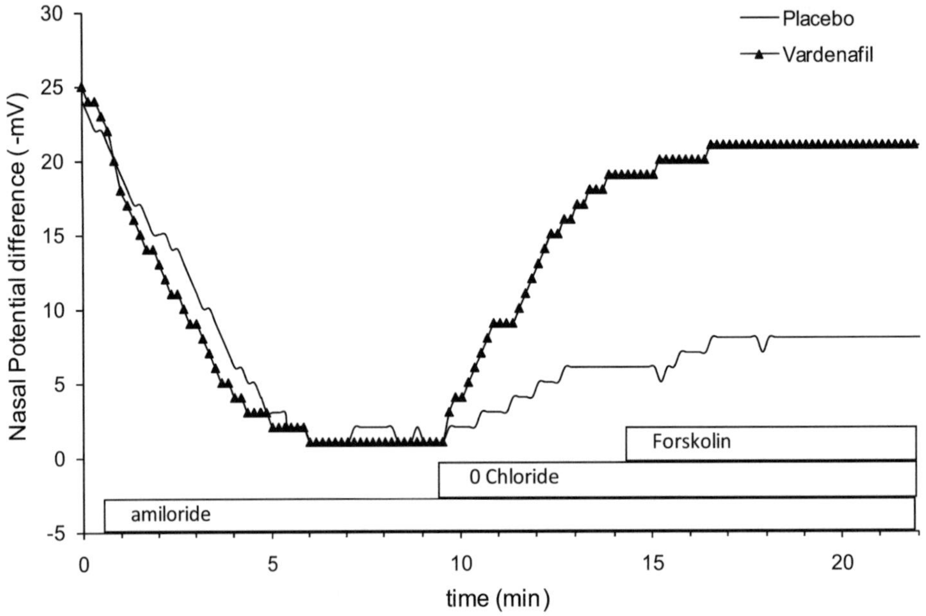

Fig. 3. Influence of vardenafil (24h after a single therapeutic dose) on ion transport evaluated by the nasal potential difference (PD) in F508del-CF mice. Chloride conductance in response to perfusion of the nasal mucosa with a solution without chloride and to forskolin is dramatically increased as compared to placebo-treated CF mice.

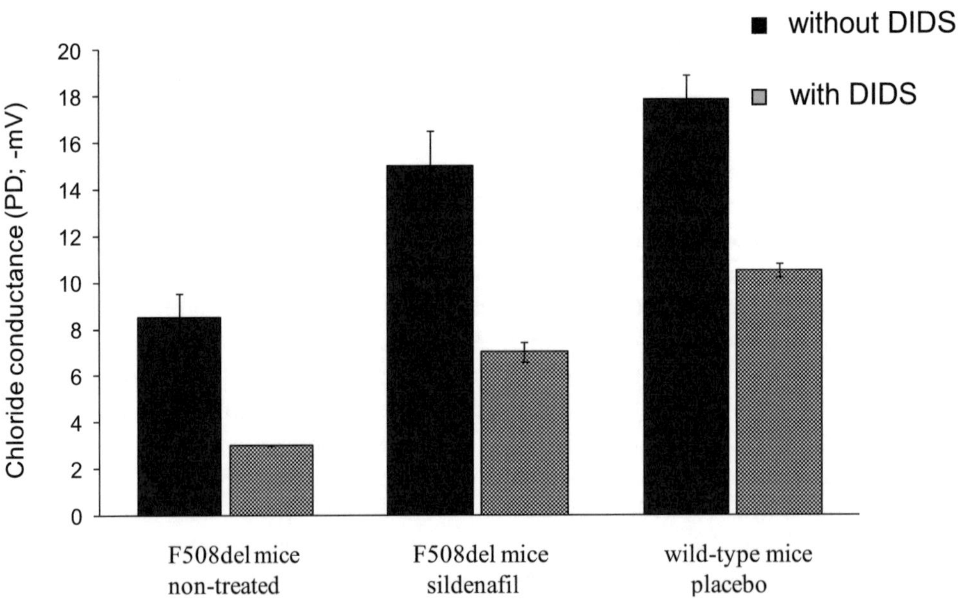

Fig. 4. Influence of sildenafil on Cftr -dependent chloride conductance evaluated by the nasal potential difference (PD) in the presence or the absence of DIDS, an inhibitor of alternative chloride conductance. Increased DIDS-insensitive conductance after sildenafil treatment reflects activation of Cftr function.

More recently, using a nebulizer setup specifically developed for mice (Figure 5), we have demonstrated that administration of PDE5 inhibitors through a single inhalation exposure is able to locally activate Cftr protein and correct the basic defects in CF [10] and that the effect lasts for at least 8 h (Figure 6). Our data have identified the inhalational route as a potential therapy for PDE5 inhibitors in CF. Consistent with our results, it has recently been demonstrated that the inhalation route of administration for vardenafil is associated with an acceptable safety profile. Apart from brief coughing on inspiration, no clinically significant changes in blood pressure or heart rate and no serious adverse events were recorded [133]. Inhalation drug therapy has several potential advantages over oral and intravenous routes, including rapid onset of pharmacological action, minimized systemic adverse effects and reduced effective drug doses compared to the same drug delivered orally [134]; this greatly highlights the impact of our work for translational science.

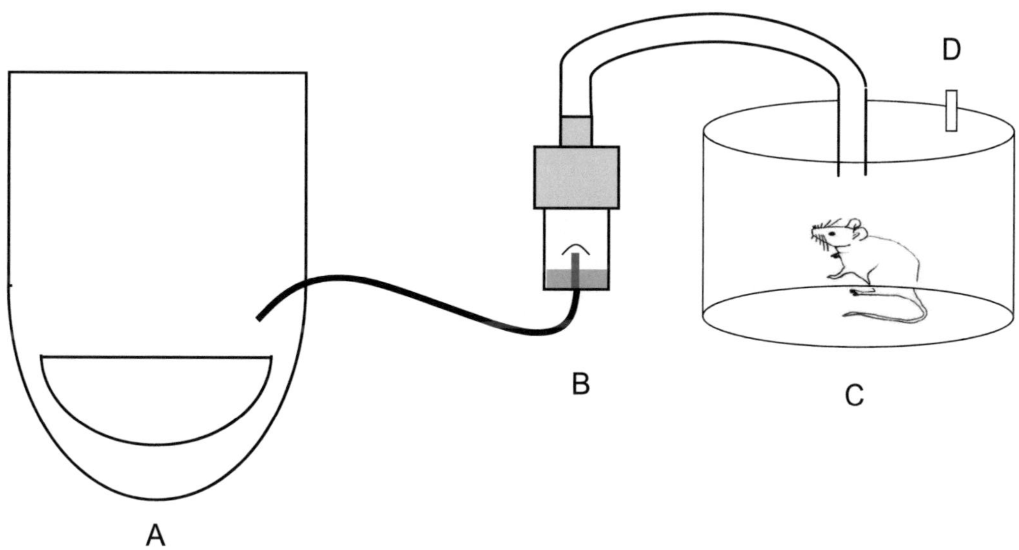

Fig. 5. Schematic representation of the whole-body immersion inhalation chamber setup we developed for a single mouse. (A) compressor, (B) nebulizer, (C) inhalation chamber with (D) expiratory gate.

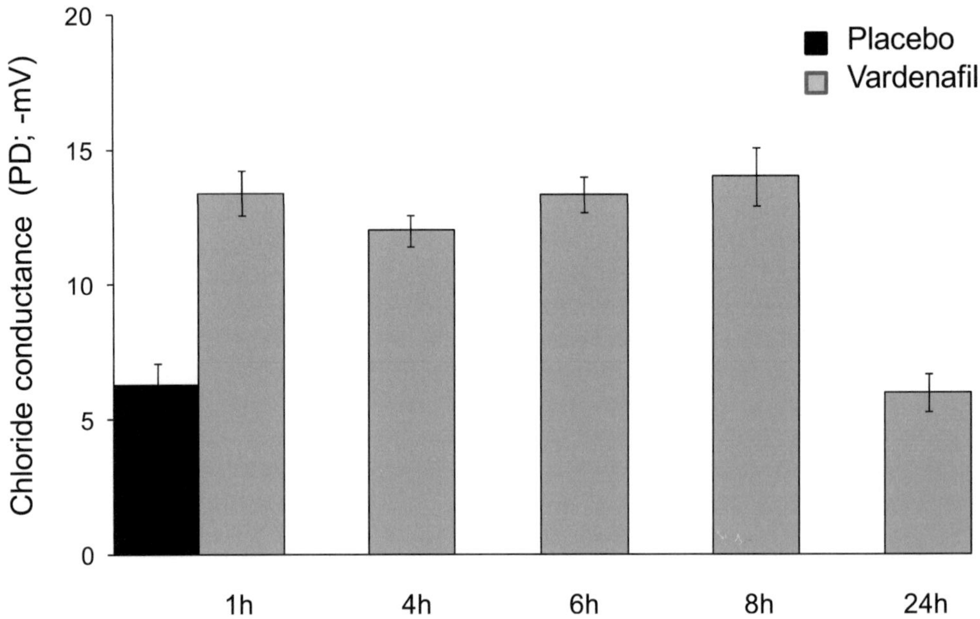

Fig. 6. Duration of the correcting effect of inhaled vardenafil on chloride conductance, evaluated by nasal potential difference (PD) in F508del-CF mice 1, 4, 6, 8 and 24h after a single nebulisation with placebo or with vardenafil. The correcting effect of vardenafil lasts at least 8 h after inhalation.

7. Intraperitoneal administration of PDE5 inhibitors administration at clinical doses attenuates exaggerated inflammatory responses in CF in vivo conditions

Another important goal of mutation-specific CF treatment is attenuation of exaggerated lung inflammatory responses [134-137]. As lung inflammation plays a major role in morbi-mortality in CF, identifying a therapeutic strategy that combines ability to correct the basic ion transport defect and to reduce dysregulated inflammatory responses is very exciting and promising. It has been reported that sildenafil reduces neutrophil lung infiltration in murine airways infected with *P. aeruginosa* [138]. In addition, toxicological studies have shown that sildenafil pretreatment attenuates acrolein-triggered airway inflammation associated with mucin overproduction [139].

More recently, we have found that vardenafil, selected as a representative PDE5 inhibitor for its longer-lasting Cftr activating effect, modulates the vicious circle of lung inflammation and attenuates the expression of pro-inflammatory cytokines and chemokines and cell infiltrates in the bronchoalveolar lavage (BAL) of CF and wild-type mice [140] Our data indicate that intraperitoneal administration of a single pharmacological dose (0.14 mg/kg body weight) of vardenafil is followed by a reducing response in cell infiltrate and in the biosynthesis of several biomarkers of the inflammatory response. Most notably, levels of CCL-2 (chemokine C-C motif ligand), a cytokine playing a key role in the contribution of macrophages in the inflammatory response [136], are significantly reduced in the BAL fluid after vardenafil treatment, particularly in CF animals (Figure 7).

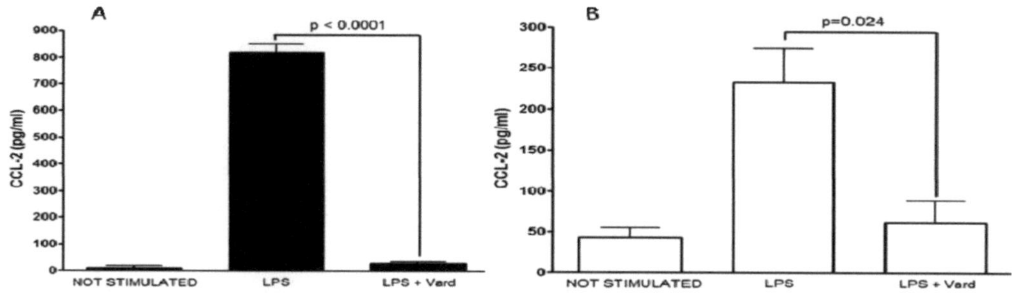

Fig. 7. Anti-inflammatory effect of *in vivo* treatment, by intraperitoneal injection, of a single therapeutic dose of vardenafil (vard) to F508del-CF (A) and wild-type (B) mice on the lipopolyssaccharide (LPS of *P. aeruginosa*) induced inflammatory response. Biosynthesis of CCL-2 is significantly reduced in the bronchoalveolar lavage (BAL) of vardenafil-treated CF and non-CF animals.

The mechanism of action of vardenafil as an anti-inflammatory agent in CF as well as the target-effector cells involved in these responses are under investigation by our group. Altogether, our data indicate that PDE5 inhibitors have a strong therapeutic potential for treating CF. A clinical trial aimed at investigating the safety and efficacy of sildenafil in CF lung disease is listed on www.clinicaltrials.gov (NCT00659529).

8. Conclusions

There is still no cure for CF. The CF patient may benefit from today's privileged strategy which consists on targeting a pharmacological mutation-specific treatment. Currently candidate molecules suitable for CFTR pharmacotherapy are either being sought after or under investigation. Based on the high prevalence of *F508del-CFTR* mutation – more than two-thirds of patients with CF carry at least one copy of the allele -, strategies to rescue the functional status of the mutated protein will benefit most of the CF population. As PDE5 inhibitors such as sildenafil, vardenafil and tadalafil are able to correct transepithelial ion transport abnormalities and to limit exaggerated inflammatory responses related to the presence of F508del-CF protein, the drugs are promising compounds for fundamental pharmacotherapy in CF. Since the drugs are in clinical use, therapeutic approaches to address F508del-CFTR defects by PDE5 inhibitors could be considered as a 'low-hanging fruit' strategy in the drug discovery tree. The fact that such compounds have been approved for other therapeutic indications could speed up their development as CF therapeutics, as compared to other agents that are under investigation only for CF therapy and for which further exploratory studies are needed before being streamed towards clinical testing.

In summary, CFTR correction with PDE5 inhibitors is a promising therapeutic approach based on functional correction of F508del-CFTR activity and on a possible anti-inflammatory action in F508del mice. The effects of these compounds on other CF mutation classes remain to be assessed.

9. Acknowledgements

TL is an associate researcher with the Fonds de la Recherche Scientifique Médicale (FRSM). BL is a PhD fellow with the Fonds Spéciaux de Recherche (FSR; Université catholique de Louvain). SN is a postdoctoral fellow with the FSR and Marie Curie Actions of the European Commission. We thank Gregory Reychler for his assistance in the development of the inhalation chamber setup. Supported by grants of the French CF Association (Vaincre la Mucoviscidose), the FRSM, FSR and the Foundation St Luc (St Luc University Hospital and Université catholique de Louvain).

10. References

[1] Kerem B, Rommens JM, Buchanan JA, Markiewicz D, Cox TK, Chakravarti A, Buchwald M, Tsui LC (1989) Identification of the cystic fibrosis gene: Genetic analysis. *Science* 245:1073-1080.

[2] Riordan JR, Rommens JM, Kerem B, Alon N, Rozmahel R, Grzelczak Z, Zielenski J, Lok S, Plavsic N, Chou JL, et al (1989). Identification of the cystic fibrosis gene: Cloning and characterization of complementary DNA. *Science* 245:1066-1073.

[3] Rowe SM, Miller S, Sorscher EJ (2005) Cystic fibrosis. *N Engl J Med* 352:1992-2001.

[4] Davis PB (2006) Cystic fibrosis since 1938. *Am J Respir Crit Care Med* 173:475-482.

[5] Lukacs GL, Mohamed A, Kartner N, Chang XB, Riordan JR, Grinstein S (1994). Conformational maturation of CFTR but not its mutant counterpart (Delta F508) occurs in the endoplasmic reticulum and requires atp. *EMBO J* 13:6076-6086.

[6] Amaral MD (2004) CFTR and chaperones: processing and degradation. *J Mol Neurosci* 23:41-8.

[7] Dormer RL, Harris CM, Clark Z, Pereira MM, Doull IJ, Norez C, Becq F, McPherson MA (2005) Sildenafil (Viagra) corrects DeltaF508-CFTR location in nasal epithelial cells from patients with cystic fibrosis. *Thorax* 60:55-59.

[8] Robert R, Carlile GW, Pavel C, Liu N, Anjos SM, Liao J, Luo Y, Zhang D, Thomas DY, Hanrahan JW (2008) Structural analog of sildenafil identified as a novel corrector of the F508del-CFTR trafficking defect. *Mol Pharmacol* 73:478-489.

[9] Lubamba B, Lecourt H, Lebacq J, Lebecque P, De Jonge H, Wallemacq P, Leal T (2008). Preclinical evidence that sildenafil and vardenafil activate chloride transport in cystic fibrosis. *Am J Respir Crit Care Med* 177:506-515.

[10] Lubamba B, Lebacq J, Reychler G, Marbaix E, Wallemacq P, Lebecque P, Leal T (2011) Inhaled phosphodiesterase type 5 inhibitors restore chloride transport in cystic fibrosis mice. *Eur Respir J* 37:72-78.

[11] Beavo JA, Rogers NL, Crofford OB, Hardman JG, Sutherland EW, Newman EV (1970) Effects of xanthine derivatives on lipolysis and on adenosine 3',5'-monophosphate phosphodiesterase activity. *Mol Pharmacol* 6:597-603.

[12] Cheung WY (1970) Cyclic nucleotide phosphodiesterase. *Adv Biochemical Psychopharmacol* 3:51-65.

[13] Conti M (2000) Phosphodiesterases and cyclic nucleotide signaling in endocrine cells. *Mol Endocrinol* 14:1317-1327.

[14] Soderling SH, Beavo JA (2000) Regulation of cAMP and cGMP signaling: new phosphodiesterases and new functions. *Curr Opin Cell Biol* 12:174-179

[15] Francis SH, Turko IV, Corbin JD (2001) Cyclic nucleotide phosphodiesterases: relating structure and function. *Prog Nucleic Acid Res Mol Biol* 65:1-52.

[16] Mehats C, Andersen CB, Filopanti M, Jin SL, Conti M (2002) Cyclic nucleotide phosphodiesterases and their role in endocrine cell signaling. *Trends Endocrinol Metabol* 13:29-35.

[17] Xu RX, Rocque WJ, Lambert MH, Vanderwall DE, Luther MA, Nolte RT (2004) Crystal structures of the catalytic domain of phosphodiesterase 4B complexed with AMP, 8-Br-AMP, and rolipram. *J Mol Biol* 337:355-365.

[18] Zhang HT, Zhao Y, Huang Y, Dorairaj NR, Chandler LJ, O'Donnell JM (2004) Inhibition of the phosphodiesterase 4 (PDE4) enzyme reverses memory deficits produced by infusion of the MEK inhibitor U0126 into the CA1 subregion of the rat hippocampus. *Neuropsychopharmacology* 29:1432-1439.

[19] Yan C, Zhao AZ, Bentley JK, Loughney K, Ferguson K, Beavo JA (1995) Molecular cloning and characterization of a calmodulin-dependent phosphodiesterase enriched in olfactory sensory neurons. *Proc Natl Acad Sci USA* 92:9677-9681.

[20] Loughney K, Martins TJ, Harris EA, Sadhu K, Hicks JB, Sonnenburg WK, Beavo JA, Ferguson K (1996) Isolation and characterization of cDNAs corresponding to two human calcium, calmodulin-regulated, 3',5'-cyclic nucleotide phosphodiesterases. *J Biol Chem* 271:796-806.

[21] Yu SM, Hung LM, Lin CC (1997) cGMP-elevating agents suppress proliferation of vascular smooth muscle cells by inhibiting the activation of epidermal growth factor signaling pathway. *Circulation* 95:1269-1277.

[22] Rosman GJ, Martins TJ, Sonnenburg WK, Beavo JA, Ferguson K, Loughney K (1997) Isolation and characterization of human cDNAs encoding a cGMP-stimulated 3',5'-cyclic nucleotide phosphodiesterase. *Gene* 191:89-95.

[23] Rivet-Bastide M, Vandecasteele G, Hatem S, Verde I, Benardeau A, Mercadier JJ, Fischmeister R (1997) cGMP-stimulated cyclic nucleotide phosphodiesterase regulates the basal calcium current in human atrial myocytes. *J Clin Invest* 99:2710-2718.

[24] Sadhu K, Hensley K, Florio VA, Wolda SL (1999) Differential expression of the cyclic GMP-stimulated phosphodiesterase PDE2A in human venous and capillary endothelial cells. *J Histochem Cytochem* 47:895-906.

[25] Palmer D, Maurice DH (2000) Dual expression and differential regulation of phosphodiesterase 3A and phosphodiesterase 3B in human vascular smooth muscle: implications for phosphodiesterase 3 inhibition in human cardiovascular tissues. *Mol Pharmacol* 58:247-252.

[26] Tenor H, Hatzelmann A, Kupferschmidt R, Stanciu L, Djukanovic R, Schudt C, Wendel A, Church MK, Shute JK (1995) Cyclic nucleotide phosphodiesterase isoenzyme activities in human alveolar macrophages. *Clin Exp Allergy* 25:625-633.

[27] Tenor H, Hatzelmann A, Wendel A, Schudt C (1995) Identification of phosphodiesterase IV activity and its cyclic adenosine monophosphate-dependent up-regulation in a human keratinocyte cell line (HaCaT). *J Invest Dermatol* 105:70-74.

[28] Tenor H, Staniciu L, Schudt C, Hatzelmann A, Wendel A, Djukanovic R, Church MK, Shute JK (1995) Cyclic nucleotide phosphodiesterases from purified human CD4+ and CD8+ T lymphocytes. *Clin Exp Allergy* 25:616-624.

[29] Hamet P, Coquil JF (1978) Cyclic GMP binding and cyclic GMP phosphodiesterase in rat platelets. *J Cyclic Nucleotide Res* 4:281-290.

[30] Coquil JF, Franks DJ, Wells JN, Dupuis M, Hamet P (1980) Characteristics of a new binding protein distinct from the kinase for guanosine 3':5'-monophosphate in rat platelets. *Biochim Biophys Acta* 631:148-165.
[31] Francis SH, Corbin JD (1988) Purification of cGMP-binding protein phosphodiesterase from rat lung. *Meth Enzymol* 159:722-729.
[32] Francis SH, Lincoln TM, Corbin JD (1980) Characterization of a novel cGMP binding protein from rat lung. *J Biol Chem* 255:620-626.
[33] Sebkhi A, Strange JW, Phillips SC, Wharton J, Wilkins MR (2003) Phosphodiesterase type 5 as a target for the treatment of hypoxia-induced pulmonary hypertension. *Circulation* 107:3230-3235.
[34] Takimoto E, Belardi D, Tocchetti CG, Vahebi S, Cormaci G, Ketner EA, Moens AL, Champion HC, Kass DA (2007) Compartmentalization of cardiac beta-adrenergic inotropy modulation by phosphodiesterase type 5. *Circulation* 115:2159-2167.
[35] Zhang X, Feng Q, Cote RH (2005) Efficacy and selectivity of phosphodiesterase-targeted drugs in inhibiting photoreceptor phosphodiesterase (PDE6) in retinal photoreceptors. *Invest Ophthalmol Vis Sci* 46:3060-3066.
[36] Smith SJ, Brookes-Fazakerley S, Donnelly LE, Barnes PJ, Barnette MS, Giembycz MA (2003) Ubiquitous expression of phosphodiesterase 7A in human proinflammatory and immune cells. *Am J Physiol* 284:L279-289.
[37] Wang P, Wu P, Egan RW, Billah MM (2001) Human phosphodiesterase 8A splice variants: cloning, gene organization, and tissue distribution. *Gene* 280:183-194.
[38] Hayashi M, Kita K, Ohashi Y, Aihara E, Takeuchi K (2007) Phosphodiesterase isozymes involved in regulation of HCO3- secretion in isolated mouse duodenum in vitro. *Biochem Pharmacol* 74:1507-1513.
[39] Kobayashi T, Gamanuma M, Sasaki T, Yamashita Y, Yuasa K, Kotera J, Omori K (2003) Molecular comparison of rat cyclic nucleotide phosphodiesterase 8 family: unique expression of PDE8B in rat brain. *Gene* 319:21-31.
[40] Perez-Torres S, Cortes R, Tolnay M, Probst A, Palacios JM, Mengod G (2003) Alterations on phosphodiesterase type 7 and 8 isozyme mRNA expression in Alzheimer's disease brains examined by in situ hybridization. *Exp Neurol* 182:322-334.
[41] Glavas NA, Ostenson C, Schaefer JB, Vasta V, Beavo JA (2001) T cell activation up-regulates cyclic nucleotide phosphodiesterases 8A1 and 7A3. *Proc Natl Acad Sci USA* 98:6319-6324.
[42] Dong H, Osmanova V, Epstein PM, Brocke S (2006) Phosphodiesterase 8 (PDE8) regulates chemotaxis of activated lymphocytes. *Biochem Biophys Res Commun* 345:713-719.
[43] Vasta V, Shimizu-Albergine M, Beavo JA (2006) Modulation of Leydig cell function by cyclic nucleotide phosphodiesterase 8A. *Proc Natl Acad Sci USA* 103:19925-19930.
[44] Dov A, Abramovitch E, Warwar N, Nesher R (2008) Diminished phosphodiesterase-8B potentiates biphasic insulin response to glucose. *Endocrinology* 149:741-748.
[45] Soderling SH, Bayuga SJ, Beavo JA (1998) Cloning and characterization of a cAMP-specific cyclic nucleotide phosphodiesterase. *Proc Natl Acad Sci USA* 95:8991-8996.
[46] Soderling SH, Bayuga SJ, Beavo JA (1998) Identification and characterization of a novel family of cyclic nucleotide phosphodiesterases. *J Biol Chem* 273:15553-15558.
[47] Soderling SH, Bayuga SJ, Beavo JA (1999) Isolation and characterization of a dual-substrate phosphodiesterase gene family: PDE10A. *Proc Natl Acad Sci USA* 96:7071-7076.

[48] Fujishige K, Kotera J, Michibata H, Yuasa K, Takebayashi S, Okumura K, Omori K (1999) Cloning and characterization of a novel human phosphodiesterase that hydrolyzes both cAMP and cGMP (PDE10A). *J Biol Chem* 274:18438-18445.

[49] Loughney K, Snyder PB, Uher L, Rosman GJ, Ferguson K, Florio VA (1999) Isolation and characterization of PDE10A, a novel human 3', 5'-cyclic nucleotide phosphodiesterase. *Gene* 234:109-117.

[50] Hebb AL, Robertson HA, Denovan-Wright EM (2004) Striatal phosphodiesterase mRNA and protein levels are reduced in Huntington's disease transgenic mice prior to the onset of motor symptoms. *Neuroscience* 123:967-981.

[51] Fawcett L, Baxendale R, Stacey P, McGrouther C, Harrow I, Soderling S, Hetman J, Beavo JA, Phillips SC (2000) Molecular cloning and characterization of a distinct human phosphodiesterase gene family: PDE11A. *Proc Natl Acad Sci USA* 97:3702-3707.

[52] Hetman JM, Soderling SH, Glavas NA, Beavo JA (2000) Cloning and characterization of PDE7B, a cAMP-specific phosphodiesterase. *Proc Natl Acad Sci USA* 97:472-476.

[53] Weeks JL 2nd, Zoraghi R, Francis SH, Corbin JD (2007) N-Terminal domain of phosphodiesterase-11A4 (PDE11A4) decreases affinity of the catalytic site for substrates and tadalafil, and is involved in oligomerization. *Biochemistry* 46:10353-10364.

[54] Bender AT, Beavo JA (2006) Cyclic nucleotide phosphodiesterases: molecular regulation to clinical use. *Pharmacol Rev* 58:488-520.

[55] Bhatt-Mehta V, Schumacher RE. Treatment of apnea of prematurity. Paediatr Drugs 2003;5:195-210.

[56] Barnes PJ (2003) Theophylline: new perspectives for an old drug. *Am J Respir Crit Care Med* 167:813-818.

[57] Barnes PJ (2003) Therapy of chronic obstructive pulmonary disease. *Pharmacol Ther* 97:87-94.

[58] Barnes PJ (200) Theophylline in chronic obstructive pulmonary disease: new horizons. *Proc Am Thorac Soc* 2:334-339.

[59] Barnes PJ, Stockley RA (2005) COPD: current therapeutic interventions and future approaches. *Eur Respir J* 25:1084-1106.

[60] Muller CE, Jacobson KA (2011) Xanthines as adenosine receptor antagonists. *Handb Exp Pharmacol*:151-199.

[61] Sullivan M, Egerton M, Shakur Y, Marquardsen A, Houslay MD (1994) Molecular cloning and expression, in both COS-1 cells and S. cerevisiae, of a human cytosolic type-IVA, cyclic AMP specific phosphodiesterase (hPDE-IVA-h6.1). *Cell Signal* 6:793-812.

[62] Guerreiro S, Toulorge D, Hirsch E, Marien M, Sokoloff P, Michel PP (2008) Paraxanthine, the primary metabolite of caffeine, provides protection against dopaminergic cell death via stimulation of ryanodine receptor channels. *Mol Pharmacol* 74:980-989.

[63] Wells JN, Wu YJ, Baird CE, Hardman JG (1975) Phosphodiesterases from porcine coronary arteries: inhibition of separated forms by xanthines, papaverine, and cyclic nucleotides. *Mol Pharmacol* 11:775-783.

[64] Suvarna NU, O'Donnell JM (2002) Hydrolysis of N-methyl-D-aspartate receptor-stimulated cAMP and cGMP by PDE4 and PDE2 phosphodiesterases in primary neuronal cultures of rat cerebral cortex and hippocampus. *J Pharmacol Exp Ther* 302:249-256.

[65] Podzuweit T, Nennstiel P, Muller A (1995) Isozyme selective inhibition of cGMP-stimulated cyclic nucleotide phosphodiesterases by erythro-9-(2-hydroxy-3-nonyl) adenine. *Cell Signal* 7:733-738.

[66] Repaske DR, Swinnen JV, Jin SL, Van Wyk JJ, Conti M (1992) A polymerase chain reaction strategy to identify and clone cyclic nucleotide phosphodiesterase cDNAs. Molecular cloning of the cDNA encoding the 63-kDa calmodulin-dependent phosphodiesterase. *J Biol Chem* 267:18683-18688.

[67] Boess FG, Hendrix M, van der Staay FJ, Erb C, Schreiber R, van Staveren W, de Vente J, Prickaerts J, Blokland A, Koenig G (2004) Inhibition of phosphodiesterase 2 increases neuronal cGMP, synaptic plasticity and memory performance. *Neuropharmacology* 47:1081-1092.

[68] Rutten K, Van Donkelaar EL, Ferrington L, Blokland A, Bollen E, Steinbusch HW, Kelly PA, Prickaerts JH (2009) Phosphodiesterase inhibitors enhance object memory independent of cerebral blood flow and glucose utilization in rats. *Neuropsychopharmacology* 34:1914-1925.

[69] Reed TM, Repaske DR, Snyder GL, Greengard P, Vorhees CV (2002) Phosphodiesterase 1B knock-out mice exhibit exaggerated locomotor hyperactivity and DARPP-32 phosphorylation in response to dopamine agonists and display impaired spatial learning. *J Neurosci* 22:5188-5197.

[70] Truss MC, Stief CG, Uckert S, Becker AJ, Wefer J, Schultheiss D, Jonas U (2001) Phosphodiesterase 1 inhibition in the treatment of lower urinary tract dysfunction: from bench to bedside. *World J Urol* 19:344-350.

[71] Medina AE, Krahe TE, Ramoa AS (2006) Restoration of neuronal plasticity by a phosphodiesterase type 1 inhibitor in a model of fetal alcohol exposure. *J Neurosci* 26:1057-1060.

[72] Menniti FS, Faraci WS, Schmidt CJ (2006) Phosphodiesterases in the CNS: targets for drug development. *Nat Rev Drug Discov* 5:660-670.

[73] Filgueiras CC, Krahe TE, Medina AE (2010) Phosphodiesterase type 1 inhibition improves learning in rats exposed to alcohol during the third trimester equivalent of human gestation. *Neurosci Lett* 473:202-207.

[74] Jeon KI, Xu X, Aizawa T, Lim JH, Jono H, Kwon DS, Abe J, Berk BC, Li JD, Yan C (2010) Vinpocetine inhibits NF-kappaB-dependent inflammation via an IKK-dependent but PDE-independent mechanism. *Proc Natl Acad Sci USA* 107:9795-9800.

[75] Medina AE (2010) Vinpocetine as a potent antiinflammatory agent. *Proc Natl Acad Sci USA* 107:9921-9922.

[76] Vandecasteele G, Verde I, Rucker-Martin C, Donzeau-Gouge P, Fischmeister R (2001) Cyclic GMP regulation of the L-type Ca(2+) channel current in human atrial myocytes. *J Physiol* 533:329-340.

[77] Shin DD, Brandimarte F, De Luca L, Sabbah HN, Fonarow GC, Filippatos G, Komajda M, Gheorghiade M (2007) Review of current and investigational pharmacologic agents for acute heart failure syndromes. *Am J Cardiol* 99:4A-23A.

[78] Nohria A, Tsang SW, Fang JC, Lewis EF, Jarcho JA, Mudge GH, Stevenson LW (2003) Clinical assessment identifies hemodynamic profiles that predict outcomes in patients admitted with heart failure. *J Am Coll Cardiol* 41:1797-1804.

[79] Carev M, Bulat C, Karanovic N, Lojpur M, Jercic A, Nenadic D, Marovih Z, Husedzinovic I, Letica D (2010) Combined usage of inhaled and intravenous milrinone in pulmonary hypertension after heart valve surgery. *Coll Antropol* 34:1113-1117.

[80] Essayan DM (2001) Cyclic nucleotide phosphodiesterases. *J Allergy Clin Immunol* 108:671-680.

[81] Toward TJ, Smith N, Broadley KJ (2004) Effect of phosphodiesterase-5 inhibitor, sildenafil (Viagra), in animal models of airways disease. *Am J Respir Crit Care Med* 169:227-234.

[82] Scott AI, Perini AF, Shering PA, Whalley LJ (1991) In-patient major depression: is rolipram as effective as amitriptyline? *Eur J Clin Pharmacol* 40:127-129.

[83] O'Byrne PM, Gauvreau G (2009) Phosphodiesterase-4 inhibition in COPD. *Lancet* 374:665-667.

[84] Ghofrani HA, Osterloh IH, Grimminger F (2006) Sildenafil: from angina to erectile dysfunction to pulmonary hypertension and beyond. *Nature Rev Drug Discov* 5:689-702.

[85] Corbin JD, Beasley A, Blount MA, Francis SH (2005) High lung PDE5: a strong basis for treating pulmonary hypertension with PDE5 inhibitors. *Biochem Biophys Res Commun* 334:930-938.

[86] Wharton J, Strange JW, Moller GM, Growcott EJ, Ren X, Franklyn AP, Phillips SC, Wilkins MR (2005) Antiproliferative effects of phosphodiesterase type 5 inhibition in human pulmonary artery cells. *Am J Respir Crit Care Med* 172:105-113.

[87] Moncada S, Martin JF (1993) Evolution of nitric oxide. *Lancet* 341:1511.

[88] Prickaerts J, van Staveren WC, Sik A, Markerink-van Ittersum M, Niewohner U, van der Staay FJ, Blokland A, de Vente J (2002) Effects of two selective phosphodiesterase type 5 inhibitors, sildenafil and vardenafil, on object recognition memory and hippocampal cyclic GMP levels in the rat. *Neuroscience* 113:351-361.

[89] Baratti CM, Boccia MM (1999) Effects of sildenafil on long-term retention of an inhibitory avoidance response in mice. *Behav Pharmacol* 10:731-737.

[90] Gardner C, Robas N, Cawkill D, Fidock M (2000) Cloning and characterization of the human and mouse PDE7B, a novel cAMP-specific cyclic nucleotide phosphodiesterase. *Biochem Biophys Res Commun* 272:186-192.

[91] Sasaki T, Kotera J, Yuasa K, Omori K (2000) Identification of human PDE7B, a cAMP-specific phosphodiesterase. *Biochem Biophys Res Commun* 271:575-583.

[92] Pitts WJ, Vaccaro W, Huynh T, Leftheris K, Roberge JY, Barbosa J, Guo J, Brown B, Watson A, Donaldson K, Starling GC, Kiener PA, Poss MA, Dodd JH, Barrish JC (2004) Identification of purine inhibitors of phosphodiesterase 7 (PDE7). *Bioorg Med Chem Lett* 14:2955-2958.

[93] Vergne F, Bernardelli P, Lorthiois E, Pham N, Proust E, Oliveira C, Mafroud AK, Royer F, Wrigglesworth R, Schellhaas J, Barvian M, Moreau F, Idrissi M, Tertre A, Bertin B, Coupe M, Berna P, Soulard P (2004) Discovery of thiadiazoles as a novel structural class of potent and selective PDE7 inhibitors. Part 1: design, synthesis and structure-activity relationship studies. *Bioorg Med Chem Lett* 14:4607-4613.

[94] Zhang L, Murray F, Zahno A, Kanter JR, Chou D, Suda R, Fenlon M, Rassenti L, Cottam H, Kipps TJ, Insel PA (2008) Cyclic nucleotide phosphodiesterase profiling reveals increased expression of phosphodiesterase 7B in chronic lymphocytic leukemia. *Proc Natl Acad Sci USA* 105:19532-19537.

[95] Vang AG, Ben-Sasson SZ, Dong H, Kream B, DeNinno MP, Claffey MM, Housley W, Clark RB, Epstein PM, Brocke S (2010) PDE8 regulates rapid Teff cell adhesion and proliferation independent of ICER. *PLoS One* 5:e12011.

[96] Tsai LC, Shimizu-Albergine M, Beavo JA (2011) The high affinity cAMP-specific phosphodiesterase 8B (PDE8B) controls steroidogenesis in the mouse adrenal gland. *Mol Pharmacol* 79:639-648.

[97] Antoni FA (2000) Molecular diversity of cyclic AMP signalling. *Front Neuroendocrinol* 21:103-132.

[98] Chappe V, Mettey Y, Vierfond JM, Hanrahan JW, Gola M, Verrier B, Becq F (1998) Structural basis for specificity and potency of xanthine derivatives as activators of the CFTR chloride channel. *Br J Pharmacol* 123:683-693.

[99] Drumm ML, Wilkinson DJ, Smit LS, Worrell RT, Strong TV, Frizzell RA, Dawson DC, Collins FS (1991) Chloride conductance expressed by delta F508 and other mutant CFTRs in Xenopus oocytes. *Science* 254:1797-1799.

[100] Grubb B, Lazarowski E, Knowles M, Boucher R (1993) Isobutylmethylxanthine fails to stimulate chloride secretion in cystic fibrosis airway epithelia. *Am J Respir Cell Mol Biol* 8:454-460.

[101] Haws CM, Nepomuceno IB, Krouse ME, Wakelee H, Law T, Xia Y, Nguyen H, Wine JJ (1996) Delta F508-CFTR channels: kinetics, activation by forskolin, and potentiation by xanthines. *Am J Physiol* 270:C1544-1555.

[102] Takeuchi K, Yagi K, Kato S, Ukawa H (1997) Roles of prostaglandin E-receptor subtypes in gastric and duodenal bicarbonate secretion in rats. *Gastroenterology* 113:1553-1559.

[103] Aoi M, Aihara E, Nakashima M, Takeuchi K (2004) Participation of prostaglandin E receptor EP4 subtype in duodenal bicarbonate secretion in rats. *Am J Physiol Gastrointest Liver Physiol* 287:G96-103.

[104] Kelley TJ, Al-Nakkash L, Drumm ML (1995) CFTR-mediated chloride permeability is regulated by type III phosphodiesterases in airway epithelial cells. *Am J Respir Cell Mol Biol* 13:657-664.

[105] Kelley TJ, Al-Nakkash L, Cotton CU, Drumm ML (1996) Activation of endogenous deltaF508 cystic fibrosis transmembrane conductance regulator by phosphodiesterase inhibition. *J Clin Invest* 98:513-520.

[106] Kelley TJ, Thomas K, Milgram LJ, Drumm ML (1997) In vivo activation of the cystic fibrosis transmembrane conductance regulator mutant deltaF508 in murine nasal epithelium. *Proc Natl Acad Sci USA* 94:2604-2608.

[107] Smith SN, Middleton PG, Chadwick S, Jaffe A, Bush KA, Rolleston S, Farley R, Delaney SJ, Wainwright B, Geddes DM, Alton EW (1999) The in vivo effects of milrinone on the airways of cystic fibrosis mice and human subjects. *Am J Respir Cell Mol Biol* 20:129-134.

[108] Hogan DL, Crombie DL, Isenberg JI, Svendsen P, Schaffalitzky de Muckadell OB, Ainsworth MA (1997) CFTR mediates cAMP- and Ca2+-activated duodenal epithelial HCO3- secretion. *Am J Physiol* 272:G872-878.

[109] O'Grady SM, Jiang X, Maniak PJ, Birmachu W, Scribner LR, Bulbulian B, Gullikson GW (2002) Cyclic AMP-dependent Cl secretion is regulated by multiple phosphodiesterase subtypes in human colonic epithelial cells. *J Membr Biol* 185:137-144.

[110] Hayashi M, Kita K, Ohashi Y, Aihara E, Takeuchi K (2007) Phosphodiesterase isozymes involved in regulation of HCO3- secretion in isolated mouse duodenum in vitro. *Biochem Pharmacol* 74:1507-1513.

[111] McPherson MA, Pereira MM, Lloyd Mills C, Murray KJ, Dormer RL (1999) A cyclic nucleotide PDE5 inhibitor corrects defective mucin secretion in submandibular

cells containing antibody directed against the cystic fibrosis transmembrane conductance regulator protein. *FEBS Lett* 464:48-52.
[112] Ahn HS, Foster M, Cable M, Pitts BJ, Sybertz EJ (1991) Ca/CaM-stimulated and cGMP-specific phosphodiesterases in vascular and non-vascular tissues. *Adv Exp Med Biol* 308:191-197.
[113] Milligan PA, Marshall SF, Karlsson MO (2002) A population pharmacokinetic analysis of sildenafil citrate in patients with erectile dysfunction. *Br J Clin Pharmacol* 53 Suppl 1:45S-52S.
[114] Nichols DJ, Muirhead GJ, Harness JA (2002) Pharmacokinetics of sildenafil after single oral doses in healthy male subjects: absolute bioavailability, food effects and dose proportionality. *Br J Clin Pharmacol* 53 Suppl 1:5S-12S.
[115] Muirhead GJ, Rance DJ, Walker DK, Wastall P (2002) Comparative human pharmacokinetics and metabolism of single-dose oral and intravenous sildenafil. *Br J Clin Pharmacol* 53 Suppl 1:13S-20S.
[116] Burgess G, Hoogkamer H, Collings L, Dingemanse J (2008) Mutual pharmacokinetic interactions between steady-state bosentan and sildenafil. *Eur J Clin Pharmacol* 64:43-50.
[117] Klotz T, Sachse R, Heidrich A, Jockenhovel F, Rohde G, Wensing G, Horstmann R, Engelmann R (2001) Vardenafil increases penile rigidity and tumescence in erectile dysfunction patients: a RigiScan and pharmacokinetic study. *World J Urol* 19:32-39.
[118] Gresser U, Gleiter CH (2002) Erectile dysfunction: comparison of efficacy and side effects of the PDE-5 inhibitors sildenafil, vardenafil and tadalafil--review of the literature. *Eur J Med Res* 7:435-446.
[119] Stark S, Sachse R, Liedl T, Hensen J, Rohde G, Wensing G, Horstmann R, Schrott KM (2001) Vardenafil increases penile rigidity and tumescence in men with erectile dysfunction after a single oral dose. *Eur Urol* 40:181-188; discussion 189-190.
[120] Ormrod D, Easthope SE, Figgitt DP (2002) Vardenafil. *Drugs Aging* 19:217-227.
[121] Eardley I, Cartledge J (2002) Tadalafil (Cialis) for men with erectile dysfunction. *Int J Clin Pract* 56:300-304.
[122] Bella AJ, Brock GB (2003) Tadalafil in the treatment of erectile dysfunction. *Curr Urol Rep* 4:472-478.
[123] Staab A, Tillmann C, Forgue ST, Mackie A, Allerheiligen SR, Rapado J, Troconiz IF (2004) Population dose-response model for tadalafil in the treatment of male erectile dysfunction. *Pharm Res* 21:1463-1470.
[124] Brock GB (2003) Tadalafil: a new agent for erectile dysfunction. *Can J Urol* 10 Suppl 1:17-22.
[125] Porst H, Padma-Nathan H, Giuliano F, Anglin G, Varanese L, Rosen R (2003) Efficacy of tadalafil for the treatment of erectile dysfunction at 24 and 36 hours after dosing: a randomized controlled trial. *Urology* 62:121-125; discussion 125-126.
[126] Curran M, Keating G (2003) Tadalafil. *Drugs* 63:2203-2212; discussion 2213-2214.
[127] Pedemonte N, Lukacs GL, Du K, Caci E, Zegarra-Moran O, Galietta LJ, Verkman AS (2005) Small-molecule correctors of defective DeltaF508-CFTR cellular processing identified by high-throughput screening. *J Clin Invest* 115:2564-2571.
[128] Van Goor F, Straley KS, Cao D, Gonzalez J, Hadida S, Hazlewood A, Joubran J, Knapp T, Makings LR, Miller M, Neuberger T, Olson E, Panchenko V, Rader J, Singh A, Stack JH, Tung R, Grootenhuis PD, Negulescu P (2006) Rescue of DeltaF508-CFTR trafficking and gating in human cystic fibrosis airway primary cultures by small molecules. *Am J Physiol Lung Cell Mol Physiol* 290:L1117-1130.

[129] Carlile GW, Robert R, Zhang D, Teske KA, Luo Y, Hanrahan JW, Thomas DY (2007) Correctors of protein trafficking defects identified by a novel high-throughput screening assay. *Chem Biochem* 8:1012-1020.

[130] van Doorninck JH, French PJ, Verbeek E, Peters RH, Morreau H, Bijman J, Scholte BJ (1995) A mouse model for the cystic fibrosis delta F508 mutation. *EMBO J* 14:4403-4411.

[131] Lubamba B, Lebacq J, Lebecque P, Vanbever R, Leonard A, Wallemacq P, Leal T (2009) Airway delivery of low dose miglustat normalizes nasal potential differenece in F508del cystic fibrosis mice. *Am J Respir Crit Care Med* 179:1022-8.

[132] Sermet-Gaudelus I, De Boeck K, Casimir GJ, Vermeulen F, Leal T, Mogenet A, Roussel D, Fritsch J, Constantine S, Reha A, Hirawat S, Miller NL, Ajayi T, Elfring GL, Miller L (2010) Ataluren (PTC124) Induces CFTR Protein Expression and Activity in Children with Nonsense Mutation Cystic Fibrosis. *Am J Respir Crit Care Med* 182:1262-72.

[133] Berry B, Altman P, Rowe J, Vaisman T (2009) Comparison of pharmacokinetics of vardenafil administered using an ultrasonic nebulizer for inhalation versus a single 10-mg oral tablet. *J Sex Med* July 28 [Epub ahead of print].

[134] Dalby R, Suman J (2003) Inhalation therapy: technological milestones in asthma treatment. *Adv Drug Deliv Rev* 55: 779–791.

[135] Legssyer R, Huaux F, Lebacq J, Delos M, Marbaix E, Lebecque P, Lison D, Scholte BJ, Wallemacq P, Leal T (206) Azithromycin reduces spontaneous and induced inflammation in delta F508 cystic fibrosis mice. *Respir Res* 7:134.

[136] Meyer M, Huaux F, Gavilanes X, van den Brûle S, Lebecque P, Lo Re S, Lison D, Scholte B, Wallemacq P, Leal T (2009) Azithromycin reduces exaggerated cytokine production by M1 alveolar macrophages in cystic fibrosis. *Am J Respir Cell Mol Biol* 41:590-602.

[137] Gavilanes X, Huaux F, Meyer M, Lebecque P, Marbaix E, Lison D, Scholte B, Wallemacq P, Leal T (2009) Azithromycin fails to reduce increased expression of neutrophil-related cytokines in primary-cultured epithelial cells from cystic fibrosis mice. *J Cyst Fibros* 8:203-210.

[138] Poschet JF, Timmins GS, Taylor-Cousar JL, Ornatowski W, Fazio J, Perkett E, Wilson KR, Yu HD, de Jonge HR, Deretic V (2007) Pharmacological modulation of cGMP levels by phosphodiesterase 5 inhibitors as a therapeutic strategy for treatment of respiratory pathology in cystic fibrosis. *Am J Physiol Lung Cell Mol Physiol* 293:L712-719.

[139] Wang Y, Loo TW, Bartlett MC, Clarke DM (2007) Correctors promote maturation of cystic fibrosis transmembrane conductance regulator (CFTR)-processing mutants by binding to the protein. *J Biol Chem* 282:33247-33251.

[140] Lubamba BA, Panin N, Wauthier S, Huaux F, Lison D, Lebecque P, Wallemacq P, Leal T (2010) Anti-inflammatory effect of vardenafil in CF lung disease. *Ped Pulmonol* 45(S33):308-309.

19

Pharmacological Modulators of Sphingolipid Metabolism for the Treatment of Cystic Fibrosis Lung Inflammation

M.C. Dechecchi et al.*

Laboratory of Molecular Pathology, Laboratory of Clinical Chemistry and Haematology, University Hospital of Verona, Verona, Italy

1. Introduction

Cystic Fibrosis (CF) lung disease is characterised by progressive chronic infection and inflammation of the airways. This prolonged airway inflammatory response leads to irreversible lung damage and fibrosis which is believed to be driven by two distinct, coordinated events: *a)* a defective cystic fibrosis transmembrane regulator (CFTR) causes airway surface dehydration and increased mucus viscosity leading to chronic colonization with *Pseudomonas aeruginosa* (*P.aeruginosa*) (Boucher, 2007); *b)* mutated CFTR triggers the generation of pro-inflammatory and chemotactic cytokines orchestrated by bronchial epithelial cells, independently of infection (Rubin, 2007; Elizur et al., 2008). The chemokine IL-8, abundantly expressed at sites of chronic inflammation, seems to play a major role in driving the formation of neutrophil (PMN)-rich exudates into the lung of CF patients (Khan et al., 1995; Noah et al., 1997; DiMango et al., 1998; Puchelle et al., 2001; Joseph et al., 2005; Perez et al., 2007). Therefore, reduction of the exaggerated production of IL-8 is key therapeutic target in CF. Anti-inflammatory drugs are an attractive therapeutic tool in CF aimed to decrease the rate of decline in lung function. However, the inherent complexity of the inflammatory response combined with the obvious dependency on this response to contain infection and the side effect profiles of common anti-inflammatories, have made identifying the most suitable therapy a major priority.

---

*E. Nicolis[1], P. Mazzi[2], M. Paroni[3], F. Cioffi[4], A. Tamanini[1],V. Bezzerri[1], M. Tebon[1], I. Lampronti[5], S. Huang[6], L. Wiszniewski[6], M.T. Scupoli[4], A. Bragonzi[3], R. Gambari[5], G. Berton[2] and G. Cabrini[1]

[1]*Laboratory of Molecular Pathology, Laboratory of Clinical Chemistry and Haematology, University Hospital of Verona, Verona, Italy*

[2]*Department of Pathology, University of Verona, Italy*

[3]*Infections and Cystic Fibrosis Unit, San Raffaele Scientific Institute, Milano, Italy*

[4]*Interdepartmental Laboratory for Medical Research (LURM) and Department of Clinical and Experimental Medicine - Section of Haematology, University of Verona, Italy*

[5]*Department of Biochemistry and Molecular Biology, University of Ferrara, Ferrara, Italy*

[6]*Epithelix Sàrl, Genève, Switzerland*

Consensus is growing on sphingolipids (SLs) as novel targets to cure pulmonary disorders including CF, since modulation of cellular ceramide reduces lung inflammation (Lahiri and Futerman, 2007; Uhlig and Gulbins, 2008). The results in the area of ceramide and CF pathophysiology are very interesting, although contradicting due to the animal models used and methods of ceramide detection (Wojewodka , 2011). The accumulation of ceramide has been identified as one of the key regulators of inflammation in CF airways in different CFTR-/- mouse models (Teichgraber, 2008). On the contrary, decreased ceramide levels have been shown in CFTR ko mice (Guibault, 2008). The possible explanation for this discrepancy seems to be the special diet required for CFTR ko mice, that severely affects the concentration of SLs. Other possible causes, such as genetic determinants, could influence individual levels of SLs (Hicks, 2009). In a different study, no significant difference has been found in basal ceramide levels in immortalised CF bronchial epithelial cells and lung homogenate from CFTR ko mice compared to wild type cells and mice (Yu, 2009). Very importantly, ceramide has been demonstrated to accumulate in the lower airways of CF patients and to be positively associated with neutrophilic inflammation (Brodlie, 2010), supporting the hypothesis that reduction of ceramide may be a therapeutic target for CF lung inflammation.

Extending our previous study (Dechecchi, 2008), we have recently demonstrated that the iminosugar *N*-butyldeoxynojirimycin (miglustat), an inhibitor of the first step in glycosphingolipid (GSL) biosynthesis, reducing the *P.aeruginosa* induced immunoreactive ceramide expression, produces an anti-inflammatory effect in human bronchial epithelial cells *in vitro* and down-regulates the neutrophil chemotaxis in murine lungs *in vivo* (Dechecchi, 2011). These findings strengthen the notion that the metabolism of SLs can be manipulated as a therapeutic option for CF lung disease. With regard to new treatments for CF lung pathology, miglustat deserves great attention since it restores CFTR function in respiratory and pancreatic cells *in vitro* (Norez, 2006; Dechecchi, 2008) and in CF mice (Lubamba, 2009) and produces an anti-inflammatory effect *in vitro* and *in vivo* (Dechecchi, 2011). Notably, miglustat is a FDA-approved and EMA−designated orally bioavailable orphan drug, used in Europe and USA for the treatment of Gaucher disease and other GSL storage diseases.

In this chapter we review the pre-clinical evidence on the anti-inflammatory effect of miglustat in comparative effectiveness studies with the SL inhibitor amitriptyline and the glucocorticoid (GC) dexamethasone. Importance will be placed on the efficacy of each anti-inflammatory molecule to balance between the anti-inflammatory activity and possible impairment of the host defence.

2. CF bronchial cells seem to be resistant to the treatment with glucocorticoids

Chronic inflammation is commonly treated by a number of approaches including fast-acting symptomatic drugs, such as non-steroidal anti-inflammatory drugs (NSAIDs), glucocorticoids and slow-acting disease-modifying anti-rheumatic drugs, such as low-dose methotrexate. In the treatment of chronic lung inflammation of CF patients, corticosteroids and NSAIDs have garnered the most attention, to date. Although traditional treatments with corticosteroids and ibuprofen have demonstrated potential benefits in CF patients, their use is limited by severe adverse effects, as for high doses of prednisone, or by a narrow pharmacological window, as in the case of ibuprofen (Birke, 2001; Koehler, 2004; Konstan, 2005). The endobronchial location makes CF pulmonary inflammation potentially amenable to inhaled therapies, thus achieving much higher concentrations in the airway epithelium and limiting the adverse effects of long term systemic use. As the airway epithelium is targeted by inhaled agents, bronchial epithelial cells *in vitro* have been widely used to prove the efficacy of these drugs. The glucocorticoid dexamethasone, largely used in the treatments of inflammatory conditions is scarcely effective in reducing the expression of the chemokine IL-8 in CF bronchial epithelial cells (Figure 1). As a matter of fact, it produces inhibitory effect only at the higher dose (30 μM) (Figure1A) in CF bronchial epithelial IB3-1 cells whereas it fails to reduce the transcription of IL-8 in Cufi-1 cells (Figure 1B). Different from the results obtained in CF CuFi-1 cells, treatment with dexamethasone results in reducing the inflammatory response, in non CF NuLi-1 cells (Figure 1C). These findings suggest that CF bronchial cells seem to be resistant to GC treatment, consistent with scarce efficacy of GC treatment observed in CF patients.

3. *P.aeruginosa* stimulated IL-8 mRNA expression is reduced in CF bronchial epithelial cells treated with inhibitors of SL metabolism miglustat and NB-DGJ

The role of CFTR deficiency in promoting inflammation remains unclear. Inhibition of function of wild type CFTR by $CFTR_{inh172}$ (Perez, 2007) or correction of F508del mutated CFTR function by MPB-07 or miglustat (Dechecchi, 2007; 2008) regulates the inflammatory response to *P. aeruginosa,* suggesting that the pro-inflammatory circuitry in CF airways could be initiated from those epithelial cells lacking CFTR function. However the galactose analogue *N*-butyldeoxygalactonojirimycin (NB-DGJ), which is not a corrector of F508del-CFTR function (Norez, 2006), similarly reduces the PAO1 stimulated IL-8 mRNA expression in CF cells (Figure 2). Additionally this reduction has been obtained both in CF and non CF cells with both miglustat and NB-DGJ (Dechecchi, 2008). Therefore, miglustat affects the inflammatory response to *P. aeruginosa* through a mechanism which, at least partly, is independent of the correction of F508del-CFTR function. As far as the effect of miglustat and NB-DGJ on immune response is concerned, they could affect the host response to *P.aeruginosa* through the regulation of SL metabolism, in particular CerGlcT and/or non lysosomal glucosylceramidase, an activity shared by both compounds (Butters, 2005), thus strengthening the notion that the metabolism of SLs can be manipulated as a therapeutic option for CF lung disease.

4. Amitriptyline reduces IL-8 gene expression in CF bronchial cells

Two main routes have been defined for the generation of ceramide: hydrolysis of sphingomyelin (SM) by acid sphingomyelinase (ASM) and *de novo* biosynthesis (Hannun, 2008). Ceramide generated by ASM plays an important role in the infection by *P. aeruginosa* since it reorganizes into rafts required to internalize bacteria, induce apoptosis and regulate the cytokine response (Grassme', 2003). Treatment of CF mice by ASM inhibitors, such as amitriptyline and others tricyclic antidepressants, has been shown to reduce the degree of inflammation (Teichgraber, 2008; Becker, 2010). Notably, amitriptyline results in dose dependent inhibition of IL-8 transcription by bronchial epithelial cell lines IB3-1 and CuFi-1, infected with *P.aeruginosa* (Figure 3), consistent with the overall anti-inflammatory

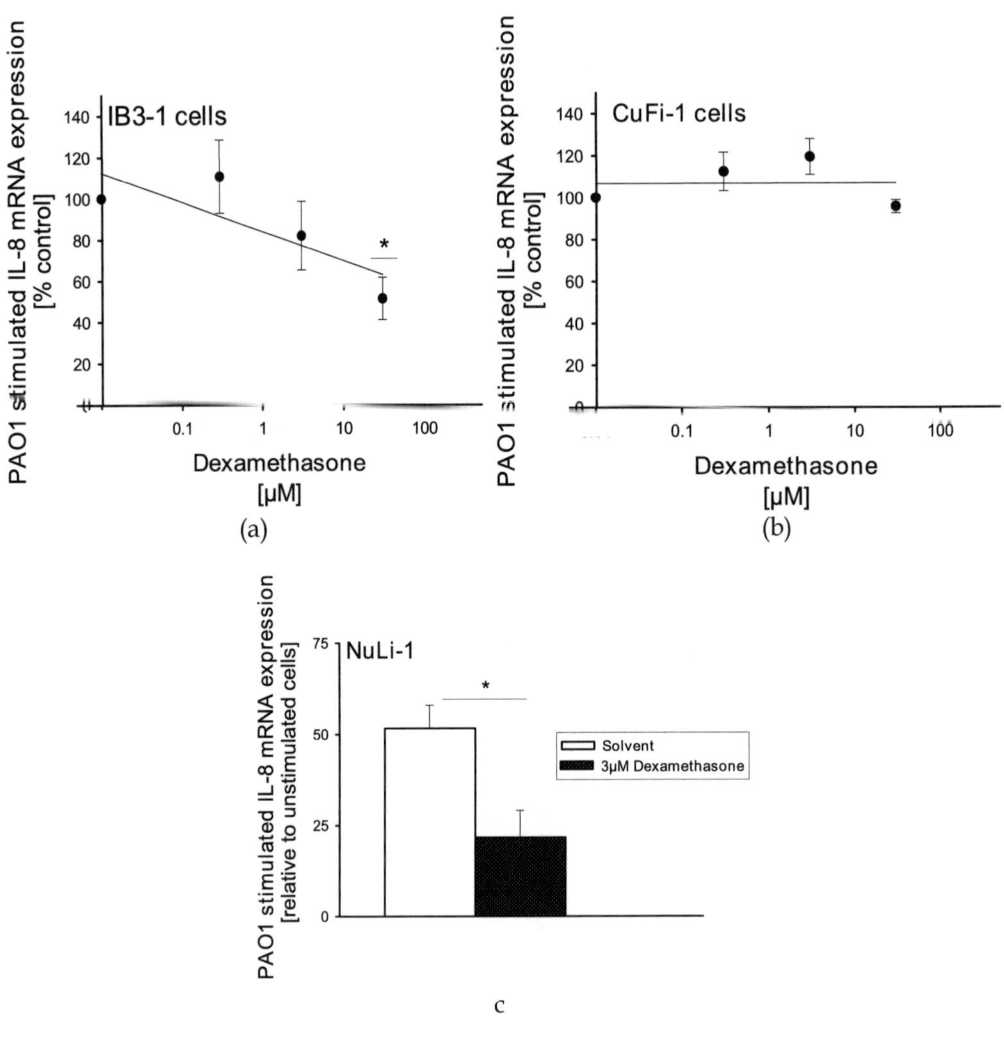

Fig. 1. Effect of dexamethasone on inflammatory response to *P.aeruginosa* in CF and non CF bronchial epithelial cells.

IB3-1 (human bronchial epithelial cell line) (Zeitlin, 1991) (*A*), CuFi-1 (F508del/F508del CFTR mutant genotype) (*B*) and NuLi-1 (*C*), (wild type CFTR) (Zabner, 2003) cell lines were treated with dexamethasone, at doses indicated in the figure, or solvent alone, for 24 hours and then infected with *P.aeruginosa* strain PAO1 (kindly provided by A. Prince, Columbia University, New York)(50CFU/cell) for 4 hours at 37° C. The inflammatory response was evaluated by studying the expression of mRNA of IL-8, measured by Real-time qPCR as described (Dechecchi, 2008) and obtained by comparing the ratio IL-8 and the housekeeping gene GAPDH between non infected and infected cells. Results are expressed as mean ± standard error of the mean (n=5). Comparisons between groups were made by using Student's *t* test. Statistical significance was defined with $p<0.05$. * , *p* value <0.05.

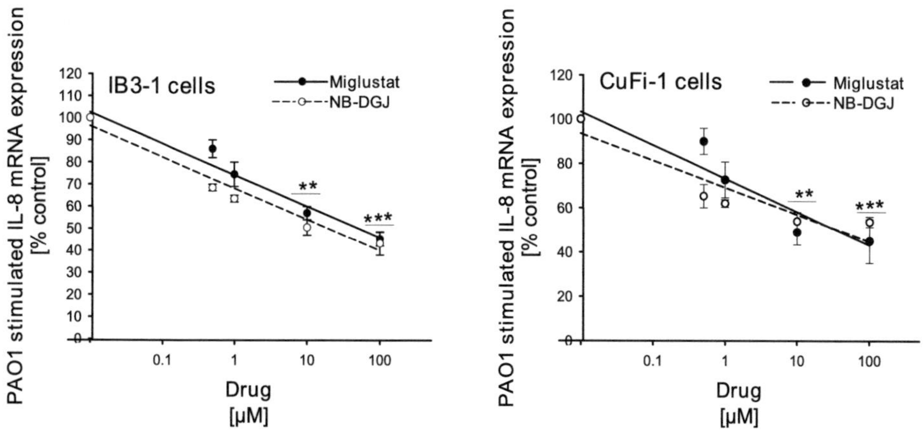

(a) (b)

Fig. 2. Result of miglustat and NB-DGJ on *P.aeruginosa* stimulated IL-8 mRNA expression in CF bronchial cell lines IB3-1 and CuFi-1 cells.

IB3-1 (*A*) and CuFi-1 (*B*) cells were treated with miglustat, NB-DGJ, at doses indicated in the figure, or solvent alone for 24 hours and then infected with PAO1 as in Figure 1. Stimulated IL-8 mRNA expression was calculated as indicated in the legend of Figure 1 and expressed as % of untreated cells. Data reported are mean ± standard error of the mean of 3 independent experiments, performed in duplicate. **, p value < 0.01; ***, p value < 0.001.

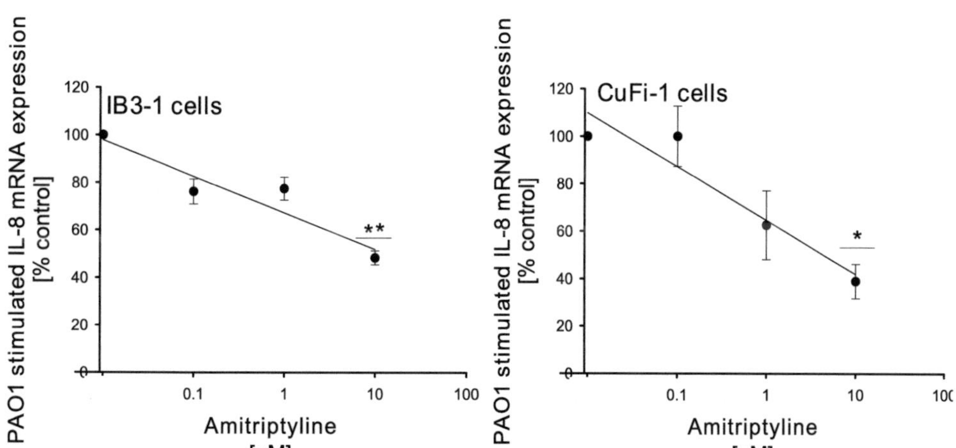

(a) (b)

Fig. 3. Result of amitriptyline on *P.aeruginosa* stimulated IL-8 mRNA expression in CF bronchial cell lines IB3-1 and CuFi-1 cells

IB3-1 (*A*) and CuFi-1 (*B*) cells were treated with amitriptyline, at doses indicated in the figure, or solvent alone for 24 hours and then infected with PAO1 as in Figure 1. Stimulated IL-8 mRNA expression was calculated as indicated in the legend of Figure 1 and expressed as % of untreated cells. Data reported are mean ± standard error of the mean of 8 (IB3-1) or 6 (CuFi-1) independent experiments, performed in duplicate. *, *p* value <0.05; **, p value < 0.01.

effect reported in CF murine lungs (Teichgraber, 2008; Becker, 2010). Interestingly, we have recently demonstrated that, besides inhibiting IL-8 transcription, both miglustat and amitriptyline reduce the *P.aeruginosa* induced immunoreactive ceramide expression (Dechecchi, 2011), by targeting different pathways of SL metabolism: CerGlcT and/or non-lysosomal glucosylceramidase (miglustat) and ASM (amitriptyline). As far as the effect on immune response is concerned, the same overall decrease of ceramide could regulate the transmembrane signaling between the receptors for pathogens and the transcription of the inflammatory genes, thus reducing inflammation.

5. Miglustat and amitriptyline inhibit the pro-inflammatory signaling downstream the receptors for *P.aeruginosa* and for pro-inflammatory cytokines

The importance of ceramide as a pro-inflammatory mediator derives from its capability to activate protein kinases and phosphatases in different downstream pathways and from the generation of second messengers (Hannun, 2008). Ceramide is produced in response to various stimulants such as cytokines, heat, UV radiation, lipopolysaccharide (LPS) and other agents thus leading to specific and overlapping events that include the activation of a common set of kinases and transcription factors. Both miglustat and amitriptyline inhibit the expression of IL-8 mRNA stimulated by either *P.aeruginosa* or TNFα or IL-1β (Figure 4), indicating that they affect the pro-inflammatory signaling downstream and in common with the receptors for *P. aeruginosa* and for these pro-inflammatory cytokines. Importantly, ceramide-induced activation of the transcription factor NF-kB and p38 kinase amplifies the production of several inflammatory mediators and adhesion molecules (Won, 2004). Therefore, it can be hypothesized that miglustat and amitriptyline, decreasing plasma membrane ceramide, generated by *P.aeruginosa* infection or pro-inflammatory cytokines, attenuate the activation of NF-kB mediated signaling cascade which in turn down-regulates the immune response.

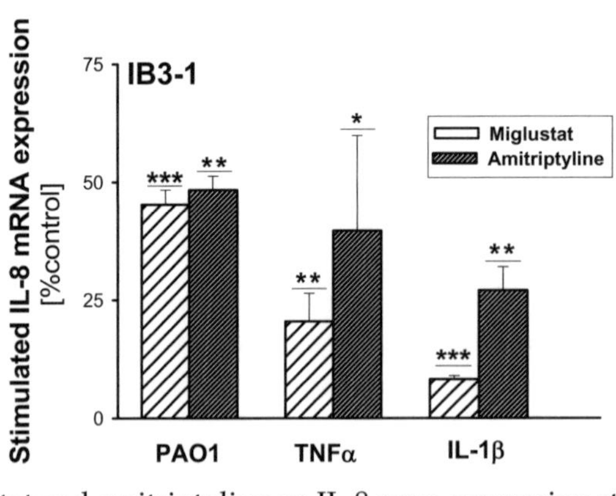

Fig. 4. Effect of miglustat and amitriptyline on IL-8 gene expression stimulated by *P.aeruginosa*, TNFα or IL-1β.

IB3-1 cells were treated with miglustat (100μM), amitriptyline (10μM) or solvent alone for 24 hours and then infected with PAO1 or stimulated by the pro-inflammatory cytokines TNF α (10ng/ml) or IL-1 β (50 ng/ml) for 4 hours at 37°C as in Figure 1. Stimulated IL-8 mRNA expression was calculated as indicated in the legend of Figure 1 and expressed as % of untreated cells. Data reported are mean ± standard error of the mean of 3 independent experiments performed in duplicate. *, *p* value <0.05; **, p value < 0.01; ***, p value < 0.001.

6. Miglustat down-regulates the expression of key genes involved in neutrophil chemotaxis in human bronchial CF epithelial cells

The infection of a host by a pathogenic microorganism initiates complex cascade of events directed toward the recruitment of defence mechanisms. Parallel analysis of gene expression provides a new tool for studying interplay of signals and transcriptional responses in biological systems. Infection of IB3-1 cells with the *P.aeruginosa* strain PAO1, for a short time (4 hours), up-regulates the expression of genes involved in the inflammatory response, mainly neutrophil chemotaxis, such as the chemokines IL-8, Gro-α/β/γ, GCP-2, the adhesion molecule ICAM-1, the cytokines IL-1α/β, IL-6, TNF-α, the antimicrobial peptide HBD-4, Toll-like receptor 2 and NFKB1 (Figure 5A). These results obtained in CF cell line correlate with findings in cultured human bronchial epithelial primary cells derived from the bronchi of CF patients (Figure 5B), which exhibit many of the morphological and functional characteristics believed to be associated with CF airway disease (Neuberger, 2011) and recall many features of the colonization of the respiratory epithelium by pathogens. As far as host defence mechanisms are concerned, bronchial epithelium is not simply a physical barrier against invading pathogens but is also an important source of inflammatory mediators, actively involved in the immune response. Therefore cultured CF bronchial cells provide a useful tool for the pre-clinical testing of novel pharmacotherapies. Indeed, miglustat has an anti-inflammatory effect in CF bronchial cells, since it reduces the expression of key genes induced by *P.aeruginosa* and IL-8 protein release (Dechecchi, 2011). Also amitriptyline has an anti-inflammatory effect in CF bronchial cell lines (Figure 5A) and at lower extent in CF primary cells (Figure 5B). Regarding the therapeutic activity of amitriptyline, it should be noted that systemic inhibition of ASM might negatively affect the host defence, as demonstrated by studies on mice completely lacking ASM which were found to be unable to control infections (Grassme', 2003). Moreover, since amitriptyline inhibits serotonin and noradrenaline uptake in presynaptic nerve ending (Maubach, 1999), it might cause severe adverse effects in long term use in CF children. As with all treatments, utility will largely depend on the balance between potential risks and benefits.

7. Miglustat up-regulates the transcription of the antimicrobial peptide HBD-4

The treatment of CF patients with drug aimed to limit the excessive inflammatory response could mean that they become vulnerable to infections. As a matter of fact, dexamethasone down-regulates the expression of HBD-4 (Figure 6), an antimicrobial peptide induced by infectious or inflammatory stimuli, that plays an important role in the host innate immune response, with strong activity against *P.aeruginosa* (Yanagi, 2005). This result is consistent with suppression of *b*-defensins by GC treatment, already reported (Jang, 2007). On the other hand, well known huge side effects of long term use of steroids limit their clinical utility in CF patients (Nichols, 2008). On the contrary, miglustat up-regulates the expression of HBD-4, both in cell lines and primary cells (Figures 5 and 6), adding ground to the suggestion that miglustat could not compromise the ability to resist infection with pathogens in CF patients. Additionally, results on the safety of miglustat obtained during the first 5 years of the clinical studies, do not report any increased susceptibility to bacterial infections in patients affected by Gaucher disease (Hollak, 2009). All this considered the proximity to a treatment of CF lung inflammation with miglustat is real and promising.

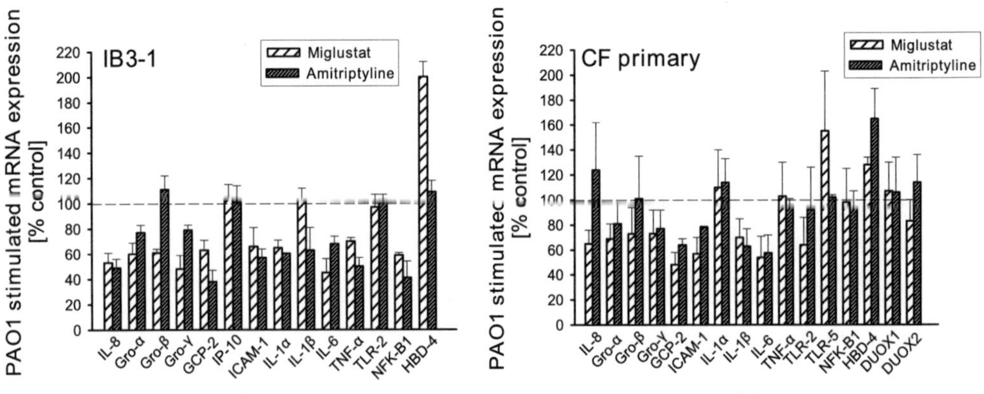

(a) (b)

Fig. 5. Inflammatory response to *P.aeruginosa* in IB3-1 and CF primary cells treated with miglustat or amitriptyline.

IB3-1 cells (*A*) and human airway epithelium reconstituted in vitro with cells isolated from CF patients and cultivated on micro-porous filters at air-liquid interface (MucilAir™, Epithelix Sàrl, Genève, Switzerland) (*B*) were treated with miglustat (100μM), amitriptyline (10μM) or solvent alone for 24 hours and then infected with PAO1. The inflammatory response was evaluated by studying the expression of several genes known to be associated with host immune defences by RNA macroarrays (TaqMan Low Density Array, Applied Biosystems, Foster City, CA) as detailed (Dechecchi, 2011). Stimulated mRNA expression was calculated as indicated in the legend of Figure 1 and expressed as % of untreated cells. (*A*) IB3-1 cells. Miglustat significantly reduces the expression of IL-8, ICAM-1, TNF-α (**, p value<0.01), gro-α/β/γ, GCP-2, IL-1α, IL-6 and NFKB1(*, *p* value<0.05) and increases the expression of HBD-4 (**, p value<0.01). Amitriptyline significantly reduces the expression of IL-8, Gro-α, ICAM-1 (**, p value<0.01), gro-γ, GCP-2, IL-1α/1β, IL-6, TNF-α and NFKB1(*, *p* value<0.05) (n=6). (*B*) CF primary cells. Miglustat significantly reduces the expression of IL-8, GCP-2, ICAM-1, TNF-α, IL-6 (*, *p* value<0.05) and increases the expression of HBD-4 (*, p value<0.05). Amitriptyline significantly reduces the expression of GCP-2, ICAM-1, IL-1β, IL-6 (*, *p* value<0.05) and increases the expression of HBD-4 (*, p value<0.05) (n=4).

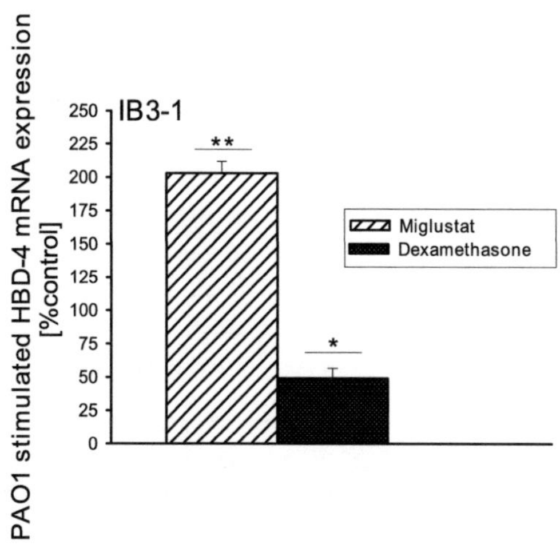

Fig. 6. *P.aeruginosa* stimulated transcription of the antimicrobial peptide HBD-4 in IB3-1 cells: result of miglustat and dexamethasone.

IB3-1 cells were treated with miglustat (100μM), dexamethasone (30μM) or solvent alone for 24 hours and then infected with PAO1 as in Figure 1. Stimulated HBD-4 mRNA expression was measured by Real-time qPCR as described (Dechecchi, 2011), calculated as indicated in the legend of Figure 1 and expressed as % of untreated cells. Data reported are mean ± standard error of the mean of 5 independent experiments performed in duplicate. **, p value<0.01 (miglustat); *, *p* value<0.05 (dexamethasone).

8. Miglustat down-regulates neutrophil chemotaxis in the early inflammatory response *in vivo*

The pressing challenge for the discovery of new drugs is to transform findings from bench studies into effective therapies. The success of results obtained with CFTR correctors and potentiators suggests that primary coltures of human airway epithelia will likely be the model system of choice for future proof of principle studies of experimental therapeutics (Neuberger, 2011). With regard to miglustat, the anti-inflammatory effect observed in CF primary cells (Dechecchi, 2011) provides a significant body of evidence concerning the utility of miglustat in modifying lung inflammation. However, an essential requirement for entering clinical trial is a thorough testing in pre-clinical animal models. As a matter of fact development of new animal models of CF such as CFTR knock-out pigs (Rogers, 2008), raises the possibility to employ these animals to evaluate new treatments. Murine models of acute and chronic infection with *P.aeruginosa,* along with mice genetically modified for the CFTR gene, are a key asset in CF research and mimic many of the characteristic features of CF lung pathology (Bragonzi, 2010). Additionally, mice with the airway specific over expression of the Na+ channel βENaC, develop a CF–like lung inflammation (Mall, 2004). These models have provided insights in the effectiveness of anti-inflammatory therapy in reducing lung damage. Interestingly, lung inflammation of βENaC over expressing mice seems to be resistant to GC treatment (Livraghi, 2009) and amitriptyline reduces the degree of inflammation in CFTR-/- mice (Teichgraber, 2008; Becker 2010). As far as the effectiveness of miglustat is concerned, it reduces the recruitment of PMN into the bronchoalveolar space induced by intranasal instillation of LPS (Figure 7A) (Dechecchi, 2011). The pharmacokinetic profile and tissue distribution of miglustat, after oral dosing in small rodents, demonstrate that it is well absorbed, exhibits a bioavailability of 40-60%, is widely distributed within the body and, notably, it is present at high concentrations in the lung 1 hour after administration (Treiber, 2007). Indeed, a treatment schedule of an oral administration with miglustat one hour before the intra tracheal inoculum with *P. aeruginosa* is effective in reducing the inflammatory response associated to acute pneumonia in terms of leukocyte recruitment and myeloperoxidase (MPO) activity in the airways (Figure 7B and Figure 7C). Taken together, these results indicate that miglustat may down-regulates neutrophil recruitment in the early phase of the inflammatory response.

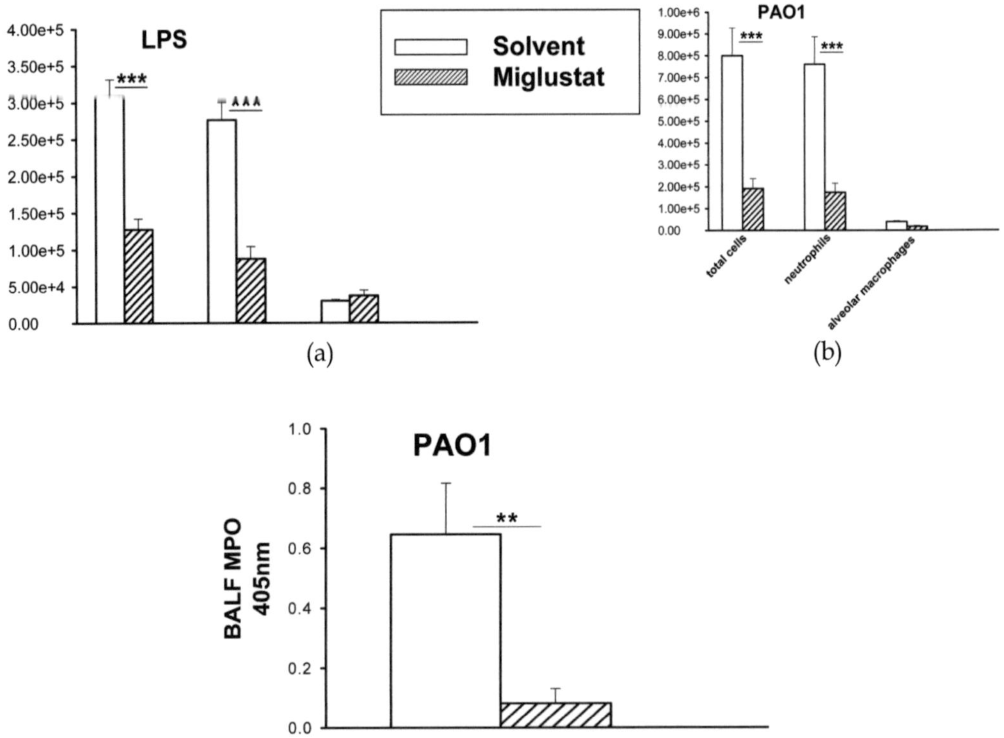

c

Fig. 7. Effect of miglustat on murine models of lung inflammation.

(*A*). Aqueous solution of miglustat (100 mg/Kg) or vehicle alone was administered once daily in wild type C57BL/6J mice by intraesophageal gavage, for a period of three consecutive days before pro-inflammatory challenge with LPS by intranasal instillation. Bronchoalveolar lavage fluid (BALF) was examined 4 hrs after challenge, as described (Dechecchi, 2011). Data reported are mean ± standard error of the mean. n=6(vehicle), n=12 (miglustat). ***, p value < 0.001. (*B* and *C*). C57BL/6 mice were infected by intra-tracheal injection with the reference *P. aeruginosa* strain PAO1 (1x10^5 CFU) one hour after oral injection with miglustat (400mg/kg), or vehicle. Mice were sacrificed 4 hours after PAO1 injection and the inflammatory response associated to PAO1-induced acute pneumonia in terms of leukocyte recruitment (*B*) and MPO activity (*C*) in the airways was analyzed as described (Bragonzi, 2009, Moalli, 2011). Data reported are mean

± standard error of the mean. n=5 (vehicle), n=6 (miglustat). ***, p value < 0.001(leukocyte recruitment); **, p value < 0.01(MPO activity).

9. Conclusions

Strategies aimed to limit the excessive inflammatory response by targeting neutrophil recruitment are a relevant approach for CF patients. In general, each anti-inflammatory molecule should balance between the anti-infective role of neutrophils and the detrimental effects that they produce in the course of chronic inflammation due to the release of proteases and reactive oxygen species. In this respect, while others anti-inflammatory based therapies have failed in humans with CF in the past, the regulation of SLs may represent a useful potential target for pharmacotherapy. This review summarizes evidence derived from the validation of the anti-inflammatory properties of miglustat in bronchial epithelial cells *in vitro* and in murine models of lung inflammation and infection *in vivo,* demonstrating a down-regulation of neutrophils chemotactic signaling. Recalling that miglustat is an orally bioavailable FDA-approved and EMA–designated orphan available drug, therapeutic trials for CF patients could be envisioned in the near future.

10. Acknowledgment

We are very grateful to A. Tamanini for helpful discussions, F. Quiri and V. Lovato for excellent technical assistance, A. Prince (Columbia University, New York) for the *P.aeruginosa* laboratory strain PAO1, In Vitro Model and Cell Culture Care of the University of Iowa for providing NuLi-1 and CuFi-1 cells.

This research was supported by Italian Cystic Fibrosis Research Foundation (grant FFC # 16/2010) with the contribution of "Assistgroup", "Latteria Montello SpA" and "Delegazione FFC di Imola" (to MCD).

11. References

Becker K.A.; Riethmüller J.; Lüth A.; Döring G.; Kleuser B.; Gulbins E. (2010). Acid Sphingomyelinase Inhibitors Normalize Pulmonary Ceramide and Inflammation in Cystic Fibrosis. Am J Respir Cell Mol Biol. 42(6):716-24

Birke F.W.; Meade C.J.; Anderskewitz R.; Speck G.A.; Jennewein H.M. (2001). In vitro and in vivo pharmacological Characterization of BIIL 284, a novel and potent leukotriene B(4) receptor antagonist. *J Pharmacol Exp Ther.* 297:458-66

Boucher R.C. (2007). Evidence for airway surface dehydration as the initiating event in CF airway disease. *J Intern Med* 261:5−16

Bragonzi A.; Worlitzsch D.; Pier G.B.; Timpert P.; Ulrich M.; Hentzer M.; Andersen J.B.; Givskov M.; Conese M.; Doring G. (2005). Nonmucoid *Pseudomonas aeruginosa* expresses alginate in the lungs of patients with cystic fibrosis and in a mouse model. *J Infect Dis* 192:410-9

Bragonzi A.; Paroni M.; Nonis A.; Cramer N.; Montanari S.; Rejman J.; Di Serio C.; Döring G.; Tümmler B. (2009). *Pseudomonas aeruginosa* microevolution during cystic fibrosis lung infection establishes clones with adapted Virulence. *Am J Respir Crit Care Med.* 180(2):138-45.

Bragonzi A. (2010). Murine models of acute and chronic lung infection with cystic fibrosis pathogens. Int J Med Microbiol. 300(8):584-93.

Brodlie M.; McKean M.C.; Johnson G.E.; Gray J.; Fisher A.J.; Corris P.A.; Lordan J.L.; Ward C. (2010). Ceramide is Increased in the Lower Airway Epithelium of People with Advanced Cystic Fibrosis Lung Disease. *Am J Respir Crit Care Med* 182 (3): 369-75

Butters T.D.; Dwek R.A. and Platt F.M. (2005). Imino sugar inhibitors for treating the lysosomal Glycosphingolipidoses. Glycobiology 15, 43R-52R.

Dechecchi M.C.; Nicolis E.; Bezzerri V.; Vella A.; Colombatti M.; Assael B.M.; Mettey Y.;Borgatti M.; Mancini I.; Gambari R.; Becq F. and Cabrini G. (2007). MPB-07 reduces the inflammatory response to *Pseudomonas aeruginosa* in cystic fibrosis bronchial cells. *Am J Respir Cell Mol Biol* 36, 615-624

Dechecchi M.C.; Nicolis E.; Norez C.; Bezzerri V.; Borgatti M.; Mancini I.; Rizzotti P.; Ribeiro C.M.; Gambari R.; Becq F.;Cabrini G. (2008). Anti-inflammatory effect of miglustat in bronchial epithelial cells. *J Cyst Fibros.* 7(6):555-65

Dechecchi M.C.; Nicolis E.; Mazzi P.; Cioffi F.; Bezzerri V.; Lampronti I.; Huang S.; Wiszniewski L.; Gambari R.; Scupoli M.T.; Berton G.; Cabrini G. (2011). Modulators of Sphingolipid Metabolism Reduce Lung Inflammation. *Am J Respir Cell Mol Biol.* Jun 9. [Epub ahead of print]

DiMango E.;Ratner A.J.; Bryan R.; Tabibi S.; Prince A. (1998) Activation of NF-kB by adherent Pseudomonas aeruginosa in normal and cystic fibrosis respiratory epithelial cells. *J Clin Invest* 101:2598-2605

Elizur A.; Cannon C.L. ; Ferkol T.W. (2008). Airway inflammation in cystic fibrosis. *Chest* 133:489–495

Grassme' H.; Jendrossek V.; Riehle A.; von Kürthy G.; Berger J.; Schwarz H.; Weller M.; Kolesnick R.; Gulbins E. (2003). Host defense against *Pseudomonas aeruginosa* requires ceramide-rich membrane rafts. Nature Medicine 9:322-330

Guilbault C.; De Sanctis J.B.; Wojewodka G.; Saeed Z.; Lachance C.; Skinner T.A.; Vilela R.M.; Kubow S.; Lands L.C.; Hajduch M.; Matouk E.; Radzioch D. (2008). Fenretinide corrects newly found ceramide deficiency in cystic fibrosis. *Am J Respir Cell Mol Biol.* 38(1):47-56

Hannun YA. and Obeid L.M. (2008). Principles of bioactive lipid signaling: lessons from sphingolipids. Nat Rew Mol Cell Biol 9:139-150

Hicks A.A.; Pramstaller P.P.; Johansson A.; Vitart V.; Rudan I.; Ugocsai P.; Aulchenko Y.; Franklin C.; Liebisch G.; Erdmann J.; Jonasson I.; Zorkoltseva I.V.; Pattaro C.; Hayward C.; Isaacs A.; Hengstenberg C.; Campbell S.; Gnewuch C.; Janssens A.C.; Kirichenko A.V.; König I.R.; Marroni F.; Polasek O.; Demirkan A.; Kolcic I.; Schwienbacher C.; Igl W.; Biloglav Z.; Witteman J.C.; Pichler I.; Zaboli G.; Axenovich T.I.; Peters A.; Schreiber S.; Wichmann H.E.; Schunkert H.; Hastie N.; Oostra B.A.; Wild S.H.; Meitinger T.; Gyllensten U.; van Duijn C.M.; Wilson J.F.; Wright A.; Schmitz G.; Campbell H.; (2009). Genetic determinants of circulating sphingolipid concentrations in European populations. *PLoS Genet.* 5:1-11

Hollak C.E.; Hughes D.; van Schaik I.N.; Schwierin B.; Bembi B. (2009). Miglustat (Zavesca) in type 1 Gaucher disease: 5- year results of a post-authorization safety surveillance programme. Pharmacoepidemiol Drug Saf. 18(9):770-7

Jang B-C.; Lim K-J.; Suh M-H.; Park J-G. and Suh S. (2007). Dexamethasone suppresses interleukin-1B-induced human β-defensin 2 mRNA expression: involvement of p38

MAPk, JNK, MKP-1 and NF-kB transcriptional factor in A549 cells. FEMS Immunol Med Microbiol 51: 171-184

Joseph T.; Look D.; Ferkol T. (2005). NF-kB activation and sustained IL-8 gene expression in primary cultures of cystic fibrosis airway epithelial cells stimulated with *Pseudomonas aeruginosa. Am J Physiol Lung Cell Mol Physiol* 288: L471-L479

Khan T.Z. ; Wagener J.S. ; Bost T. ; Martinez J. ; Accurso F.J. ; Riches D.W. ; (1995). Early pulmonary inflammation in infants with cystic fibrosis. *Am J Respir Crit Care Med* 151:1075-1082

Koehler D.R.; Downey G.P.; Sweezey N.B.; Tanswell A.K.; Hu J. (2004) Lung inflammation as a therapeutic target in cystic fibrosis. *Am J Respir Cell Mol Biol* 31:377-381

Konstan M.W.; Doring G. ;Lands L.C.; Hilliard K.A.; Koker P.; Bhattacharya .; Staab A.; Hamilton A.L. (2005). Results of a phase II clinical trial of BIIL284 BS for the treatment of CF lung disease. *Pediatric Pulmonol S* 28: 125-126

Lahiri S. and Futerman A.H. (2007).The metabolism and function of sphingolipids and glycosphingolipid. *Cell Mol Life Sci.* 64: 2270-2284.

Livraghi A.; Grubb B.R.; Hudson E.J.; Wilkinson K.J.; Sheehan J.K.; Mall M.A. O'Neal W.K. Boucher R.C.; Randell S.H. (2009). Airway and lung pathology due to mucosal surface dehydration in {beta}-epithelial Na+ channel- overexpressing mice: role of TNF-{alpha} and IL-4R{alpha} signaling, influence of neonatal development, and limited efficacy of glucocorticoid treatment.J Immunol. 182(7):4357-67

Lubamba B.; Lebacq J.; Lebecque P.; Vanbever R.; Leonard A.; Wallemacq P.; Leal T. (2009). Airway delivery of low-dose miglustat normalizes nasal potential difference in F508del cystic fibrosis mice. *Am J Respir Crit Care Med.* 179:1022-8.

Mall M.; Grubb B.R.; Harkema J.R.; O'Neal W.K.; Boucher R.C. (2004). Increased airway epithelial Na+ absorption produces cystic fibrosis–like lung disease in mice. Nat Med 10:487–493

Maubach K.A.; Rupniak N.M.; Kramer M.S.; Hill R.G. (1999). Novel strategies for pharmacotherapy of depression. Curr Opin Chem Biol. 481-8

Moalli F, Paroni M, Véliz Rodriguez T, Riva F, Polentarutti N, Bottazzi B, Valentino S, Mantero S, Nebuloni M, Mantovani A, Bragonzi A, Garlanda C. The therapeutic potential of the humoral pattern recognition molecule PTX3 in chronic lung infection caused by Pseudomonas aeruginosa. J Immunol. 2011 May 1;186(9):5425-34.

Neuberger T.; Burton B.; Clark H. and Van Goor F. (2011). Use of primary cultures of human bronchial epithelial cells Isolated from cystic fibrosis patients for the pre-clinical testing of CFTR modulators, In: Cystic Fibrosis, Methods in Molecular Biology, M.D. Amaral and K. Kunzelmann (eds), 39-54, Springer Science

Nichols D.P; Konstan M.W. and Chmiel J.F. (2008) Anti-inflammatory therapies for cystic fibrosis-related lung disease. Clinic Rev Aller Immunol 35: 135-153

Noah T.L.; Black H.R.; Cheng P.W,; Wood R.E.; Leigh M.W. (1997) Nasal and bronchoalveolar lavage fluid cytokines in early cystic fibrosis. *J Infect Dis* 175: 638-647

Norez C.; Noel S.; Wilke M.; Bijvelds M.; Jorna H.; Melin P.; DeJonge H. and Becq F. (2006). Rescue of functional delF508- CFTR channels in cystic fibrosis epithelial cells by the α-glucosidase inhibitor miglustat. FEBS Lett. 580:2081- 2086.

Perez A.; Issler A.C.; Cotton C.U.; Kelley T.J.; Verkman A.S.; Davis P.B. (2007). CFTR inhibition mimics the cystic fibrosis inflammatory profile. *Am J Physiol Lung Cell Mol Physiol* 292:L383–395

Puchelle E. ; De Bentzmann S. ; Hubeau C. ; Jacquot J. ; Gaillard D. (2001). Mechanisms involved in cystic fibrosis airway inflammation. *Pediatr Pulmonol* S23:143-5

Rogers C.S.; Stoltz D.a,; Meyerholz D.K. et al (2008). Disruption of the CFTR gene produces a model of cystic fibrosis in newborn pigs. Science 321: 1837-41

Rubin BK. (2007). CFTR is a modulator of airway inflammation. *Am J Physiol Lung Cell Mol Physiol* 292:L381–382.

Teichgraber V.; Ulrich M.; Endlich N.; Riethmüller J.;Wilker B.; De Oliveira-Munding C.C.; van Heeckeren A.M.; Barr M.L.; von Kürthy G.; Schmid K.W.; Weller M.; Tümmler B.; Lang F.; Grassme H.; Döring G.; Gulbins E (2008). Ceramide accumulation mediates inflammation, cell death and infection susceptibility in cystic fibrosis. *Nature Med* 14:382-391

Treiber A.; Morand O. and Clozel M. (2007) The pharmacokinetics and tissue distribution of the glucosylceramide synthase inhibitor miglustat in the rat. Xenobiotica 37:298-314.

Uhlig S.; Gulbins E. (2008). Sphingolipids in the lungs. *Am J Respir Crit Care Med.* 178(11):1100-14

Vicentini L.P.; Mazzi L.; Caveggion E.; Continolo S.; Fumagalli L.; Lapinet-Vera J.A.; Lowell C.A.; Berton G. (2002). Fgr deficiency results in defective eosinophil recruitment to the lung during allergic airway inflammation. *J Immunol* 168: 6446

Wojewodka G.; De Sanctis J.B. and Radzioch D. (2011). Ceramide in Cystic Fibrosis : A potential new target for therapeutic intervention. J of Lipids 2011: 1-13

Won J.S.; Im Y.B.; Khan M.; Singh A.K.; Singh I. (2004). The role of neutral sphingomyelinase produced ceramide in lipopolysaccharide-mediated expression of inducible nitric oxide synthase.J Neurochem. 88:583-93

Yanagi S.; Ashitani J.; Ishimoto H.; Date Y.; Mukae H.; Chino N.; Nakazato M. (2005). Isolation of human beta-defensin-4 in lung tissue and its increase in lower respiratory tract infection. Respir Res. 6:130

Yu H.; Zeidan Y.H.; Wu B.X.; Jenkins R.W.; Flotte T.R.; Hannun Y.A.; Virella-Lowell I. (2009). Defective acid sphingomyelinase pathway with *Pseudomonas aeruginosa* infection in cystic fibrosis. *American Journal of Respiratory Cell and Molecular Biology* 41:367-375

Zabner J.; Karp P.; Seiler M.; Phillips S.L. Mitchell C.J.; Saavedra M.; Welsh M.; Klingelhutz A.J. (2003). Development of cystic fibrosis and non cystic fibrosis airway cell lines. *Am. J. Physiol. Lung Cell Mol. Physiol.* 284:L844-L854.

Zeitlin P.L.; Lu L.; Rhim J.; Cutting G.; Stetten G.; Kieffer K.A.; Craig R.; Guggino W.B. (1991). A cystic fibrosis bronchial epithelial cell line: immortalization by adeno-12-SV40 infection. *Am. J.Respir. Cell Mol Biol* 4: 313-319.

Part 5

Disease Management

20

The Importance of Adherence and Compliance with Treatment in Cystic Fibrosis

Rosa Patricia Arias-Llorente,
Carlos Bousoño García and Juan J. Díaz Martín
Cystic Fibrosis Unit. Universitary Central Hospital of Asturias
Spain

1. Introduction

Over the last few years, the survival of cystic fibrosis (CF) patients has increased markedly. This is attributed to earlier diagnoses of the disease, the improvement of patient care involving multidisciplinary teams and more effective therapeutic options.

The therapeutic requirements of patients with CF are highly complex. Many patients require continuous care at home with many prophylactic medications, such as nebulised or oral antibiotics, pancreatic enzymes, mucolytic agents, vitamin and nutritional supplements as well as daily physiotherapy and a healthy lifestyle with adequate nutrition and exercise. These treatments are intensified and become more complicated during the exacerbation of the disease. Throughout its evolution, other pathologies associated with CF may also occur which require extra treatment regimens.

The complexity of the therapeutic requirements of these patients has added to their longevity. The life-long duration of the treatment and their complexity, have been pointed to as the main determinants of therapeutic adherence. Preventative management and symptomatic treatment are introduced in early childhood for most people with CF, and so management and treatment routines have been a daily concern for most adults for many years. (Kettler et al., 2002; Modi et al., 2006).

All of these difficulties have been identified as determinants of adherence and they are shared with the patients of other chronic diseases. Accordingly, the compliance rate in CF cases is very similar as that of the other chronically ill. In 1979, Sackett and Snow reviewed 537 studies on adherence in chronic disease cases, indicating that the range of adherence for long term preventative regimens was 33-94% with a mean adherence rate of 57% and for long term treatment the range was 41-61% with a mean adherence rate of 54%. Later, poor compliance with medical advice and prescribed treatments in the chronically ill in general is well-documented in the literature, and adherence rarely exceeds 80% and more often it is between 30% and 70%. (Abbott et al., 1996; Conway et al., 1996; Daniels et al., 2011; Kettler et al., 2002; Michaud et al., 1991; Modi et al., 2006).

2. The definition of adherence and compliance

The term compliance is applied when patients follow closely and correctly all the therapeutic indications prescribed by physicians. So, the definition of compliance is "the extent to which patients are obedient and follow the instructions, proscriptions and prescriptions of health professionals". We talk about adherence meaning the extent to which the patient responds to these indications, taking them and 'endorsing' them as his own. This refers not only to medication, but it also includes non-pharmacological measures, such as hygiene, diet controls, etc. (Kettler et al., 2002, as cited in Meichenbaum & Turk, 1987). So, adherence is defined as an "active, voluntary, collaborative involvement of the patient in a mutually acceptable course of behaviour to produce a desired preventative or therapeutic result". However, both terms receive general use and so are treated indifferently in the literature. No doubt the results of adherence are influenced by the definition adopted. Lots of different classifications of adherence - and extent of this has been described - have been assessed from different points of view. Some authors have suggested that patients should be described as fully-adherent, partially-adherent or non-compliant (Lask, 1994). Koocher differentiates the term non-compliant into three groups: those who have an inadequate understanding of the disease, those who present a psychological resistance to disease, and those who - when properly educated - choose not to be compliant (Koocher et al., 1990).

On the other hand, it has been found to be very difficult to classify an individual as compliant. Studies have found that despite compliance, significantly less than 100% could achieve the desired health outcomes (Kettler et al., 2002). However, the cut off point at which they would stop objectifying favourable results and should promote greater compliance is very difficult to define.

Poor adherence can lead to more rapid disease progression. (Abbott et al., 2001; Patterson et al., 1993). Nonetheless, there are studies that reject the existence of a conclusive association between poor compliance and disease progression (Abbott et al., 1994). However, a lack of compliance may increase the number of consultations and hospital admissions with a consequent increase in health spending. In addition, it may hinder the knowledge of the effectiveness of treatments. On the other hand, it is believed that total adherence may not be necessary, as the complete fulfilment of all of the components of a treatment does not guarantee good health. (Abbott et al., 2001). It is known that a patient with poor compliance may stay well, perhaps because of individual responses to different treatments. It is reasonable, therefore, be able to find a balance between the two sides, but is not an easy task for the specialist in relation to these patients.

3. The measurement of adherence

The measure of treatment adherence is not an easy task. We must find a balance between the errors obtained using certain procedures - such as personal interview - and the difficulty in performing other more objective technical procedures.

The methods most commonly used to study adherence in patients with CF include:

3.1 Personal interview

The most frequently used method is to ask directly or take a survey of the patient as to whether the treatment takes place and to what extent it does so. However, patients often tend to overestimate their compliance (Abbott et al., 1996; Conway et al., 1996, Kettler et al., 2002) and frequently this does not reflect the opinion of the specialist. This data can be compared by asking the opinion of the medical team responsible for the patient or else their family. Although this is the easiest and most accessible system for assessing adherence to all kinds of treatments, it cannot be denied that the results are not entirely objective.

3.2 Therapeutic response

Using this method of measuring adherence in such a complex disease as CF and the many variants of treatment can lead to errors. In particular, knowledge of the desired effect achieved by taking a certain drug is almost impossible given the significant interaction between the different treatments.

3.3 Serum or urinary excretion of drugs or their metabolites

The first thing to note is that this is an invasive method and as such it is highly uncomfortable for the patient, who would have to undergo a large number of extractions in order to verify their genuine compliance. This problem is compounded by the pharmacokinetic variations of the substances studied, and it allows the analysis of only certain medications and reports only those drugs that have been recently consumed by the patient.

3.4 Monitoring with electronics, such as aerosol dispensers or nebulisers, that record the date and time of each dispensation

This data would be periodically downloaded for analysis so as to give an idea of adherence. Amongst its advantages it is worth noting that it allows us to guess the behaviour of patients, it is non-invasive, and it allows the collection of data over a long period of time without the patient having to attend hospital. On the other hand, this type of monitoring has its limitations. With its high cost we must also add the fact that data provide information about the use of a medication removed from dispenser. However, it is reasonable to assume that most patients who make the effort to remove medication from the dispenser in the prescribed way will also consume the medication. This technology is limited when used for evaluating physical therapy, and it gives no information on adherence to such treatment regimens as exercise or diet (Kettler et al., 2002; McNamara et al., 2009; Modi et al., 2006).

4. Predictors of compliance

Once the degree of compliance of a patient is measured, it is interesting to know the reasons for why compliance might not be adequate and identify the motivations for good adherence. Understanding the factors that may be related to adherence will enable us to act on them to some degree and so improve compliance and impact upon the course of the disease.

Described below are the factors that have often been studied as predictors of compliance in the literature.

4.1 The relationship between the patient and health professionals

In a chronic disease with a complex treatment such as CF, the relationship of patients with their health professionals is very important. This can have a positive or negative impact on compliance, and so it should foster an environment of trust that allows for good communications between them. Numerous studies have shown that those who believe that it is important to follow your doctor's instructions and those who have confidence in the benefits of their treatment are more compliant. (Abbott et al., 2001; Patterson et al., 1993) The level of adherence has been linked with the knowledge of the specifics associated with prescribed medical treatments. Therefore, the physician must strive to convey adequate information which is detailed yet easy to understand. After all, in many cases the patient has not properly understood the reason for each prescription, as made clear by the fact that 12%-32% of mothers do not fully understand the medical advice concerning their child (Ievers et al., 1999).

Such appropriate information must convince patients that their actions when performing the treatment will impact on the course of their disease. The fact of involving the patient will give us with the ability to schedule a treatment plan together with them and which allows us to improve adherence. To do this, we must recognise that there is no single treatment for all patients and it should be individualised and simplified wherever possible.

Moreover, the maintenance of adequate adherence to prescribed treatments is very important for care monitoring and the provision of adequate supervision, and we should always try not to judge and accept that a lack of enforcement is, to a certain extent, normal with this type of disease (Conway et al., 1996; Lask et al., 1994).

4.2 The severity of the disease

The perception of the severity of the disease differs between doctors and patients. From the doctor’s point of view, the patients underestimate the severity of their disease and overestimate their care.

Some authors suggest that adherence is worse amongst those patients with more severe cases due to a lack of positive reinforcement in that they do not notice any beneficial effect resulting from adherence to their treatment (Kettler et al., 2002). However, the severity of the disease has often been evaluated as a possible predictor of adherence in CF cases with conflicting results (Abbott et al., 1994, 1996, 2001; Conway et al., 1996; Gudas et al., 1991; Kettler et al., 2002).

4.3 Social and family relationships

It is very important that patients with CF receive good socio-familial support. Strong family cohesion and adequate social support have been associated with better adherence to treatment. A special importance is attached to the family in the care of patients during childhood, where the burden of treatment compliance during this time of life is maintained by the parents (Battistini et al., 1998; Eddy et al., 1998; Foster et al., 2001; Moise et al., 1987).

However, there are other difficult times, such as adolescence, where receiving strong family support and positive reinforcement is central to maintaining good adhesion to the different treatments that have to meet the needs of these patients. The stresses between parents and children, and poor relationships between parents, are associated with low compliance and could have an adverse impact on the disease and health status of children with CF (Dziuban et al., 2010; Eddy et al., 1998; Foster et al., 2001; Smith et al., 2010).

4.4 Types of treatment

There is wide agreement in the literature over the differences in adherence to the different components of the treatment of patients with CF. While the adherence to antibiotic therapy (80-95%) and intake of enzymes (65-90%) is high, we cannot say the same for habitual physiotherapy, exercise and the taking of vitamins and nutritional supplements, for which compliance is found to be about 40-55%. The high compliance found in relation to certain aspects of the treatment of patients with CF probably reflects the short-term benefit associated with a given treatment or else any immediate unpleasant symptoms which may result from non-compliance. An example of this would be the appearance of steatorrhea as a consequence of ending the intake of pancreatic enzymes in patients with exocrine pancreatic insufficiency. (Abbott et al., 1994; Conway et al., 1996; Daniels et al., 2011; McNamara et al., 2009).

4.5 Age

Treatment adherence tends to decrease with age. Younger children show greater compliance, perhaps because during this time the responsibility for treatment lies with their parents. However, later on during adolescence, adherence decreases when the patient takes responsibility for their own treatment (Bucks et al., 2009; Dziuban et al., 2010; Gudas et al., 1991; Zindani et al., 2006).

The overall compliance of adolescents with CF is around 50%. Several factors, such as the family environment, staff perceptions about their illness, shame of displaying their problem in front of friends, and their relationship with their doctor are all classically associated with compliance, which is difficult to predict at this age due to the multiple factors involved (Michaud et al., 1991). All these factors occur at the time when the adolescent is transferred to the adult specialist (Kettler et al., 2002), and many patients experience suspicion and insecurity which also often tends to affect adherence.

In chronic diseases, the normal behaviour of denial and a reduction of anxiety tend to increase with age in facilitating emotional adjustment in adulthood. So, while these attitudes improve the mental health of these patients they also often negatively affect their adherence (Lask, 1994).

4.6 Epidemiological factors

Demographic factors such as sex, level of educational, knowledge of the disease, socioeconomic status and occupation, and clinical factors such as the age of diagnosis and the frequency of clinical visits, have all been evaluated as possible predictors of adherence in CF cases, and have met with conflicting results (Abbott et al., 1994, 1996, 2001; Dziuban et al., 2010; Gudas et al., 1991; Oerman et al., 2000).

4.7 Ways of coping with the disease

Psychological factors are beginning to emerge as strong predictors of adherence. Classically, it was said that the incidence of mental health disorders in people with CF is recognisably similar to that of the general population. However, high levels of stress are common and require recognition and attention (Abbott et al., 2001; Dziuban et al., 2010; Kettler et al., 2002).

A large percentage of patients with CF and their parents reported elevated symptoms of depression. In a recent study, rates of depressive symptoms were elevated in children with CF and their parents (29% for children, 35% for mothers and 23% for fathers). In addition, child depressive symptoms were significantly associated with lower rates of adherence to airway clearance (Smith et al., 2010).

Moise claims that there are lower levels of psychological distress and better adjustment in patients who use avoidance as a way of coping with illness, and those who use more direct methods and are positive (Moise et al., 1987).

It is well-documented that poor psychological well-being can influence a detrimental physiological function and a disease's progression, morbidity and mortality (Abbott et al., 2001). Perhaps it should be admitted that a degree of non-compliance is normal in these patients.

Concern about their illness and the perception that they have little personal control over its course has been shown to be a facilitator of adherence. The way of coping with CF has a potential influence on the direction and course of their disease. In particular, denial has been associated with rebellion and persistent non-compliance, while the adopting of an attitude of optimism and hope is associated with greater compliance (Abbott et al., 1996, 2001; Dziuban et al., 2010).

Currently, there is a major dilemma amongst health professionals with regard to promoting good mental health, whether they should allow denial and avoidance strategies for the patient to cope with the disease, or else whether they should promote compliance, which is dependent upon the recognition of the disease and the need for treatment.

5. Treatment compliance in children and adults with CF

The irregular adherence to treatment of patients with CF can alter the course of their illness. There are a number of important consequences of a failure to comply in treating CF, namely: deaths from cardiovascular diseases and infections, hospital admissions, increased visits, additional diagnostic testing requirements, additional alternative or unnecessary treatments, the home storage of medications and increased health spending. Knowledge of these aspects which motivate a patient in meeting certain treatments, and the discovery of the reasons given to justify the failure of others, can help the physician to promote adherence among their patients and influence the course of their disease.

In 2008, we published a study designed to determine treatment compliance and how it was perceived by patients, parents and by a team of specialists in CF. We also analysed the relative importance given to each of the prescribed treatments and the reasons that were given for non-adherence, and we investigated the possible predictors of therapeutic compliance. We also looked at the reasons for non-adherence, so as to determine possible predictors of therapeutic compliance (Arias-Llorente et al., 2008).

5.1 Patients and methods

5.1.1 Patients

Thirty-four CF patients controlled by the outpatient CF clinic of the University Central Hospital of Asturias and which attended periodic revisions (one each trimester) participated in the study. Up until the age of 14 they are controlled by paediatric gastroenterologists and pneumologists and by an adult specialist from that age on.

5.1.2 Study protocol

Data was collected by reviewing the clinical histories of the patients and it included epidemiologic data (age, gender, age at the diagnosis of CF, the timing of the evolution of the disease and CFTR mutation), a respiratory evaluation (the treatment received at the time of the interview, spirometric values, Bhalla score, lung transplantation) and a digestive evaluation (body mass index (BMI), nutritional index (NI), blood levels of alkaline phosphatase, transaminases, gamma-glutamyl transpeptidase, fat soluble vitamins, folic acid, albumin, β-carotene, faecal elastase, and immunoreactive trypsin, 72-hour faecal fat) and global evaluation (associated co-morbidities, Shwachman-Kulczycki score).

5.1.3 Questionnaire

A self-administered questionnaire was given to each patient when attending a routine visit to be answered in the clinic. Patients older than 12 years completed the questionnaire themselves, while it was filled out by the parents of younger patients. The questionnaire included four different subsets of questions, one for each of the different treatments usually given to CF patients, namely: physiotherapy, respiratory medication (including DNase, antibiotics and inhaled corticosteriods), digestive medication (including pancreatic enzymes, vitamins, deoxycholic acid and antacids) and nutritional supplements.

For each subset of therapeutic options, the CF patients were asked multiple questions on treatment compliance, the frequency of treatment, the importance attached to the treatment, their personal opinion about their own treatment compliance and the reasons given for non-compliance. At the end of the questionnaire, the CF patients score (from 0 to 100%) their global therapeutic compliance, considering all the treatments received.

According to the score obtained by the questionnaire, patients were then grouped according to their compliance or non-compliance for each of the therapeutic options and globally.

In addition, the paediatric and adult gastroenterologists, pneumologists and nurses of the CF clinic were also asked to subjectively classify the treatment compliance of the CF patients in terms of compliance and non-compliance.

5.2 Results

Thirty-four CF patients (21 of which were female) with an age range of 1.6 to 40.6 years (mean 14.5) were included in the study. Fourteen patients were under 10 years of age, 11 between 10 and 20, and 9 were older than 20. The average time of the evolution of the disease was 12.2 years (range from 1.3 to 40.6).

5.2.1 Adherence for each type of treatment

At the time of the study the average number of digestive and respiratory medications to be taken by the patients were 3.5 (range 0 to 7) and 4.5 (range 1 to 9) respectively.

Treatment compliance was greater for digestive (88.2%) and respiratory medication (61.8%), compared to physiotherapy (41.2%) and nutritional supplements (59%). This data is shown in Table 1, as well as that extracted from the views of the health professionals with regard to adherence of the patients to each type of treatment. The questionnaire results show a global compliance of 59%, whereby only 56% were compliant according to the opinion of the clinicians. Moreover, when the patient was directly asked, at the end of the questionnaire, to indicate their adherence to the therapy in their opinion, the treatment compliance was higher both for each type of treatment and globally.

	QUESTIONNAIRE	SPECIALISTS	PATIENTS
Physiotherapy	41.2%	35.3%	62.%
Respiratory	61.8%	59%	75.8%
Nutritional	59%	56%	77.7%
Digestive	88.2%	70.4%	91.2%
Global	59%	56%	84.8%

Table 1. The percentage of therapeutic adherence for each type of treatment based upon a questionnaire and specialist opinions and the perception of patients.

In conclusion, CF patients had a greater treatment adherence when prescribed digestive and respiratory medications as opposed to physiotherapy and nutritional supplements.

5.2.2 Degree and frequency of compliance

All of the CF patients take their digestive medications daily, although 64.7% admitted that they only consume pancreatic enzymes during principal meals and not during snacks. 50% of the CF patients indicated daily treatment compliance with respiratory medication and nutritional supplements. On the other hand, 14.7% only took their respiratory medications when they felt worse and 5.8% never took them, and nearly 30% of the patients said that they never consume their nutritional supplements.

The data from our questionnaire about physiotherapy is quite remarkable. Only 38.2% admitted to practising physiotherapy daily, while nearly 45% of patients reported as having physiotherapy only when they felt worse, occasionally or else never.

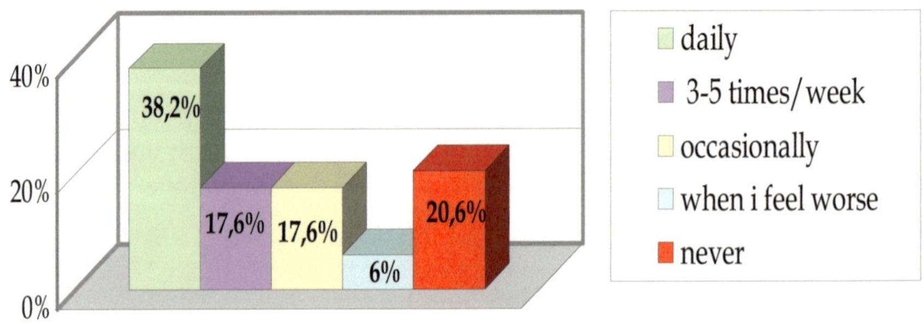

Fig. 1. Frequency of practice of physiotherapy (percentage of patients).

5.2.3 The importance given to different types of treatment and their impact on quality of life

The importance attached by patients to each type of treatment (average scores between 1 and 10): physiotherapy, 7.17; respiratory medication, 8; digestive, 9.4; nutritional support, 6.2) influenced compliance, and the treatments with the highest score saw the best level of adherence.

CF patients considered their digestive medication to be indispensable (94.1%) compared to respiratory medications, physiotherapy and nutritional supplements (70.6%, 59% and 44.1% respectively).

Type of treatment effect on quality of life was evaluated by the CF patients, and Table 2 shows the results of this evaluation. While 85.3% of the patients thought that digestive medications significantly improve their quality of life, half of the CF patients considered that physiotherapy plays little or no role on their perceived quality of life.

	Much	Enough	Little	Nothing
Physiotherapy	35.2%(25–45)	17.6%(5–31)	17.6%(5–31)	29.4% (14–44)
Respiratory	26.5% (11–41)	29.4% (14–44)	11.7% (3–28)	14.7% (3–27)
Digestive	38.2% (20–52)	44.1% (27–61)	2.9% (0.08–17)	8.8% (2–27)
Nutritional	11.7% (3–28)	38.2% (20–52)	11.7% (3–28%)	14.7% (3–27)

Table 2. The impact of treatments on quality of life of the patients (95% confidence interval limits in brackets).

5.2.4 Satisfaction

Patient satisfaction about their own treatment adherence was significantly higher for digestive medication, with 70.6 % of the CF patients considering that they were taking the correct dose of digestive medication, while only 8.8% considered that they should have been more compliant. By way of contrast, only 29.4% of the CF patients considered that they were practising as much physiotherapy as they needed, in comparison to 41.2% who thought that they should practise more frequently.

5.2.5 Reasons for poor compliance

The main reason given for not taking digestive medications was forgetfulness. However, the most repeated excuses for not complying with respiratory medication and nutritional supplements were the belief that they didn't need the medications (11.7% and 14.7% respectively), together with a lack of time for respiratory medication (8.8%) and the unpleasant taste or texture for nutritional supplements (14.7%).

The reasons given for not doing physiotherapy exercises included not having enough time (23.5%), not needing the treatment (20.6%) and substitution by other exercises (20.6%). Actually, the median time that our patients employ in practising physiotherapy is noticeably less than the ageing of sickness evolution (7.6 years vs. 12.2 years). A considerable number of patients believe that physiotherapy is not necessary after receiving lung transplantation.

	% patients
Physiotherapy	
Not enough time	29.4%
I don´t think need it, I feel well without treatment.	20.6%
Exercise instead	20.6%
I don´t believe that it does my any good	14.7%
It interferes with my social life	11.8%
Simply forget	8.8%
Transplantation	5.9%
Respiratory medication	
I don´t think need it	11.7%
Not enough time	8.8%
Only when I feel worse	8.8%
It interferes with my social life	5.9%
Simply forget	5.9%
Exercise instead	2.9%
Nutritional supplements	
I don´t think need it	14.7%
I don´t like the taste or texture	14.7%
Simply forget	8.8%
I don´t believe in it	5.9%

Table 3. The predominant reasons for poor compliance with different treatments (percentage of patients).

5.2.6 Differences between compliant and non-compliant CF patients

It was objectified that treatment adherence decreases with age. We have observed that 23.8% of patients younger than 15 years were non-compliant, while this percentage rose to 69.2% for those older than 15 years, up to 89% for those older than 20 years. Non-compliant patients were significantly older (the average age of compliant patients was 10.4 years; that of non-compliant patients was 20.5 years, $p=0.008$) and had a longer time of evolution for their disease (compliant 9.4 years; non-compliant 16.8 years, $p = 0.025$). In our study, we have observed that adherence to treatment decreases with the severity of the CF disease (Shwachman score compliant 83.2 vs. non-compliant 73.9 points, $p = 0.048$).

No gender differences were observed. Moreover, compliant CF patients attached more importance to all of the different therapeutic options than non-compliant CF patients (Table 4). Nutritional parameters were also analysed, and compliant CF patients displayed significantly higher albumin values than non-compliant patients. No differences were observed for any of the other biochemical factors studied. No age-adjusted differences were observed in BMI. No differences were observed for faecal fat, NI, and spirometric values.

	COMPLIANT Mean (SD)	NON-COMPLIANT Mean (SD)	P
Physiotherapy	9.5 (2)	5 (0.7)	0.000
Respiratory	8.8 (1.5)	6.4 (3)	0.010
Digestive	9.7 (0.7)	7 (1.7)	0.001
Nutritional	8.6 (1.4)	4.3 (3.1)	0.000

Table 4. The importance attached to different therapeutic options by CF patients on a scale from 1 to 10 points.

5.3 Discussion

identified as determinants of adherence to different treatments. At the time of our study, the average number of digestive and respiratory medications to be taken by patients was 3.5 (range 0 to 7) and 4.5 (range 1 to 9) respectively. These medications numbered too many even when compared with other studies, where there are even lists with more than twenty different treatments (Marciel et al., 2010). The explanation for this difference may be that the average age of patients is greater where there is a more prolonged progression of the disease and a possibly more serious illness. Whilst - in our study - the average age of the patients was 14.5 years, the mean time of the evolution of the disease was 12.2 years, and 58.8% of the controlled patients in our unit presented a good global prognostic score according to the Shwachman-Kulczycki scale, and even 26.4% were qualified as excellent.

If these treatments are added to the need for other medications for associated pathologies and daily physiotherapy practice, they can give us an idea of how complicated the treatment was and the time spent on it. Given the long duration and arduous nature of these regimens, the maintenance of good compliance over prolonged periods will be a difficult task for the specialist responsible. Moreover, there are many other factors which may influence a decline in adherence: the perception of the disease which the patient has at any time, their different ways of coping with the disease (which can change throughout life), family, economic or social problems, a lack of trust in the responsible physician, erroneous beliefs about the benefits of different treatments, etc.

As such, the patients who were considered to be particularly compliant could also go through phases of declining adherence. For this reason, it is very important not to relax during the monitoring of these chronic patients and to be alert to any problems that may affect their adherence to their treatment (Duff & Latchford, 2010). During this time, the team of specialists should try to understand and motivate the patient.

Accordingly, there are works that strive to determine not only the degree of compliance of these patients, but also its variation over time and the reasons for this. Using this type of information, it is possible to identify which aspects of the treatment can be improved and to work together with families so as to individualise treatments. For example, a study designed to determine adherence to nebulised antibiotics by monitoring the routine data downloads of an adaptive aerosol delivery nebuliser in children with CF found considerable variation in adherence, both between and within patients, and even over the course of the day (evening adherence was better than morning adherence). Treatment regimens were changed for 8/28 patients, based upon the data on adherence obtained by this study (McNamara et al., 2009).

Treatment adherence in CF cases, as with many other chronic diseases, has been around 50% and has rarely exceeded 80% (Abbott et al., 1996; Conway et al., 1996; Daniels et al., 2011; Kettler et al., 2002; McNamara et al., 2009). According to the data obtained by the questionnaire score, overall treatment compliance with the CF group controlled in our unit was 59%. Also, patients were asked directly as to what their level of compliance was, it was much higher both overall and for each type of treatment. Indeed, half of the patients believe that they comply with the therapeutic indications made by the specialist by at least 90%, a better level of adherence than the indicated by the results obtained by the questionnaire score.

The fact that patients tend to overestimate their adherence to treatment is usually reflected in the literature. By way of contrast, the opinion of health professionals suggests a generally lower level of adherence (Abbott et al., 2001; Conway et al., 1996; Daniels et al., 2011; Modi et al., 2006). Moreover, it is usually the case that the perception of the severity of the disease also differs between physician and patient. A recent study assessed the agreement between rates of adherence to prescribed nebulisers when measured by self-reports, clinician reports and electronic monitoring suitable for long-term use, and differences in adherence were found. Here, median self-reported adherence was 80% whilst median clinician reported adherence was down to 50%-60% (Daniels et al., 2011). This was also observed in our study, as adherence to treatment as assessed by the team of specialists was lower than both the overall and for each type of treatment. So, according to our data, only 70% of those patients who believed themselves to be compliant (according to the questionnaire results) are also considered to be so by their specialised doctors.

However, self-reporting and clinician reporting of adherence does not provide accurate measurement of adherence when compared with more objective measurement methods. In this case, adherence is usually less than as shown in the study mentioned above, where the level of adherence measured by nebuliser downloads was 36% (Daniels et al., 2011).

We are aware that the results of our study are based on subjective data obtained after a personal interview with parents and/or patients, which are then contrasted with the opinions of the clinicians belonging to the CF unit. There are also studies that clearly show that clinical impressions are not accurate enough to determine the real therapeutic adherence of patients, and so it would be also convenient to use a more objective method (Marciel et al., 2010; Modi et al.; 2006; Shemesh et al., 2004). It has been mentioned that the level of adherence could vary according to the subjectivity of the method employed, such as with a personal questionnaire, even if the results are corrected with the opinions of the medical professionals or other objective measures, such as blood-serum levels, the urinary excretion of medications or their metabolites, or the monitoring of adherence with electronic recording devices or the dispensers of medications (Conway et al., 1996; Modi et al., 2006; Rand et al., 1992; Teichman et al., 2000). Nevertheless these methods have their own inconveniences. With regard to the drug levels in serum or urine, we must emphasise that they are invasive methods and they may only represent yet another test for patients, due to the multiple samples needed to check their compliance, in addition to the pharmacokinetic variations of the substance are to be studied. Regarding electronic monitoring, the data obtained only provides information about the use of a medication dispenser, but not about whether the patient is actually taking the medication removed from the dispenser; moreover, this type of monitoring remains too expensive. This could also limit other evaluations concerning such aspects as diet, exercise and physiotherapy (Kettler et al., 2002; Rand et al., 1992).

In addition to finding differences in treatment compliance according to the methods discussed above, there are many works that refer to differences in adherence to the different components of the treatment carried out by patients with CF. Traditionally, it is said that adherence is low - between 40% and 55% - to nutritional supplements and physiotherapy. Meanwhile, treatment compliance to pancreatic enzymes and respiratory antibiotics increases to between 75% and 90% (Abbott et al., 2001; Daniels et al., 2011; Kettler et al., 2002; Modi et al., 2006).

In our study, and with regard to the types of treatment, most patients performed digestive medication (88.2% of patients), followed by respiratory medication (61.8%). Meanwhile 59% of patients were considered compliant with respect to nutritional support whilst only 41.2% were compliant with physiotherapy. In our case, the number of patients who were compliant towards digestive medication is similar to the results shown elsewhere (Abbott et al., 1994, 1996, 2001; Daniels et al., 2011; Modi et al., 2006) as well as the fact that only a third of patients took pancreatic enzymes at every meal, including snacks (Michaud et al., 1991). However, the level of adherence to respiratory medication was less than in others studies, which is perhaps explained by the fact that we did not analyse specific compliance with every aspect of respiratory treatment. If we had taken into consideration the individual's adherence to bronchodilators, antibiotics or inhaled corticosteroids, the adherence to treatment would probably have been greater.

When we asked patients about the importance that they attach to the different types of treatment (on a scale from 1 to 10 points), the highest score was assigned to digestive medication (9.4 points), corresponding with the most valued treatment in terms of compliance and its impact on quality of life. As such, 85.3% of the patients thought that digestive medication significantly improved their quality of life. As described in previous publications, our patients displayed better compliance with those treatments that they believed to be more important (Abbott et al., 2001; Patterson et al., 1993) and to have more repercussions for their quality of life (Conway et al., 1996; Czjkowski et al., 1987).

In accordance with the details above, the two types of treatments that most patients seemed to consider essential were digestive and respiratory medications (94.1% and 70.6% respectively). This idea, coupled with the higher compliance observed in these treatments, is collected in earlier studies and it may reflect the short-term benefits of these and the precocity of the appearance of unpleasant symptoms as a result of non-compliance (Abbott et al., 1994, 1996, 2001; Conway et al., 1996; Kettler et al., 2002). Thus, adherence to pancreatic enzyme typically is high in order to avoid steatorrhea and the main reason for not taking this medication is "forgotten" and only one person says no need to take it despite having malabsorption.

At the opposite end are nutritional supplements and physiotherapy. It is of concern that uniquely 44.1% consider nutritional supplements to be an essential treatment in clear concordance to the main reason given for not taking nutritional supplements: "I don't think I need it". And finally, only 59% of the patients believe physiotherapy is an essential treatment, in clear opposition to what physicians think. In fact, the type of treatment which we found to reflect a greater discrepancy between the opinions of doctors and patients was physiotherapy. This way of thinking agrees with patients' perception of their slight repercussions for their quality of life (half of the CF patients felt that physiotherapy played little or no role in their treatment) and the different degrees of importance attached to physiotherapy by compliant and non-compliant patients (9.5 points vs. 5 points, $p<0.001$). In this connection, the data of our questionnaire concerning physiotherapy is remarkable since the practise of physiotherapy was particularly deficient with regard to the number of subjects doing it and its frequency; however, this is also found in the literature (Abbott et al., 1996; Bernard & Cohen, 2004; Passero et al., 1981). The number of patients who practised daily physiotherapy only reached 38.2%, similar to other results in CF clinics (Abbott et al., 2001; Oerman et al., 2000), and 20% even say that they never practice physiotherapy.

On the other hand, the beginning of physiotherapy should be instituted at the time of the diagnosis of CF, a finding which is not supported by the average time that our patients have been practising (mean ± SD: 7.6±6.1 years), which is strikingly lower than the average time of the disease (12.2±8.9 years).

Therefore, the main reasons claimed for non-compliance are a lack of time, the erroneous belief that they don't need it or that they can substitute them with other exercise. As such, the perception that there are no beneficial effects with the treatment is wholesale problem for physiotherapy (Bernard & Cohen, 2004; Conway et al., 1996; Czjkowski et al., 1987; Shemesh et al., 2004; Teichman et al., 2001), and it has been published as being substituted with exercise in 20% of cases, just as we found (20.6%).

A particular time when there is a risk of a decrease in adherence occurs, typically, after lung transplantation. Accordingly, we must emphasise that half of our transplanted patients have given up physiotherapy techniques afterwards, giving this hopeful event as the very reason for their lack of adherence. Even if it is known that medical opinions obviously contrast with this attitude, there is a recognised decrease in their therapeutic fulfilment after a lung transplantation which continues over time. It may be that they experience a better sense of wellbeing and so could hypothesise that they didn't need it anymore. At this time, it is essential to provide them with clear information and to take care in following up with adequate supervision so as to reorient and help them eradicate these erroneous beliefs (Foster et al., 2001; Lask, 1994; Kettler et al., 2002; Oerman et al., 2000; Teichman et al., 2000).

Such beliefs about the benefits of and need for each type of treatment significantly influence in the treatment adherence.

In terms of patient satisfaction about their own adherence, it should be noted that is noticeably higher with the digestive intake of medication, such that 70.6% think that they should take this type of medication and only 8.8% think they should take more. At the other extreme is physiotherapy, where only 29.4% of patients believe that they should practise physiotherapy at all and 41% think that they should do it more often. If we compare this data with those described in previous works, it confirms a trend (Abbott et al., 1994). This is to say that patients are more satisfied with their compliance with digestive or respiratory medication than with their practise of physiotherapy. It is a paradoxical result because, although very few are happy with the practise of physiotherapy, there are few who think that they should do it more often.

There are several factors which should be taken into account as possible predictors of adherence in CF cases, with contradictory results: demographic data such as sex, age, level of education, knowledge of sickness, socio-economic status, socio-familial relations and profession, as well as clinical factors such as age at diagnosis, the severity of the CF or the frequency of checkups at CF clinics (Bernard & Cohen 2004; Jaffe & Bush, 2001; Kettler et al., 2002; Oerman et al., 2000; Passero et al., 1981; Zindani et al., 2006). Our study found a statistically significant difference both in terms of the average age of each patient group, (compliant at 10.4 years and non-compliant at 20.5 years) and the time of the evolution of the disease (compliant at 9.5 years and non-compliant at 16.8 years). The fact that adherence to treatment tends to diminish with age has also been mentioned in the earlier studies (Conway et al., 1996; Gudas et al., 1991). In childhood, a high level of compliance is frequently observed, which is probably explained due to the fact that during this period of life the responsibility lies with the parents (Battistini et al., 1998; Foster et al., 2001). Family cohesion and adequate social support have both been associated with better adherence to treatment (Eddy et al., 1998; Foster et al., 2001; Hamutcy et al., 2002; Teichman 20009). In addition, the ways of coping with the disease by the mechanisms of denial and avoidance - which have been described as negative predictors of adherence to treatment - tend to increase with age amongst these chronically ill patients as they facilitate their emotional adjustment into adulthood (Kettler et al., 2002; Lask, 1994).

A special time when compliance with treatment tends to decrease significantly is during adolescence, as was also found in our study, whereby parents release their progeny. This notion is reflected repeatedly in the literature for years (Bernard & Cohen, 2004; Bucks et al., 2009; Conway et al., 1996; Mc Laughlin et al., 2008; Passero et al., 1998). So, in a study done in Montreal University 20 years ago on compliance with treatment amongst adolescents affected by chronic illness, such as CF, it was concluded that there was a global adherence of 50%; nevertheless only 11% of the subjects demonstrated the successful accomplishment of all of the therapeutic components (Michaud et al., 1991). In another study at Michigan University several years later, it has been shown that there is a significant difference between those patients who are less than 12 years old and those who are over twelve year old with regard to the intake of liposoluble vitamins amongst CF patients (Jaffe & Bush, 2001).

Adolescence means that the patients are presented with several other challenges apart from their illness, such that all of a sudden they are supposed to take control of themselves; perhaps they are prone to diminish its importance, or perhaps they display a reluctance to chat with their peers about their 'big' problem, or perhaps, even, they adopt a "hide and run" policy. They apologise, arguing with such reasons as "it interferes with my social life," "I don't want my friends to know that I suffer from CF," as we have confirmed. Another reason in the decrease in self-accomplishment could be the transfer from paediatricians to adult medical staff (McLaughlin et al., 2008; Michaud et al., 1991), since initially it could mean a degree of instability and lack of reliance that is traduced into less adherence.

For all of these reasons, there is often a growing recognition of need for support for their transition into adult-oriented healthcare. There is significant variability in the transitional support provided to young adults with CF (Mc Laughlin et al., 2008; Scal & Ireland; 2005). The first problem is the age of transition, because while in many centres the transfer of care for CF occurs at a median age of 19 years, in other programs it has been reported that the introduction of the concept of transition takes place before the age of 15 years (Anderson 2002). In our CF unit, up until the age of 14 (younger than 15 years) they are controlled by paediatric gastroenterologists and pneumologists, and by an adult specialist from that age onwards. The second problem relates to the different methods of transition that have been used. Few programmes provide educational materials about transition to patients and families, and fewer than half provide a transition time-line or designate a specific team member to be responsible for the key elements of transition (Mc Laughlin et al., 2008; Marciel et al., 2010).

With regard to the severity of the disease, as determined by the score on the Shwachman-Kulczycki scale, significant differences were found between the compliant and non-compliant groups. We have observed that adherence to treatment decreases with the severity of CF. Some authors explain this phenomenon by reasoning to a lack of positive reinforcement whereby patients do not note a beneficial effect with their adherence to treatment (Hamutcy et al., 2002). However, there are also other authors who describe the opposite, with results relating disease severity with adherence to treatment (Oerman et al., 2000; Zindani et al., 2006).

In summary, we can say that there are differences in the degree of compliance by these patients with the various components of the treatment carried out. There is greater adherence to digestive and respiratory medications than to physiotherapy and nutritional supplements. We found a decrease in adherence according to age, the longer the history of the disease and the greater its severity. In addition, the treatments which were evaluated by patients as most important and as having the greatest impact on their quality of life witnessed the most adherence.

6. Conclusion

We can conclude that the global compliance with treatment is similar to that of other works, with a tendency of patients to overestimate their accomplishments as compared with the opinions of clinical staff. There are differences in the level of adherence to the various treatments, and this is realised by these patients.

Of all the treatments that patients carry out, it was felt that the treatment which had the greatest impact on their quality of life, that which most considered to be essential and with which they were personally the most satisfied, involved gastrointestinal medicaments. Nevertheless, the practise of physiotherapy was highly deficient with regard to the number of subjects performing it and the frequency with which they did it, influenced by the general belief that it does not make much difference and that it has little repercussion for their quality of life.

We have confirmed a decrease in therapeutic adherence with age, the longer the duration of evolution and the severity of the illness. There was no influence from the gender of the patients, their nutritional parameters, or from the data on pulmonary function. The treatments mostly appreciated by the patients as most essential were coincident with a higher level of adherence, emphasising the need for careful and continuous information, and the modification of erroneous beliefs.

7. Acknowledgment

We would like to extend our deepest appreciation to the children and their families and the adults with CF of our unit.

8. References

Abbott, J., Dodd, M., Bilton, D. & Webb, A.K. (1994). Treatment compliance in adults with cystic fibrosis, *Thorax* Vol. 49(2): 115-120.

Abbott, J., Dodd, M. & Webb, A.K. (1996). Health perceptions and treatment adherence in adults with cystic fibrosis, *Thorax* Vol. 51(12): 1233-1238.

Abbott, J., Dodd, M., Gee, L. & Webb, A.K. (2001). Ways of coping with cystic fibrosis: implications for treatment adherence, *Disabil Rehabil.* Vol. 23(8): 315-324.

Anderson, D.L, Flume, P.A, Hardy, K.K & Gray, S (2002). Transition programs in cystic fibrosis centres: perceptions of patients, *Pediatr Pulmonol.* Vol.33 (5):327- 331.

Arias-Llorente, R.P; Bousoño, C. & Diaz, J.J. (2008). Treatment compliance in children and adults of cystic fibrosis, *J. Cyst. Fibrosis* Vol. 7: 359-367.

Battistini, A., Grzincich, G.L., Pisi, G., Bocchi, U., Marvasi, R., Costantini, I., et al. (1998) Respiratory physio-Kinesitherapy in cystic fibrosis: the parents` viewpoint, *Pediatr Med. Chir.* Vol. 10 (1): 1-14.

Bernard, R.S. & Cohen, L.L. (2004). Increasing adherence to cystic fibrosis treatment: a systematic review of behaviour techniques, *Pediatr Pulmonol.* Vol.. 37(1): 8-16.

Bucks, R.S., Hawkins, K., Skinner, T.C., Horn, S., Seddon, P & Horne, R. (2009). Adherence to treatment in adolescents with cystic fibrosis: the role of illness perceptions and treatment beliefs, *J. Pediatr Psychol.* Vol. 34(8): 893-902.

Conway, S.P., Pond, M.N., Hamnett, T. & Watson, A. (1996) Compliance with treatment in adult patients with cystic fibrosis, *Thorax* Vol. 51(1): 29-33.

Czajkowski, D. & Koocher, G. (1987) Medical compliance and coping with cystic fibrosis, *J. Child Psychol. Psychiatry* Vol. 23: 311-319.

Daniels, T., Goodacre, L., Sutton, C., Pollard, K., Conway, S. & Peckham, D. (2011). Accurate assessment of adherence: Self and clinical report versus electronic monitoring of nebulisers, *Chest* (Epub ahead of print).

Duff, A.J. & Latchford G.J (2010). Motivational interviewing for adherence problems in cystic fibrosis, *Pediatr Pulmonol* Vol.45(3): 211-220.

Dziuban, E.J., Saab-Abazeed, L. Chaudhry, S.R., Streetman, D.S. & Nasr, S.Z. (2010). Identifying barriers to treatment adherence and related attitudinal patterns in adolescents with cystic fibrosis, *Pediatr Pulmonol.* Vol. 45(5): 450-458.

Eddy, M.E., Carter, B.D., Kronenberger, W.G., Conradsen, S., Eid, N.S., Bourland, S.L. & Adams, G. (1998). Parent relationships and compliance in cystic fibrosis, *J. Pediatr Health Care* Vol. 12(4):196-202.

Foster, C., Eiser, C., Oades, P., Sheldon, C., Tripp, J., Goldman, P., Rice, S. & Trott, J. (2001). Treatment demands and differential treatment of patients with cystic fibrosis and their siblings: patient, parent and sibling accounts, *Child Care Health Dev.* Vol. 27(4): 349-364.

Gudas, L.J., Koocher, G.P. & Wypij, D. (1991) Perceptions of medical compliance in children and adolescent with cystic fibrosis, *J. Dev. Behav Pediatr.* Vol 12(4): 236-242.

Hamutcy, R., Rowland, J.M., Horn, M.V., Kaminsky, C., McLaughlin, E.F., Starnes, V.A. & Woo, M.S. (2002) Clinical Finding and Lung Pathology in children with Cystic Fibrosis, *Am. J. Respir. Crit. Care Med.* Vol. 165: 1172-1175.

Ievers, C.E, Brown, R.T, Drotar, D., Caplan, D., Pishevar, B.S and Lambert, RG. (1999). Knowledge of physician prescriptions and adherence to treatment among children with cystic fibrosis and their mothers. *J Dev Behav Pediatr.* Vol.20(5):335-343.

Jaffe, A. & Bush, A. (2001). Cystic fibrosis: review of the decade, *Monaldi Arch. Chest. Dis.* Vol. 56(3): 240-247.

Kettler, L.J., Sawyer, S.M., Winefield, H.R. & Greville H.W. (2002). Determinants of adherence in adults with cystic fibrosis, *Thorax* Vol. 57: 459-464.

Lask, B. (1994). Non-adherence to treatment in cystic fibrosis, *J. R. Soc. Med.* Vol. 87 (supl 21): 25-27.

Marciel, K.K.,Saiman, L.,Quittell, L.M., Dawkins, K. & Quittner, A.L. (2010). Cell phone intervention to improve adherence: cystic fibrosis care team, patient, and parent perspectives, *Pediatr. Pulmonol.* Vol 45(2):157-164.

McLaughlin, S.E., Diener-West M., Indurkhya, A., Rubin, H., Heckman R. & Boyle M.P. (2008). Improving transition from paediatric to adult cystic fibrosis care: lessons from a national survey of current practices, *Pediatrics* Vol.121(5):1160-1166.

McNamara, P.S., McCormmack, P., McDonald, A.J., Heaf, L. & southern, K.W. (2009). Open adherence monitoring using routine data download from an adaptive aerosol delivery nebuliser in children with cystic fibrosis, *J. Cyst. Fibrosis* Vol. 8(4): 258-263.

Michaud, P.A., Frappier, J.Y. & Pless, I.B. (1991). Compliance in adolescents with chronic disease, *Arch. Fr. Pediatr.* Vol 48(5): 329-336.

Modi, A.C., Lim, C.S., Yu, N., Geller, D., Wagner, M.H. & Quittner, A. (2006). A multi-method assessment of treatment adherence for children with cystic fibrosis, *J. Cyst. Fibros.* Vol. 5(3): 177-185.

Moise, J.R, Drotar, D., Doershuk, C.F. & Stern RC. (1987). Correlates of psychosocial adjustment among young adults with cystic fibrosis, *J. Dev. Behav. Pediatr.* Vol.;8(3):141-148.

Oerman, C.M., Swank, P.R. & Sockrider, M.M. (2000). Validation of an instrument measuring patient satisfaction with chest physiotherapy techniques in cystic fibrosis, *Chest* Vol. 118(1): 92-97.

Passero, M.A., Remor, B. & Salomon, J. (1981). Patient-reported compliance with cystic fibrosis therapy, *Clin. Pediatr.* Vol. 20: 264-268.

Paterson, J.M., Budd, J., Goetz, D. & Warwick, W.J. (1993). Family correlates of a ten year pulmonary health trend in cystic fibrosis, *Pediatrics* Vol. 91: 383-389

Rand, C.S., Wise, R.A., Nides, M., et al. (1992). Metered-dose inhaler adherence in a clinical trial, *Am. Rev. Respir. Dis.* Vol. 146: 1559-1564.

Scal, P. & Ireland, M. (2005).Addressing transition to adult health care for adolescents with special health care needs, *Pediatrics* Vol. 115 (6):1607–1612.

Shemesh, E., Shneider, B.L., Savitzky, J.K., Arnott, L. et al. (2004). Medication adherence in paediatric and adolescent liver transplant recipients, *Pediatrics* Vol. 113(4): 825-832

Smith, B.A., Modi, A.C, Quittner, A.L. & Wood, B.L. (2010). Depressive symptoms in children with cystic fibrosis and parents and its effects on adherence to airway clearance, *Pedriatr Pulmonol.* Vol. 45(8): 756-763.

Teichman, B.J., Burker, E.J., Weiner, M. & Egan, T.M. (2000). Factors associated with adherence to treatment regimens after lung transplantation, *Prog. Transplant.* Vol. 10(2): 113-121.

Zindani, G.N., Streetman, D.D., Streetman, D.S. & Nasr, S.Z. (2006). Adherence to treatment in children and adolescent patients with cystic fibrosis, *J. Adolesc. Health* Vol. 38(1): 13-17.

21

Improving the Likelihood of Success in Trials and the Efficiency of Delivery of Mucolytics and Antibiotics

Carlos F. Lange
Dept. of Mechanical Engineering, University of Alberta
Canada

1. Introduction

The use of models estimating the dosage delivered to a lung region to help design delivery systems for new drugs is well established (e.g. Finlay et al. (1997)). This approach, also called *in silico* testing, however has not yet received regulatory acceptance (Forbes et al. (2011)). A far less common application of lung deposition models is in the estimation of the concentration of the inhaled drug in the liquid layer that coats the human airways, also know as the airway surface liquid (ASL).

One case when the lung concentration of the inhaled drug is more relevant than the total deposited dosage is in the treatment of the effects of cystic fibrosis. To enhance the mucociliary clearance and to promote normal lung function in cystic fibrosis patients, mucolytic agents have been developed for aerosol delivery to the lung. These drug compounds are considered topically active, since their efficacy depends on reaching a proper concentration level, as determined by *in vitro* and *ex vivo* experiments. When designing clinical trials and treatment protocols, the total dosage delivered by inhalation needs to ensure that such concentration levels are reached in the mucus layer in each lung generation.

With the continuing emergence of multiply antibiotic-resistant organisms, the need to develop new, more powerful antibiotics remains evident. For determining an effective dose of a new antibiotic, it is common practise to use a series of clinical trials with different doses of the new drug starting from a small amount and moving to higher amounts gradually. However, resource limitations sometimes constrain the initial trial to a single dose, imposing the condition that this single attempt be effective before additional funds are made available. A requirement for efficacy of antibiotics is that the *in vivo* drug concentration be sustained at a level that ensures minimum inhibitory concentration (MIC), since otherwise resistance may be promoted.

Antibiotics and mucolytics are drugs that exhibit concentration dependence in their efficacy. Therefore, ensuring appropriate concentration of these drugs in the relevant body fluid is important for obtaining the desired therapeutic and physiological result. Until recently there had been no suitable method available to predict the amount of inhaled drug required to ensure efficacious concentration levels in the airway surface liquid (ASL).

Now, the combination of a lung deposition model with a novel model of the ASL layer allow for an estimate of the local average drug concentration in each lung generation k after inhalation

$$C_{k,\mathrm{ASL}} = \frac{m_{k,\mathrm{drug}}}{(V_{k,\mathrm{ASL}} + V_{k,\mathrm{aerosol}})} \tag{1}$$

The main focus of this chapter is to present a recently developed model that estimates local concentration of inhaled pharmaceutical aerosols in the ASL and to explain, with examples, how such a model can assist in the development of new inhaled drugs that are topically active, i.e. that depend on reaching proper concentration levels locally in the lung. Examples of recent use of this model are Desai et al. (2003); Sweeney et al. (2005); Wang et al. (2003).

2. Modelling drug deposition in the lung

To estimate the local concentration of a drug in the lung, it is necessary to estimate first the amount of drug deposited in each lung generation.

The modelling of deposition of inhaled aerosols over the years has evolved from simple and limited algebraic models (James et al. (1991)) to more complex and accurate empirical (Martonen et al. (1994)), one-way coupled (Ferron et al. (1988)), and two-way coupled hygroscopic models (Finlay & Stapleton (1995)), based on the Lagrangian approach. All these models treat the lung as unidimensional, calculating deposition on a typical or average aerosol path. While Lagrangian models can well represent the inhalation and deposition from continuous nebulizers, single breath inhalers and smart nebulizers derive their enhanced performance from time dependent effects that can only be accurately captured by Eulerian models. Eulerian deposition models have been available for many years (Egan & Nixon (1985); Roth et al. (2003); Taulbee & Yu (1975)) and recently have also incorporated one-way coupled hygroscopicity (Mitsakou et al. (2005)). However, they have not found widespread use, probably because of the relative complexity of their implementation.

The application of Computational Fluid Dynamics (CFD) to model aerosol deposition in a three-dimensional representation of the airways is relatively recent. Initially, the simulations were constrained to specific stretches of the airway path, such as the trachea and a few generations of the lung, or the alveolar region (Dailey & Ghadiali (2007)). These simulations offer some insight into the local effects of geometry on the flow, such as the tracheal rings, the shape of the carinal ridge or the size change of the alveoli. However, these analyzes are limited by the lack of upstream information about the flow.

Of all components required to predict lung deposition, arguably the most important and most challenging is the correct prediction of extrathoracic losses. These losses, compounded by inhalability losses in the case of infants and small children using masks, define the dosage actually delivered to the lung, assuming the device output is known. As DeHaan & Finlay (2001; 2004) demonstrated with dry powder inhalers, extrathoracic deposition can depart quite significantly from the baseline case of particles inhaled from a smooth, wide, straight tube with approximately constant inhalation rate studied by Stahlhofen et al. (1983). While we now understand much better the flow and deposition mechanisms occurring in the oropharyngeal region following the analysis of Heenan et al. (2004), the large scatter of data caused by intersubject variabilities even during controlled inhalation conditions (Stahlhofen et al. (1983)) would preclude any accurate prediction of extrathoracic losses. Fortunately, a comprehensive study of the effects of intersubject variability by Grgic et al.

(2004) led to the discovery of a universal form of the Stokes parameter allowing for a more accurate prediction of the oropharyngeal deposition in a wide variety of realistic mouth-throat geometries. This mathematical relationship can potentially be used to predict lung dosages from inhalers, instead of the currently used delivered dose.

One-dimensional, dynamical lung deposition models, though heavily simplified with respect to the airway geometry, can incorporate all the fundamental physical processes that affect particle size and deposition at a small fraction of the computational effort of CFD. Naturally, these 1-D models cannot resolve local deposition patterns, such as required by a tumour, but they can be properly tuned to give accurate results for delivery of drugs that target an entire lung region. The treatment of lung diseases associated with cystic fibrosis, such as bacterial infections and mucolytic treatments, are examples of cases that target a single lung region, namely the tracheobronchial region. Advanced one-dimensional models can provide this regional deposition information with high accuracy, as demonstrated by Finlay, Lange, Li & Hoskinson (2000). For these reasons, 1-D models seem better suited for the use in the modelling of local concentration of deposited drugs in the lung.

3. Modelling mucus and the Airway Surface Liquid layer

The model of the Airway Surface Liquid (ASL) layer, developed at the University of Alberta by the author in collaboration with W. Finlay and M. King (Finlay, Lange, King & Speert (2000); Hasan & Lange (2007); Lange et al. (2001)) is the first and, to this date, the only model of its kind. The model approximates the amount of liquid matter present in each lung generation, which, in conjunction with the local dosage provided by the deposition model, allows for the estimate of the local concentration of the inhaled drug.

A previous attempt to estimate concentration of deposited aerosols was performed by Böhm et al. (2003). They used an empirical estimate of lung deposition and a simple assumption of a constant thickness of the ASL layer in a single generation. An approach closer to the one proposed here was employed by Kimmel et al. (2001) to study transient clearance and mucus concentration in rats. But the mucus layer thickness was considered constant throughout the tracheobronchial region.

The ASL model distinguishes two layers with essentially different physical properties: the periciliary liquid layer (PCL), a watery layer (sol) covering the airway epithelium, and the mucus layer, a viscoelastic gel that floats on top of the PCL (see Fig. 1).

The volume of liquid in each layer is modelled separately. The sum of the two gives the total ASL volume in each generation, $V_{k,\mathrm{ASL}}$. For the calculation of the volume we assume a continuous annular layer of liquid along each generation. Figure 2 shows a schematic cross-sectional view of an airway.

The dimensions of the airways are obtained from the lung geometry model by Finlay (2001), which has been shown to correlate well with *in vivo* regional deposition experiments (Finlay, Hoskinson & Stapleton (1998)). The geometry assumes a symmetric branching airway system, starting from the extrathoracic region (mouth cavity, pharynx and larynx), followed by the trachea, and branching symmetrically into two main bronchi, then into four lobar bronchi, and so on. Each new branch segment is called a generation, k. The trachea is considered the first generation ($k = 0$), and the main bronchi are $k = 1$, so that the number of airways in each generation is always 2^k.

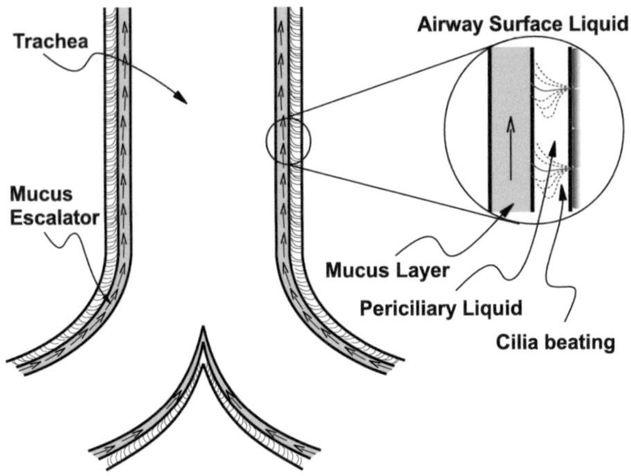

Fig. 1. Schematic of the airways with ASL layer and mucociliary escalator.

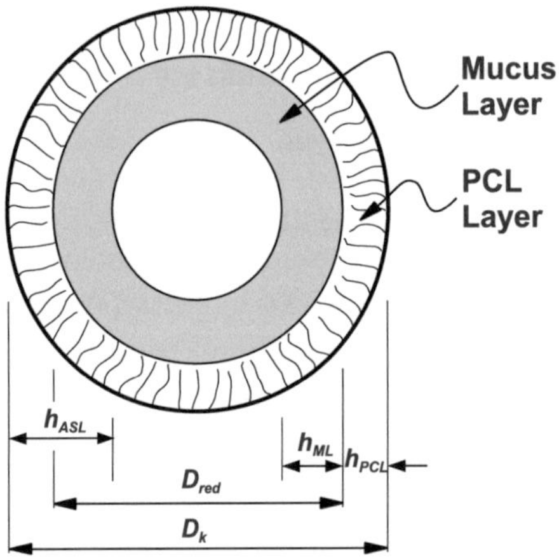

Fig. 2. Airway cross-section with PCL and mucus layers.

In contrast with the classical lung model, Weibel A (Weibel (1963)), which considers generations 0–16 to form the tracheobronchial region, Finlay's model sets the transition between the tracheobronchial region and the more distal alveolar region at the generation 14. This distinction is relevant, because mucociliary transport exists only in the conductive airways, starting at the terminal bronchioles, which are the most distal ciliated airways. While the calculation of the deposited dosage, described above, utilizes the complete lung geometry, the ASL layer is only defined in the tracheobronchial region. The dimensions of the airways in each tracheobronchial generation are reproduced from Finlay (2001) in Table 1.

The ASL model uses the same average airway diameter and length in generation k as the deposition model, D_k and L_k. With these geometric characteristics, the volume of ASL in generation k can be calculated as

$$V_{k,\mathrm{ASL}} = \pi\, L_k\, 2^k\, \left(D_k\, h_{k,\mathrm{ASL}} - h_{k,\mathrm{ASL}}^2\right) \tag{2}$$

where the thickness of the ASL layer, $h_{k,\mathrm{ASL}}$, needs to be determined and is defined as

$$h_{k,\mathrm{ASL}} = h_{k,\mathrm{PCL}} + h_{k,\mathrm{ML}} \tag{3}$$

Generation	Length [cm]	Diameter [cm]
0	12.456	1.810
1	3.614	1.414
2	2.862	1.115
3	2.281	.885
4	1.780	.706
5	1.126	.565
6	.897	.454
7	.828	.364
8	.745	.286
9	.653	.218
10	.555	.162
11	.454	.121
12	.357	.092
13	.277	.073
14	.219	.061

Table 1. Airway dimensions in the tracheobronchial tree (from Finlay (2001)).

i.e., it is the sum of $h_{k,\text{PCL}}$ and $h_{k,\text{ML}}$, the thicknesses of the PCL and mucus layers, respectively.

In certain cases, such as in the inhalation of mucolytics, it is the volume of mucus only that is required. In this case, the same assumptions as above give

$$V_{k,\text{ML}} = \pi\, L_k\, 2^k \left(D_{k,\text{red}}\, h_{k,\text{ML}} - h_{k,\text{ML}}^2 \right) \tag{4}$$

where $D_{k,\text{red}}$ is the airway diameter reduced by the PCL layer thickness

$$D_{k,\text{red}} = D_k - 2\, h_{k,\text{PCL}} \tag{5}$$

Since the airway geometry follows the deposition model and is known, all that is required to estimate the volumes of mucus and ASL are the layer thicknesses. In the following sections the calculation of the PCL and mucus layer thicknesses is described.

3.1 Thickness of PCL layer

The PCL layer is formed by a watery liquid that facilitates the beating of the cilia and keeps the thicker mucus layer afloat at an exact distance to be reached by the tip of the cilia during their forward beating (Widdicombe (1997)). Although the regulation mechanism of the PCL layer thickness in the airways is still the subject of controversy (Matsui et al. (1998)), it is recognized that this regulated thickness is well approximated by the length of the cilia.

Measurements of cilia lengths in humans were performed by Serafini & Michaelson (1977) and are given in Table 2.

Two curve fits were tested to approximate the Serafini and Michaelson measurements with a smooth curve along the entire tracheobronchial region. The fitted functions that estimate the cilia length at generation k, and by extension the thickness of the PCL layer, are

$$h_{k,\text{PCL}} = 5.911\, \mathrm{e}^{-k/13.4048} \qquad \text{(fit1)} \tag{6}$$

Generation	Length [μm]
0	6.03
3	4.70
5	3.87
6	3.72
7	3.60

Table 2. Human ciliary length in various lung generations from measurements.

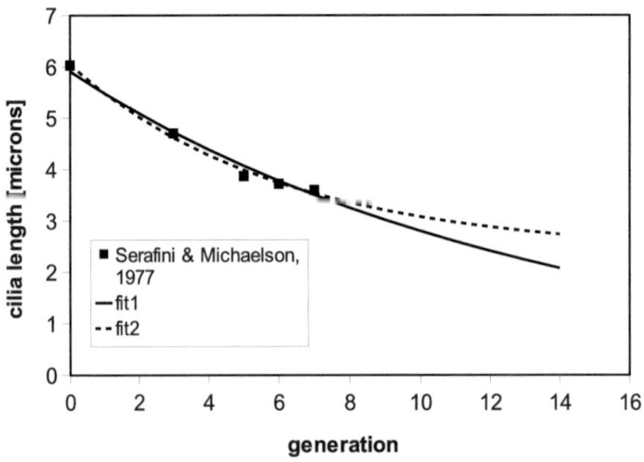

Fig. 3. Experimental and curve fitted values of cilia length in humans.

Generation	$h_{k,\mathrm{PCL}}$ [μm]
0	6.04
1	5.49
2	5.02
3	4.61
4	4.27
5	3.99
6	3.74
7	3.53
8	3.36
9	3.21
10	3.08
11	2.97
12	2.88
13	2.81
14	2.74

Table 3. Human ciliary length and PCL thickness in various lung generations.

$$h_{k,\mathrm{PCL}} = 2.3717 + 3.6724\,\mathrm{e}^{-k/6.0837} \qquad \text{(fit2)} \tag{7}$$

A plot of the raw data and of both curves can be seen in Fig. 3.

Curve fit "fit2" was selected as best fit and the corresponding values of thickness of the PCL layer, based on eq. 7 above, are shown in Table 3.

3.2 Mucus layer thickness

The mucus layer is essentially a gel formed by secretions from goblet cells located in the airway epithelium and also from submucosal glands in the larger airways (Widdicombe (1997)). The thickness of the mucus layer is estimated assuming a continuous layer of constant thickness in each generation, using mass conservation, and modelling the average mucus velocity and production rate for each generation.

The mucus layer is constantly driven by the coordinated beating of airway cilia from the distal generations to the trachea forming the so-called mucus escalator, as illustrated in Fig. 1. The 14th generation is assumed to be the most distal tracheobronchial generation, as described above, where mucus production starts. In reality, as there is no sharp transition from the alveolar region to the tracheobronchial region, the mucus production also does not start always at the 14th generation. In addition, in the more distal generations the mucus layer is not yet fully continuous, but there are probably patches of mucus until the cumulative production ensures full coverage of the airways. For lack of a better alternative, the present model assumes that mucus production starts at generation 14 and forms a continuous annular layer from the onset.

Mucus is actually continuously produced along the conductive airways. The amount produced at a generation k joins the cumulative amount produced at all previous (more distal) generations up to that generation, as the mucus is transported towards the trachea. The amount of mucus that flows through generation k is the accumulated amount produced up to this point, i.e. the sum of all mucus produced by generations $k+1$ to 14, plus the locally produced amount ($\dot{p}_k$). This local total production is called $\dot{P}_k$.

The flow rate of mucus through all airways of a generation is equal to the product of the annular cross-sectional area of the mucus layer, $A_{k,\mathrm{ML}}$, and the mucociliary transport velocity at this generation (clearance velocity), U_k, i.e.

$$\dot{P}_k = A_{k,\mathrm{ML}}\, U_k = 2^k\, \pi\, \left(D_{k,\mathrm{red}}\, h_{k,\mathrm{ML}} - h_{k,\mathrm{ML}}^2\right)\, U_k \tag{8}$$

where $D_{k,\mathrm{red}}$ is defined in eq. 5, and the cumulative production rate $\dot{P}_k$ at generation k is defined by the recursive formula

$$\dot{P}_k = \dot{p}_k + \dot{P}_{k+1} \tag{9}$$

where $\dot{p}_k$ is the local production rate at generation k. The estimates of $\dot{p}_k$ are described below in section 3.3.

Equation 8 is a quadratic polynomial in terms of $h_{k,\mathrm{ML}}$

$$2^k\, \pi\, U_k\, h_{k,\mathrm{ML}}^2 - 2^k\, \pi\, U_k\, D_{k,\mathrm{red}}\, h_{k,\mathrm{ML}} + \dot{P}_k = 0 \tag{10}$$

whose only physical solution is

$$h_{k,\mathrm{ML}} = \frac{2^k\, \pi\, U_k\, D_{k,\mathrm{red}} - \sqrt{(2^k\, \pi\, U_k\, D_{k,\mathrm{red}})^2 - 4\,(2^k)\, \pi\, U_k\, \dot{P}_k}}{2\,(2^k)\, \pi\, U_k} \tag{11}$$

Rearranging the terms and defining the reduced airway radius corresponding to $R_{k,\mathrm{red}} = D_{k,\mathrm{red}}/2$, eq. 11 can be rewritten

$$h_{k,\mathrm{ML}} = R_{k,\mathrm{red}} - \sqrt{R_{k,\mathrm{red}}^2 - \frac{\dot{P}_k}{2^k \, \pi \, U_k}} \tag{12}$$

Hence, the average thickness of the mucus layer in a generation can be determined, if the cumulative production up to that generation ($\dot{P}_k$) and the local clearance velocity (U_k) are known. Their determination in this model is described in the following sections.

Equation 12 provides also a condition to test for airway clogging. If the result from the two terms inside the square root is negative, this means that the clearance velocity is too slow to transport the required mucus flow rate through the whole airway cross-section, which would cause the airways to clog. Although airway clogging actually occurs in severe disease states, the present model is not designed to deal with clogging and parameter sets resulting in clogging should be disregarded.

3.3 Distributed mucus production

For the distribution of the mucus production along the conducting airways there are no human data currently available. As an approximation for the distribution of mucus secretion in humans, the airway surface density of total secretory material measured by Plopper et al. (1989) in various lung generations of the rhesus monkey was adopted. The rhesus monkey is considered in many aspects one of the animals closest to humans, and their similarity in terms of airway surface morphology is well established (Jeffery (1983)).

The volume of total secretory product in the surface epithelium and in submucosal glands per unit airway area measured by Plopper et al. (1989) in specific generations of the monkey's lung was as shown in Table 4.

Generation	Total
0	3.671
3	4.179
6	3.086
11	2.169
13	1.039
15	0.656

Table 4. Distribution of total mucus secretory product in rhesus monkey [$\times 10^{-3}$ mm^3/mm^2] (from Plopper et al. (1989)).

By assuming that the total secretory product per unit airway area is proportional to the amount actually produced per unit area, and by assuming these values scale to humans simply with the airway surface area, i.e. the same rates per unit area apply, these distributed rates were transferred and directly applied to the human lung model. To obtain intermediate values for the missing generations, two straight lines were fit to the data. The first curve fit was a simple interpolation between the first two points. For the second curve fit the value at generation 15 was disregarded. Not only is generation 15 beyond the assumed end of the tracheobronchial region, but also its inclusion would cause the resulting curve fit to end too abruptly at generation 14. With the actual, adjusted values shown in Table 5 the resulting curve tends to zero at generation 16, which agrees better with the adopted lung model (see Fig. 4).

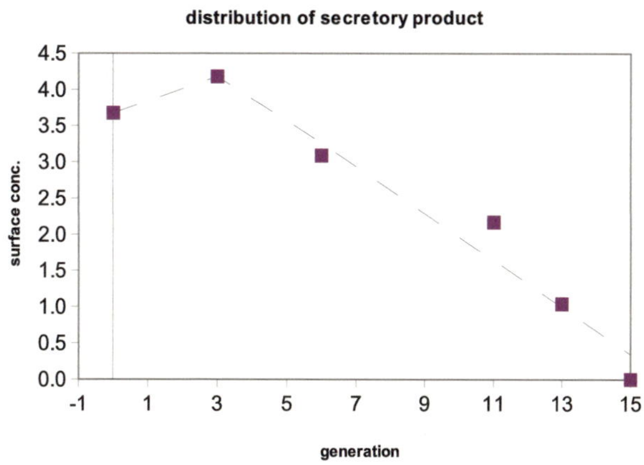

Fig. 4. Distributed mucus production (volumetric surface production [$\times 10^{-3}$ mm^3/mm^2]) and curve fits (eqs. 13 and 14).

Generation	Adjusted Surf. Production
0	3.671
3	4.179
6	3.086
11	2.169
13	1.039
15	0.000

Table 5. Distribution of volumetric mucus production in humans [$\times 10^{-3}$ mm^3/mm^2].

The fitted curves shown in Fig. 4 and used to calculate the distributed local mucus production per unit area $\dot{p}_k''$ correspond to the following functions

$$\text{For generations } 0-3: \qquad \dot{p}_k'' = 0.1693\,k + 3.671 \tag{13}$$

$$\text{For generations } 3-14: \qquad \dot{p}_k'' = -0.3238\,k + 5.203 \tag{14}$$

where k is the generation and the result is in $\times 10^{-3}$ mm^3/mm^2. Table 6 shows the corresponding values in each generation.

The distributed local mucus production per unit area $\dot{p}_k''$ is combined with the dimensions of the adopted lung geometry model to result in reference values of average mucus production rates in each generation, according to the following equation

$$\dot{p}_{k,\text{ref}} = \dot{p}_k'' \left(2^k\,\pi\,L_k\,D_k\right) \tag{15}$$

Equation 15 combined with eq. 9 result in a reference profile of distributed mucus production in the airways, $\dot{P}_{k,\text{ref}}$. Since the production rate of mucus varies from person to person and can also vary with time for the same individual, this reference profile of mucus production is used to scale the actual production profile according to the value of actual total daily production of the subject, $\dot{P}_{\text{tot}}$. A reasonable daily production amount for a healthy, non-smoking adult is 10 ml/day. Typically, a range of values is used in the calculations with 5 ml/day being a reasonable minimum for an adult, and 30 ml/day or greater being considered hypersecretion,

Generation	Surface Production
0	3.67
1	3.84
2	4.01
3	4.18
4	3.91
5	3.58
6	3.26
7	2.94
8	2.61
9	2.29
10	1.97
11	1.64
12	1.32
13	0.99
14	0.67

Table 6. Distribution of volumetric mucus production $\dot{p}_k''$ in humans [$\times 10^{-3}$ mm^3/mm^2].

requiring therapy (Hardy & Anderson (1996)). In fact, patients with severe bronchorrhea have been reported to produce in average more than 60 ml/day (Tamaoki et al. (1994)).

The actual cumulative production values are obtained by modifying the reference values with a scaling factor, namely the ratio between the prescribed total daily production and the cumulative reference production at the trachea (gen. 0)

$$\dot{P}_k = \left(\frac{\dot{P}_{\text{tot}}}{\dot{P}_{0,\text{ref}}} \right) \dot{P}_{k,\text{ref}} \tag{16}$$

Equation 16 provides the actual cumulative production required in eq. 12.

3.4 Mucus clearance velocity

The airway mucus is a highly viscoelastic fluid that is transported by the lung clearance mechanism (cilia beating) from the terminal bronchioli to the trachea. Due to its viscoelasticity, the mucus forms a continuous layer that flows with almost no mixing. Inhaled particles trapped in this layer are transported smoothly and continuously towards the trachea, where they are swallowed. This mucociliary clearance process can be treated as a series of "escalators" that transport mucus and whatever it is carrying from one generation to the next with constant velocity within each generation.

If a tracer substance is inhaled and its clearance measured, the time to clear the trachea (the first generation to be cleared) would be $\tau_0 = L_0/U_0$, where U_0 is the constant mucus transport velocity at the trachea. The amount of tracer deposited in the main bronchi, the next generation to be cleared, would require the time to travel through the bronchi, $\tau_1 = L_1/U_1$, plus the time to travel through the trachea τ_0 to be cleared. This process is illustrated in Fig. 5. In general, measuring from the time when the first particles deposited in generation k begin

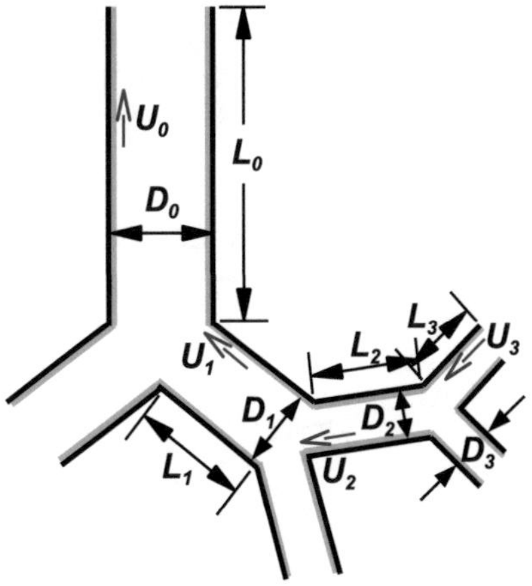

Fig. 5. Schematic of the mucociliary escalator.

to be cleared until the time when the last particles from that generation are cleared results in

$$\sum_{i=0}^{k} \tau_i - \sum_{j=0}^{k-1} \tau_j = \sum_{i=0}^{k} \frac{L_i}{U_i} - \sum_{j=0}^{k-1} \frac{L_j}{U_j} = \frac{L_k}{U_k} = \tau_k \tag{17}$$

By combining cumulative deposition data from the lung deposition model and the *in vivo* clearance data from Stahlhofen et al. (1980) the time τ_k required to clear each generation was determined. Fig. 6 illustrates this process.

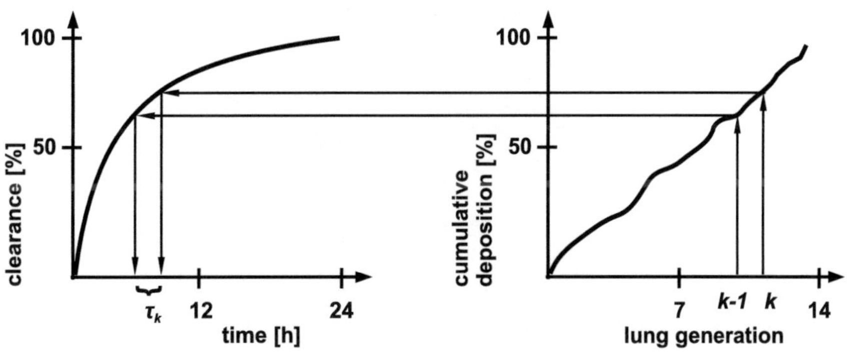

Fig. 6. Time to clear generation k obtained from comparison between cumulative deposition and clearance data.

Four cases measured by Stahlhofen et al. (1980) (breathing pattern A (op. cit., Fig. 8): subject 1 and d_a=9.5 μm, subject 4 and d_a=9.1 μm; breathing pattern B (op. cit., Fig. 9): subject 1 and d_a=7.5 μm, subject 4 and d_a=7.3 μm) were calculated with the 1-D deposition model from Finlay & Stapleton (1995), using the lung geometry dimensions from Finlay (2001). Note that the length of the trachea was shortened by 3 cm, because of the way the tracheobronchial region was imaged in Stahlhofen et al. (1980). The resulting velocity profiles were scaled with a reference clearance velocity at the trachea ($U_{0,\text{ref}} = 5.5$ mm/min) and averaged so that a standard reference clearance velocity profile was generated. This reference profile of mucus transport velocities in each generation ($U_{k,\text{ref}}$) is shown in Table 7. Figure 7 shows a comparison of the present reference velocity profile with other similar profiles estimated by Lee et al. (1979), Yu et al. (1986) and Cuddihy & Yeh (1988). All profiles were scaled to a tracheal clearance velocity of 5.5 mm/min.

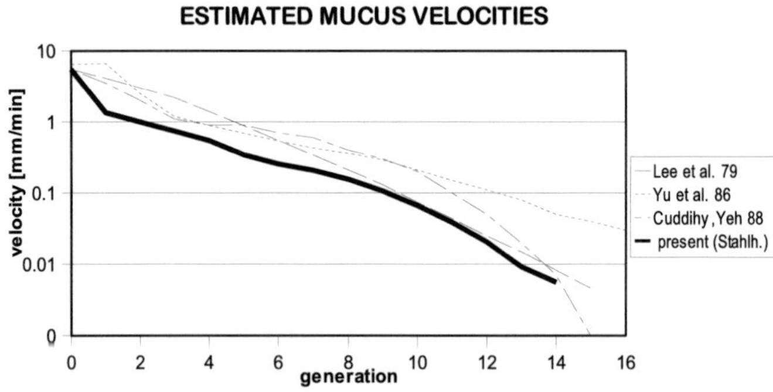

Fig. 7. Comparison of clearance velocity profiles (all profiles scaled to U_0=5.5 mm/min).

Generation	Clearance Velocity
0	5.5000
1	1.3415
2	0.9943
3	0.7439
4	0.5477
5	0.3425
6	0.2551
7	0.2073
8	0.1554
9	0.1063
10	0.0667
11	0.0389
12	0.0206
13	0.0092
14	0.0056

Table 7. Clearance velocity profile ($U_{k,\text{ref}}$ in [mm/min], constant in each generation).

Similarly to the variability in the daily mucus production rate, the clearance velocity also shows variation between individuals and for a single individual, depending on their physical activity, for instance. The linear velocity of mucus flow in the trachea in young nonsmokers has been measured by marker particle clearance as typically 10–15 mm/min (Wanner et al. (1996)). CF patients have been assessed with tracheal clearance velocities that range from essentially zero up to these normal values Yeates et al. (1975).

Here again the actual clearance velocities used in the model are obtained by scaling the entire profile with the ratio between the prescribed tracheal velocity $U_{0,\text{set}}$ and the reference value $U_{0,\text{ref}}$ as follows

$$U_k = \left(\frac{U_{0,\text{set}}}{U_{0,\text{ref}}}\right) U_{k,\text{ref}} \tag{18}$$

Equation 18 provides the actual clearance velocities required in eq. 12.

Using the clearance velocity profiles shown in Fig. 7 and a distributed mucus production based on eqs. 13 and 14, scaled to a total of 10 ml/day, a comparison of estimated mucus layer thicknesses can be calculated. The results are shown in Fig. 8.

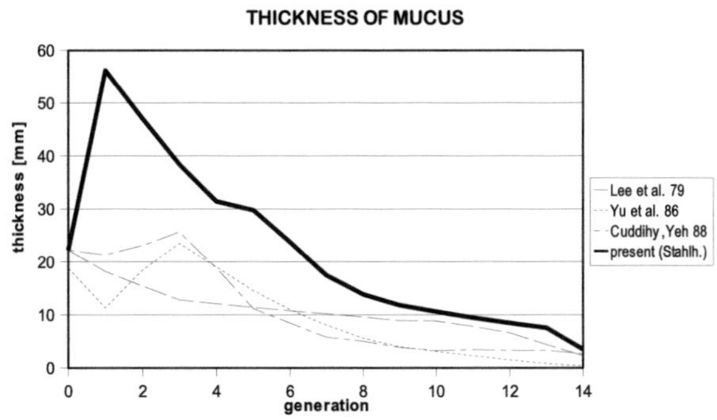

Fig. 8. Comparison of mucus layer thicknesses based on clearance velocities from Fig. 7 and 10 ml/day distributed production.

Combining the thicknesses of the mucus and the PCL layers, the total volume of ASL in each generation can be finally calculated using eq. 2.

4. Modelling local lung concentration of topically active drugs

Once the mass of drug deposited in each generation is obtained with the aerosol deposition model, and the volume of ASL in each generation is obtained with the ASL model, local concentration values can be estimated.

Pharmaceutical aerosols are often an aqueous solution or suspension and the water they carry contributes to the dilution of the drug in the ASL. In addition to knowing the mass of drug deposited in each generation, $m_{k,\text{drug}}$, it is important to also keep track of the mass of water deposited together with the drug, $m_{k,\text{water}}$. If the aerosol is hygroscopic, evaporation may take place in the first few generations and condensation may occur deeper in the more distal airways. The deposition model should account for these changes. We can convert the deposited mass of drug and water to the corresponding volume of deposited aerosol, using

$$V_{k,\text{aerosol}} = \frac{m_{k,\text{drug}}}{\rho_{\text{eff}}} + \frac{m_{k,\text{water}}}{\rho_{\text{water}}} \tag{19}$$

where ρ_{eff} and ρ_{water} are the effective density of the drug formulation and of water, respectively.

All the required information is now available to estimate the average concentration of the drug in the mucus layer, $C_{k,\text{ML}}$, or in the total ASL layer, $C_{k,\text{ASL}}$, in each generation

$$C_{k,\text{ML}} = \frac{m_{k,\text{drug}}}{(V_{k,\text{ML}} + V_{k,\text{aerosol}})} \tag{20}$$

$$C_{k,\text{ASL}} = \frac{m_{k,\text{drug}}}{(V_{k,\text{ASL}} + V_{k,\text{aerosol}})} \tag{21}$$

To account for inter-subject variability and other uncertainties, ranges of physiological values should be used, resulting in minimum and maximum expected concentration values. Table 8 lists a range of physiological values that can be used.

	unit	Min.	Nominal	Max.
Tracheal Clearance Velocity	mm/min	5	10 to 15	20
Daily Mucus Production	ml/day	5	10	60

Table 8. Range of physiological values of input quantities to the model.

The result of the model is a series of concentration curves for each scenario. These local concentrations are then compared with efficacy levels and toxicity levels of the drug, to verify if they are within those limits. The type of delivery device and the prescribed dosage can be adjusted to optimize the predicted concentration levels, thus increasing the likelihood of a successful outcome.

5. Advances in delivery devices

Recent advances of drug delivery devices have increased substantially their efficiency and their ability to adjust the dose delivered to the lung. From the low cost vented jet nebulizers to the more sophisticated breath-actuated, also known as smart nebulizers, the current generation of inhalers allows for the efficient delivery of large doses with an increasing ability to control the amount delivered. Both aspects are important when delivering antibiotics to the lung. Efficient delivery of a large dose may be required to ensure MIC levels are reached. At the same time, control over the dosage is required to ensure that toxicity levels of the antibiotic are not exceeded.

Despite the development of competing types of devices for drug delivery to the lung, from metered dose inhalers to dry powder inhalers, jet nebulizers have never been completely replaced. They are still capable of delivering the largest dosages to the lung. The ability to contain high volume fills makes them uniquely adapted for this purpose. Many types of continuous output nebulizers are on the market today. Among them, valved vented (also called breath enhanced) jet nebulizers reduce the amount of drug lost during exhalation by delivering aerosol preferentially during inhalation. Less affordable, but more compact, ultrasonic nebulizers find widespread use in many clinical settings. Finlay, Stapleton & Zuberbuhler (1998) compared various traditional nebulizers and found a large variation in the predicted lung dosage between the devices.

Nebulizers have experienced a revival through the introduction of so-called "smart nebulizers" (Smaldone (2002)). This is a relatively informal classification that includes all the liquid atomizers, which either use or control the breathing pattern for targeted drug delivery. The technologies used for liquid atomization may vary, but these smart nebulizers have in common the attempt to link aerosol generation with the patient inhalation. Examples of smart nebulizers based on jet nebulization are the breath actuated AeroEclipse® (MMC), the Prodose AAD® System (Profile/Respironics), and the AKITA® system (InAMed). Other smart nebulizers or liquid atomizers use different nebulization technologies. Aerodose® (Aerogen) and eFlow® (Pari) are examples of vibrating orifice based nebulizers, which are capable of more precise dosing. All these new devices incorporate breath actuation and some level of drug delivery control and feedback. Ideally, these monitoring capabilities of the delivered dosage and control of aerosol emission in smart nebulizers could be coupled with an embedded processing unit that estimates the actual deposited dose in the lung, allowing for individually adjusted treatment with the highest probability of successful outcome, as suggested by Lange & Finlay (2006).

This desirable ability to ensure that a prescribed dosage is effectively delivered to the lung is particularly important in the case of antibiotic treatment of lung infections in cystic fibrosis, to reduce the risk of promoting drug resistance through low concentration levels of antimicrobial in the ASL.

6. Applications of the model

The ASL concentration model described above could be in the future incorporated into the control and feedback systems of smart nebulizers, coaching individual patients to inhale the precise dosage required to reach the MIC as estimated by the model.

Currently, the ASL concentration model can be of vital assistance to the design of clinical trials to increase the chances of a positive outcome by ensuring proper concentration levels are achieved in the lung during the tests. An example of how this model can be used to improve the outcome of clinical trials was described by Hasan & Lange (2007). Two antibiotics were compared, using data from the literature. One of the two was tobramycin, an inhaled antibiotic, which is widely used by CF patients. The other example was taurolidine, which was considered for use against *B. cepacia* in CF patients, but failed to produce results in its first clinical trial with delivery by inhalation.

Using the same input parameters described in Hasan & Lange (2007) for the case of tobramycin, corresponding to the study of Ramsey et al. (1999), the estimates of ASL concentration of the antibiotic were recalculated with increased accuracy by taking into account hygroscopic effects in the aerosol size distribution. The new estimates, shown in Fig. 9, result in slightly increased concentrations, which confirm the prediction that concentration levels well exceeded the value of 0.08 mg/mL, or ten times higher than the *in vitro* MIC value, recommended for *in vivo* efficacy against *P. aeruginosa*. These concentration levels were predicted for all 16 scenarios within the range of input parameters studied, while Fig. 9 only shows a few representative cases, including the maximum and minimum curves of the range.

A different outcome befell a clinical trial of taurolidine, a promising drug candidate against *P. aeruginosa* and *B. cepacia* in CF. The outcome of the randomized double-blinded placebo-controlled crossover trial by Ledson et al. (2002), showed no improvement in sputum *B. cepacia* colony counts. As a consequence of this result, development of the inhaled form of this new drug was halted.

Using model input data that matched as closely as possible the study by Ledson et al. (2002), the above-described model estimated ASL concentration levels that in many cases did not exceed the *in vitro* MIC values of 0.4 mg/mL (see Fig. 10), when it is known that *in vivo* concentrations need to be much higher for successful antimicrobial effect.

The higher end of the predictions reached approximately 5 times the *in vitro* MIC, but this scenario (high mucociliary clearance velocity and low mucus production) corresponds more likely to a non-CF patient, such as the single case reported by Ledson et al. (2000). Taking this higher concentration (2 mg/mL) as a new required level, one could use the ASL concentration model to help design a hypothetical trial that would ensure such levels were reached in the

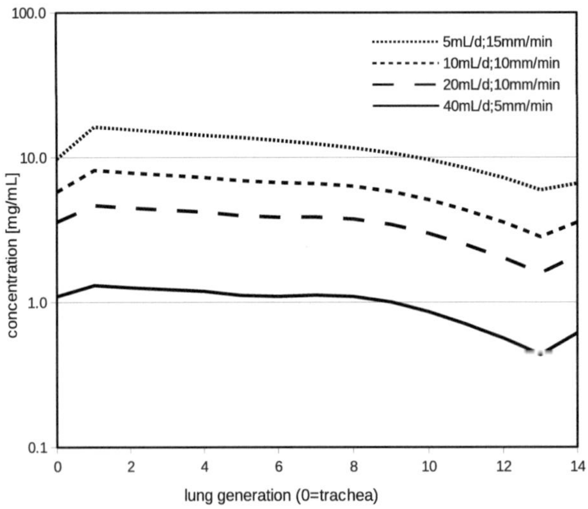

Fig. 9. Estimated ASL concentration of tobramycin in clinical trial.

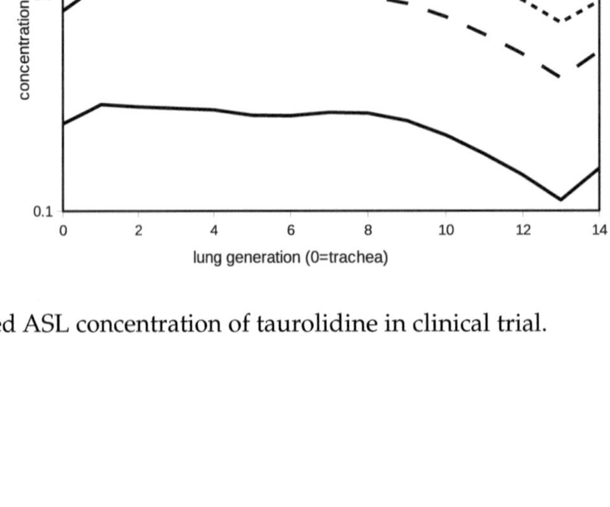

Fig. 10. Estimated ASL concentration of taurolidine in clinical trial.

majority of the cases. Figure 11 demonstrates such a scenario, which could be achieved with a slightly larger nebulizer fill and a significantly larger concentration of taurolidine in the solution.

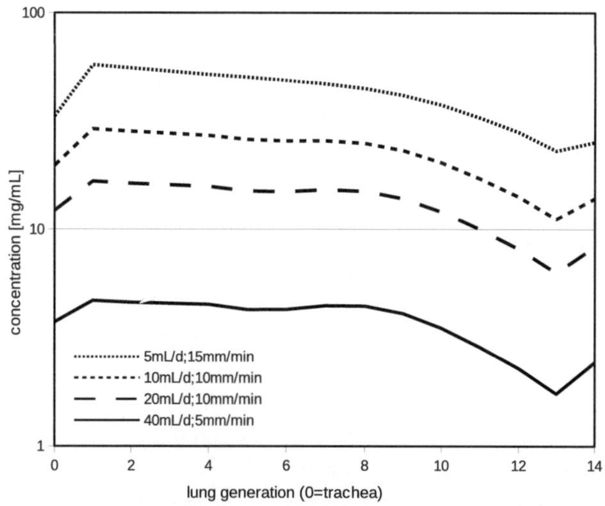

Fig. 11. Estimated ASL concentration of taurolidine in a hypothetical trial that were designed with assistance of the ASL concentration model.

Although a new trial design with higher ASL concentrations would still not be guaranteed to succeed, it would at least stand a better chance of a positive outcome that would allow the continuation of the new drug development.

We conclude that the ASL concentration model is an important tool in the design of clinical trials of inhaled drugs that require a certain concentration level in the lung mucus or the ASL for efficacy.

Similarly, in later stages of the development of a new inhaled drug, the ASL concentration model can greatly assist in the selection of the most appropriate drug delivery device and in establishing the most adequate treatment protocols.

7. Acknowledgements

The mucus and ASL models were developed by the author under the supervision of W. Finlay and in close collaboration with M. King. Their contribution is gratefully acknowledged.

8. References

Böhm, R., Nikodemova, D. & Holy, K. (2003). Use of various microdosimetric models for the prediction of radon induced damage in human lungs, *Radiat. Prot. Dosim.* 104(2): 127–137.

Cuddihy, R. G. & Yeh, H. C. (1988). *Respiratory tract clearance of particles and substances dissociated from particles*, Springer, Berlin, chapter 11, pp. 169–193.

Dailey, H. L. & Ghadiali, S. N. (2007). Fluid-structure analysis of microparticle transport in deformable pulmonary alveoli, *J. Aerosol Sci.* 38: 269–288.

DeHaan, W. H. & Finlay, W. H. (2001). *In vitro* monodisperse aerosol deposition in a mouth and throat with six different inhalation devices, *J. Aerosol Med.* 14(3): 361–367.

DeHaan, W. H. & Finlay, W. H. (2004). Prediciting estrathoracic deposition from dry powder inhalers, *J. Aerosol Sci.* 35(3): 309–331.

Desai, T. R., Tyrrell, G. J., Ng, T. & Finlay, W. H. (2003). In vitro evaluation of nebulization properties, antimicrobial activity and regional airway surface liquid concentration of liposomal polymyxin B sulfate, *Pharm. Res.* 20: 442–447.

Egan, M. J. & Nixon, W. (1985). A model of aerosol deposition in the lung for use in inhalation dose assessments, *Radiation Protection Dosimetry* 11(1): 5–17.

Ferron, G. A., Kreyling, W. G. & Haider, B. (1988). Inhalation of salt aerosol particles – II. Growth and deposition in the respiratory tract, *J. Aerosol Sci.* 19(5): 611–631.

Finlay, W. H. (2001). *The Mechanics of Inhaled Pharmaceutical Aerosols: An Introduction*, Academic Press, London.

Finlay, W. H., Hoskinson, M. & Stapleton, K. W. (1998). Can models be trusted to subdivide lung deposition into alveolar and tracheobronchial fractions?, *Respiratory Drug Delivery VI*, Interpharm Press, Buffalo Grove, IL, USA, pp. 235–242.

Finlay, W. H., Lange, C. F., King, M. & Speert, D. P. (2000). Lung delivery of aerosolized dextran, *Am. J. Respir. Crit. Care Med.* 161: 91–97.

Finlay, W. H., Lange, C. F., Li, W.-I. & Hoskinson, M. (2000). Validating deposition models in disease: what is needed?, *J. Aerosol Med.* 13: 381–385.

Finlay, W. H. & Stapleton, K. W. (1995). The effect on regional lung deposition of coupled heat and mass transfer between hygroscopic droplets and their surrounding phase, *J. Aerosol Sci.* 26(4): 655–670.

Finlay, W. H., Stapleton, K. W. & Zuberbuhler, P. (1997). Predicting regional lung dosages of a nebulized suspension: Pulmicort® (budesonide), *Part. Sci. Technol.* 15: 243–251.

Finlay, W. H., Stapleton, K. W. & Zuberbuhler, P. (1998). Variations in predicted regional lung deposition of salbutamol sulphate between 19 nebulizer models, *J. Aerosol Med.* 11: 65–80.

Forbes, B., Asgharian, B., Dailey, L. A., Ferguson, D., Gerde, P., Gumbleton, M., Gustavsson, L., Hardy, C., Hassall, D., Jones, R., Lock, R., Maas, J., McGovern, T., Pitcairn, G. R., Somers, G. & Wolff, R. K. (2011). Challenges in inhaled product development and opportunities for open innovation, *Adv. Drug Deliv. Rev.* 63: 69–87.

Grgic, B., Finlay, W. H., Burnell, P. K. P. & Heenan, A. F. (2004). *In vitro* intersubject and intrasubject deposition measurements in realistic mouth-throat geometries, *J. Aerosol Sci.* 35(1): 1025–1040.

Hardy, K. A. & Anderson, B. D. (1996). Noninvasive clearance of airway secretions, *Respir. Care Clin. N. Am.* 2: 323–345.

Hasan, M. A. & Lange, C. F. (2007). Estimating *in vivo* airway surface liquid concentration in trials of inhaled antibiotics, *J. Aerosol Med.* 20(3): 282–293.

Heenan, A. F., Finlay, W. H., Grgic, B., Pollard, A. & Burnell, P. K. P. (2004). An investigation of the relationship between the flow field and regional deposition in realistic extra-thoracic airways, *J. Aerosol Sci.* 35: 1013–1023.

James, A. C., Stahlhofen, W., Rudolf, G., Egan, M. J., Nixon, W., Gehr, P. & Briant, J. K. (1991). The respiratory tract deposition model proposed by the ICRP task group, *Radiation Protection Dosimetry* 38(1): 159–165.

Jeffery, P. K. (1983). Morphologic features of airway surface epithelial cells and glands, *Am. Rev. Respir. Dis.* 128: S14–S20.

Kimmel, E. C., Reboulet, J. E. & Carpenter, R. L. (2001). A typical path model of tracheobronchial clearance of inhaled particles in rats, *Toxicol. Ind. Health* 17: 277–284.

Lange, C. F. & Finlay, W. H. (2006). Liquid atomising: nebulizing and other methods of producing aerosols, *J. Aerosol Med.* 19(1): 28–35.

Lange, C. F., Hancock, R. E. W., Samuel, J. & Finlay, W. H. (2001). *In vitro* aerosol delivery and regional airway surface liquid concentration of a liposomal cationic peptide, *J. Pharm. Sci.* 90(10): 1647–1657.

Ledson, M. J., Cowperthwaite, C., Walshaw, M. J., Gallagher, M. J., Williets, T. & Hart, C. A. (2000). Nebulized taurolidine and *B. cepacia* bronchiectasis, *Thorax* 55: 91–93.

Ledson, M. J., Gallagher, M. J., Robinson, M., Cowperthwaite, C., Williets, T., Hart, C. A. & Walshaw, M. J. (2002). A randomized double-blinded placebo-controlled crossover trial of nebulized taurolidine in adult cystic fibrosis patients infected with *Burkholderia cepacia*, *J. Aerosol Med.* 15(1): 51–57.

Lee, P. S., Gerrity, T. R., Hass, F. J. & Lourenco, R. V. (1979). A model for tracheobronchial clearance of inhaled particles in man and a comparison with data, *IEEE Trans. Biomed. Eng.* BME-26(11): 624–629.

Martonen, T. B., Yang, Y. & Hwang, D. (1994). Hygroscopic behaviour of secondary cigarette smoke in human nasal passages, *S.T.P. Pharma Sciences* 4: 69–76.

Matsui, H., Randell, S. H., Peretti, S. W., Davis, C. W. & Boucher, R. C. (1998). Coordinated clearance of periciliary liquid and mucus from airway surfaces, *J. Clin. Invest.* 102(6): 1125–1131.

Mitsakou, C., Helmis, C. & Housiadas, C. (2005). Eulerian modelling of lung deposition with sectional representation of aerosol dynamics, *J. Aerosol Sci.* 36: 75–94.

Plopper, C. G., Heidsiek, J. G., Weir, A. J., St. George, J. A. & Hyde, D. M. (1989). Tracheobronchial epithelium in the adult rhesus monkey: a quantitative histochemical and ultrastructural study, *Am. J. Anat.* 184: 31–40.

Ramsey, B. W., Pepe, M. S., Quan, J. M., Otto, K. L., Montgomery, A. B., Warren, J. W., Vasilijev, K. M., Borowitz, D., Bowman, C. M., Marshall, B. C., Marshall, S. & Smith, A. L. (1999). Intermittent administration of inhaled tobramycin in patients with cystic fibrosis, *New Eng. J. Med.* 340(1): 23–30.

Roth, A. P., Lange, C. F. & Finlay, W. H. (2003). The effect of breathing pattern on nebulizer drug delivery, *J. Aerosol Med.* 16(3): 325–339.

Serafini, S. M. & Michaelson, E. D. (1977). Length and distribution of cilia in human and canine airways, *Bull. Europ. Physiopath. Resp.* 13: 551–559.

Smaldone, G. C. (2002). Smart nebulizers, *Respir. Care* 47: 1434–1441.

Stahlhofen, W., Gebhart, J. & Heyder, J. (1980). Experimental determination of the regional deposition of aerosol particles in the human respiratory tract, *Am. Ind. Hyg. Assoc. J.* 41(6): 385–398a.

Stahlhofen, W., Gebhart, J., Heyder, J. & Scheuch, G. (1983). New regional deposition data of the human respiratory tract, *J. Aerosol Sci.* 14: 186–188.

Sweeney, L. G., Wang, Z., Loebenberg, R., Wong, J. P., Lange, C. F. & Finlay, W. H. (2005). Spray-freeze-dried liposomal ciprofloxacin powder for inhaled aerosol drug delivery, *Int. J. Pharm.* 305: 180–185.

Tamaoki, J., Chiyotani, A., Tagaya, E., Sakai, N. & Konno, K. (1994). Effect of long term treatment with oxitropium bromide on airway secretion in chronic brochitis and diffuse panbronchiolitis, *Thorax* 49: 545–548.

Taulbee, D. B. & Yu, C. P. (1975). A theory of aerosol deposition in the human respiratory tract, *J. Appl. Physiol.* 38(1): 77–85.

Wang, Z., Cheng, H. T., Roa, W. & Finlay, W. H. (2003). Farnesol for aerosol inhalation: nebulization and activity against human lung cancer cells, *J. Pharm. Sci.* 6: 95–100.

Wanner, A., Salathé, M. & O'Riordan, T. G. (1996). Mucociliary clearance in the airways, *Am. J. Respir. Crit. Care Med.* 154: 1868–1902.

Weibel, E. R. (1963). *Morphology of the human lung*, Acedemic Publishers, New York.

Widdicombe, J. G. (1997). Airway surface liquid: concepts and measurements, *in* D. F. Rogers & M. I. Lethem (eds), *Airway Mucus: Basic Mechanisms and Clinical Perspectives*, Birkhäuser, Basel, chapter 1, pp. 1–17.

Yeates, D. B., Sturgess, J. M., Kahi, S. R., Levison, H. & Aspin, N. (1975). Mucociliary transport in trachea of patients with cystic fibrosis, *Arch. Dis. Childhood* 51: 28–33.

Yu, C. P., Hu, J. P., Yen, B. M., Spektor, D. M. & Lippmann, M. (1986). *Models for mucociliary particle clearance in lung airways*, Lewis, Chelsea, Michigan, chapter 39, pp. 569–578.

22

Airways Clearance Techniques in Cystic Fibrosis: Physiology, Devices and the Future

Adrian H. Kendrick
Department of Respiratory Medicine, University Hospitals, Bristol England

1. Introduction

The appearance of the lungs of a cystic fibrosis (CF) patient at post mortem is typically one of consolidation, with areas of bronchiectasis filled with mucopurulent material and of mucus plugging of the small airways (Yankaskas et al., 2004). The airways of the upper respiratory tract have increased secretion production, whilst in the lower respiratory tract there is increased mucus production and an increase in sputum. This sputum is usually thick and tenacious, becoming thicker and more abundant during an exacerbation and leading to progressive lung damage. It is therefore essential that in patients with CF the process of airway clearance is enhanced, where needed, to attempt to reduce these long-term effects.

The purpose of this chapter is to outline 1) the normal structure and function of the airways, 2) the process of mucus clearance in normal airways, 3) the effects that CF has on both the physiology and mucus clearance, 4) the current understanding of airway clearance device in terms of how they work and their application and finally 6) to look towards the future.

2. Structure and function in normal airways

The structure of the airways, and hence the function of the airways is affected by disease (Ranga & Kleinerman, 1978). Understanding the structure of the normal airways and how CF changes the airway function is essential in understanding the potential application of airway clearance techniques in clinical practice.

2.1 Normal airway structure

The airways start at the trachea and terminate at the alveolar sacks where gas exchange takes place (Fig 1).

There are about 23 branches of the airways from trachea to alveoli. The first 15 generations do not play a role in gas exchange and constitute the anatomical dead space (~150 ml). Gas exchange commences from generation 15 onwards, with alveolar ducts appearing at generations 19 - 22. Generation 23 is the last generation of the airways, constituting the alveolar sacs. The total number of alveoli ranges from 200 to 600 million (mean 300 million), the number correlating with the standing height of the subject (Angus & Thurlbeck, 1972).

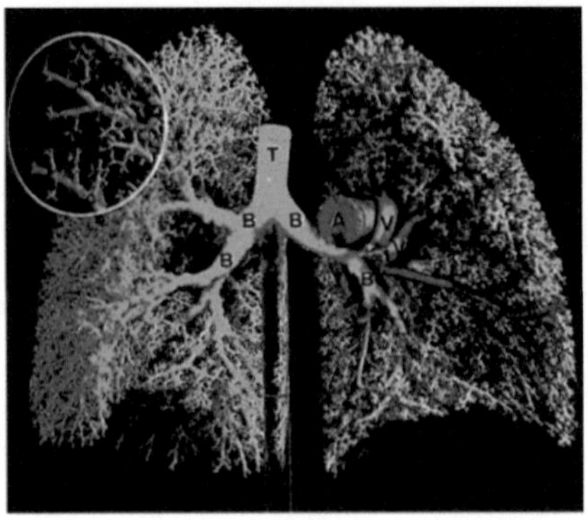

Fig. 1. Resin cast of a human lung showing the branching pattern of the bronchial tree (B) which originates from the trachea (T). In the left lung, the pulmonary arteries (A) and veins (V) are marked. The inset shows the peripheral airway branching at higher power. Reproduced with permission from Wiebel ER, The Pathway for Oxygen: Structure and Function in the Mammalian Respiratory System. Harvard University Press, London, England, 1984

The bronchi contain cartilage which maintains airway patency, whilst the bronchioli have no cartilage (Fig 2). Histologically, the airway epithelium becomes thinner towards the alveoli, where the distance between the air in the alveoli and blood in the pulmonary capillaries is about 0.2 µm.

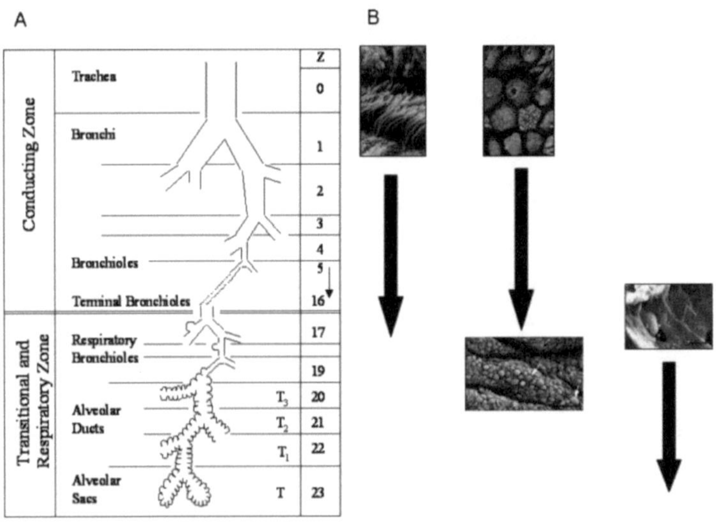

Fig. 2. A) Organization of the airway tree, divided into conducting zones, the transitional and respiratory zones where alveolar begin to appear before leading to the alveolar ducts and sacs. Based on Weibel ER. Morphometry of the human Lung. Heidelberg: Springer. New York Academic, 1963. B) Ciliated epithelia cells and goblet cells occur in the larger airways, decreasing towards the smaller airways. Goblet cells are replaced in the transitional and conducting zones by Clara cells. Pores of Kohn appear in the alveolar walls and are important in terms of collateral ventilation.

Ciliated epithelial cells decrease in number and shape from the large airways towards the small airways. Goblet cells abound in the larger airways, with around 6000 mucus secreting cells.mm^{-2}, and are responsible, along with the submucosal secretory cells, for producing the thick layer of mucus that lines all but the smallest of conducting airways. Mucin is rapidly released from the mucus-secreting cells in response to a range of stimuli including direct chemical irritation, inflammatory cytokines and neural activity (Rogers, 1994). The number of Goblet cells and their secretions increases significantly in CF.

In the smaller airways, Goblet cells are replaced by Clara cells which constitute about 80% of the cell population. Clara cells may play a role in the *Cystic Fibrosis transmembrane conductance regulator* (CFTR) gene-dependant regulation of epithelial electrolyte and water secretion in addition to their roles of surfactant production, protection against oxidative stress and suppression of inflammation (Kulaksiz et al, 2002). CFTR expression is significantly greater in the respiratory and terminal bronchioles compared to the proximal airways and alveoli (Engelhardt et al, 1994). Smooth muscle in the airway wall gradually increases so that in the terminal bronchioles it constitutes around 20% of the wall thickness.

2.2 Normal function

The normal lung maintains sterility below the first bronchial division despite breathing in 450 l.h^{-1} at rest of air contaminated with viruses and bacteria. To move this volume of gas, the ventilatory pump must create negative and positive pressures within the thorax for air to enter and leave, respectively. In addition, the pump must provide a system of distributing the inhaled gas to the alveoli, where blood supplied to the alveoli by the pulmonary circulation will come into contact with the alveolar gas. Hence, for gas exchange to take place 1) the lungs must be ventilated, 2) the pulmonary circulation must be perfused, and 3) the ventilation and perfusion must be matched.

The airways present a major challenge to the movement of air from the atmosphere to the alveoli. The airways narrow with each branching, decreasing from about 18 mm in the trachea, to 0.7 mm at generation 14 and 0.3 mm at the alveolar ducts. Hence, there is a significant increase in the surface area for gas exchange, which may be as great as 143 m^2 in the average male (Weibel, 1984).

As the airways narrow, the resistance (pressure ÷ flow) to airflow increases along a single airway. In reality though, the highest resistance is found in the large central airways, whilst the resistance in the peripheral airways accounts for only 20% of the total resistance due to the increased cross-sectional area of the millions of peripheral airways in parallel. In the large airways, where air moves by bulk flow, a turbulent airflow pattern predominates, thus increasing resistance, whilst in the peripheral airways, diffusion is the predominant means for moving gas (Fig 3).

As the respiratory bronchioles and alveolar ducts contribute little to the overall resistance of the lungs as a whole, the distribution of gas within these units is determined principally by the compliance of the lungs (C_L)—a measure of stiffness or floppiness of the object ($C_L = \Delta\text{volume} \div \Delta\text{pressure}$). In normal lungs, the pressure-volume relationship is such that each tidal breath occurs at the steep part of the relationship, where compliance is high (Fig 4).

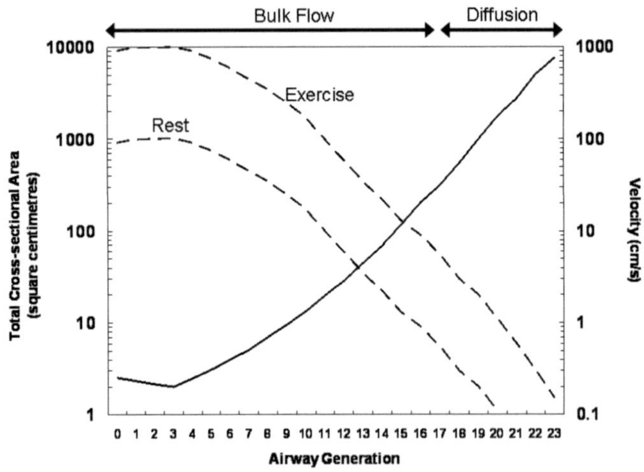

Fig. 3. The relationship of airway cross-sectional area and airflow velocity to airway generation in the human lung. As the airways branch, the total cross-sectional area increases from 2.5 cm^2 in the trachea, to around 13 cm^2 at the tenth generation (1024 airways) with a final cross-sectional area of around 300 cm^2 in the acinar region. The airflow velocity falls by more than 100-fold from the trachea down to the acinus (1 m.s^{-1} to 1 cm.s^{-1}). In exercise, the airflow velocity may be up to ten times greater and so greater airflow is observed within the acinus. Data from various sources.

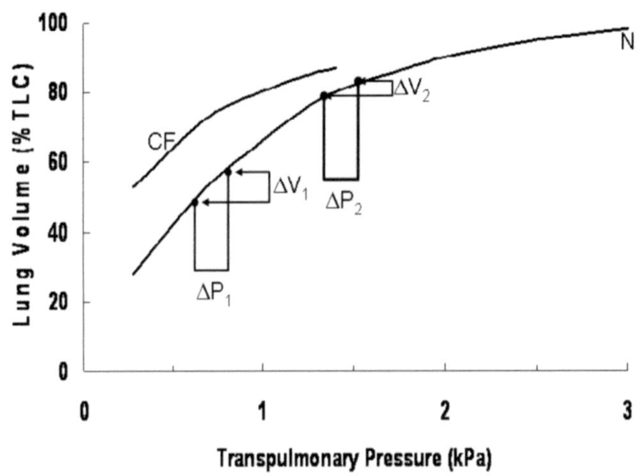

Fig. 4. Schematic of pressure volumes curves in normal subjects (N) and in patients with CF. In normal subjects, for the change in pressure ($\Delta P_1 = \Delta P_2$) there is a greater change in volume at ΔP_1 than for ΔP_2 demonstrating that the compliance of the lungs is greater at ΔP_1 than at ΔP_2. Normal tidal breathing occurs on the steeper portion of the pressure-volume curve. In CF, the pressure volume curve is altered - there is normal compliance of the lungs over the normal tidal volume range, but reduced compliance at high lung volumes (summary data from Mansell et al, 1974)

When we breathe in close to maximum, the pressure-volume relationship is much flatter (more pressure needed to increase a given volume) and so it is much harder to breathe, making the work of breathing greater. On the other hand, when we breathe fully out, the pressure-volume curve is much steeper, indicating that full exhalation is not limited by lung compliance. One key point on this curve is the end-expiratory lung volume (EELV) or functional residual capacity (FRC). This is the equilibrium point in the relationship between the outward pull of the chest wall and the inward collapse of the lungs, where the relative magnitudes are equal, but opposite.

If we apply this observation to an individual alveolus, then the larger it is at the start of tidal inhalation, the stiffer (less compliant) it is and so less air enters the alveoli. This is observed by looking at the distribution of inspired air, which goes preferentially to the more complaint lung bases. In addition to the compliance, ventilation is further distributed within the alveolar units by the pores of Kohn, which connect the alveoli within a lobe; this is referred to as collateral ventilation. (Desplechain et al, 1983). This should permit equilibrium of gas pressures in different lung regions, but this only appears to apply in diseased lungs, as in normal lungs the flow resistance of the collateral pathways is high, and so movement of gas via this route is minimal. (Macklem, 1971). These pores allow transfer of gas between alveoli and function to minimize the collapse of lung units if a more central airway becomes blocked. (Hogg et al, 1969).

One aspect of ventilation that is affected by respiratory disease is the work of breathing. (Campbell et al, 1957; Milic-Emili, 1991). During the passive expiration of a normal resting tidal breath, the work of breathing is performed entirely by the inspiratory muscles. Approximately 50% of the work during inspiration is dissipated as heat in overcoming the frictional forces that oppose inspiration. The remaining 50% is stored as potential energy in the deformed elastic tissues of the lungs and chest wall, as they are at a point above the EELV and hence are not in equilibrium. This potential energy is available for expiration and is dissipated as heat in overcoming the frictional forces that resist expiration.

Energy that is stored in the deformed elastic tissue allows the work of expiration to be transferred to the inspiratory muscles. The actual work performed by the respiratory muscles is very small (~ 3 $ml.min^{-1}$ O_2), compared to the average resting oxygen uptake of 250 $ml.min^{-1}$, and so accounts for only about 1 - 2% of the resting metabolic rate.

The work of breathing overcomes two main problems—the elastic recoil of the lungs and chest wall, and the airway resistance to gas flow. The total work of breathing is the sum of the elastic and resistive work and may be related to lung volume or breathing frequency (Fig 5). It is likely that each individual selects the most appropriate breathing frequency in order to minimize the work of breathing.

3. Mucus clearance mechanisms

When the lungs are ventilated they are exposed to a vast range of particulate matter, bacteria and viruses. The main defence mechanism against these is the viscous mucus layer, which provides a physical protective barrier to chemical damage of the epithelium (Foster, 2002; Rubin, 2002).

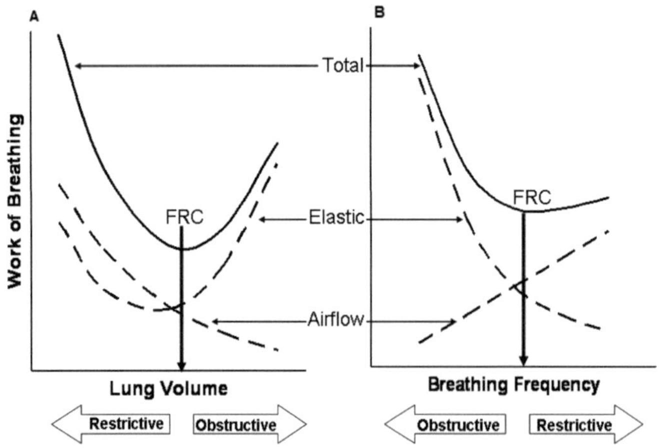

Fig. 5. Schematic diagram of the relationships of work of breathing against lung volume (A) and breathing frequency (B). The total work of breathing is the summation of the elastic properties of lungs and chest wall and airway resistance components. In normal subjects, there will be an optimal lung volume and optimal breathing frequency which is probably set for each individual. The effects of obstructive and restrictive lung disorders are shown for both relationships.

Airway mucus is a complex substance that lines the respiratory tract. Bacteria and other airborne particles become trapped in this sticky mucus and then are swept upwards and outwards by the tiny hair-like structures - cilia. The interaction between normal mucus, cilia and associated structures make up the mucociliary clearance system (MC).

Many inhaled irritants simply dissolve in the mucus, whilst inhaled particles are deposited in the airways either by impaction or sedimentation. These particles are then degraded by the proteases in the mucus or removed intact by the mucus. In the smaller airways sedimentation occurs due to the low airflow, so the particles are deposited and removed by macrophages.

For bacteria and viruses, the first line of defence is the physical removal by the mucus. Within the mucus, humoral defences include immunoglobulins, protease inhibitors and endogenous antibiotics. The airway provides numerous defence mechanisms to prevent microbial colonization by the large numbers of bacteria and viruses present in ambient air. Important components of this defence are the antimicrobial peptides and proteins present in the airway surface fluid—the mucin-rich fluid covering the respiratory epithelium (Rose & Voynow, 2006; Voynow & Rubin, 2009). Recently, evidence has indicated that within the airways of normal subjects is an endogenous antibiotic—human defensins, which is believed to play an important role as part of the airway defence mechanisms (Schneider et al, 2005). Human β-defensin gene (*HBD-2*) represents the first human defence that is produced following stimulation of epithelial cells by contact with micro-organisms, such as *Pseudomonas aeruginosa,* or cytokines, such as tumour necrosis factor-α (*TNF-*α) and Interleukin-1β (*IL-1*β) (Laube et al, 2006). Cellular immunity is also in evidence throughout the epithelium with macrophages, neutrophils and lymphocytes commonly occurring during infections in the normal lung.

Respiratory health is dependent on consistent clearance of airway secretions (Wanner et al, 1996; Houtmeyers et al, 1999). A healthy MC moves respiratory secretions to central airways, with the final clearance achieved by a combination of coughing and swallowing.

3.1 Cough and expiratory flow

Cough may be increased in respiratory infection and assists in clearing the airways from generations 7 - 8 upwards, augmenting the MC when overwhelmed by copious secretions.

Cough is a normal reflex mechanism that commences with a brief rapid inspiration usually greater than the resting tidal volume, this volume being sufficient for expiratory activity. (Ross et al, 1955; Bennett et al, 1990; Bennett & Zeman, 1994). The glottis closes for about 200 ms. There is an associated sharp rise in both pleural and abdominal pressure to between 6.6 to 13.3 kPa, resulting from expiratory muscle and diaphragmatic contraction; lung volume is held constant. Glottal closure limits expiratory muscle shortening, so promoting the isometric contraction of the expiratory muscles. This allows the expiratory muscles to maintain a much more advantageous force-length relationship, resulting in the generation of greater positive intra-abdominal and intrathoracic pressures, which may be up to 40 kPa.

Once the glottis is opened, the expiratory phase of cough occurs. The high intrathoracic pressures developed during the compressive phase promote high expiratory flow rates. Initially, there is a very brief blast of turbulent flow. This initial peak of expiratory flow lasts for between 20 ms to 50 ms and the cough Peak Expiratory Flow (cPEF) may exceed 720 $l.min^{-1}$ (Fig 6). This burst of air is due to the additive effects of the gas expired from the distal parenchymal units and the gas displaced by the more central airways, which are compressed by the high intrathoracic pressures. (Knudson et al, 1974). Although glottal closure enhances this phase of cough, it is not essential for an effective cough. (Von Leden & Isshiki, 1965). After the initial explosive burst of air, a period of between 200 to 500 ms occurs with much lower expiratory flows of between 180 to 240 $l.min^{-1}$. During this period, lung volume, transpulmonary pressure and cough expiratory flows all decrease.

As expiratory flow rate decreases, the airflow velocity changes—the relationship being dependent on the cross-sectional area of the airways (velocity = flow ÷ cross-sectional area). As shown in Fig 3, the peripheral airways have the largest cross-sectional area, whilst the larger bronchi and trachea have a much lower cross-sectional area. Hence as the cross-sectional area of the airways decreases, the velocity of air increases for a given expiratory flow rate. In other words, the velocity of the gas increases as the air moves from the peripheral to the central airways.

Gas velocity may be further enhanced in the central airways due to dynamic airway compression, where the airway narrows due to the pressure surrounding it being greater than the pressure within it. Narrowing the airway reduces the cross-sectional area, and so velocity increases for a given flow rate.

In normal airways, and during resting tidal breathing, the velocity of air is around 500 $cm.s^{-1}$ down to the airway generations 7 to 8 (Fig 3). At the peak of cough the velocity of air may exceed 16,000 $cm.s^{-1}$. The cough lasts for approximately 0.5s: up to 1 litre of air may be expelled and the cough is ended either by glottal closure or respiratory muscle relaxation, with a consequent fall in pleural pressure (Fig 6). Often there are further small coughs, which diminish in intensity as lung volume declines towards residual volume.

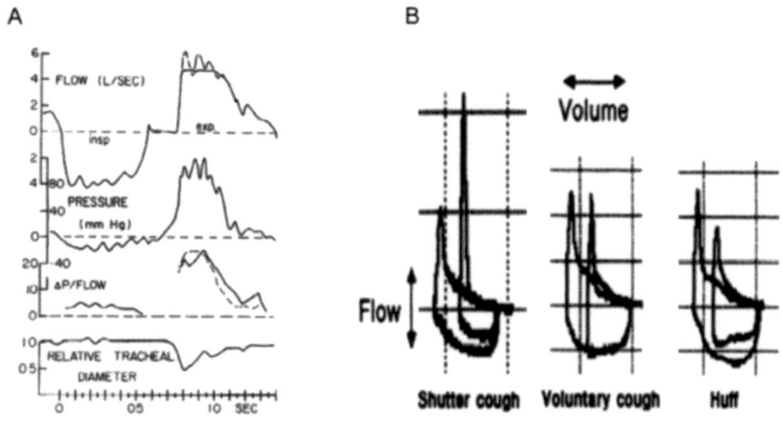

Fig. 6. A) Measurements taken during a cough and the preceding inspiration of a healthy male subject. From top to bottom: volume flow of air; oesophageal pressure; resistance to airflow (ΔP/flow). The inspiratory phase lasts about 0.65 seconds and resulted in an intake of about 2.5 litres of air. Following a short period of glottal closure (about 0.2 sec.) about the same volume of air was expelled within 0.5 sec. During inspiration, the change in intrapleural pressure measured using the oesophageal balloon rarely exceeded - 20 mmHg but, during expiration, the change reached between +100 to 140 mmHg. Maximum inspiratory flow rates were 3 - 4 $l.s^{-1}$ and expiratory flow rates reached maxima of 5 - 6.5 $l.s^{-1}$. (From Ross et al, 1955 with permission). B) Coughs performed by a subject, either voluntary, shutter, or huff, was recorded by having the subject cough into a rolling seal spirometer. On average an airway pressure of +70 cmH_2O was required. Finally, the partial forced expiration or huff was performed in the same manner but without glottal closure. These manoeuvres are superimposed upon the subject's normal flow volume curve (From Bennett & Zeman, 1990 with permission)

In relation to mucous clearance, the actual velocity of airflow through the airways alters the kinetic energy (KE) available. As $KE = mv^2 \div 2$, ($\therefore KE \propto v^2$), where m is the mass of the object and v the velocity, a doubling of the velocity will result in a fourfold increase in the KE. So, the effects of dynamic compression are such that a narrowing of the airways results in an increase in velocity, which in turn results in increases in kinetic energy, thus enhancing the removal of mucus adhering to the airway wall. Zahm et al (1991), using a simulated cough device, found that the displacement of artificial mucus following a simulated cough was greater at smaller airway diameters. Hasani et al (1994) observed that during expiratory flow, mucus transport was more efficient in the central rather than the peripheral airways.

In order to understand how airway clearance devices may be used to assist in the removal of these secretions, we need to understand how cough works in reality. Cough is effective in removing mucus and particulates if the secretions lining the airways are dispersed into the expiratory gas. The high velocity of airflow interacts with the bronchial secretions, resulting in '*two-phase air-liquid flow*' by which energy is transferred from the air to the liquid, resulting in a shearing effect on the liquid secretions, thus aiding the expectoration of sputum (Clarke et al, 1970; Kim et al, 1986). At velocities of between 1000 – 2500 $cm.s^{-1}$ an annular type of two-phase flow occurs, whilst at a velocity of > 2500 $cm.s^{-1}$ a mist flow with aerosol formation occurs (Fig 7).

A number of factors may be observed -

1. Airways are collapsible structures and so may vibrate and their walls may approximate each other, further aiding the loosening of mucus and promoting clearance (McCool & Leith, 1987);
2. Shearing and expectoration are affected by the viscosity, elasticity and surface tension of the bronchial secretions in a highly complex manner. (Scherer, 1981).
3. Waves of mucus have been observed in the range of airflow occurring during a cough (King et al, 1985) which may further enhance particle clearance (Kim et al, 1983);
4. The physical properties of mucus also affect cough efficiency. Mucus clearance is directly proportional to the depth of the mucus, and is inversely proportional to its viscosity and elasticity (King et al, 1985; King, 1987; King et al 1989; King et al, 1990; Albers et al, 1996)
5. Through use of radiographic methods to measure flow and tracheal cross-section during coughing, an index of 'scrubbing action' has been derived (Harris & Lawson, 1968). In healthy subjects during the first cough, around 59% of the scrubbing action occurs, with only 26% and 16% for the second and third coughs in a sequence of coughs.
6. During a forced expiration, high expiratory flow develops within about 100 ms and results in a high shear rate. Mucus transport varies inversely with shear rate, referred to as pseudoplastic flow or shear thinning. This observed decrease in viscosity can be explained by a temporary realignment of macromolecular glycoproteins due to the applied force (Lopez-Vidriero, 1981). Therefore, repeated forced expirations with short time intervals between each forced expiration may result in a reduction of the mucus viscosity and hence improve mucus transport (Zahm et al, 1991).

In healthy individuals, the rate of mucus secretion is carefully balanced with mucus clearance. The consistency of mucus is maintained such that it is thick enough to trap bacteria and other inhaled particles but thin enough to be moved easily by cilia. When airways are kept free of bacteria, other particles and excess mucus, airways remain open and permit normal gas exchange.

When mucus secretion and mucus clearance are not in balance, excessive airway mucus can cause serious problems. Excess, often sticky mucus may accumulate in the airways, resulting in an increase in the work of breathing. Regardless of the causes, the consequences for the patients are the same—a vicious cycle of recurrent, worsening episodes of inflammation, pulmonary infection, increased production of excess mucus, and airway obstruction, lung damage and respiratory failure.

The consequences of uncleared airway secretions in the airways are a clear link between mucus hypersecretion/secretion retention, exacerbation of illness, hospitalization, a sharply declining one second forced expiratory volume (FEV_1) and death (Annesi & Kauffmann, 1986; Lange et al, 1990; Prescott et al, 1995; Vestbo et al, 1996). The recognition of the clinical significance of excessive, abnormal, or retained airway secretions provides the rationale for improving mucociliary clearance as a logical treatment goal in order to avoid mucus retention and to prevent or break the life-destroying cycle of recurrent infection and progressive pulmonary deterioration.

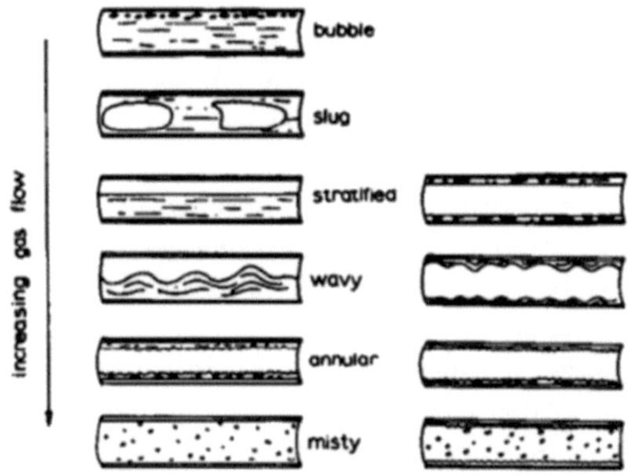

Fig. 7. Effects of gas flow rates on a mixture of gas and liquid flowing through a horizontal tube. At low flows, bubbles of gas may be dispersed in the liquid (bubble flow). As the gas flow rate increases, the bubbles become larger and fill most of the tube cross section; these gas 'slugs" alternate with volumes of liquid and are displaced toward the top of the tube (slug flow). At higher flows the gas slugs merge randomly, leading to the liquid occupy the lower part of the tube with a fairly smooth surface (stratified flow), which as the flow-rate increases further lead to marked surface roll waves appear (wavy flow). With continued increases in flow rates the film of liquid is covered by a dense array of small waves and the surface may appear smoother although there is extreme agitation of the liquid (annular flow). At extreme flow rates, the liquid waves are entrained and blow through the tube in the form of droplets (mist flow). (From Clarke et al, 1970 with permission).

4. Cystic fibrosis

There are a number of significant changes that occur in patients with CF in terms of the respiratory physiology and the mucociliary clearance mechanisms.

4.1 Respiratory physiological changes in CF

The changes that occur to the normal physiology are principally airflow obstruction, which worsens as the disease progresses. In patients with virtually normal spirometry, evidence of mild airways disease is observed by changes in airflow within the small airways, as measured by the Maximal Expiratory Flow (MEF) with 25% of the Forced Vital Capacity (FVC) remaining[1]. This is known as the $MEF_{25\%FVC}$ (Zapatal et al, 1971). In terms of gas exchange function there is widening of the alveolar-arterial PO_2 ($AaPO_2$) and an increased dead space to tidal volume ratio (V_D/V_T) (Lamarre et al, 1972). Whilst the total lung capacity (TLC) is often normal (Reis et al, 1988), the static pressure-volume curve (compliance) shows a loss of recoil pressures at low lung volumes with normal recoil pressures at high lung volumes. (Mansell et al, 1974). This results in a normal compliance of the lungs over the normal tidal volume range, but reduced compliance at high lung volumes (Fig 4).

[1]The $MEF_{25\%FVC}$ is obtained from a maximal expiratory flow volume curve. The subject inhales fully and then forcibly exhales. The volume of air exhaled in total is the forced vital capacity (FVC). With 25% of the FVC remaining, the flow rate at this point can be obtained and hence is the $MEF_{25\%FVC}$. In the US this is referred to as the forced expiratory flow (FEF) after 75% of the FVC has been exhaled ($FEF_{75\%FVC}$).

Despite malnutrition being common in CF patients, respiratory muscle weakness is not common, and, if present, is generally mild. (Mier et al, 1990). This is important as cough is common in CF with median rates being 21.2 coughs.h^{-1} (interquartile range [IQR] 14 - 34.9) at the time of exacerbation, but reducing to a median of 9.0 coughs.h^{-1} (IQR 5.8–12.8). (Smith et al, 2006) The other major abnormality of note is that exercise capacity is often limited by the combined effects of airflow obstruction and muscle wasting due to malnutrition. (Lands et al, 1992). As indicated above, the small airways may have reduced function (↓$MEF_{25\%FVC}$).

The causes of this small airways disease are possibly the result of significant increases in the inner wall and the smooth muscle areas of the peripheral airways. (Tiddens HA, et al, 2000) Changes in the airway dimensions of CF patients compared to chronic obstructive lung disease (COPD) patients showed that, for airways of 1.9 mm diameter (12th generation), there was an approximately fivefold increase in the smooth muscle area and a threefold increase in the inner wall area without epithelium. In the larger airways (35 mm diameter) there was a ~1.5 increase in smooth muscle area with an almost identical inner wall area without epithelium. These changes may also be related to age (Soboya & Tausig, 1986). Finally, the work of breathing is increased, although the increase is not solely explained by changes in lung function and lung mechanics (Fig 8), but also by the effects of TNF-α and CFTR (Bell et al, 1996).

These pathological studies demonstrate the variability of the destructive processes in the lungs of CF patients. Airway wall thickening is a marked feature of CF and is likely to extend into the small airways and be associated with airways inflammation and obstruction.

4.2 Mucus and mucociliary clearance in CF

In CF, there is increased mucus retention and bacterial colonization, due to the viscous nature of the mucus. However, there is inhibition of antimicrobial peptide activity or gene expression can result in an increased susceptibility to infections where the CF phenotype leads to reduced antimicrobial capacity of peptides in the airway. (Goldman et al, 1997; Rosenstein & Zeitlin, 1998). Thus in CF, bacterial colonization and mucus hypersecretion occur as a consequence, leading to progressive lung damage (Tiddens et al, 2000)

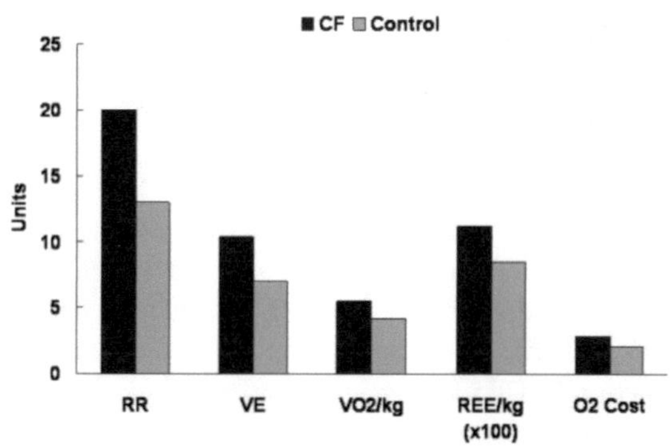

Fig. 8. Summary data on resting energy expenditure and oxygen cost of breathing in control subjects and patients with CF. The data shown (means only) shows that CF patients have a significantly higher respiratory rate (RR; breaths.min^{-1}: $p<0.05$), minute ventilation (VE; l.min^{-1}: $p<0.001$); oxygen uptake/kg (VO_2/kg; l.min^{-1}.kg^{-1}: $p<0.001$) and resting energy expenditure/kg (REE; kJ.min^{-1}.kg^{-1}: $p<0.001$) and O_2 cost (ml.l^{-1} VE). (From Bell et al, 1996).

Patients with CF have impaired airway clearance due to the following problems:

1. **Ineffective ciliary clearance**: Normal cilia beat in a coordinated unidirectional fashion to mobilize mucus and clear particulate matter from the airways. Damaged cilia perform this function inadequately or not at all;
2. **Excessive or abnormal mucus production**: CF results in excess mucus production and the mucus is abnormally thick and sticky. Large quantities of mucus, or mucus with altered physical properties, may overwhelm the mucociliary apparatus, inhibiting normal airway clearance (Rose & Voynow, 2005; Voynow & Rubin, 2009);
3. **Ineffective cough**: Cough function may be weak or ineffective if the muscles have become weak or fatigued;
4. **Obstructive lung disease**: The airway size is decreased as a result of structural changes, bronchospasm and excess mucus, limiting the ability to exhale. These effects result in much slower clearance of mucus than in normal subjects, (Regnis et al, 1994; Matthys & Kohler, 1986; Yeates et al, 1976; Wood et al, 1975) with a correlation between the lung function and mucociliary clearance (Robinson et al, 2000; Fig 9).

Because at-risk individuals are prone to recurrent episodes of respiratory inflammation, infection and, eventually, irreversible lung damage, improvement of MC is an essential goal of any treatment plan. Importantly, it is a goal that can be achieved by the individual and must include effective airway clearance therapy.

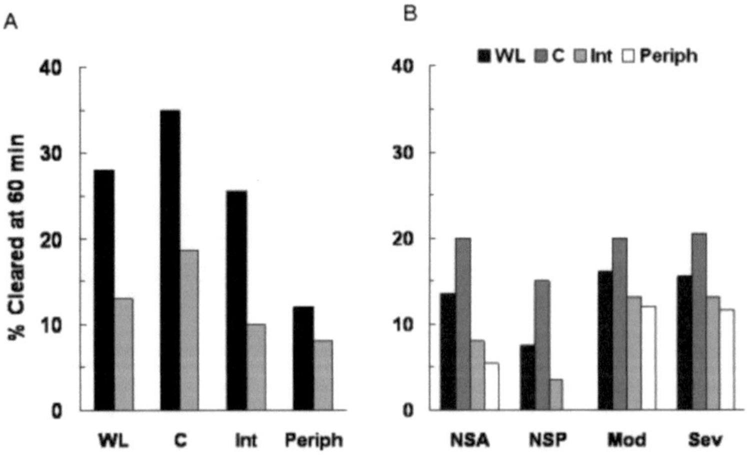

Fig. 9. Percentage of radioactivity cleared from different regions of the right lung at 60 minutes in normal subjects (black columns) and in patients with CF (grey columns). In A), the differences are observed for the whole lung (WL), Central (C), Intermediate (Int) and peripheral (Periph) airways. In B), the same regions as in A) are shown in relation to the degree of airway dysfunction in CF patients - normal small airway function (NSA; $FEV_1 \geq$ 80%pred and $FEF_{25-75} \geq$ 80%pred)[2], normal spirometry (NSP; $FEV_1 \geq$ 80%pred and $FEF_{25-75} <$ 80%pred), moderate (Mod; 40% $\leq FEV_1 <$ 80%pred) and severe (Sev; $FEV_1 <$ 40% pred) lung disease. There is no data for NSP - peripheral. Redrawn from Robinson et al, 2000)

[2]The FEF25-75% is the flow rate during a maximal forced exhalation and represents the averaged flow rates between 75% and 25% of the FVC.

5. Airway clearance devices

A number of adjunctive techniques and devices have been used to assist those who are unable, for whatever reason, to clear pulmonary secretions effectively and have been extensively reviewed (Cystic Fibrosis Trust, 2003; Yankaskas et al 2004; Kendrick, 2007; van der Schans, 2007; Bott et al, 2009; Flume et al, 2009; Daniels, 2010).

5.1 Criteria for airway clearance devices

The key to any device used to clear secretions is that it meets a number or criteria, based on the physiology. These criteria are:

1. Increase absolute peak expiratory flow (PEF) to move secretions towards the oropharynx;
2. Use of two-phase gas-liquid flow, both in closed and open airways. In the latter, mucus transport can be achieved by expiratory airflow during forced expiration, as well as tidal breathing. The peak expiratory flow/peak inspiratory flow ratio (PEF/PIF) needs to be > 1.1 to achieve this (Kim et al, 1986; Kim et al, 1986a; Kim et al, 1987) and the frequency of oscillation needs to be between 3 - 17 Hz, with the ideal frequency being around 13 Hz (Gross et al, 1985)
3. Decrease the mucus visco-elasticity in the airway, and hence improve mucus transport (App et al, 1998)
4. Elicit spontaneous coughs by mechanical stimulation of the airways to remove mucus from the trachea, inner and intermediate regions of the lungs (Laube et al, 2006; Hasani et al 1994)
5. Increase expectorated mucus volume (Konstan et al, 1994).

However, what all of these are dependent upon is the mechanical properties of the lungs of CF patients, which may deteriorate with disease progression (Arora & Gal, 1981; van der Schans, 1997). This might mean alternative approaches have to be adopted, and although these above criteria are the "ideal" criteria, there are alternative approaches which use different criteria and which may work as well or better. What is important is that we understand the criteria that each device achieves, how it may be adapted to an individual patient's needs and that changing the device as the disease progresses should always be an option worth considering.

5.2 Physiological aspects of airway clearance devices

Perhaps surprisingly, there are virtually no studies that have investigated exactly how these devices work from the physiological viewpoint and hence our understanding of how we are applying these devices into clinical practice is limited. Recently, McCarren et al (2006a, b, c) have provided evidence of how a variety of techniques work physiologically. These three studies conclude:

1. Chest wall circumference changed by 0.8 cm, the frequency of vibration was 5.5 Hz, the PEF was 58.2 $l.min^{-1}$ and the PEF/PIF ratio was 0.75, all of which are well below the ideal criteria for removing mucus (McCarren et al 2006a). What this study demonstrated was that the PEF during vibration was 50% greater than from a relaxed TLC manoeuvre and was composed of the flow rate due to a) elastic recoil, b) chest wall compression and c) chest wall oscillation. When summed, these three contributors

equated to the PEF observed during vibration, the proportional contributions being 67%, 15% and 14%, respectively;

2. There were clear relationships between the external chest wall force applied, chest wall circumference, intrapleural pressure (Fig 10) and expiratory flow (McCarren 2006b). Similar to the previous reference (McCarren et al 2006a), the intrapleural pressure observed was composed of the sum of the lung recoil, compression and oscillation components, the proportional contributions being 75%, 13% and 12%, respectively.

These two studies (McCarren et al 2006a; McCarren et al 2006b) have demonstrated some important relationships between the mechanics of the lung and the potential to remove sputum. The flow rates generated by vibration would be insufficient to augment secretion clearance by annular flow, since the PEF/PIF ratio was 0.75 and needs to exceed 1.1 (Kim et al, 1987). Why the inspiratory flow bias occurred is unclear, but may be related to the way in which physiotherapists ask the patient to take a deep breath. The frequency of vibration is also much lower than the ideal of between 11-15 Hz (Gross et al, 1985). It is currently unknown whether this vibration frequency would have a significant influence on the sputum rheology, but any decrease that may occur is likely to enhance the ability of cilia to move mucus (Wanner et al, 1996).

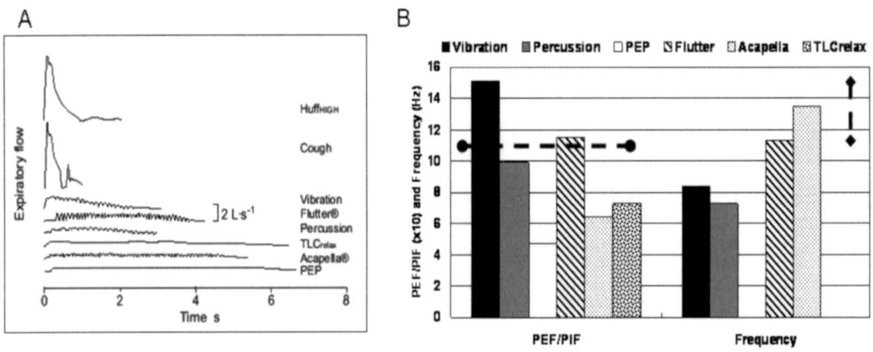

Fig. 10. A) The time course of the expiratory flow of the interventions in one subject. The eight traces have been separated vertically for clarity. $Huff_{HIGH}$: huff from high lung volumes; TLC_{relax}: total lung capacity passive expiration; PEP: positive expiratory pressure. B) Summary of data comparing measured data for PEF/PIF ratio and frequency of oscillation in various methods of airway clearance. The vertical dashed line is the ideal frequency range for the methods, whilst the horizontal dashed line is the minimum ideal PEF/PIF ratio. From McCarren et al, 2006b, with permission.

In normal subjects, expiratory flows are enhanced by lung recoil due to the additional forces applied to the chest wall during vibration by manual compression and oscillation. Where there is increased mucus and more viscous secretions, the airways will have a reduced airway radius and airway resistance will be increased.

Physiologically, these observations can be explained using Poiseuille's Equations (Resistance $\propto$ 1/airway radius^4 and Flow $\propto$ radius^4). If the airway narrows (smaller radius), there will be an increase in the resistance to airflow, and a reduction in airflow. Furthermore, Poiseuille's Equation includes a term for viscosity (η) on the denominator, and therefore changes in the viscosity of the mucus will potentially further alter the resistance and flow rates of air.

The third study in CF patients, (McCarren et al, 2006c) investigated vibration, percussion, PEP device, flutter, VRP valve and Acapella PEP. In addition, forced expiratory manoeuvres were voluntary cough and huff from high lung volumes ($huff_{HIGH}$). The important new measurements were inspiratory and expiratory flow rates recorded during the manoeuvres and the oscillation frequency determined by frequency spectral analysis. The key findings of this study were -

1. The PEF of vibration (1.58 ± 0.73 $l.s^{-1}$) was greater by 1.4 (flutter: 1.13 ± 0.3 $l.s^{-1}$) to 3.6 times (PEP: 0.44 ± 0.15 $l.s^{-1}$), but cough PEF was 4.67 ± 1.19 $l.s^{-1}$and $huff_{HIGH}$ PEF was 5.04 ± 2.3 $l.s^{-1}$;
2. The frequency of oscillation ranged 6.5–18.3 Hz, with flutter and Acapella devices having the higher oscillation frequencies (Fig 10).

None of these devices achieved the ideal combination. Vibration did not achieve the critical PEF/PIF of > 1.1, nor the critical optimal frequency (8.4 Hz). PEF was reduced due to the added resistance presented to expiration. However, the added resistance may result in stabilization of collapsible airways and allow for collateral ventilation to occur between alveoli via the Pores of Kohn, resulting in an increase in gas volume behind the mucus and hence aiding the movement of the secretions (Fink, 2002; Delaunois, 1989). As with the devices assessed, cough and $huff_{HIGH}$ do not achieve the ideal intervention status, as they do not oscillate airflow; increasing cilia beat frequency and/or decrease mucus viscosity.

Previous studies looking at the oscillation frequency using bench testing have noted that, for the Acapella and Flutter devices, the frequencies range from 8 - 25 Hz (Acapella blue), 13 - 30 Hz Acapella green) and 15 - 29 Hz (Flutter) (Volsko et al, 2003). More recently, Alves et al (2008) has demonstrated that the angle of use of the Flutter VRP1 may influence the outcome and treatment application.

With the limited physiological studies, the remaining question that has been answered to some extent is whether or not these devices alter sputum rheology (App et al, 1998). Using the flutter device and comparing changes in the characteristics of sputum, this study showed that the elastic properties of CF sputum samples were affected significantly by application of oscillations generated by the flutter at 15 and 30 min (Fig 11). The median frequency of the flutter-generated oscillations was 19 Hz.

These findings suggest that applied oscillations are capable of decreasing mucus visco-elasticity within the airways at frequencies and amplitudes achievable with the flutter device, and provide direct evidence of changes in the visco-elasticity of sputum.

Whilst the ideal frequency may be around 13 Hz, there is new evidence that suggests that a combination of 1) a higher frequency causing the airways to vibrate, resulting in the loosening (shearing) of the mucus from the airways, and 2) applying minimal positive pressure (+ 1 cmH_2O) via the Pores of Kohn and hence through the use of collateral ventilation, aids mucus clearance (Clini, 2009). This is clearly demonstrated in Fig 12 using lung ventilation scintography (Fazzi et al, 2009)

One of the other ways of removing excess sputum from the airways is by increasing airflow along the airways. During normal tidal breathing the airflow can be artificially increased by applying a venturi effect within a breathing circuit, and this increase in the velocity of the air can enhance the movement of sputum. This is achieved because the movement of air above a layer of mucus develops a shearing force over the surface of this liquid layer. When the shearing force exceeds the surface tension in the mucous layer, the mucus starts to move in the direction of the air flow (Kim et al, 1987). As the mucus moves up the bronchial tree, it will eventually be swallowed. Importantly, this effect can be achieved with minimal discomfort and without the need to cough. Where a patient's clinical condition is deteriorating and they have fatigued muscles, the cough PEF may well be reduced to the extent that clearing secretions is inhibited significantly. A device that removes excessive airway secretions only under tidal breathing conditions would obviate the need for cough.

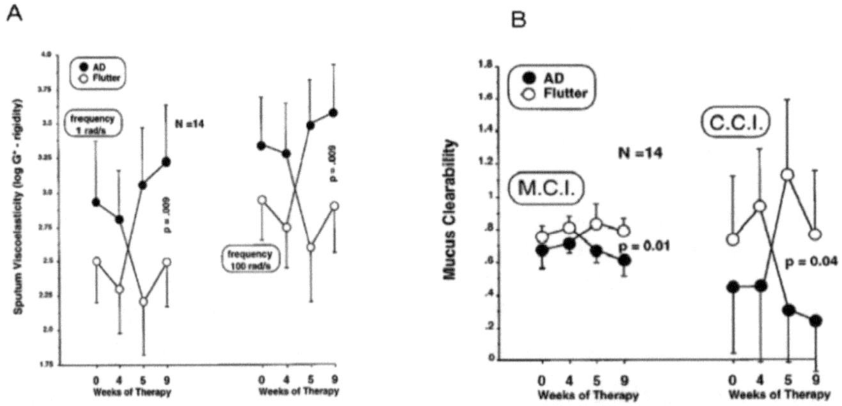

Fig. 11. Studies using Autogenic Drainage (AD) and Flutter therapy after an acute session at the start and end of 4 weeks of therapy, followed by a crossover to 4 weeks of treatment with the other therapy. A) Changes in sputum visco-elasticity and B) Mucus clearability indices, where the mucociliary clearance index (M.C.I.) and cough clearability index (C.C.I.) were calculated from sputum viscoelastic data. From App et al, 1998, with permission.

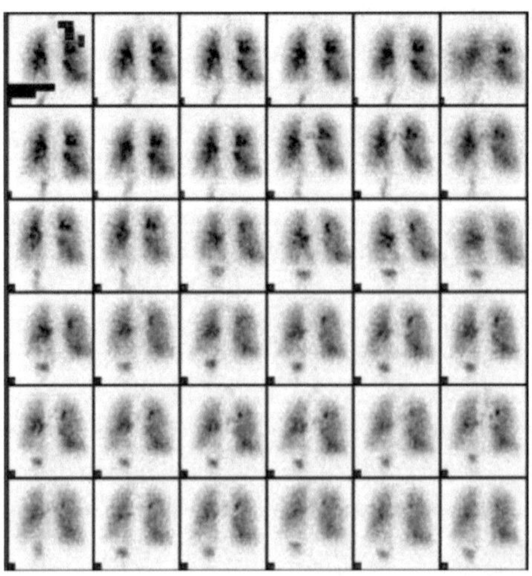

Fig. 12. Dynamic ventilation obtained using lung ventilation scintography (anterior scan) over 30 min during Temporary Positive Expiratory pressure (TPEP) therapy in a patient with COPD. Note how the central deposition of mucus plugs (dark areas) progressively clears over time. From Fazzi et al, 2008.

5.3 Do airway clearance techniques work in reality? (Cochrane reviews)

The range of techniques has recently been evaluated in six Cochrane reviews (Van der Schans, et al, 2000; Elkins et al, 2004; Main et al, 2005; Moran et al, 2009; Morrison & Agnew, 2009; Robinson et al, 2010). The conclusions from these Cochrane reviews are that: -

1. Airway clearance is important in the short term for patients with CF, but the long-term effects of no airway clearance is unknown;
2. Conventional chest physiotherapy is as effective as other forms of airway clearance;
3. Patients like their independence, and therefore any technique which they themselves can use is preferred;
4. Oscillation devices were no more or no less effective than other forms of physiotherapy;
5. There is not enough evidence to conclude, one way or the other, that Active Cycle of Breathing Techniques (ACBT) are any better or worse than any other technique.
6. Non-Invasive Ventilation (NIV) appears to help patients clear sputum more easily than other airway clearance techniques, and particularly in those patients who have difficulty in expectorating sputum.

What is somewhat disheartening in all of these reviews is the almost complete lack of really good quality research, and it is important to ensure data is collected appropriately and the primary and secondary outcome measures are available in order to fully understand the effects of any intervention.

These findings are confirmed in the review by McCool and Rosen (2006) where much of the level of evidence for airway clearance devices is fair to low and the benefits were intermediate to conflicting.

What is consistent in these studies is that, regardless of the device used, or the way in which the trial was conducted, there appears to be little change in the observed primary, and in many cases secondary, outcome measures. However, what makes these studies difficult to compare is the complete lack of commonality between recruitment, methodology, primary and secondary outcome measures, severity of disease, etc. This makes setting evidence-based practice guidelines interesting and limited in their conclusiveness.

5.4 Mathematical modelling

Whilst considerable work has been undertaken with studies on patients, other work has looked at bench testing and modelling some of the airway clearance techniques.

High Frequency Chest Compression (HFCC) has been investigated in such a way. Milla et al. (2004) investigated the actual waveform used in HFCC, which previously had been a sine wave. Changing to a triangular waveform significantly increased sputum production (4%-41%, mean 20%). From this small study of eight patients, the authors concluded that further investigation in patients using the sine and triangular waveform should be undertaken to determine the best frequencies for each waveform, disease and patient. They also pointed out that the original, and now neglected, square wave should be reassessed.

In a subsequent study (Milla et al, 2006), they investigated which frequency was appropriate to use for HFCC in order to 'tune' the device with the patient. In 100 patients, they found that the highest airflows for the sine waveform occurred between 13 - 20 Hz, with the largest volumes occurring between 6 – 10 Hz. For the square waveform, the highest flows and volumes occurred between 6 – 14 Hz. The authors provided a 'tuning' protocol for prescribing frequencies with the various HFCC machines, because they are different from one another.

Sohn et al (2005) used a computational model to investigate the non-linear effects of airway resistance, lung capacitance, and inertness of air on respiratory airflow, with airways resistance contributing the greatest effect.

Bench testing of other devices has been limited to oscillating Positive Expiratory Pressure (PEP) devices (Volsko et al, 2003) and HFCC (Lee et al, 2008). In the study of Volsko et al (2003), there was a statistically significant difference, but probably not a clinically significant difference between mean pressure, pressure amplitude and frequency over a range of experimental conditions. At medium flows, there were similar pressure waveforms, and hence overall similar performance characteristics.

Lee et al (2008) investigated the effects of different frequency and pressure waveforms using three different HFCC devices, bench tested using a mannequin. They concluded that a better understanding of the differences in frequency and pressure amplitude when applying devices to patients would allow clinicians and patients to optimize the efficacy of HFCC.

5.5 Which device to use?

Whatever technique is used to aid airway clearance, its application to a given patient must be such that we achieve a balance between the treatment demands and the patient's lifestyle. It is known that there are adherence issues as a result of the increasing time and effort required by patient self-management strategies, particularly when adults have to try and balance family, work, education etc with managing a chronic disease (Boyle, 2003). Whilst adherence to antibiotic treatment is high (80% - 95%), adherence to physiotherapy is low (40% - 55%; Kettler et al, 2002: 30%; Myers & Horn, 2006). Of note, airway clearance techniques, in adult CF patients, are perceived as a higher treatment burden with only 49% of patients performing airway clearance (Sawicki et al, 2009).

In selecting which airway clearance technique or combination of techniques to use, there are a number of key questions that should be taken into consideration –

1. Is the technique appropriate for the patient's clinical state and environment?
2. Is the technique compatible with the patient's lifestyle?
3. What does the patient like and dislike about each technique appropriate for use at that stage of their clinical status?
4. Does the patient perceive that the technique actually works?
5. What is the balance between the cost of the technique and the benefits, efficacy and preference of the technique?

Taking all of these questions into account and listening to the patient and their needs and preferences should allow the most appropriate airway clearance technique to be used, with or without the addition of behavioural techniques that increase adherence (Bernard & Cohen, 2004).

6. The future

Parents of children and adult patients want treatments that will help them achieve optimal health and quality of life goals. To make appropriate choices, they require accurate information, including a clear description of the theory and technique of available airway clearance methods. Additionally, they need information to allow them rule out treatments that are likely to be unsuitable based on particular physical or mental limitations and upon the psychological, social and economic circumstances of the entire family. Useful decision making criteria may include: -

1. What the patient and medical team want to achieve;
2. The clinical effectiveness of the technique;
3. Medical contraindications;
4. The ease of teaching/learning the technique by the patients and/or by the carer;
5. The likely acceptability and hence adherence with the technique;
6. The likely effort/work required by the technique compared to its likely benefit;
7. The patient's age, motivation, cognitive ability, concentration level and caregiver situation;
8. The degree of independence that a given technique gives the patient from the carer or the medical teams.

Airway clearance techniques are an essential part of the management of patients with CF. However, our understanding of how these devices work from bench testing and from physiological studies is limited to a very small number of studies. The studies themselves have used different populations (adults, children, mixed), with a range of disease severity and in general used the FEV_1 as the primary outcome measure. Whilst the FEV_1 is useful for assessing the respiratory well-being of patients, it presents only a limited picture of airway function. The $FEF_{25\%-75\%}$ has been used, and is thought to be sensitive to abnormalities in the small airway (McFadden & Linden, 1972; Landau et al, 1973). This, however, is only true when both the elastic recoil of the lungs and airways resistance are normal (Woolcock, 1998).

This may not be the case in CF, and is probably overlooked when interpreting results. The other key point about the $FEF_{25\%-75\%}$ is that it is very dependent on a true FVC being achieved on every occasion, which in itself may also be a significant variable. Furthermore, if the FVC increases or decreases then interpretation of this index becomes difficult. An alternative is to use the $MEF_{25\%FVC}$ which is similarly believed to be sensitive to small airway abnormalities. Again, however, if the FVC changes, the $MEF_{25\%FVC}$ cannot be compared post intervention to pre-intervention. Both these indices need careful analysis pre-to-post intervention and this can be achieved by using the iso-volume method of assessment (Boggs et al, 1982a; Boggs et al, 1982b).

Assessing the inhomogeneity of ventilation can be assessed either by nitrogen washout (Paiva & Engel, 1981) or by the use of the Lung Clearance Index (LCI) and the mixing ratio using the inert gas sulphur hexafluoride (SF6). The second method has been shown to be a more sensitive index than spirometry, (Gustafsson et al, 2003) does not require the respiratory gymnastics needed for forced expiratory manoeuvres and also appears to be age independent (Aurora et al, 2004), thereby making it highly useful for longitudinal studies. It is being increasingly used in both adult and paediatric CF patients (Horsley et al, 2008; Horsley, 2009; Kieninger et al (2011).

Whilst these physiological measurements are important guides to the course of disease, they do not present the whole picture. As stated above, what matters to the patient is how much independence they have and how much they themselves can actually do. Techniques which give the patient greater independence in the management of their own disease may well improve adherence to treatment and therapies. Including in studies, measures of patient adherence and patient acceptability are equally important.

Few studies have investigated health-related quality-of life measures, the number of exacerbations or hospital days per year, the costs or harm associated with intervention, or mortality rates. These need to be included along with the appropriate physiological measurements in any properly randomized control trial of airway clearance techniques to ensure that we fully understand how these techniques benefit or otherwise patients with CF. Furthermore, in our increasingly cost sensitive society, there needs to be a cost-benefit analysis included.

There are new techniques emerging and modifications of existing techniques which will improve the already difficult lives of patients with CF. As observed in all of the Cochrane reviews there is a clear need for properly controlled randomized trials and sensible and carefully selected primary and secondary outcomes that present the whole picture, provide the much needed evidence-based information needed to understand and apply these techniques. It is therefore incumbent on all researchers and clinicians working with CF patients to ensure that this good quality research is undertaken and published.

7. References

Albers GM, Tomkiewicz RP, May MK, et al (1996). Ring distraction technique for measuring surface tension of sputum: relationship to sputum clearability. *J Appl Physiol*, 81, 2690 - 2695.

Alves L, Pitta F, Brunetto AF (2008). Performance analysis of the Flutter VRP1 under different flows and angles. *Respir Care*, 53, 316 - 323.

Angus GE, Thurlbeck WM (1972). Number of alveoli in the human lung. *J Appl Physiol*, 32, 483 - 485.

Annesi I, Kauffmann F (1986). Is respiratory mucus hypersecretion really an innocent disorder? A 22-year mortality survey of 1,061 working men. *Am Rev Respir Dis*, 134, 688 - 693.

App EA, Kieselmann R, Reinhardt D, et al (1998). Sputum rheology changes in cystic fibrosis lung disease following two different types of physiotherapy. Chest, 114, 171 - 177.

Arora NS, Gal TJ (1981). Cough dynamics during progressive expiratory muscle weakness in healthy curanized subjects. *J Appl Physiol*, 51, 494 - 498

Aurora P, Gustafsson PM, Bush A, et al (2004). Multiple breath inert gas washout as a measure of ventilation distribution in children with cystic fibrosis. *Thorax*, 59, 1068 - 1073.

Bell SC, Saunders MJ, Elborn JS, Shale DJ (1996). Resting energy expenditure and oxygen cost of breathing in patients with cystic fibrosis. *Thorax*, 51, 126 - 131

Bennett WD, Foster WM, Chapman WF (1990). Cough-enhanced mucus clearance in the normal lung. *J Appl Physiol*, 69, 1670 - 1675

Bennett, WD, Zeman KL (1994). Effect of enhanced supra-maximal flows on cough clearance. *J Appl Physiol*, 77, 1577 - 1583

Bernard RS, Cohen LL (2004). Increasing adherence to cystic fibrosis treatment: a systematic review of behavioural techniques. *Pediatr Pulmonol*, 37, 8 - 16.

Boggs PB, Bhat KD, Vekovius WA, Debo MS (1982). Volume-adjusted maximal mid-expiratory flow (Iso-volume $FEF_{25-75\%}$): definition of "Significant" responsiveness in healthy, normal subjects. *Ann Allergy*, 48, 137 - 138

Boggs PB, Bhat KD, Vekovius WA, Debo MS (1982). The clinical significance of volume-adjusted maximal mid-expiratory flow (Iso-volume $FEF_{25-75\%}$) in assessing airway responsiveness to inhaled bronchodilator in asthmatics. *Ann Allergy*, 48, 139 - 142.

Bott J, Blumenthal S, Buxton M, et al (2009). Guidelines for the physiotherapy management of the adult, medical, spontaneously breathing patient. Joint BTS/ACPRC Guideline. *Thorax*, 64, Suppl 1, 1 - 52.

Boyle MP (2003). So many drugs, so little time: the future challenge of cystic fibrosis care. *Chest*, 123, 3 - 5.

Campbell EJM, Westlake EK, Cherniack RM (1957). Simple methods of estimating oxygen consumption and the efficiency of the muscles of breathing. *J Appl Physiol*, 11, 303 - 308.

Clarke S, Jones JG, Oliver DR (1970). Resistance to two-phase gas-liquid flow in airways. *J Appl Physiol*, 29, 464 - 471.

Clini E (2009). Positive expiratory pressure techniques in respiratory patients: old evidence and new insights. *Breathe*, 6, 153 - 159.

Cystic Fibrosis Trust (2003). Association of Chartered Physiotherapists in Cystic Fibrosis. Clinical Guidelines for the Physiotherapy Management of Cystic Fibrosis. Kent: Cystic Fibrosis Trust.

Daniels T (2010). Physiotherapeutic management strategies for the treatment of cystic fibrosis in adults. *Journal of Multidisciplinary Healthcare*, 3, 201 - 212.

Delaunois L (1989). Anatomy and physiology of collateral respiratory airways. *Eur Respir J*, 2, 893 - 904

Desplechain C, Foliguet B, Barrat E, et al (1983). The Pores of Kohn in pulmonary alveoli. *Bull Eur Physiopathol Respir*, 19, 59 - 68.

Elkins M, Jones A, van der Schans CP (2004). Positive expiratory pressure physiotherapy for airway clearance in people with cystic fibrosis. Cochrane Database of Systematic Reviews, Issue 2. Art. No.: CD003147. DOI: 10.1002/14651858.CD003147.pub3.

Engelhardt JF, Zepada M, Cohn JA, Yankaskas JR, Wilson JM (1994). Expression of cystic fibrosis gene in adult human lung. *J Clin Invest*, 93, 737 - 749.

Fazzi P, Girolami G, Albertelli R, et al (2008). IPPB with temporary expiratory (TPEP) in surgical patients with COPD. *Eur Respir J*, 32, Suppl 52, 577s

Fazzi P, Albertelli R, Grana M, Paggiaro PL (2009). Lung ventilation scintography in the assessment of obstructive lung diseases. *Breathe*, 5, 252 - 262.

Fink JB (2002). Positive pressure techniques for airway clearance. Respir Care, 47, 786 - 796

Flume PA, Robinson KA, O'Sullivan BP, et al (2009). Cystic Fibrosis pulmonary guidelines: airway clearance therapies. *Respir Care*, 54, 522 - 537.

Foster WM (2002). Mucociliary transport and cough in humans. *Pulm Pharmacol Ther*, 15, 277 - 282.

Goldman MJ, Anderson GM, Stolzenberg ED, et al (1997). Human *β-defensin-1* is a salt-sensitive antibiotic in the lung that is inactivated in cystic fibrosis. *Cell*, 88, 553 - 560.

Gross D, Zidulka A, O'Brien C, et al (1985). Peripheral mucociliary clearance with high-frequency chest wall compression. *J Appl Physiol*, 58, 1157 – 1163.

Gustafsson PM, Aurora P, Linblad A (2003). Evaluation of ventilation maldistribution as an early indicator of lung disease in children with cystic fibrosis. *Eur Respir J*, 22, 972 – 979.

Harris RS, Lawson TV (1968). The relative mechanical effectiveness and efficiency of successive voluntary coughs in healthy young adults. *Clin Sci*, 34, 569 - 577

Hasani A, Pavia D, Agnew JE, Clarke SW (1994). Regional lung clearance during cough and forced expiration technique (FET): effects of flow and viscoelasticity. *Thorax* 49, 557 - 561.

Hogg JC, Macklem PT, Thurlbeck WM (1969). The resistance of collateral channels in excised human lungs. *J Clin Invest*, 48, 421 - 431

Horsley AR, Macleod KA, Robson AG, et al (2008). Effects of cystic fibrosis lung disease on gas mixing indices derived from alveolar slope analysis. *Respir Physiol*, 162, 197 - 203.

Horsley A (2009). Lung clearance index in the assessment of airways disease. *Respir Med*, 103, 793 - 799.

Houtmeyers E, Gosselink R, Gayan-Ramirez G, Decramer M (1999). Regulation of mucociliary clearance in health and disease. *Eur Respir J*, 13, 1177 – 1188.

Kendrick AH. (2007). Airway clearance techniques in cystic fibrosis: physiology, devices and the future. *J R Soc Med*, 100, Suppl 47, 3 – 23.

Kettler LJ, Sawyer SM, Winfield HR, Greville HW. (2002). Determinants of adherence in adult cystic fibrosis. *Thorax*, 57, 459 – 464.

Kieninger E, Singer F, Fuchs O, et al (2011). Long-term course of lung clearance index between infancy and school-age in cystic fibrosis subjects *J Cyst Fibros*, 10, 487 - 490.

King M, Brock G, Lundell C. (1985). Clearance of mucus by simulated cough. *J Appl Physiol*, 58, 1776 – 1785.

King M. (1987). The role of mucus viscoelasticity in cough clearance. *Biorheology*, 24, 89 – 97.

King M, Zahm JM, Pierrot D, Vaquez-Girod S, Puchelle E (1989). The role of mucus gel viscosity spinnability and adhesive properties in clearance by simulated cough. *Biorheology*, 26, 747 – 752.

King M, Zidulka A, Phillips DM, Wight D, Gross D, Chang HK (1990). Tracheal mucus clearance in high-frequency oscillation: effect of peak flow rate bias. *Eur Respir J*, 3, 6 – 13.

Kim CS, Brown LK, Lewars GG, Sackner MA (1983). Deposition of aerosol particles and flow resistance in mathematical and experimental airway models. *J Appl Physiol*, 55, 154 - 163.

Kim CS, Rodriguez CR, Eldridge MA, Sackner MA (1986) Criteria for mucus transport in the airways by two-phase gas-liquid flow mechanism. *J Appl Physiol*, 60, 901 – 907.

Kim CS, Greene MA, Sankaran S, Sackner MA (1986a). Mucus transport in the airways by two-phase gas-liquid flow mechanism: continuous flow model. *J Appl Physiol,* 60, 908 - 917.

Kim CS, Iglesias AJ, Sackner MA (1987). Mucus clearance by two-phase gas-liquid flow mechanism: asymmetric periodic flow model. *J Appl Physiol,* 62, 959 - 971.

Knudson RJ, Mead J, Knudson DE (1974). Contribution of airway collapse to supramaximal expiratory flows. *J Appl Physiol,* 36, 653 - 667.

Konstan MW, Stern RC, Doershuk CF (1994). Efficacy of the Flutter device for airway mucus clearance in patients with cystic fibrosis. *J Pediatr,* 124, 689 - 693.

Kulaksiz H, Schmid A, Hanschied M, Ramaswamy A, Cetin Y (2002). Clara cells impact in air-side activation of CFTR in small airways. *Proc Natl Acad Sci,* 99, 6796 - 6801.

Lamarre A, Reilly BJ, Bryan AC, Levison H (1972). Early detection of pulmonary function abnormalities in cystic fibrosis. *Pediatrics,* 50, 291 - 298.

Landau LI, Hill DJ, Phelan PD (1973). Factors determining the shape of maximum expiratory flow-volume curves in childhood asthma. *Aust N Z J Med,* 3, 557 - 564

Lands LC, Heigenhauser GJF, Jones NL (1992). Analysis of factors limiting maximal exercise performance in advanced cystic fibrosis. *Clin Sci,* 83, 391 - 397.

Lange P, Nyboe J, Appleyard M, Jensen G, Schnohr P. (1990). Relation of ventilatory impairment and of chronic mucus hypersecretion to mortality from obstructive lung disease and from all causes. *Thorax,* 45, 579 - 585

Laube DM, Yim S, Ryan LK, Kisich KO, Diamond G (2006). Antimicrobial peptides in the airway. *Curr Top Microbiol Immunol,* 306, 153 - 182.

Lee YW, Lee J, Warwick WJ (2008). The comparison of three high-frequency chest compression devices. *Biomed Instrum Technol,* 42, 68 - 75.

Lopez-Vidriero MT (1981). Airway mucus; production and composition. *Chest,* 80 (Suppl), 799 - 804.

Macklem PT (1971). Airway obstruction and collateral ventilation. *Physiol Rev,* 51, 368 - 436.

Main E, Prasad A, van der Schans CP (2005). Conventional chest physiotherapy compared to other airway clearance techniques for cystic fibrosis. Cochrane Database of Systematic Reviews, Issue 1. Art. No.: CD002011. DOI: 10.1002/14651858.CD002011.pub2.

Mansell A, Dubrawsky C, Levison H, Bryan AC, Crozier DN (1974). Lung elastic recoil in cystic fibrosis. *Am Rev Respir Dis,* 109, 190 - 197.

Matthys H, Kohler D (1986). Bronchial clearance in cystic fibrosis. *Eur J Respir Dis,* 146, 311 - 318.

McCarren B, Alison JA, Herbert RD (2006a). Vibration and its effect on the respiratory system. *Aust J Physiother,* 52, 39 - 43

McCarren B, Alison JA, Herbert RD (2006b). Manual vibration increases expiratory flow rate via increased intrapleural pressure in healthy adults: and experimental study. *Aust J Physiother,* 52, 267 - 271

McCarren B, Alison JA (2006c). Physiological effects of vibration in subjects with cystic fibrosis. *Eur Respir J,* 27, 1204 - 1209.

McCool FD, Leith DE. (1987). Pathophysiology of cough. *Clin Chest Med,* 2, 189 - 195.

McCool FD, Rosen MJ. (2006). Non-pharmacologic airway clearance therapies: ACCP evidence-based clinical practical guidelines. *Chest*, 129, 250S - 259S

McFadden ER, Linden DA. (1972). A reduction in maximum mid-expiratory flow rate. A spirographic manifestation of small airway disease. *Am J Med*, 52, 725 - 737

Mier A, Ridington A, Brophy C, Hudson M, Green M (1990). Respiratory muscle function in cystic fibrosis. *Thorax*, 45, 750 - 752.

Milic-Emili J (1991). Work of breathing. In: Crystal RG, West JB, Eds. The Lung: Scientific Foundations. New York: Raven, 1065 - 1075.

Milla CE, Hansen LG, Weber A, Warwick WJ (2004). High-frequency chest compression: effect of the third generation compression waveform. *Biomed Instrum Technol*, 38, 322 - 328.

Milla CE, Hansen LG, Warwick WJ (2006). Different frequencies should be prescribed for different high frequency chest compression machines. *Biomed Instrum Technol*, 40, 319 - 324

Moran F, Bradley JM, Piper AJ (2009). Non-invasive ventilation for cystic fibrosis. Cochrane Database of Systematic Reviews, Issue 1. Art. No.: CD002769. DOI: 10.1002/14651858.CD002769.pub3.

Morrison L, Agnew J (2009). Oscillating devices for airway clearance in people with cystic fibrosis. Cochrane Database of Systematic Reviews, Issue 1. Art. No.: CD006842. DOI: 10.1002/14651858.CD006842.pub2.

Myers LB, Horn SA (2006). Adherence to chest physiotherapy in adults with cystic fibrosis. *J Health Psychol*, 11, 915 - 926.

Paiva M, Engel LA (1981). The anatomical basis for the sloping N_2 plateau. *Respir Physiol*, 44, 325 - 337

Prescott E, Lange P, Vestbo J (1995). Chronic mucus hypersecretion in COPD and death from pulmonary infection. *Eur Respir J*, 8, 1333 - 1338.

Ranga V, Kleinerman J (1978). Structure and function of small airways in health and disease. *Arch Pathol Lab Med*, 102, 609 - 617.

Regnis JA, Robinson M, Bailey DL, et al (1994). Mucociliary clearance in patients with cystic fibrosis and in normal subjects. *Am J Respir Crit Care Med*, 150, 66 - 71.

Reis AL, Sosa G, Prewitt L, Friedman PJ, Harwood IR (1988). Restricted pulmonary function in cystic fibrosis. *Chest*, 94, 575 - 579.

Robinson KA, Mckoy N, Saldanha I, Odelola OA (2010). Active cycle of breathing technique for cystic fibrosis. Cochrane Database of Systematic Reviews, Issue 11. Art. No.: CD007862. DOI: 10.1002/14651858.CD007862.pub2.

Robinson M, Eberl S, Tomlinson C, Daviskas E, Regnis JA, Bailey DL, Torzillo PJ, Menache M, Bye PT (2000). Regional mucociliary clearance in patients with cystic fibrosis. *J Aerosol Med*, 13, 73 - 86.

Rogers DF (1994). Airway goblet cells: responsive and adaptable frontline defenders. *Eur Respir J*, 7, 1690 - 1706.

Rose MC, Voynow JA (2006). Respiratory Tract Mucin Genes and Mucin Glycoproteins in health and Disease. *Physiol Rev*, 86, 245 - 278.

Rosenstein BJ, Zeitlin PL (1998). Cystic Fibrosis. *Lancet*, 351, 277 - 282

Ross BB, Gramiak R, Rahn H. (1955). Physical dynamics of the cough mechanism. *J Appl Physiol*, 8, 264 - 268.

Rubin BK (2002). Physiology of airway mucus clearance. *Respir Care*, 47, 761 - 768.

Sawicki GS, Seller DE, Robinson WM (2009). High treatment burden in adults with Cystic Fibrosis: Challenges to Disease Self-Management. *J Cyst Fibros*, 8, 91 - 96.

Scherer PW (1981). Mucus transport by cough. *Chest*, 805, 830 - 833.

Schneider JJ, Unholzer A, Schaller M, Schäfer-Korting M, Korting HC (2005). Human Defensins. *J Mol Med (Berl)*, 83, 587 - 585.

Smith JA, Owen EC, Jones AM, Dodd ME, Webb AK, Woodcock A (2006). Objective measurement of cough during pulmonary exacerbations in adults with cystic fibrosis. *Thorax*, 61, 425 - 429.

Soboya RE, Tausig LM. (1986). Quantitative aspects of lung pathology in cystic fibrosis. *Am Rev Respir Dis*, 134, 290 - 295

Sohn K, WJ Warwick, Lee YW, Lee J, Holte JE (2005). Investigation of non-uniform airflow signal oscillation during high frequency chest compression. *Biomed Eng Online* 2005 [http://www.biomedicalengineering-online.com/content/4/1/34]

Tiddens HA, Koopman LP, et al (2000). Cartilaginous airway wall dimensions and airway resistance in cystic fibrosis. *Eur Resp J*, 15, 735 - 742.

van der Schans CP (1997). Forced expiratory manoeuvres to increase transport of the bronchial mucus: a mechanistic approach. *Monaldi Arch Chest Dis*, 52, 367 - 370.

van der Schans CP, Prasad A, Main E (2000). Chest physiotherapy compared to no chest physiotherapy for cystic fibrosis. Cochrane Database of Systematic Reviews, Issue 2. Art. No.: CD001401. DOI: 10.1002/14651858.CD001401

van der Schans CP (2007). Conventional chest physical therapy for Obstructive Lung Disease. *Respir Care*, 52, 1198 - 1206.

Vestbo J, Prescott E, Lange P (1996). Association of chronic mucus hypersecretion with FEV_1 decline and chronic obstructive pulmonary disease morbidity. Copenhagen City Heart Study Group. *Am J Respir Crit Care Med*, 153, 1530 - 1535

Volsko TA, DiFiore JM, Chatburn RL (2003). Performance comparison of two oscillating positive expiratory pressure devices: Acapella versus Flutter. *Respir Care,* 48, 124 - 130.

Von Leden H, Isshiki N (1965). An analysis of cough at the level of the larynx. *Arch Otolaryngol*, 81, 616 - 625.

Voynow JA, Rubin BK. (2009). Mucins, mucus and sputum. *Chest,* 135, 505 - 512.

Wanner A, Salathe´ M, O'Riordan TG (1996). Mucociliary clearance in the airways. *Am J Respir Crit Care Med* 154, 1868 - 1902

Weibel ER (1984). The Pathway of Oxygen. Cambridge, Mass: Harvard University Press.

Wood RE, Wanner A, Hirsch J, Di Sant'Agnese (1975). Tracheal mucociliary transport in patients with cystic fibrosis and its stimulation by terbutaline. *Am Rev Respir Dis,* 111, 733 - 738.

Woolcock AJ (1998). Effects of drugs on small airways. *Am J Respir Crit Care Med*, 157 (Suppl 5), S203 - S207

Yankaskas JR, Marshall BC, Sufian B, Simon RH, Rodman D (2004). Cystic fibrosis adult care: consensus conference report. *Chest*, 125, 1 (Suppl), 1S - 39S.

Yeates DB, Sturgess JM, Kahn SR, Levison H, Aspin N. (1976). Mucociliary transport in trachea of patients with cystic fibrosis. *Arch Dis Child,* 51, 28 - 33.

Zahm JM, King M, Duvivier C, Pierrot D, Girod S, Puchelle E. (1991). Role of simulated repetitive coughing in mucus clearance. *Eur Respir J,* 4, 311 - 315.

Zapatal A, Motoyama EK, Gibson LE, Bouhuys A. (1971). Pulmonary mechanics in asthma and cystic fibrosis. *Pediatrics,* 48, 64 - 72.

23

The Physiotherapist's Use of Exercise in the Management of Young People with Cystic Fibrosis

Allison Mandrusiak and Pauline Watter
The University of Queensland, Division of Physiotherapy
Australia

1. Introduction

The aim of this chapter is to provide an overview of how physiotherapists (physical therapists) can use exercise in their management of young people with cystic fibrosis (CF), assisting the multidisciplinary team to optimise outcomes for this population. While many resources provide management information about the CF health condition, the focus is often on medical management. However, physiotherapists play an integral role in the multidisciplinary team being at the coalface of daily intervention for this population. Consequently, their role - supported by contemporary evidence - must be considered in the holistic approach to management. In this chapter we will briefly discuss the physiotherapists' general management of people with CF, with the focus directed towards the role of exercise in this management regimen.

This chapter explores the benefits of exercise to this population, and considers the factors limiting exercise performance in young people. A review of the previous studies of exercise intervention programs for people with CF in inpatient and outpatient settings will be provided, and issues affecting adherence and clinical applicability will be discussed. A novel exercise program the *Cystic Fibrosis Fitness Challenge* was developed by Mandrusiak & Watter et al. (2009c) and was specifically designed to address the limitations described in the literature. Aspects of this program and its accompanying *FitKit*$_{TM}$ will be presented in this chapter, with an exploration of how the International Classification of Function, Disability and Health – Children and Youth (ICF-CY) (World Health Organization, 2007) was used to frame the selection of performance measures and program elements. Relationships between exercise and other physiotherapy measures commonly reported for this population will also be considered, since applying the ICF framework, we can expect to find relationships between measures within and between domains. For example, impaired cardiorespiratory function may relate to reduced exercise tolerance, which then may be associated with limited activity and restricted participation. However, weak muscles due to decreased activity may also contribute to limited activity, suggesting that management needs to consider impairment, limitations and restrictions holistically rather than as separate issues.

1.1 The ICF framework for describing performance in young people with cystic fibrosis: A basis of design for exercise intervention

This chapter is scoped within the framework of the International Classification of Functioning, Disability and Health - Children and Youth (ICF-CY) (World Health Organization, 2007) which is an extension of the original framework developed in 2001 (World Health Organization, 2001). Because CF is a multifactorial health condition and usually utilizes a team management approach, the ICF-CY provides an excellent framework for a holistic description of assessments, to direct intervention and identify overlaps and gaps in management. In conjunction with family- or client-centred practice, this contemporary approach considers the client with the health condition of CF and their family as the center of management. Of specific interest to physiotherapists in their management of those with CF, relevant *body structures and functions* would include respiratory function, muscle strength and range of motion, *activities* would include motor skills and functional capacity, and *participation* would include activities of daily life at school, home and in leisure pursuits. Further, *contextual factors* include environmental and personal factors (for example, age, gender, inpatient/outpatient status and attitudes towards exercise) and are also considered within this framework. The theoretical underpinnings of the ICF framework state that performance on measures *within* a domain may be related, and further that relationships may exist in measures of performance *between* domains. This implies that changes in respiratory function (*body structures and functions* domain) may be associated with changes in muscle strength (*body structures and functions* domain). Such associations will guide selection of both assessment measures and interventions. As a between-domain example, improvements in respiratory function are expected to relate to improvements in distance walked in the six-minute walk test (*activities* domain) or sports played at school (*participations* domain). Overall, it is proposed that these interactions will provide an important foundation for comprehensive investigation of the performance of young people with CF, and for exploring the impact of contextual factors on their function (Mandrusiak et al., 2009b). Understanding these relationships will provide a strong evidence-base to direct physiotherapy.

2. The focus of the physiotherapist in the management of individuals with cystic fibrosis

The physiotherapist is considered a cornerstone member of the CF multidisciplinary team, and conventionally their management aims to reduce the respiratory impairments related to this health condition by clearing thick, tenacious secretions from the airways (Farbotko et al., 2005). To achieve this, physiotherapy has traditionally focused on airway clearance techniques, and more recently, attention has been given to the integral role of exercise to enhance management and achieve better outcomes across the now extended lifespan of those with CF. In addition, now that we understand the range of impairments that include musculoskeletal issues such as impaired strength (de Meer et al., 1999; de Jong et al., 2001; Hussey et al., 2002) and range of motion (Mandrusiak et al., 2010) , which limit activity and restrict participation in those with CF, physiotherapists are better placed to provide broad based intervention at all levels of the ICF to facilitate optimal outcomes and reduce barriers to participation by these affected children.

The theoretical basis for airway clearance techniques is included elsewhere in this text and will not be considered here. 'Passive' techniques of postural drainage, percussion and vibration, were traditionally the mainstay of respiratory physiotherapy management. These applications were "done to" the individual with CF, and while these techniques continue to play an important role, more active techniques are now available such as the active cycle of breathing technique and positive expiratory pressure devices, as well as inhalation therapy and thoracic mobility exercises (McIlwaine, 2007). This now emphasizes the role of the individual with CF and the family (especially in the case of the young person) in being an active member of the management team and proactively participating in their own treatment, using a "done with the client" or "selected by the client" philosophy. With this trend to encompass more dynamic techniques as a consequence of emerging evidence, physiotherapy now emphasizes the importance of physical exercise as an adjunct to traditional airway clearance techniques. In CF, exercise has other benefits addressing the unique complications which are emerging as longevity improves, such as impairments in posture and bone mineral density. A diagram of the ICF-CY representing the physiotherapists' perspective of possible interventions relevant to the young person with CF is provided below (Figure 1).

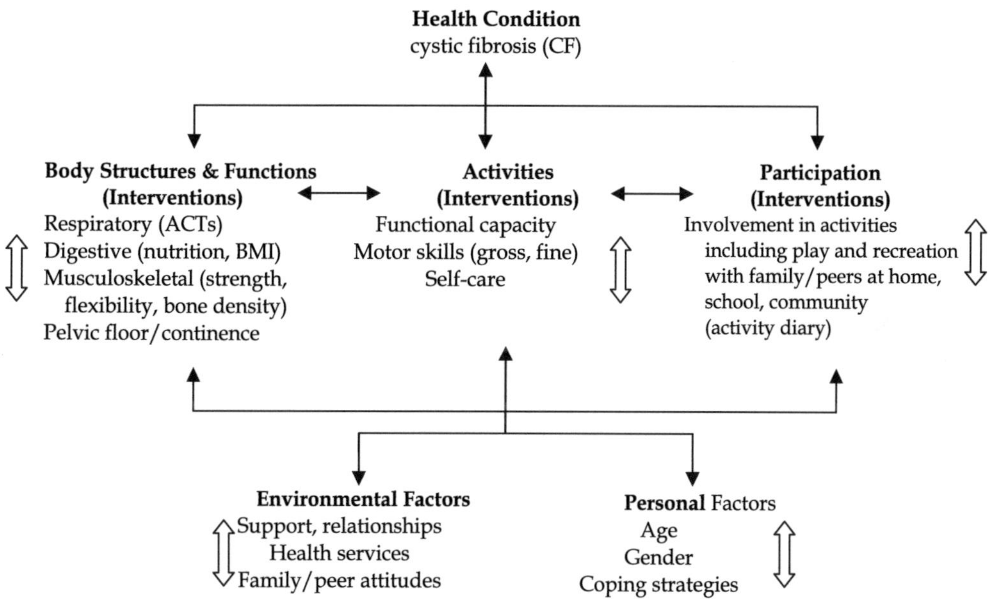

Fig. 1. The ICF-CY (World Health Organisation, 2007): adapted to include possible interventions relevant to the young person with CF.

2.1 Benefits of exercise for people with cystic fibrosis

On the most basic level, exercise is regarded as a natural daily activity for young people, and allows participation in the typical play activities of childhood as well as life-long leisure activities. Ideally, those with CF would be able to partake in exercise with its attendant benefits, and consequently engagement in exercise should be an expectation or goal as well as part of their management. Beyond this basic premise, research and evaluation in the clinical setting has earned exercise its place in the routine management of people with CF (Dodd & Prasad, 2005). Exercise has long been promoted as an essential element of the care for people with CF because exercise intolerance has always been a trait of disease progression (Orenstein and Higgins, 2005). It is therefore crucial to recognize that participation in regular physical activity is a positive prognostic factor in this population (Nixon et al., 1992). Consequently, promoting exercise for people with CF has become an integral aspect of practice, and its prescription must be based on best evidence.

Cooper (1998 p143) believes the physiological influences of exercise suggest its *"profound and important role as therapy"* for people with CF, and exercise programs show potential to be *"an elegant and natural way to stimulate and/or promote the expression of beneficial genes"*. More globally, the psychosocial changes from exercise validate its *"multidimensional impact for people with CF"* (Klijn et al., 2004 p1303). Thus the possibility of potentially modifying the clinical course of the CF health condition by an *"intervention as simple, cheap, safe and enjoyable as exercise remains appealing"* (Barker et al., 2004 p351).

A recent overview of Cochrane systematic reviews performed by Bradley and Moran (2008) summarised the evidence for physical training (exercise) for people with CF. Seven trials using randomised parallel-group design were included, with a total of 231 participants including children and adults. Three studies included children only (Selvadurai et al., 2002; Klijn et al., 2004; Turchetta et al., 2004), and two notable studies included adults and children (Cerny, 1989; Schneiderman-Walker et al., 2000). Overall, these trials showed some evidence of benefits of short- and long-term physical training for people with CF, and this was also the conclusion provided by other reviews in the field (Smidt et al., 2005; Bradley et al., 2006; Shoemaker and Hurt, 2008).

While the effectiveness of exercise intervention programs for this population has traditionally been determined by reduced impairment in body structures and functions (particularly respiratory function) and reduced activity limitations (such as greater six-minute walk distance), the role of exercise for promoting more holistic changes in function is increasingly being recognised. With increased longevity of people with CF, the prevalence of secondary musculoskeletal complications is increasing (Massery, 2005) and must be considered as part of their presentation. This supports the important role of physiotherapy beyond affecting airway clearance, and strengthens the need for an holistic approach which incorporates exercise for prevention or management of secondary musculoskeletal changes (Dodd & Prasad, 2005; Lannefors, 2004; Massery, 2005) to enhance client outcomes. This approach would include addressing range of motion, muscle strength, power and endurance, as well as strong promotion of physical activity. The ICF-CY provides a framework against which such parameters and relationships can be considered.

Further, improving a child's activity and participation are recognized as important goals of exercise intervention for this population, to maintain fitness and thus curtail the cycle of deconditioning associated with this health condition (Stanghelle, 1988; Stevens and Williams, 2007). Importantly, participation in regular physical activity is associated with many holistic benefits, such as improved quality of life and wellbeing (Boas, Danduran, & McColley, 1999; Orenstein, Nixon, Ross, & Kaplan, 1989; Selvadurai et al., 2002). The ICF-CY model facilitates exploration of the impact of exercise intervention on these wider aspects of functioning.

2.2 Providing exercise opportunities across inpatient and outpatient settings: Research supporting advances in practice

Although the performance of exercise is now an integral component of the management of young people with CF, the most effective style of exercise program across inpatient and outpatient settings is yet to be established. During hospitalization, young people with CF are often segregated to minimize cross-infection of respiratory pathogens (Cystic Fibrosis Trust, 2001; Koch et al., 2003), and this presents practical challenges for physiotherapy exercise intervention (Hind et al., 2008). In consequence, it is clear that physiotherapy exercise programs must be adaptable to the limited space at the hospital bedside for performance by individuals in isolation who cannot participate in group exercise sessions or share exercise equipment in the gym. Development of tailored programs which provide a variety of physical activities has been identified as an important aspect to enhance adherence to exercise in this population (Holzer et al., 1984; Blomquist et al., 1986; Stanghelle, 1988; Salh et al., 1989; Abbott et al., 1996; Britto et al., 2000; Schneiderman-Walker et al., 2000; Moorcroft et al., 2004; Turchetta et al., 2004), and such programs must be evidence-based to target issues characteristic of young people with CF.

Developing attractive and efficacious inpatient programs is a challenge in itself, but as highlighted by Moorcroft, Dodd, Morris and Webb (2004) and Dodd and Prasad (2005), transferring exercise programs to the outpatient setting and sustaining them in the long term is also a challenge in the CF population. Physical activity and prescribed exercises are a permanent part of living for those with CF and compliance leading to optimal outcomes is difficult to sustain. Despite these challenges, a range of literature supports the incorporation of outpatient exercise programs in the management of young people with CF. As CF is a lifelong health condition, and the benefits of exercise are well established, strategies to enhance exercise performance across the lifespan are imperative. However, the impact on health resources and clients' distances from established hospital centres make it difficult to facilitate long term supervised hospital-based outpatient exercise programs (Schneiderman-Walker et al., 2000), and sustainable programs based outside of the hospital are needed (Moorcroft et al., 2004).

During outpatient periods, there is support for home-based exercise programs rather than hospital-based programs (Bar-Or, 2000; Bernard & Cohen, 2004; Moorcroft et al., 2004; Schneiderman-Walker et al., 2000; Turchetta et al., 2004). These need to be engaging for the young person with CF, especially if s/he is to continue with these activities as an outpatient once discharged from hospital acute care. Further, it is believed that exercise programs in hospital are not attractive for young people, and that home-based programs are more acceptable (Turchetta et al., 2004). Physical activity should be enjoyable and natural, rather than bear the stigma of therapy, and this may be better achieved in the home environment (Bar-Or, 2000). Further, it is likely that home-based exercise programs save the family time and expense (Bar-Or, 2000) and are more feasible (Bernard and Cohen, 2004). Therefore, research is warranted to establish effective home-based outpatient exercise programs, and facilitate client transition into these programs from the inpatient setting.

2.2.1 Recommendations for exercise programs for young people with cystic fibrosis: Linkages to development of a novel exercise program

A summary of systematic reviews of exercise across a range of populations (Smidt et al., 2005) indicated that targeted and individualized exercise programs were more beneficial than standardized programs. In a Position Statement published by the *Australian Physiotherapy Association* (Taylor et al., 2006) the important skills of the physiotherapist for prescribing exercise are highlighted as three major dimensions: management of disorders of movement, knowledge of exercise regimens and dosages, and clinical reasoning skills to ensure that exercises are optimal for the individual. Specifically for young people with CF, exercise programs should be tailored to individual needs, as there is considerable variability in terms of disease severity, fitness, enthusiasm and preference for types of activities (Webb & Dodd, 1999; Prasad and Cerny, 2002).

To address the aforementioned needs, the *Cystic Fibrosis Fitness Challenge* (*CFFC*) developed by Mandrusiak & Watter et al. (2009c) is a targeted exercise program for use in inpatient and outpatient settings, based on recommendations from the field. Part of this innovative exercise program is a portable exercise tool (*FitKit*™) that is adaptable to limited space environments such as at the hospital bedside in the inpatient setting. The design aspects of this novel program and tools are presented in Section 2.3.

Although specific guidelines are not currently reported, it is recommended that all people with CF should be encouraged to exercise 'several times per week' (Yankaskas et al., 2004), and across the lifespan (Thoracic Society of Australia and New Zealand 2007). Specifically, exercise for *young people* with CF should be viewed as fun as well as therapy and its role should be regarded equally from the young person's point of view as well as a clinical mandate from the multidisciplinary team (Webb & Dodd, 1999). Exercises must be stimulating, age-appropriate and enjoyable, and varied to avoid monotony as well as to avoid overuse injuries (Stanghelle, 1988). Further, prescription of exercise programs should be timely, and appropriate for different settings including within the hospital and the home (Lannefors, 2004). The exercise program must be realistic and allow for the treatment demand and time pressures faced by young people with CF and their families each day, and thus the program must integrate into their lifestyle (Moorcroft et al., 2004). Enthusiasm from the multidisciplinary team members towards exercise and a flexible approach to encouraging physical activities should not be underestimated (Moorcroft et al., 2004).

Educational dialogue is also recommended, as knowledge of the CF health condition and reasons for treatment are associated with increased adherence (Gardner, 2004; Hinton et al., 2002; Prasad & Cerny, 2002). Educational resources must be age-appropriate and thus attractive and colourful (Hinton et al., 2002; Gardner, 2004). These recommendations were integrated into the design of the resources and delivery of the *CFFC* described in Section 2.3.

The ideal elements of exercise programs for this population are presented in the literature, and include: endurance and strength training for the upper and lower limbs; aerobic and anaerobic activities; interval training; weight bearing activities; and flexibility exercises (Webb & Dodd, 2000; Selvadurai et al., 2002; Klijn et al., 2004; Dodd & Prasad, 2005; Bradley et al., 2006; Sahlberg, 2008). As well as addressing the function across these multiple areas, providing a variety of activity types makes it possible to individually tailor the program according to the young person's preferences, thereby improving exercise participation (Klijn et al., 2004). These elements were considered and incorporated into the *CFFC* program.

As recommended by Rogers, Prasad and Doull (2003), intensity of exercise performance should be derived from results of exercise testing. The *"Clinical Guidelines for the Physiotherapy Management of Cystic Fibrosis: Recommendations of a Working Group"* (Cystic Fibrosis Trust, 2002) recognize that no specific information exists for exercise program intensity and duration for people with CF, and that general recommendations for the 'normal' population are used. These include an intensity of 70-85% of peak heart rate (Orenstein et al., 1981), starting with a duration of exercise classified as 'tolerable' and progressing to 20 to 30 minutes, three- to four-days per week. However, these *Clinical Guidelines* also highlight the differences between children and adults, in relation to exercise ability, indicating that prescriptions for adults may not be appropriate for young people. These differences include: differences in growth, muscle and fat; higher respiratory rate and heart rate; inferior cooling mechanisms; increased energy expenditure and increased reliance on fat metabolism (Cystic Fibrosis Trust, 2002). In young people, strength training must be properly performed, planned and not over-strenuous, as growing bones are sensitive to stress (especially repetitive loading) and the epiphysial plate is susceptible to injury before full growth is complete (Behm et al., 2008). To further minimize these risks it is important to provide a variety of activities to ensure joints are not subjected to repetitive stress (Stanghelle, 1988). Therefore, exercise programs for young people with CF should be specifically designed for this age group, and not just based on those designed for adults.

The health condition of CF affects quality of life in adults mainly due to dyspnea and limitations in exercise capacity which lead to limitations in physical functioning (de Jong et al., 1997). Thus, programs which aim to improve exercise capacity and thus reduce dyspnea may impact positively on quality of life, and it is important to incorporate these strategies into programs for younger people with CF to optimise quality of life across the lifespan.

2.2.2 Fostering adherence to exercise programs in young people with cystic fibrosis

While maintaining adherence to medications and dietary schedules is difficult in the young person with CF and considered elsewhere in this text, our focus as physiotherapists is on fostering adherence to respiratory physiotherapy programs and exercise programs especially as the child with CF enters adolescence and may expect to experience greater autonomy. Overall, people with CF prefer exercise to other components of therapy (Abbott, Dodd, Bilton, & Webb, 1994; Moorcroft et al., 2004; Moorcroft, Dodd, & Webb, 1998), regarding it as a socially acceptable 'normal activity'(Prasad and Cerny, 2002; Orenstein and Higgins, 2005), and an area over which they have control (Abbott et al., 1996). Importantly, adherence to exercise is higher than adherence to respiratory physiotherapy (Schneiderman-Walker et al., 2000). Thus, the integral role of exercise for people with CF is strengthened by its positive perception, which is important to maintaining interest and adherence across the lifespan.

Despite this reported positive perception towards exercise as therapy, the issue of treatment adherence is a growing concern for multidisciplinary CF teams (Kettler et al., 2002). This discrepancy represents a missing link between viewing exercise positively, and adhering to exercise programs. Adherence is a complex and multidimensional issue (Hobbs et al., 2003) and a detailed review is beyond the scope of this chapter. Instead, key literature in the field of adherence to exercise in young people with CF is presented, to provide strategies for the intervention exercise programs presented here.

Non-adherence to exercise programs may lead to wasted resources, reduced quality of life, missed days at school/work, and higher health care costs (Ireland, 2003; Modi and Quittner, 2003) and thus focusing attention on increasing exercise adherence in this population is critical (Bernard and Cohen, 2004). As children progress into adolescence, the desire to have more control over their lives and a tendency to rebel against authority often result in problems with adherence (Gudas et al., 1991). While strategies to improve adherence in adolescents with CF are integral, it is critical to instill knowledge about exercise during early childhood to enhance adherence into later life stages (Bernard and Cohen, 2004). People tend to look to the short- rather than the long-term benefits of treatment to decide whether to continue (Abbott et al., 1994), so strategies that track progress and improvement in exercise performance, such as log books, pedometry and field tests, may enhance perception of the short-term benefits, and thus enhance adherence.

The multidisciplinary CF team should provide universal support, continued encouragement and education to reinforce the message to the young person and their family that exercise is an important part of treatment (Boas et al., 1999; Dodd & Prasad, 2005; Prasad & Cerny, 2002). Specifically, the role of the physiotherapist for people with CF has been described as that of educator, clinician, researcher and manager (Ireland 2003). The role of educator is particularly important, as empowering patients through education positively affects adherence to treatment and thus health outcomes (Gudas et al., 1991; Hinton et al., 2002; Prasad and Cerny, 2002; Ireland, 2003; Gardner, 2004). Patients are influenced by their own internal belief system; any information or required action needs to make sense and be justifiable to them (Carr et al., 1996). To this end, there is an increasing focus on informing patients and involving them in healthcare decisions (Hinton et al., 2002), and patients should be 'fully involved in any decision-making process during treatment planning' (Chartered Society of Physiotherapy 2000: 8.1). Therefore, using exercise programs that include educational strategies and incorporate the individual in tailoring the exercise program are essential for the physiotherapist to enhance adherence across the lifespan.

An older study by Carr et al. (1996) found that many people with CF (>16 years) did not perceive physiotherapists as having a role in tailoring exercise programs for them. Further, it is reported that exercise prescriptions are often presented in a general manner, without clear specifications of parameters such as frequency and duration (Hobbs et al., 2003). Lannefors (2004) advised that recommending patients to be "physically active" is not enough, and that more active guidance and continuing encouragement is needed. These important findings and the developing evidence base suggest now that physiotherapists need to take a more active involvement in promoting exercise, and in individualizing and monitoring the effects of these programs to strengthen their role in management. Currently, best practice physiotherapy would enhance knowledge of the young person and their family to facilitate ongoing compliance.

The role of parents in influencing their child's participation in exercise is well documented. Lack of parental support towards physical activity may lead to a reduction in regular exercise (Boas et al., 1999), and considering the established relationship between fitness and prognosis (Nixon et al., 1992; Pianosi et al., 2005), this issue of parent education is of particular relevance. Attitudes toward exercise may be acquired as part of life experience and social support, and with parental encouragement to participate are especially important factors (Baker and Wideman, 2006). Further, parents with an ethos of active personal lifestyle facilitate the young person to be active (Dodd & Prasad, 2005). Education of the family is paramount: a study by Boas et al. (1999) reported that parents of young people with CF perceived fewer benefits of, and greater barriers to exercise than parents of healthy young people, and that less than half of parents in the CF group understood the long term benefits of exercise or knew that exercise performance was related to long term prognosis. However, this education may be improving, as a recent questionnaire provided to 50 young people with CF (8-18 years) and their parents showed they had "substantial exercise knowledge" (Higgins et al., 2007). Overall, there is a need for ongoing comprehensive education of the young person and their family regarding the role of exercise, to achieve optimal outcomes of intervention.

Behavioural strategies to increase adherence to exercise in young people with CF have shown some promise (Bernard & Cohen, 2004; Tuzin et al., 1998). These strategies include self-monitoring, exercising with a partner, behavioural contracting, goal-setting, contingency management, and praise and differential attention. Some of these strategies were incorporated to optimise adherence to the *CFFC* exercise program described in Section 2.3.

As outlined in a review by Dodd and Prasad (2005), there are several perceived barriers to exercise, including unsupportive parental attitudes towards exercise (Boas et al., 1999) and unacceptability of rigid training programs (Gulmans et al., 1999). Further, the daily treatment burden and fatigue associated with the CF health condition make adherence to recommended exercise programs more difficult (Prasad and Cerny, 2002), and this population receives relatively little positive reinforcement for efforts to adhere to treatment (Kettler et al., 2002). This is a driver for physiotherapists when individualizing exercise programs for this population, to ensure integration of physical activity into daily life instead of imposing 'extra' treatment, and to provide appropriate positive reinforcement for participation in exercise. As per the ICF-CY, parents have best impact when facilitatory behaviours towards exercise are displayed.

Specific recommendations for optimising adherence to exercise programs developed for young people with CF are presented in the literature. It is recognised that young people participate more consistently in programs that include a variety of activities, recreational elements and fun (Blomquist et al., 1986), particularly individualized programs which employ activities based on personal preference and perceived competence (Abbott et al., 1996; Britto, Garrett, Konrad, Majure, & Leigh, 2000; Holzer et al., 1984; Moorcroft et al., 2004; Salh et al., 1989; Schneiderman-Walker et al., 2000; Turchetta et al., 2004). In contrast, when the program is regimented, prescribed at an incorrect intensity or not age-appropriate, adherence tends to be poor (Gulmans et al, 1999). Further, programs delivered with specific information about optimal frequency and duration will enhance adherence (Hobbs et al., 2003). An individualised program will facilitate incorporation of regular exercise into their daily life and an already demanding treatment routine (Klijn et al., 2004; Moorcroft et al., 2004). These suggestions to enhance adherence were considered in the development of the exercise program presented later in this chapter.

In summary, addressing adherence issues is paramount to the effectiveness of exercise programs, particularly in a population already burdened by many daily treatments. The multidisciplinary CF team, particularly physiotherapists, must provide support and enthusiasm to promote exercise performance. Educational dialogue is paramount, and should be targeted at the level of the young person with CF and their family. Individualized exercise programs that provide a variety of activities based on the young person's preference and competence, and that allow tracking of personal progress, are more likely to succeed. Overall, this highlights the importance of promoting effective and tailored exercise regimes for young people with CF, and it is vital to include strategies aimed at improving and encouraging adherence.

2.3 A novel approach to facilitating exercise for young people with cystic fibrosis

As outlined above, exercise is a central feature of management in youth with CF due to its positive effects in reducing impairments in cardiorespiratory and musculoskeletal structures and functions, increasing activity and facilitating participation, acknowledging that individual contextual factors may also impact. In response to current clinical challenges and to recommendations in the literature, we developed a novel program (the *Cystic Fibrosis Fitness Challenge* (*CFFC*), and accompanying *FitKit*™) to facilitate performance of exercise integrated into daily life for young people with CF, and design aspects of this program are presented in this section.

The *FitKit*™ (Figure 2) was developed as a portable, tailored resource designed to facilitate exercise performance in a variety of settings - the bedside, gym, inpatient and outpatient - representing an effective tool for physiotherapists working with young people with CF. The portable design of the *FitKit*™ and overall *CFFC* is particularly appropriate in the hospital setting, to support exercise performance where space issues are increasingly common due to segregation of patients for infection control. A variety of exercise elements was included in this program, supported by previous studies in the field, and by findings from earlier studies by Mandrusiak and Watter et al. (2009c) into the presentation of young people with CF in the context of the ICF-CY. A pool of 100 activities presented on colour-coded Activity Cards was developed to address each of the exercise components of aerobic, anaerobic, strength and flexibility. The program facilitator pre-selected the Activity Cards suitable for each participant, and then worked with the participant to select those that they enjoyed, at the same time achieving the therapeutic goals. The *CFFC* involved a 30-60 minute session each weekday over the course of a usual 10-14 day inpatient period, and independently 3-5 days per week at home (outpatient period). Clear guidelines were developed to guide the program facilitators to achieve optimal implementation of the *CFFC*.

A Physical Activity Log (PAL) was designed for participants to record activities performed in each session, during inpatient and outpatient phases of management. Demonstrations for completing the PAL during the inpatient period were provided by the program facilitator, progressing towards self-completion prior to discharge. Information documented in the PAL included exercise type, intensity (for example, heart rate, level of perceived exertion or breathlessness), duration / repetitions, enjoyment level of the activity, limiting factors, pedometry score, and quality and quantity of the sputum expectorated. A sticker system was integrated whereby participants received a gold star for vigorous intensity activities, and a coloured star for moderate intensity activities. This system provided visual feedback and positive reinforcement regarding the intensity and appropriateness of activities performed, and encouraged participants to monitor and progress performance. Also, the PAL provided visual reminders to the participant to ensure adequate hydration during each session. Educational strategies were incorporated into the resources in the *FitKit*™ to increase awareness within this population about the role of exercise (Gudas et al., 1991; Hinton et al., 2002; Prasad and Cerny, 2002; Ireland, 2003; Gardner, 2004) during inpatient and outpatient periods, with emphasis on monitoring exercise intensity (heart rate, and to be aware of exertion and breathlessness levels) to ensure inclusion of activities of vigorous intensity. Overall, the *FitKit*™ is feasible, utilizing inexpensive and readily available resources and equipment (Figure 2), which has significant clinical implications (Orenstein & Higgins, 2005).

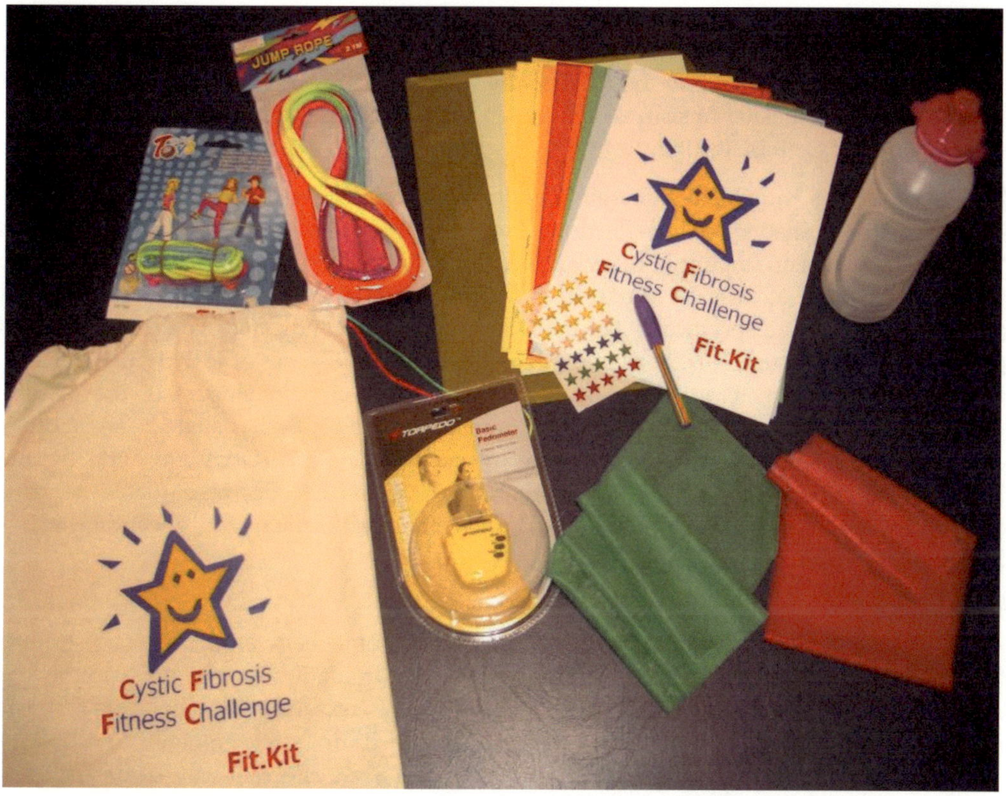

Fig. 2. The portable *FitKit*™ used in the *Cystic Fibrosis Fitness Challenge* program

The *CFFC* program provides an evidence-based novel approach to facilitating performance of physiotherapy exercise programs, across both inpatient and outpatient settings. A randomised controlled trial (Mandrusiak & Watter et al., 2009c) showed the effectiveness of this program during inpatient (10-14 days) and outpatient (8-12 weeks) phases of management in a group of young people with CF 7-17 years of age (n=31).

To summarize the recommendations that have been integrated into the design and delivery of this program, the *CFFC* provided a variety of age-appropriate activities that can be tailored to individual preferences across inpatient and outpatient (home) settings, incorporating education, communication and behavior modification strategies. The overall aim is to enhance integration of physical activity into daily life, and thus achieve long term adherence and optimal outcomes. Individualized exercise programs that provide a variety of activities based on the young person's preference and competence, and that allow tracking of personal progress, are more likely to succeed, and these elements were embedded into the design of the *CFFC* and *FitKit*™.

2.4 Overview of the role of exercise testing for young people with cystic fibrosis: What do physiotherapists measure?

A holistic range of measures which map to all of the ICF domains described above are provided by various professionals in the team managing those with CF, including measures of respiratory function, diet, medication, musculoskeletal function, as well as activity and quality of life. The physiotherapist is not necessarily involved in collecting them all, but is most likely to collect data about body structures and functions such as respiratory function tests and musculoskeletal measures, activity and functional exercise capacity. The focus of this section is on exercise testing.

Exercise testing is the global assessment of the response to exercise, and is an important parameter that is inadequately reflected by resting respiratory function tests (Baraldi and Carraro, 2006). It is an important outcome measure (Stevens and Williams, 2007) which may be more sensitive to disease progression and survival than respiratory function tests (McIlwaine, 2007), and specifically, aerobic fitness is a reliable indicator of disease status and prognosis (Nixon et al., 1992). For young people with CF, measures of activity performance and exercise testing can provide valuable information about the impact of the disease, functional limitations and trends over time (Rogers et al., 2003; Barker et al., 2004), and it is employed as an outcome variable in some intervention studies (Orenstein and Higgins, 2005). Further, Rogers et al. (2003) suggest that regular exercise testing accentuates the value of exercise to young people with CF and their families, which may encourage active lifestyles.

The guidelines for the *Association of Chartered Physiotherapists in Cystic Fibrosis* (in Rogers et al., 2003) recommend that all young people with CF should have annual exercise testing. Measurements of exercise capacity should provide the foundation for any prescription and adaptation of exercise programs (Rogers et al., 2003). Currently, exercise capacity is assessed using a range of laboratory- and clinically-based tools including cycle ergometry, walk tests, step tests and shuttle tests. Debate remains as to the most effective way of determining exercise capacity (Rogers et al., 2003), and some of the most commonly used measures are discussed below.

2.4.1 Maximal and submaximal tests of capacity

Maximum oxygen consumption (VO_2max) is the best index of aerobic capacity, and is significantly correlated with subsequent survival in people with CF (Pianosi et al., 2005). VO_2max is the "gold standard" measure of cardiorespiratory fitness, and maximal tests are performed in a laboratory using cycle ergometry or treadmills (Bruce, 1971). However, a number of factors limit the application of maximal tests to young people. Firstly, most daily activities are not performed at maximal levels and instead are at moderate intensities interspersed with short bursts of high intensity activities (Bailey et al., 1995), thus using maximal tests may not provide a realistic simulation of a young person's physical capacity (Chetta et al., 2001; Rogers et al., 2003; Solway, Brooks, Lacasse, & Thomas, 2001). Secondly, maximal tests are tiring and the physiological stress of testing, as well as the possible safety risks and expense to the patient, may outweigh the information gained (Nixon et al., 1996), and many young people with CF are reluctant to perform them (Rogers et al., 2003). Thirdly, data from maximal exercise tests may not be reproducible (Stevens and Williams, 2007). Finally, these tests are usually performed by specialist respiratory personnel and require sophisticated laboratory equipment that may need to be modified for young people and may not be available in all institutions (Orenstein, 1998; McIlwaine, 2007). In view of these issues, maximal exercise testing is currently outside the scope of routine clinical physiotherapy practice (Thoracic Society of Australia and New Zealand, 2007), and is not discussed further here.

According to Braggion (1989), submaximal field tests are better tools than maximal cycle ergometry or treadmill tests to evaluate a range of parameters including cardiorespiratory adaptations to exercise, motor aspects of performance (including agility, muscle strength and range of motion), and motivation to perform. Further, while field-based exercise tests do not always determine a person's maximal exercise response, they can give valuable clinical information on factors that limit activity performance on a day-to-day basis (Noonan and Dean, 2000; Narang et al., 2003; Rogers et al., 2003). Field tests are attractive to clinicians and researchers as they provide easy to administer and inexpensive forms of exercise assessment using typical activities of daily living such as walking (Orenstein, 1998). These can be undertaken outside of formal testing laboratories which may promote a less stressful environment for the young person (Cox et al., 2006) and some are useful in the research context where portable tools can provide follow-up information without the need for repeated visits to hospital facilities. Further, there is some evidence that young people with CF prefer field tests to formal exercise tests (Selvadurai et al., 2003). However, it is important to recognize that some information which is detected by more complex exercise tests may be missed by simple field tests (Narang et al., 2003).

In summary, young people rarely engage in sustained, heavy exercise, suggesting that traditional maximal exercise tests may not represent their patterns of daily physical activity (Cooper, 1995). Submaximal tests may better simulate childhood activities and thus provide insight into their functional capacity. These performance measures must be simple and convenient to use in order to be applicable to a variety of settings, such as the clinic, the hospital bedside and in the field (Narang et al., 2003), and such tests include walk tests, step tests and jump tests.

2.4.1.1 Walk tests

A variety of walk tests exist, but the six-minute walk test (6MWT) (Butland et al., 1982) is endorsed as the safest and easiest to administer, and it is better tolerated and better reflects activities of daily living than other walk tests such as the shuttle walk test (American Thoracic Society, 2002). It is an important clinical assessment tool, since it provides a composite assessment of respiratory, cardiac and metabolic systems during exercise (Li et al., 2005). It is self-paced and assesses the submaximal level of functional capacity, where the participant chooses their own level of intensity (American Thoracic Society, 2002). This self-paced nature may more closely reflect functional performance than externally paced exercise tests such as shuttle tests (Solway et al., 2001). Further, the use of a standard time (six-minutes) rather than a predetermined distance provides a better measure of endurance (McGavin et al., 1976).

Butland et al. (1982) revised the original 12 Minute Walk Test, to better accommodate patients with respiratory disease for whom walking for 12 minutes is too exhausting. The resulting 6MWT was found to perform as well as the 12 minute walk test, and is now a widely used measure for young people with CF, as it is reproducible (Gulmans et al., 1996; Balfour-Lynn et al., 1998; Cunha et al., 2006; Mandrusiak et al., 2009a), valid (Gulmans et al., 1996) and easy to perform in young people with CF (Cunha et al., 2006). It has been studied in a range of CF cohorts including inpatients (Mandrusiak et al., 2009a) and outpatients (Butland et al., 1982; Cunha et al., 2006; Gulmans et al., 1996).

The primary measurement is distance walked in six-minutes (6MWD), but data can also be collected about oxygen saturation (SpO_2), heart rate (HR) and breathlessness (Enright, 2003). Also, 'work' can be calculated as distance walked (m) x body weight (kg) (Chuang et al., 2001) and is recommended instead of distance as it more accurately indicates true performance (Cunha et al., 2006).

As summarised by Noonan and Dean (2000), the 6MWT can be employed as a one-time measure of functional capacity, or to measure change in functional capacity over time or in response to intervention. In people with CF, the 6MWT has been validated, being compared with cycle ergometry (Gulmans et al., 1996) and the 3min step test (Balfour-Lynn et al., 1998). A significant improvement in 6MWD was found in young people with CF at completion of hospital treatment for acute respiratory infection (Upton et al., 1988). Although no minimal clinically important difference (MCID) (Guyatt et al., 2002) for 6MWD has been established for the CF population, in adults with chronic obstructive pulmonary disease an improvement of 70 meters walked after an intervention is necessary to be 95% confident that the improvement was significant (Redelmeier et al., 1997).

Li et al. (2005) found a significant correlation between the 6MWD and VO_2max on the treadmill in typical children. It was also reported that in people with CF, 6MWD correlated with VO_2max, physical work capacity and the minimum arterial oxygen saturation (SaO_2) (Nixon et al., 1996), as well as with forced expiratory volume in one second (FEV_1) (Geiger et al., 2007).

Geiger et al. (2007) presented a modified 6MWT in which the participant pushed a measuring wheel, to establish reference values of healthy young people (n=528; 3-17 years). Li et al. (2005) presented height-specific reference values from a cohort of healthy (Chinese) children (n=1445; 7-16 years). 6MWD was related to height in some studies (Nixon et al., 1996; Cunha et al., 2006) but was not in other studies (Bradley et al., 1999), and correlated with weight by Gulmans et al. (1996). Although complete data has not been developed and consensus is not reached on all issues, it is important to consider factors relating to growth when comparing repeated results for young people with CF over time, and also comparing young people with CF to normative values.

A limitation of the 6MWT is that it requires an uninterrupted corridor of at least 30 meters, so is not adaptable to all settings. Consequently, this test may not be suitable for performance at the hospital bedside or in the home, where possible space limitations may not ensure standardized administration. Hence, tests that correlate with the 6MWT but require less space may present attractive alternatives. However, where applicable, the 6MWT appears to be the preferred tool for assessing exercise capacity in young people with CF.

2.4.1.2 Shuttle tests

The modified shuttle walk test as described by Selvadurai et al. (2003) is a symptom-limited exercise test, in which the participant moves from end to end of a 10m course in time with the 'beeps' from a pre-recorded tape. This test is valid in young people with CF (Cox et al., 2006), sensitive to change after hospitalization (Bradley et al., 1999, 2000) and correlates with VO_2max (Rogers et al., 2003). It is a natural activity and easy to administer, but does require 10 meters of uninterrupted space, and its practicality in the clinic setting has been questioned (Balfour-Lynn et al., 1998). Thus, motor tasks which allow more efficient delivery, and are adaptable to a range of clinical environments such as the hospital bedside or the outpatient clinic cubicle, may provide a suitable alternative.

2.4.1.3 Step tests

The three-minute step test is an externally paced, simple and portable test which is independent of effort and validated for use in children over six-years of age (Balfour-Lynn et al., 1998). It detects improvement in exercise capacity following hospitalization (Pike et al., 2001), but its use may be limited in those with well preserved lung function and fitness levels due to a potential ceiling effect (Selvadurai et al., 2003). It is also clear that actual workload will vary according to step height and weight and height of the participant (Selvadurai et al., 2003).

2.4.1.4 Jump tests

Mandrusiak et al. (2009a) established test-retest reliability of two jump tests (Astride Jumps and Forwards-Backwards Jumps) for young people with CF in the inpatient setting, using motor measures (number of jumps, time to fatigue) and physiological measures (heart rate, oxygen saturation via pulse oximetry, Borg Rating of Perceived Breathlessness (Burdon et al., 1982), and 15 Count Breathlessness Score (Prasad et al., 2000)). These jump tests are reflective of the natural activity pattern of typical young people, which is characterized by short bursts of high intensity activity (Bailey et al., 1995), and are particularly appropriate for the clinical setting as they are portable and easy to administer in limited space environments such as at the hospital bedside or outpatient clinic room. The score is the number of jumps performed before fatigue, and this score has been shown to improve significantly after hospitalization in 33 young people with CF (7-17 years) (Wilson et al., 2005). Work is being conducted to establish references for Australian children for such simple activities used in daily life.

In summary, measures of physical performance and exercise capacity are integral to the management of young people with CF. Tests for this population should be non-invasive, simple and quick to administer, inexpensive and applicable to a variety of settings (Cooper, 1998), and reflective of typical activities of childhood. In our experience, children tolerated and enjoyed the 6MWT and jump tests, and these are user-friendly field tests.

3. Conclusion

This chapter concerns the integral role of exercise in the management of young people with CF, providing a contemporary overview of current research and practice as well as the existing limitations and gaps to direct future research. The innovative *Cystic Fibrosis Fitness Challenge* and *FitKit*$_{TM}$ developed by the chapter authors presented a working example of how the ICF-CY framework can direct selection of performance measures and guide development of a program, as well as assessment of effectiveness of the intervention. This contemporary information supports the evidence base for the role of exercise in the management of those with CF and is an essential aspect of the physiotherapy role within the multidisciplinary team.

4. Acknowledgment

The Authors wish to express their sincere gratitude to the staff at the Physiotherapy Department of the Royal Children's Hospital (Brisbane, Australia) and the young people with CF and their families, for their integral role in the studies on which parts of this chapter is based. Some of this work was funded by the Australian Cystic Fibrosis Research Trust PhD Studentship Grant.

5. References

Abbott, J., M. Dodd, D. Bilton, and A.K. Webb. 1994. Treatment Compliance in Adults with Cystic-Fibrosis. *Thorax*. 49:115-120.

Abbott, J., M. Dodd, and A.K. Webb. 1996. Health perceptions and treatment adherence in adults with cystic fibrosis. *Thorax*. 51:1233-1238.

American Thoracic Society. 2002. ATS statement: guidelines for the six-minute walk test. ATS Committee on Proficiency Standards for Clinical Pulmonary Function Laboratories. *American Journal of Respiratory and Critical Care Medicine*. 166:111-117.

Bailey, R.C., J. Olson, S.L. Pepper, J. Porszasz, T.J. Barstow, and D.M. Cooper. 1995. The level and tempo of children's activities: an observational study. *Medicine and Science in Sports and Exercise*. 27:1033-1041.

Baker, C., and L. Wideman. 2006. Attitudes Toward Physical Activity in Adolescents With Cystic Fibrosis: Sex Differences After Training: A Pilot Study. *Journal of Pediatric Nursing*. 21:197 - 210.

Balfour-Lynn, I.M., S.A. Prasad, A. Laverty, B.F. Whitehead, and R. Dinwiddie. 1998. A step in the right direction: Assessing exercise tolerance in cystic fibrosis. *Pediatric Pulmonology*. 25:278-284.

Bar-Or, O. 2000. Home-based exercise programs in cystic fibrosis: Are they worth it? *Journal of Pediatrics*. 136:279-280.

Baraldi, E., and S. Carraro. 2006. Exercise testing and chronic lung diseases in children. *Paediatric Respiratory Reviews*. 7 Suppl 1:S196-198.

Barker, M., A. Hebestreit, W. Gruber, and H. Hebestreit. 2004. Exercise testing and training in German CF centers. *Pediatric Pulmonology*. 37:351-355.

Behm, D.G., A.D. Faigenbaum, B. Falk, and P. Klentrou. 2008. Canadian Society for Exercise Physiology position paper: resistance training in children and adolescents. *Applied*

Physiology, Nutrition, And Metabolism = Physiologie AppliquÃ©e, Nutrition Et MÃ©tabolisme. 33:547-561.

Bernard, R.S., and L.L. Cohen. 2004. Increasing adherence to cystic fibrosis treatment: A systematic review of behavioral techniques. *Pediatric Pulmonology*. 37:8-16.

Blomquist, M., U. Freyschuss, L. Wiman, and B. Strandvik. 1986. Physical activity and self-treatment in cystic fibrosis. *Archives of Disease in Childhood*. 61:362-367.

Boas, S.R., M.J. Danduran, and S.A. McColley. 1999. Parental attitudes about exercise regarding their children with cystic fibrosis. *International Journal of Sports Medicine*. 20:334-338.

Bradley, J., J. Howard, E. Wallace, and S. Elborn. 1999. Validity of a modified shuttle test in adult cystic fibrosis. *Thorax*. 54:437-439.

Bradley, J., J. Howard, E. Wallace, and S. Elborn. 2000. Reliability, repeatability, and sensitivity of the modified shuttle test in adult cystic fibrosis. *Chest*. 117:1666-1671.

Bradley, J., and F. Moran. 2008. Physical training for cystic fibrosis. *Cochrane Database of Systematic Reviews*. doi:DOI: 10.1002/14651858.CD002768.pub2.

Bradley, J., F. Moran, and J. Elborn. 2006. Evidence for physical therapies (airway clearance and physical training) in cystic fibrosis: An overview of five Cochrane systematic reviews. *Respiratory Medicine*. 100:191-201.

Braggion, C., M. Cornacchia, A. Miano, F. Schena, G. Verlato, and G. Mastella. 1989. Exercise Tolerance and Effects of Training in Young Patients with Cystic Fibrosis and Mild Airway Obstruction. *Pediatric Pulmonology*. 7:145-152.

Britto, M.T., J.M. Garrett, T.R. Konrad, J.M. Majure, and M.W. Leigh. 2000. Comparison of physical activity in adolescents with cystic fibrosis versus age-matched controls. *Pediatric Pulmonology*. 30:86-91.

Bruce, R.A. 1971. Exercise testing of patients with coronary heart disease: principles and normal standards. *Ann Clinical Research*.323-332.

Burdon, G.W., E.F. Juniper, K.J. Killian, F.E. Hargreave, and E.J.M. Campbell. 1982. The perception of breathlessness in asthma. *American Review of Respiratory Disease*. 126:825-828.

Butland, R.J.A., J. Pang, E.R. Gross, A.A. Woodcock, and D.M. Geddes. 1982. 2-Minute, 6-Minute, and 12-Minute Walking Tests in Respiratory-Disease. *British Medical Journal*. 284:1607-1608.

Carr, L., R. Smith, J. Pryor, and C. Partridge. 1996. Cystic Fibrosis Patients' Views and Beliefs About Chest Clearance and Exercise -- A pilot study. *Physiotherapy*. 82:621-627.

Cerny, F.J. 1989. Relative Effects of Bronchial Drainage and Exercise for in-Hospital Care of Patients with Cystic-Fibrosis. *Physical Therapy*. 69:633-639.

Chuang, M.L., I.F. Lin, and K. Wasserman. 2001. The body weight-walking distance product as related to lung function, anaerobic threshold and peak VO2 in COPD patients. *Respiratory Medicine*. 95:618-626.

Cooper, D.M. 1995. Rethinking Exercise Testing in Children - a Challenge. *American Journal of Respiratory and Critical Care Medicine*. 152:1154-1157.

Cooper, D.M. 1998. Exercise and cystic fibrosis: The search for a therapeutic optimum. *Pediatric Pulmonology*. 25:143-144.

Cox, N.S., J. Follett, and K.O. McKay. 2006. Modified shuttle test performance in hospitalized children and adolescents with cystic fibrosis. *Journal of Cystic Fibrosis*. 5:165-170.

Cunha, M.T., T. Rozov, R.C. de Oliveira, and J.R. Jardim. 2006. Six-minute walk test in children and adolescents with cystic fibrosis. *Pediatric Pulmonology*. 41:618-622.

Cystic Fibrosis Trust. 2001. Standards for the clinical care of children and adults with cystic fibrosis *In*, London

Cystic Fibrosis Trust. 2002. Clinical guidelines for the physiotherapy management of cystic fibrosis: Recommendations of a working group. 17-20 pp.

de Jong, W., A.A. Kaptein, C.P. vanderSchans, G.P.M. Mannes, W.M.C. vanAalderen, R.G. Grevink, and G.H. Koeter. 1997. Quality of life in patients with cystic fibrosis. *Pediatric Pulmonology*. 23:95-100.

de Jong, W., W.M.C. Van Aalderen, J. Kraan, G.H. Koeter, and C.P. van der Schans. 2001. Skeletal muscle strength in patients with cystic fibrosis. *Physiotherapy Theory and Practice*. 17:23-28.

de Meer, K., V.A.M. Gulmans, and J. van der Laag. 1999. Peripheral muscle weakness and exercise capacity in children with cystic fibrosis. *American Journal of Respiratory and Critical Care Medicine*. 159:748-754.

Dodd, M.E., and S.A. Prasad. 2005. Physiotherapy management of cystic fibrosis. *Chronic Respiratory Disease*. 2:139-149.

Enright, P.L. 2003. The Six-Minute Walk Test. *Respiratory Care*. 48:783-785.

Farbotko, K., C. Wilson, P. Watter, and J. MacDonald. 2005. Change in physiotherapy management of children with cystic fibrosis in a large urban hospital. *Physiotherapy Theory and Practice*. 21:13-21.

Gardner, L. 2004. Teaching young children about cystic fibrosis. *Pediatric Nursing*. 16:34-36.

Gudas, L.J., G.P. Koocher, and D. Wypij. 1991. Perceptions of medical compliance in children and adolescents with cystic fibrosis. *Journal of Developmental and Behavioural Pediatrics*. 12:236-242.

Gulmans, V.A.M., K. de Meer, H.J.L. Brackel, J.A.J. Faber, R. Berger, and P.J.M. Helders. 1999. Outpatient exercise training in children with cystic fibrosis: Physiological effects, perceived competence, and acceptability. *Pediatric Pulmonology*. 28:39-46.

Gulmans, V.A.M., N. vanVeldhoven, K. deMeer, and P.J.M. Helders. 1996. The six-minute walking test in children with cystic fibrosis: Reliability and validity. *Pediatric Pulmonology*. 22:85-89.

Guyatt, G.H., D. Osoba, A.W. Wu, K.W. Wyrwich, and G.R. Norman. 2002. Methods to explain the clinical significance of health status measures. . *Mayo Clinical Proc.* 77:371-383.

Higgins, L.W., D.M. Orenstein, and C.E. Baker. 2007. Development of an exercise knowledge test for children with cystic fibrosis. *Pediatric Pulmonology*. 42:359.

Hind, K., J.G. Truscott, and S.P. Conway. 2008. Exercise during childhood and adolescence: A prophylaxis against cystic fibrosis-related low bone mineral density? Exercise for bone health in cystic fibrosis. *Journal of Cystic Fibrosis*. 7:270 - 276.

Hinton, S., S. Watson, R. Chesson, and S. Mathers. 2002. Information needs of young people with cystic fibrosis. *Paediatric Nursing*. 14:18-21.

Hobbs, S.A., J.B. Schweitzer, L.L. Cohen, A.L. Hayes, C. Schoell, and B.K. Crain. 2003. Maternal attributions related to compliance with cystic fibrosis treatment. *Journal of Clinical Psychology in Medical Settings*. 10:273-277.

Holzer, F.J., R. Schnall, and L.I. Landau. 1984. The Effect of a Home Exercise Program in Children with Cystic-Fibrosis and Asthma. *Australian Paediatric Journal*. 20:297-301.

Hussey, J., J. Gormley, G. Leen, and P. Greally. 2002. Peripheral muscle strength in young males with cystic fibrosis. *Journal of Cystic Fibrosis*. 1:116-121.

Ireland, C. 2003. Adherence to Physiotherapy and Quality of Life for Adults and Adolescents with Cystic Fibrosis. *Physiotherapy*. 89:397-407.

Kettler, L.J., S.M. Sawyer, H.R. Winefield, and H.W. Greville. 2002. Determinants of adherence in adults with cystic fibrosis (Occasional Review). *Thorax*. 57:459-454.

Klijn, P.H.C., A. Oudshoorn, C.K. van der Ent, J. van der Net, J.L. Kimpen, and P.J.M. Helders. 2004. Effects of anaerobic training in children with cystic fibrosis - A randomized controlled study. *Chest*. 125:1299-1305.

Koch, C., B. Frederiksen, and N. Hoiby. 2003. Patient cohorting and infection control. *Seminars in Respiratory and Critical Care Medicine*. 24:703-716.

Lannefors, L. 2004. Influences on posture [Cystic Fibrosis Conference symposium session summary]. *Pediatric Pulmonology*. 38:155-157.

Li, A.M., J. Yin, J.T. Au, H.K. So, T. Tsang, E. Wong, T.F. Fok, and P.C. Ng. 2007. Standard reference for the six-minute-walk test in healthy children aged 7 to 16 years. *American Journal of Respiratory and Critical Care Medicine*. 176:174-180.

Li, A.M., J. Yin, C.C.W. Yu, T. Tsang, H.K. So, E. Wong, D. Chan, E.K.L. Hon, and R. Sung. 2005. The six-minute walk test in healthy children: reliability and validity. *European Respiratory Journal*. 25:1057-1060.

Mandrusiak, A., D. Giraud, J. MacDonald, C. Wilson, and P. Watter. 2010. Muscle length and joint range of motion in children with cystic fibrosis compared to matched-controls. *Physiotherapy Canada*. 62:141-146.

Mandrusiak, A., C. Maurer, J. MacDonald, C. Wilson, and P. Watter 2009a. Functional capacity tests in young people with cystic fibrosis. *New Zealand Journal of Physiotherapy*. 37:112-115.

Mandrusiak, A., J. MacDonald, and P. Watter. 2009b. The International Classification of Functioning, Disability and Health: an effective model for describing young people with cystic fibrosis. *Child: care, health and development*. 35:2-4.

Mandrusiak, A., J. MacDonald, C. Wilson., J. Paratz., P. Watter. 2009c. Effect of a targeted exercise program on function, activity and participation of young people with cystic fibrosis: using the ICF model as a basis of design. Doctoral Thesis, The University of Queensland, Australia.

Massery, M. 2005. Musculoskeletal and neuromuscular interventions: a physical approach to cystic fibrosis. *Journal of the Royal Society of Medicine*. 98:55-66.

McGavin, C.R., S.P. Gupta, and G.J.R. McHardy. 1976. 12-Minute Walking Test for Assessing Disability in Chronic-Bronchitis. *British Medical Journal*. 1:822-823.

McIlwaine, M. 2007. Chest physical therapy, breathing techniques and exercise in children with CF. *Paediatric Respiratory Reviews*. 8:8-16.

Modi, A.C., and A.L. Quittner. 2003. Validation of a Disease-Specific Measure of Health-Related Quality of Life for Children with Cystic Fibrosis. *Journal of Pediatric Psychology*. 28:535-546.

Moorcroft, A.J., M.E. Dodd, J. Morris, and A.K. Webb. 2004. Individualised unsupervised exercise training in adults with cystic fibrosis: a 1 year randomised controlled trial. *Thorax*. 59:1074-1080.

Narang, I., S. Pike, M. Rosenthal, I.M. Balfour-Lynn, and A. Bush. 2003. Three-minute step test to assess exercise capacity in children with cystic fibrosis with mild lung disease. *Pediatric Pulmonology*. 35:108-113.

Nixon, P.A., M.L. Joswiak, and F.J. Fricker. 1996. A six-minute walk test for assessing exercise tolerance in severely ill children. *Journal of Pediatrics*. 129:362-366.

Nixon, P.A., D.M. Orenstein, S.F. Kelsey, and C.F. Doershuk. 1992. The Prognostic Value of Exercise Testing in Patients with Cystic-Fibrosis. *New England Journal of Medicine*. 327:1785-1788.

Noonan, V., and E. Dean. 2000. Submaximal exercise testing: clinical application and interpretation. *Physical Therapy*. 80:782-807.

Orenstein, D.M. 1998. Exercise testing in cystic fibrosis. *Pediatric Pulmonology*. 25:223-225.

Orenstein, D.M., B.A. Franklin, C.F. Doershuk, H.K. Hellerstein, K.J. Germann, J.G. Horowitz, and R.C. Stern. 1981. Exercise Conditioning and Cardiopulmonary Fitness in Cystic-Fibrosis - the Effects of a 3-Month Supervised Running Program. *Chest*. 80:392-398.

Orenstein, D.M., and L.W. Higgins. 2005. Update on the role of exercise in cystic fibrosis. *Current Opinion in Pulmonary Medicine*. 11:519-523.

Pianosi, P., J. LeBlanc, and A. Almudevar. 2005. Peak oxygen uptake and mortality in children with cystic fibrosis. *Thorax*. 60:50-54.

Pike, S.E., S.A. Prasad, and I.M. Balfour-Lynn. 2001. Effect of intravenous antibiotics on exercise tolerance (3-min step test) in cystic fibrosis. *Pediatric Pulmonology*. 32:38-43.

Prasad, S.A., and F.J. Cerny. 2002. Factors that influence adherence to exercise and their effectiveness: Application to cystic fibrosis. *Pediatric Pulmonology*. 34:66-72.

Prasad, S.A., S.D. Randall, and I.M. Balfour-Lynn. 2000. Fifteen-count breathlessness score: An objective measure for children. *Pediatric Pulmonology*. 30:56-62.

Redelmeier, D.A., A.M. Bayoumi, R.S. Goldstein, and G.H. Guyatt. 1997. Interpreting small differences in functional status:The six-minute walk test in chronic lung disease patients. *American Journal of Respiratory and Critical Care Medicine*. 155:1278-1282.

Rogers, D., S.A. Prasad, and I. Doull. 2003. Exercise testing in children with cystic fibrosis. *Journal of the Royal Society of Medicine*. 96:23-29.

Sahlberg, M. 2008. Physical exercise in cystic fibrosis - studies on muscle strength, oxygen uptake and lung function in young adult patients. University of Gothenburg, Gothenburg, Sweden.

Salh, W., D. Bilton, M. Dodd, and A.K. Webb. 1989. Effect of Exercise and Physiotherapy in Aiding Sputum Expectoration in Adults with Cystic-Fibrosis. *Thorax*. 44:1006-1008.

Schneiderman-Walker, J., S.L. Pollock, M. Corey, D.D. Wilkes, G.J. Canny, L. Pedder, and J.J. Reisman. 2000. A randomized controlled trial of a 3-year home exercise program in cystic fibrosis. *Journal of Pediatrics*. 136:304-310.

Selvadurai, H.C., C.J. Blimkie, N. Meyers, C.M. Mellis, P.J. Cooper, and P.P. van Asperen. 2002. Randomized controlled study of in-hospital exercise training programs in children with cystic fibrosis. *Pediatric Pulmonology*. 33:194-200.

Selvadurai, H.C., P.J. Cooper, N. Meyers, C.J. Blimkie, L. Smith, C.M. Mellis, and P.P. Van Asperen. 2003. Validation of shuttle tests in children with cystic fibrosis. *Pediatric Pulmonology*. 35:133-138.

Shoemaker, M.J., and H. Hurt. 2008. The evidence regarding exercise training in the management of cystic fibrosis: A systematic review. *Cardiopulmonary Physical Therapy Journal*. 19:75-83.

Smidt, N., H.C.W. de Vet, L.M. Bouter, and J. Dekker. 2005. Effectiveness of exercise therapy: a best-evidence summary of systematic reviews. *Australian Journal of Physiotherapy*. 51:71-85.

Solway, S., D. Brooks, Y. Lacasse, and S. Thomas. 2001. A qualitative systematic overview of the meaurement properties of functional walk tests used in the cardiorespiratory domain. *Chest*. 119:256-270.

Stanghelle, J.K. 1988. Physical Exercise for Patients with Cystic-Fibrosis - a Review. *International Journal of Sports Medicine*. 9:6-18.

Stevens, D., and C.A. Williams. 2007. Exercise testing and training with the young cystic fibrosis patient. *Journal of Sports Science and Medicine*. 6:286 - 291.

Taylor, N., K. Dodd, N. Shields, and A. Bruder. 2006. APA Position Statement: Evidence regarding therapeutic exercise in physiotherapy. *In*, Australian Physiotherapy Association website. 1-5.

Thoracic Society of Australia and New Zealand. 2007. Physiotherapy for cystic fibrosis in Australia: A consensus statement. *The Thoracic Society of Australia and New Zealand*.125.

Turchetta, A., T. Salerno, V. Lucidi, F. Libera, R. Cutrera, and A. Bush. 2004. Usefulness of a program of hospital-supervised physical training in patients with cystic fibrosis. *Pediatric Pulmonology*. 38:115-118.

Upton, C.J., J.C. Tyrrell, and E.J. Hiller. 1988. 2 Minute Walking Distance in Cystic-Fibrosis. *Archives of Disease in Childhood*. 63:1444-1448.

Webb, A.K., and M.E. Dodd. 1999. Exercise and sport in cystic fibrosis: benefits and risks. *British Journal of Sports Medicine*. 33:77-78.

Webb, A.K., and M.E. Dodd. 2000. Exercise and training for adults with cystic fibrosis. *In* Cystic FIbrosis. M.E. Hodson and D.M. Geddes, editors. Arnold, London. 433-448.

Wilson, C., J. MacDonald, C. Harrison, A. Mandrusiak, A. Chang, P. O'Rourke, and P. Watter. 2005. Activity outcomes characterised within the International Classification of Functioning and Disability in young people with cystic fibrosis. *In* Sixth Australian and New Zealand Cystic Fibrosis Conference. Adelaide, Australia. 53.

World Health Organization. 2007. International classification of functioning, disability, and health—children and youth. World Health Organization, Geneva.

World Health Organization. 2001. International classification of functioning, disability, and health. World Health Organization, Geneva.

Yankaskas, J.R., B.C. Marshall, B. Sufian, and et al. 2004. Cystic fibrosis adult care: Consensus conference report. *Chest*. 125.

24

Exercise Performance and Breathing Patterns in Cystic Fibrosis

Georgia Perpati
Adult Cystic Fibrosis Unit, Athens Hospital of Chest Diseases, Greece

1. Introduction

Cystic fibrosis (CF) patients often experience exercise limitations. Although exercise capacity in CF patients has been extensively investigated over the past 15 years, factors contributing to exercise limitation in such patients have not been fully characterized.

The prognostic value of various exercise indices is considered in numerous clinical studies. However, whether exercise rehabilitation programs will improve the long term prognosis for CF patients remains controversial.

2. Cardiopulmonary exercise testing (CPET): Physiology of exercise

Ventilation, pulmonary gas transfer, cardiac output and peripheral blood flow, all increase in response to the metabolic demands of working muscles.

The pattern of breathing can be described by the following equation:

$$V_E = V_T \times f_b \qquad (1)$$

where V_E is pulmonary ventilation, V_T the tidal volume (the volume of air inhaled and exhaled during one respiratory cycle) and f_b the frequency of breathing. In normal subjects during exercise the increase in V_E is achieved by increases in V_T at low and moderate work load, up to 50-60% of vital capacity (Jones and Rebuck , 1979). This is achieved by gradual increases in end inspiratory lung volume to about 80% of total lung capacity (TLC) and reductions in end expiratory volume to about 40% of TLC (Cotes, 1979).

At higher exercise intensity the increase of ventilation is achieved through rise in frequency of breathing. Obviously, in smaller lung volumes, like in children, the f_b commonly seen is at higher levels , not rare up to 60 br/min.

Furthermore, the breathing pattern during exercise includes additional variables, as inspiratory flow (V_I) and the duty cycle (T_i / T_{tot}). In these terms, the above mentioned equation could be written as:

$$V_E = V_I \times T_i / T_{tot} \times 60/f_b \qquad (2)$$

Also, the V_D / V_T ratio (physiological dead space) normally is 25 to 35% at rest and in exercise falls to 5 to 20%, due to V_T increase (Jones et al., 1966).

Oxygen consumption depends on work rate levels. The characteristics of oxygen uptake kinetics (VO_2) differ with exercise intensity (Webb and Dodd, 1995). When exercise is performed at a given work rate below lactate threshold (LT) there is a linear dynamic relationship between VO_2 and the work rate. When exercise is performed at work rate above LT, the VO_2 kinetics become more complex and there is an additional slow component either drives to the max VO_2 levels (VO_2 max) or delay steady state VO_2 (then the highest VO_2 value is characterized as VO_2 peak) (Xu and Rhodes, 1999).

Also, in healthy population, cardiac output *(Q)* during exercise is linearly related to oxygen uptake (Smith et al., 1988, Wasseman et al., 1997). It is important to note that at low exercise intensity (up to 30% of VO_2 max) approximately 50% of energy demands covered by carbohydrates as the other 50% use lipids as source of energy (Borsheim and Bahr, 2003). At higher exercise levels, the energy sources used remain under investigation.

The anaerobic threshold (AT) is the point reached during exercise of increasing intensity, at which aerobic processes give way to anaerobic processes. At this point oxygen intake is unable to meet energy needs and for additional work the energy provided by anaerobic glycolysis. There are various methods have been used to estimate the AT, like measurement of lactate production in plasma accompanies increase in ventilation or measurements of carbon dioxide output and ventilation as indicators of blood lactate increases (Wasserman, 1987, 1994, Zoladz et al 1998).

VO_2 t / slope is an index expresses the oxygen debt and used to describe the early phase of recovery after exercise. VO_2 t / slope has been evaluated in congestive heart failure, chronic obstructive pulmonary disease, cystic fibrosis, beta thalassaemia etc. (Nanas, 1999,2009, Vogiatzis 2005, Pouliou 2001, Koike, 1995). In healthy subjects all these changes during exercise, express their ability for a normal response to exercise. However, in this adaptive capacity should be taken into account some factors affect it like gender, age and physical activity.

CPET is an important tool for evaluation of exercise performance in healthy individuals and additionally utilized in clinical practice to assess a patient's level of intolerance to exercise and the possible underlying causes for this.

During the test, patients are subjected to symptom-limited incremental exercise and breath by breath monitoring of cardiopulmonary variables mentioned above (VO_2, V_E, VCO_2, f b, VO_2 t / slope, HR, *Q* etc). Moreover they undergo assessment of perceptional responses (eg dyspnea, leg fatigue), measurements of arterial oxygen desaturation, lung volumes and muscle pressures. The incremental exercise period should last 10 - 12 minutes. The measures are reproducible and useful for diagnostic and prognostic purposes (Jones, 1997).

3. Ventilatory response and oxygen kinetics during maximal exercise and early recovery in patients with cystic fibrosis (CF)

One of the earliest observed abnormalities of pulmonary function in CF is an increase in the physiological dead space related to disease severity (Godfrey et al., 1971). This high resting ratio increases further with exercise due to a limited V_T and severe mismatching of ventilation and perfusion (Cerny et al 1982). Ventilation is higher for a given workload.

When Forced Expiratory Volume in first second (FEV_1) is > 60%, the CF patients can exercise almost as the healthy population, while patients with severe disease have limited capacity to increase their tidal volume during exercise and in order to maintain alveolar ventilation they heighten f_b.

As airways obstruction progresses the tidal expiratory flow limitation (EFL), accompanied by decreased inspiratory time (T_i) and lower inspiratory time to total respiratory cycle time (T_i / T_{tot}), leads to raised f_b and essentially to air trapping. EFL has been associated with chronic dynamic hyperinflation during tidal breathing where end-expiratory lung volume is greater than the relaxation volume of the respiratory system.

This dynamic hyperinflation affects the function of respiratory muscles by diaphragm flattening and shortening of the auxiliary and intercostals muscles. Inspiratory muscles overworked on large volumes become unable to pay off the oxygen debt and with exercise progress will fatigue prematurely (Hirsch et al., 1989, Coates et al., 1988).

Oxygen uptake kinetics are slowed in cystic fibrosis. During exercise, ventilation rises in a linear fashion until oxygen consumption reaches a level of 60-70% of VO_2 max, but in CF patients the VO_2 max usually is not reached and at earlier point the oxygen supply becomes inadequate to meet demand and begins anaerobic metabolism and lactic acid accumulation. The recovery is also slower, as it expressed by increased VO_2 t / slope (Webb and Dodd, 1995, Pouliou et al, 2001, Perpati et al., 2010).

The mechanisms causing prolonged oxygen kinetics on early phase of exercise recovery, has not been fully understood although has been observed in deconditioning, heart failure, COPD and CF. A possible cause is a slow recovery of energy stores of the peripheral skeletal muscles (Harris et al., 1976). In the muscles of patients with chronic respiratory impairment the oxidative phosphorylation impaired and there is an early activation of anaerobic glycolysis. Another mechanism that should be considered in the prolonged VO_2 recovery is the oxygen cost of breathing. In CF patients there is a basic physiologic defect leading to enlarged dead space and it is present even in the most mildly affected patients. Progressive airway obstruction reduces vital capacity resulting in VT limitation. In compensation, decreased inspiratory time and increased end-expiratory volume are observed in order to preserve adequate inspiratory and expiratory flow rates. Airway obstruction causes prolongation of expiratory flow rate and in association with the increased breathing frequency results in air trapping. The work and oxygen cost of breathing are increased at high lung volumes and finally exercise is discontinued.

Studies to assess cardiac output in CF patients during steady state exercise found that cardiac function did not influence exercise performance. Although a limitation in diastolic reserve has been observed and there is a rapid rise in the heart rate, the cardiovascular responses are relatively normal for a given workload. However there are some recent data conclude that in CF patients with severe disease, CF related diabetes and older CF patients there is abnormal haemodynamic response to exercise (Hull et al., 2011). As for gas exchange abnormalities, it has been demonstrated that in patients with mild to moderate disease oxygen desaturation is not present during exercise.

The first time that exercise limitation in CF patients had been correlated with pulmonary mechanics rather than circulatory factors and hypoxia was in 1971 (Godfrey et al). Later, Browning et al. investigating 11 adult patients with CF showed that there was a correlation between disease severity and respiratory rate during exercise (Browning et al., 1990). Coates et al also found that there is decreased V_T and T_i, don't lead necessary to respiratory failure although there is a carbon dioxide rise at the onset (Coates et al., 1988). Lands et al. in a study with 14 patients found VE max and VO_2 max decreased during exercise without V_E/VO_2 and V_E/VCO_2 difference between patients and healthy controls. In the same study VO_2 max correlated with FEV_1 (Lands et al., 1992). Nixon and Webb confirmed that VO_2 max was statistically significant prognostic index for disease severity and survival (Nixon et al., 1995). Pouliou et al. describe prolonged oxygen kinetics at early recovery in adult patients with CF (Pouliou et al., 2001). Perpati et al. described breathing pattern in CF patients during maximal CPET and evaluated the correlation between resting respiratory variables and exercise capacity in CF participants (Perpati et al., 2010). They investigated 18 adult patients and 11 healthy subjects who underwent pulmonary function test at rest and symptom-limited treadmill CPET. The main ventilatory response indices at rest, peak exercise and recovery, for each group, are presented at Table 1. Patient's ability to increase V_T and V_E was limited in comparison with healthy subjects. CF patients showed similar ability to increase f_b from rest to peak exercise in comparison with healthy subjects, however they exhibited a prolonged rapid breathing after exercise along with shortened inspiratory time. VO_2 peak was lower in patients and in the same group recovery was longer, as it is expressed by lower VO_2 /t slope.

	Patients			Healthy subjects		
	Rest	Peak	Recovery	Rest	Peak	Recovery
V_E (lt/min)	12.5±2.4	57.2±19	14.4±6.7	11.3±2	81.3±13.2	20.5±5.8
V_T (lt)	0.56±0.1	1.53±0.6	0.72±0.3	0.57±0.2	1.88±0.4	1.2±0.3
f_b (breaths/min)	23±6	38±9	32±8	19±4	44±8	22±5
T_I (s)	1.2±0.3	0.8±0.2	0.9±0.2	1.5±0.3	0.7±0.1	1±0.2
V_T/T_I (lt/s)	0.5±0.2	1.9±0.6	0.8±0.3	0.4±0.1	2.7±0.4	1.2±0.3
VO_2	4.93±1.8	29.12±7	5.77±3.3	4.03±1.1	35.54±7.3	4.82±1.9
V_D/V_T	0.35±0.2	0.16±0.02	0.19±0.04	0.36±0.2	0.10±0.02	0.16±0.04
V_E/VO_2		25.65±5.5			19.9±5.88	
V_E/VCO_2		28.51±5.3			26.62±3.14	
VO_2/t-slope		0.59±0.25			0.95±0.18	

Table 1. CPET indices at rest, peak exercise and recovery for patients with cystic fibrosis and healthy subjects

4. Factors limiting maximal exercise performance in cystic fibrosis: The role of resting lung function, nutrition and disease severity

As mentioned above, it appears that the role of pulmonary mechanics is crucial to exercise limitation. The resting lung function and thus the disease severity have been associated with exercise performance as it is expressed by VO_2 max and VO_2 t / slope.

In serial studies there is a significant correlation between these variables and FEV1 (Moorcroft et al., 1997, Nixon et al., 1992, Pouliou et al., 2001). Moreover, recent data confirm that oxygen uptake at maximal exercise and early recovery are correlated to resting respiratory variables including inspiratory capacity (IC) and explore its role as predictor of exercise capacity (Perpati et al., 2010). The significant correlations of VO_2 peak and VO_2/t-slope to resting lung function are listed in Table 2. In a multivariate stepwise regression analysis, using peak VO_2 as the dependent variable and the pulmonary function test measurements as independent variables respectively, the only significant predictor emerged was IC. VO_2/t-slope was also lower in CF patients and showed significant correlation with IC. In a final stepwise regression analysis including all independent variables of the resting pulmonary function tests, the only predictor selected for VO_2 peak and VO_2/t-slope was IC (Figure 2).

Parameters	VO_2 peak		VO_2/t-slope	
	r	*p* value	*r*	*p* value
FEV_1, % pred	0.575	0.013	0.774	0.0001
FVC, % pred	0.602	0.008	0.663	0.003
FEV_1/FVC, %	0.513	0.029	0.678	0.002
IC, ml	0.608	0.007	0.859	0.0001

Table 2. Significant correlations of VO_2 peak and VO_2/t-slope to various resting respiratory parameters.

Although pulmonary disease correlates with exercise tolerance, especially in those CF patients with an FEV_1 less than 50% of predicted, nutritional status and muscle function may also play an important role for maintaining anaerobic and aerobic exercise. Several studies with mild or moderate pulmonary disease reported increases in lactate levels and early occurrence of the lactate threshold during incremental exercise, indicating an increase in muscle metabolism and suggesting that peak exercise is not limited by ventilation, but rather by non pulmonary factors that lead to leg fatigue (Moorcroft et al., 2005, Mc Loughlin et al., 1997, Nikolaizik et al., 1998)

In a study included 104 CF who performed progressive cycle ergometry to a symptom limited maximum, the conclusion was that the main factor limiting exercise in mild to moderate disease is peripheral muscle effort (Moorcroft et al., 2005). Reduced muscle performance may be due to poor nutritional status or reduced habitual activity. There are some data to support the hypothesis that the cause is an intrinsic muscle defect.

However, clearly there is a strong relationship between nutrition and muscle function (Elkin et al., 2000). In patients with CF and advanced lung disease, nutritional status plays a significant role in determining exercise capacity but poor nutrition is not correlated with pulmonary function and resting O_2 partial pressure (PaO_2). Malnutrition leads initially to loss of body fat and then to lean tissue wasting and can have adverse metabolic and structural effects on skeletal muscles. Leading to loss of leg muscle mass and decreased respiratory muscle strength, malnutrition can impair exercise performance.

The data of studies exploring the effect of nutritional supplementation on exercise tolerance are controversial. This fact support the hypothesis that exercise limitation in CF patients is the result of multiple combined effects of airways obstruction, nutritional status and metabolic processes.

5. The prognostic value of exercise testing in patients with cystic fibrosis

FEV_1, maximum oxygen consumption (VO_2 peak) during CPET and the Schwachman score (SS) are commonly used to assess functional capacity and disease severity in CF patients. Pouliou et al. explored the relationship between oxygen kinetics during early recovery after maximal CPET and the severity of the disease. They showed that VO_2 t / slope is closely correlated to FEV_1 and SS (Figure 1).

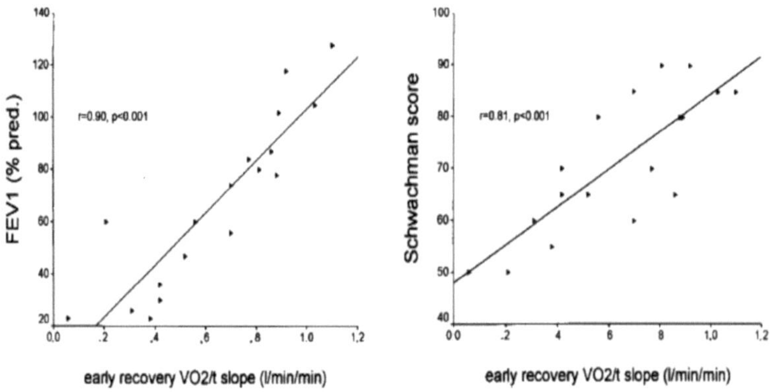

Fig. 1. Correlation between VO_2 t / slope and disease severity.

To the knowledge that resting respiratory variables have a significant correlation to VO_2 peak and to VO_2 t/slope, recent data have been reported about the potential role of IC as of independent predictor of exercise capacity (Perpati et al., 2010).

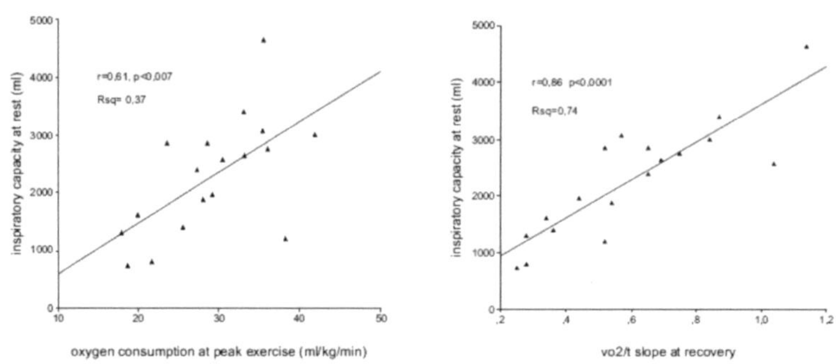

Fig. 2. Correlation between inspiratory capacity and oxygen kinetics at peak exercise and early recovery.

In studies designed to determine the prognostic value of CPET in CF patients higher levels of aerobic fitness are associated with a significantly lower risk of dying. Better aerobic fitness may simply be a marker for less severe illness, however measurement of VO_2 peak appeared to be valuable for predicting prognosis. A multicenter retrospective study analysed 3-year outcomes indicated that there is higher risk of death in patients with lower FEV_1, BMI, diabetes mellitus and higher alveolar arterial gradient for oxygen at peak exercise. Prospective studies needed to confirm the prognostic value of CPET in long term survival and compare its prognostic value with that of FEV_1, especially in patients with mild to moderate disease.

5.1 Submaximal cardiopulmonary exercise testing in cystic fibrosis patients

Submaximal exercise testing is considered a promising exercise capacity testing, especially in patients with limited performance because of fatigue due to disease severity. Submaximal CPET is more tolerable for CF patients as the test is terminated when oxygen uptake approached 75 % of the VO_2 peak. There are a few data showing that VO_2 kinetics during submaximal CPET are a more sensitive index of beneficial effects of exercise training than VO_2 peak and AT in healthy subjects. However, the experience with submaximal CPET in CF patients is generally limited (Hebestreit et al., 2005, Braggion et al., 1989).

In contrast there is a large experience over time with 6 min walk test (6MWT) as a useful tool assessed exercise capacity in patients with CF, mainly for severe disease and children (Gulmans et al., 1996, Nixon et al, 1996, Upton et al., 1988, Butland et al., 1982). The 6MWT is a practical, simple test that measures the maximal distance that a patient can walk at his or her own pace in six minutes. This self paced test is performed in an indoor corridor (or alternatively on a treadmill). The walking course should be 30 m long. The 6MWT provides a global assessment of functional capacity and although it doesn't give specific information and therefore has limited diagnostic capacity, it can be an excellent tool for severe ill patients as it resembles to everyday life activities. Many lung transplant centers use it at the time of assessment prior to transplantation, to determine baseline at start of program, at 6 weeks and every 3 months or to reflect functional changes and after transplantation at 6 weeks, 3 months and formal assessments. This is used in processes of patients referral for transplantation, training protocol design and rehabilitation potential estimation, as severe exercise intolerance could also be a factor precluding transplantation.

6. Perspectives in clinical practice: Rehabilitation programs

CF lung disease is often associated with physical inactivity and deconditioning. The effectiveness of exercise training program in CF patients has been studied in randomized controlled trials. The objective change in exercise capacity was reported as an improvement in VO_2 peak in two studies. Also there are studies reported change in peak heart rate, desaturation during exercise and annual decline in FVC at three years. Controversially, there are studies showing no significant differences in peak minute ventilation or annual decline of FEV_1, although there is a trend for FEV_1 improvement. If exercise training including anaerobic exercises can improve muscle strength and muscle size resulting in weight gain remains also under consideration. Further, in terms of quality of life, positive effects towards perceived feasibility have been noted (Turchetta eta l., 2004, Selvadurai et al., 2002, Schneiderman-Walker et al., 2000, Orenstein et al., 1981).

In a recent systematic Cohrane review of trials investigating the effect of exercise training programs on exercise endurance in patients with CF, the authors conclude that there is limited evidence that regular exercise training is associated with improved aerobic and anaerobic capacity, higher pulmonary function and enhanced airway mucus clearance (Bradley, Moran., 2008). Further research is needed to assess relative benefits of rehabilitation program for these patients.

In another review, Williams et al. present general exercise and training recommendations for children and adolescents with CF including cycling, walking, gymnastics and day to day activities for about 30 min, 3-5 times per week intermittently (Williams et al., 2010). For patients with mild to moderate disease they add activities like swimming, tennis and climbing. In all cases is suggested to avoid activities like bungee-jumping, high diving, scuba diving and hiking in high altitude. The potential risks is associated with more intensive exercise includes dehydration, hypoxemia, hemoptysis, pneumothorax, arrhythmias and fractures in presence of CF related bone disease (Goldbeck et al., 2011).

However, improvements in exercise endurance require individual dosages of training stimuli and vary among individuals.

Prior to transplantation, an individualized pulmonary rehabilitation program is prescribed in order to increase or maintaining mobility and functional capacity, decrease dyspnea and hospitalizations, monitoring oxygen saturation and maintaining morale. Postoperative rehabilitation's goals is safe discharge of functional patients and accelerate recovery in outpatients setting. The training focuses on shoulder range of motion, stretching, strengthening and aerobics to increase endurance (Helm D., 2007).

7. Conclusions

Exercise testing is an important outcome variable in CF patients, correlated with disease severity and survival, exploring the ventilator and cardiac responses to progressively increasing workload and indentifying factors related to this ability for exercise. As there is no perfect test for that, is suggested (Orenstein, 1998) each Cystic Fibrosis Center to adopt the most appropriate for its patients needs and use it consistently.

Looking at pulmonary rehabilitation as a program of medical practice implies methods of improvement the patient's functional ability, in terms of medical, mental, emotional and social potential, we will have to explore further the effect of an individualized approach in designed exercise training protocols and encourage physical training as a part of multimodality treatment of CF.

8. References

Børsheim E, Bahr R. Effect of exercise intensity, duration and mode on post-exercise oxygen consumption. Sports Med. 2003;33(14):1037-60.

Bradley J and Moran F. Physical Training for Cystic Fibrosis. Cochrane Database of Systematic Reviews, no 1, Article ID CD002768, 2008.

Braggion C, Cornacchia M, Miano A, et al. Exercise tolerance and effects of training in young patients with cystic fibrosis and mild airway obstruction. Pediatr Pulmonol. 1989;7(3):145-52.

Browning B, D'Alonso GE, Tobin MJ. Importance of respiratory rate as an indicator of respiratory dysfunction in patients with cystic fibrosis. Chest June 1990;97(6):1317e21.

Butland RJ, Pang J, Gross ER, et al. Two-, six-, and 12-minute walking tests in respiratory disease. Br Med J (Clin Res Ed). 1982 May 29;284(6329):1607-8.

Coates AL, Canny G, Zinman R, et al. The effects of chronic airflow limitation, increased dead space, and the pattern of ventilation on gas exchange during maximal exercise in advanced cystic fibrosis. Am Rev Respir Dis 1988; 138:1524 –1531

Elkin SL, Williams L, Moore M, et al. Relationship of skeletal muscle mass, muscle strength and bone mineral density in adults with cystic fibrosis. Clin Sci (Lond). 2000 Oct;99(4):309-14.

Godfrey S, Mearns M. Pulmonary function and response to exercise in cystic fibrosis. Arch Dis Child 1971; 46:144–151.

Goldbeck L, Holling I., Schlack R. et al. The impact of an inpatient family-oriented rehabilitation program on parent-reported psychological symptoms of chronically ill children. Klin Paediatr.2011; 223 (2): 79-84

Gulmans VA, van Veldhoven NH, de Meer K, Helders PJ. The six-minute walking test in children with cystic fibrosis: reliability and validity. Pediatr Pulmonol. 1996 Aug;22(2):85-9.

Harris RC, Edwards RHT, Hultman E, et al. The time course of phosphoryl-creatine resynthesis during recovery of the quadriceps muscle in man. Pflugers Arch 1976; 367:137–142

Hebestreit H, Hebestreit A, Trusen A, Hughson RL. Oxygen uptake kinetics are slowed in cystic fibrosis. Med Sci Sports Exerc. 2005 Jan;37(1):10-7.

Hirsch JA, Zhang SP, Rudnick MP, et al. Resting oxygen consumption and ventilation in cystic fibrosis. Pediatr Pulmonol. 1989;6(1):19-26.

Helm D. Physiotherapy. Lung Transplantation Manual, UHN, 2007: Chapter 10; 80-84.

Hodson and Geddes, Saunders 2nd edition, 2000.

Jones NL, McHardy GJR et al. Physiological dead space and alveolar-arterial gas pressure differences during exercise. . Clin Sci 1966; 31:19-29

Jones NL, Rebuck AS. Tidal volume during exercise in patients with diffuse fibrosing alveolitis. Bull Eur Physiopathol Respir 1979;15: 321-327

Jones NL. Clinical Exercise Testing. 4th edition, 1997.

Koike A, Yajima T, Adachi H, et al. Evaluation of exercise capacity using submaximal exercise at a constant work rate in patients with cardiovascular disease. Circulation. 1995 Mar 15;91(6):1719-24.

Lands LC, Heigenhauser GJ, Jones NL. Analysis of factors limiting maximal exercise performance in cystic fibrosis. Clin Sci 1992;83:391e7.

Mc Loughlin P, McKeogh D., Byrne P. et al. Assessment of fitness in patients with cystic fibrosis and mild lung disease. Thorax 1997; 52: 425-430.

Moorcroft J, Dodd ME, Webb AK. Exercise testing and prognosis in adult cystic fibrosis. Thorax 1997;52:291e3.

Moorcroft J, Dodd ME, Morris J, Webb AK. Symptoms, lactate and exercise limitation at peak cycle ergometry in adults with cystic fibrosis. Eur Respir J 2005; 25: 1050-1056.

Nanas S, Nanas J, Kassiotis CH, et al. Respiratory muscles performance is related to oxygen kinetics during maximal exercise and early recovery in patients with congestive heart failure. Circulation 1999; 100:503–508

Nanas S, Vasileiadis I, Dimopoulos S, et al. New insights into the exercise intolerance of beta-thalassemia major patients. Scand J Med Sci Sports. 2009 Feb;19(1):96-102.

Nikolaizik, Knopfli, Leister et al. The anaerobic threshold in cystic fibrosis: comparison of V-slope method, lactate turn points and Conconi test. Pediatr. Pulmonol.1998; 25: 147-153.

Nixon PA, Orenstein DM, Kelsey SF, et al. The prognostic value of exercise testing in patients with cystic fibrosis. NEJM 1992; 327:1785e8.

Nixon P, Joswiak M, Fricker F. A six minute walk test for assessing exercise tolerance in severely ill children. J Paediatr. 1996; 129: 362-366

Orenstein DM, Franklin BA, Doershuk CF et al. Exercise conditioning and cardiopulmonary fitness in cystic fibrosis. The effects of a three-month supervised running program. . Chest. 1981 Oct;80(4):392-8.

Orenstein DM. Exercise Testing in Cystic Fibrosis. Editorial. Pediatric Pulmonology, 1998; 25: 223-225.

Perpati G., S. Nanas, E. Pouliou et al. Resting respiratory variables and exercise capacity in adult patients with cystic fibrosis. Respiratory Medicine 2010 (104) 1444 -1449.

Pouliou E, Nanas S, Papamichalopoulos A, et al. Prolonged oxygen kinetics during early recovery from maximal exercise in adult patients with cystic fibrosis. Chest 2001 Apr;119(4): 1073e8.

Selvadurai, Blimkie, Meyers et al. Randomized controlled study of in-hospital exercise training programs in children with cystic fibrosis, Pediatric Pulmonology, 2002: vol.33, no3, pp194-200.

Smith SA, Russell AE, West MJ et al Automated non-invasive measurement of cardiac output: comparison of electrical bioimpedance and carbon dioxide rebreathing techniques. Br Heart J. 1988 Mar;59(3):292-8.

Schneiderman-Walker, Pollock, Corey at al. A randomized controlled trial of a 3-year home exercise program in cystic fibrosis. Journal of Pediatrics, 2000: vol.136, no3: 304-310.

Turschetta A., Salerno T., Lucidi V., et al. Usefulness of a program of hospital supervised physical training in patients with cystic fibrosis. Pediatric Pulmonology, 2004:vol.38, no2, pp115-118.

Upton CJ, Tyrrell JC, Hiller EJ. Two minute walking distance in cystic fibrosis. Arch Dis Child. 1988 Dec;63(12):1444-8.

Vogiatzis I., Georgiadou O., Golemati S. et al. Patterns of dynamic hyperinflation during exercise and recovery in patients with severe chronic obstructive pulmonary disease. Thorax. 2005 Sep;60(9):723-9.

Wasserman K. Determinants and detection of anaerobic threshold and consequences of exercise above it. Circulation. 1987 Dec;76(6 Pt 2):VI29-39. Review.

Wasserman K. et al. Dynamics of oxygen uptake for submaximal exercise and recovery in patients with chronic heart failure. Chest. 1994 Jun;105(6):1693-700

Wasserman K. et al. Cardiac output estimated noninvasively from oxygen uptake during exercise. J Appl Physiol. 1997 Mar;82(3):908-12.

Webb AK, Dodd ME. Exercise and cystic fibrosis. J R Soc Med 1995; 88(suppl 25):30–36

Williams CA, Benden C, Stevens D, Radtke T. Exercise training in children and adolescents with cystic fibrosis: theory into practice. Int J Pediatr. 2010;2010. pii: 670640. Epub 2010 Sep 19.

Xu F, Rhodes EC. Oxygen Uptake kinetics during exercise. Sports Med 1999; 27(5): 313-27.

Zoladz JA, Duda K, Majerczak J. VO2/power output relationship and the slow component of oxygen uptake kinetics during cycling at different pedaling rates: relationship to venous lactate accumulation and blood acid-base balance. Physiol Res. 1998;47(6):427-38.